Therapeutic
Modalities

The Art and Science

Second Edition

Therapeutic Modalities
The Art and Science
Second Edition

Kenneth L. Knight, PhD, ATC, FACSM
Jesse Knight Professor of Exercise Sciences
Department of Exercise Sciences
College of Life Sciences
Brigham Young University
Provo, Utah

David O. Draper, EdD, ATC, LAT
Professor of Exercise Sciences
Department of Exercise Sciences
College of Life Sciences
Brigham Young University
Provo, Utah

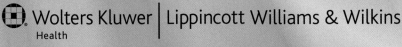
Wolters Kluwer | Lippincott Williams & Wilkins
Health

Philadelphia • Baltimore • New York • London
Buenos Aires • Hong Kong • Sydney • Tokyo

Acquisitions Editor: Emily Lupash
Product Manager: Matt Hauber
Marketing Manager: Sarah Schuessler
Production Project Manager: Cynthia Rudy
Designer: Terry Mallon
Photographer: Mark A. Philbrick
Graphic Artist: Kim Battista
Prepress Vendor: SPi Global

Library of Congress Cataloging-in-Publication Data

Knight, Kenneth L.
   Therapeutic modalities : the art and science / Ken Knight, David Draper. — 2nd ed.
       p. ; cm.
   Includes bibliographical references and index.
   ISBN 978-1-4511-0294-9
   I. Draper, David O. II. Title.
   [DNLM: 1. Physical Therapy Modalities. 2. Orthopedic Procedures—methods. WB 460]
   615.8'2—dc23

                                                                2012033918

Printed in China

DISCLAIMER

Care has been taken to confirm the accuracy of the information present and to describe generally accepted practices. However, the authors, editors, and publisher are not responsible for errors or omissions or for any consequences from application of the information in this book and make no warranty, expressed or implied, with respect to the currency, completeness, or accuracy of the contents of the publication. Application of this information in a particular situation remains the professional responsibility of the practitioner; the clinical treatments described and recommended may not be considered absolute and universal recommendations.

The authors, editors, and publisher have exerted every effort to ensure that drug selection and dosage set forth in this text are in accordance with the current recommendations and practice at the time of publication. However, in view of ongoing research, changes in government regulations, and the constant flow of information relating to drug therapy and drug reactions, the reader is urged to check the package insert for each drug for any change in indications and dosage and for added warnings and precautions. This is particularly important when the recommended agent is a new or infrequently employed drug.

Some drugs and medical devices presented in this publication have Food and Drug Administration (FDA) clearance for limited use in restricted research settings. It is the responsibility of the health care provider to ascertain the FDA status of each drug or device planned for use in their clinical practice.

To purchase additional copies of this book, call our customer service department at (800) 638-3030 or fax orders to (301) 223-2320. International customers should call (301) 223-2300.

Visit Lippincott Williams & Wilkins on the Internet: http://www.lww.com. Lippincott Williams & Wilkins customer service representatives are available from 8:30 am to 6:00 pm, EST.

9 8 7 6 5 4 3 2

RRS1401

**TO OUR STUDENTS, PATIENTS, AND COLLEAGUES—
FOR STRETCHING OUR THINKING**

Preface

We are excited to share this updated and expanded second edition of *Therapeutic Modalities: The Art and Science*. We appreciate the kind remarks regarding the first edition and the helpful suggestions for improving it.

The use of therapeutic modalities, like clinical practice in all the health professions, is an art—an art influenced by experience and tradition as well as by science and theory. It would be easier if using therapeutic modalities were based entirely on scientific fact, but this is not the case. When research is inadequate, the clinician must rely on tradition and experience to guide application. Hence we have subtitled this textbook *The Art and Science*.

Clinicians need to understand both the how and the why of therapeutic modality use to be thinking, decision-making professionals rather than technicians. Although there is a theoretical basis for each modality application, the robustness of the theories varies. Some theories have a solid science base, whereas others are derived mostly from tradition. The lack of a scientific basis does not mean a theory is wrong, but that it might be uncertain. We have made a great effort to help readers understand the basis of the theories without overwhelming them with detail and depth. Studying the development of various theories will help students sharpen their critical-thinking skills. Only then will they become professionals and have the ability to make proper decisions about which modality to use when, to keep up with future developments, and to evaluate intelligently the claims of manufacturers.

The Audience

This introductory text is intended primarily for undergraduate students and others new to therapeutic modalities. We feel, however, that the book has much to offer to graduate students, clinicians, and those who may not be current with all the latest research and techniques in the field.

What's New in this Edition?

- A new chapter, Evidence-Based Medicine, the first comprehensive work on EBM in the athletic training literature

- Extensive revision and expansion of the chapters on Healing, Pain Principles, Pain Application, and Massage
- Clarification and minor additions to the chapters on Record Keeping, Thermotherapy Application, Cryotherapy Application, Diathermy, and Traction
- Reordering of parts so that Electrotherapy follows Thermotherapy
- 511 new references, a 65% increase over the 789 references in the first edition
- 135 new definitions in the glossary
- Case studies in the Principles chapters that illustrate how we have clinically applied the principles being presented
- "Critical Thinking" queries have been retitled as "Concept Check" to reflect their reality.
- Discovery and learning activities (labs and application checks) to enhance reader comprehension are now on a Website rather than in a separate clinical activities manual.

What has not Changed?

- The most important question ever asked, "Why?"
- Our conversational tone
- Our efforts to tell a complex story in a simple way
- Liberal use of illustrations to illustrate principles—more than 280 photos, charts, and graphs in this edition
- Reliance on our extensive clinical and research experience, research that has been stimulated by clinical questions and geared to answer those clinical questions

Evidence-Based Medicine

Our efforts to expand the information on evidence-based medicine (EBM) previously in Chapter 1 lead to a lengthy new chapter (Chapter 2) with 233 references. We celebrate the EBM concept and movement, but are dismayed by the misunderstanding and misinterpretation of it. In part, misunderstanding is the result of the lack of a single source that summarizes the philosophy, development, and application of evidence in general, as well as evidence-based medicine. There has been a great effort in athletic training, as in all branches of health care, to integrate EBM into clinical practice. Many of these efforts have been done in isolation. Without an overriding physiological understanding of EBM and its related concepts, students and many clinicians have struggled to fully implement its concepts.

Our efforts to bring understanding resulted in a more comprehensive chapter than anticipated. Even we will not cover all the topics in a therapeutic modalities class, nor do we anticipate they will be presented in any other single class. Yet all of the concepts in this chapter are necessary. They must be assimilated. We suggest they be part of many, if not all, athletic training didactic and clinical classes, so the concepts are learned and practiced line upon line, precept upon precept. Thus this chapter should be used throughout the curriculum.

Like much of medicine, the principles and practices of evidence-based medicine are not topics to be merely learned, rather concepts to be internalized and lived.

Pain

The greatly expanded pain principles chapter includes discussions of the multidimensional nature of pain perception and differentiates between pain, pain experience, suffering, disability, and pain tolerance. We have also developed the concepts of neuropathic pain, idiopathic pain, learned pain, pain models, and the multitude of factors used to classify pain. These help in discussing pain with others who may use different classification systems, but more importantly they enhance understanding the neuromatrix theory of pain and therefore how to manage pain.

Perhaps the most exciting enhancement in these chapters is the concepts of learned pain and mirror therapy. We have known for years that pain often persists long after the cause of the pain is healed, but we could not explain why it occurs. The concept of learned pain provides a physiological mechanism for this phenomenon. Coupled with understanding the effect of mirror therapy on modulating phantom limb pain, it gives direction to the concept of resetting central control, that is, reprogramming of the brain. Although there may not be an application of mirror therapy with sports injuries, understanding its concepts helps manage chronic or persistent pain through resetting central control.

References

Our extensive use of references is based on our philosophy that they are important to a text because they:
- ensure that the material in the text is grounded, and in agreement with contemporary thinking on the topic.
- direct readers to where they can find additional information on the topic.
- allow readers to explore in more detail the historical development of thinking about topics.

Student and Instructor Resources

Additional resources for students and instructors can be found on the companion Website at http://thePoint.lww.com. See the inside front cover of this text for details.

DISCOVERY AND LEARNING ACTIVITIES

Discovery and learning activities (labs and application checks) are now online rather than in a separate *Clinical Activities* manual. This will make it easier to update these activities, and will allow individual instructors who have developed their own clinical activities to post them on the Website for their students, as well as making them available for students of other universities.

FULL TEXT ONLINE

The fully searchable online e-book is available at the companion Website, http://thePoint.lww.com. Use the code on the inside front cover to access it.

ADDITIONAL RESOURCES FOR INSTRUCTORS

We understand the demand on an instructor's time, so to help make your job easier, you will have access to Instructor Resources upon adoption of *Therapeutic Modalities: The Art and Science,* Second Edition. The instructor's resource center at http://thePoint.lww.com includes the following materials:
- A test generator with approximately 500 multiple choice, true–false, and fill-in-the-blank questions
- PowerPoint slide presentations
- An image bank that contains all of the figures and tables from the textbook

User's Guide

This User's Guide introduces you to the many features of *Therapeutic Modalities: The Art and Science*. Taking full advantage of these features, you not only read about therapeutic modalities, you become engaged in activities that help you learn and put your knowledge into practice.

The authors have loaded the chapters with features that help you understand the key points and apply your new skills in choosing and implementing therapeutic modalities.

Opening Scenes start each chapter with a short scenario posing a situation related to the chapter contents.

Closing Scenes at the end of the chapter complete the vignette, helping you see how content is put into practice.

1

Therapeutic Modalities:
What They Are and Why They Are Used

Chapter Outline

Defining and Classifying Therapeutic Modalities
Maximizing the Effectiveness of Therapeutic Modalities
Art and Science
Knobology
Application: Evidence Versus Opinion, Rumor Versus Reality, Fact Versus Fiction
Clinical Decision Making
Selecting a Therapeutic Modality
Whose Decision?
Selection Criteria

Rehabilitation and Therapeutic Modalities
Rehabilitation Defined
Four Erroneous Concepts About Rehabilitation
A Systems Approach to Rehabilitation
Twelve Principles of Orthopedic Injury Rehabilitation
The 10 Core Goals of Orthopedic Injury Rehabilitation
The Psychology of Rehabilitation
Preparation for Using Therapeutic Modalities

OPENING SCENE

A father enlisted his young son to help remove a small dead tree from their yard. The eager boy got a small hatchet from the garage and began feverishly chopping away at tree limbs (Fig. 1.1). Although he worked very hard, his progress was slow. The father appeared with a power saw and quickly cut off the limbs and trunk. He said, "Son, it's important to work hard—but it's even more important to work smart. We could use that little hatchet and work hard all day chopping up these limbs, or we can work smart and use the right tool to finish the job in just minutes."

FIGURE 1.1 You can get the job done with the wrong tool, but it takes longer and the result might not be as successful.

2

---

16   Part I • In Perspective

3. *Once you finish your formal education, take the opportunity to attend and actively participate in continuing education seminars. Some professions will require you to maintain continuing education units (CEUs). The National Athletic Trainers' Association (NATA) requires its members to obtain 75 hours of additional learning every 3 years. Currently the American Physical Therapy Association (APTA) does not require this, but some individual state regulations do. There are numerous opportunities for continuing education at many professional meetings, including the NATA, APTA, and American College of Sports Medicine (ACSM) annual meetings.*
4. *Most professional organizations sponsor a peer-reviewed journal that is sent to all members. For example, the*

apeutic modality information than *Physical Therapy*. Make it a habit to study the journal of your primary professional organization, and periodically peruse the journals of related health professions. They represent the most current science and clinical practice in your specialty. Reading and implementing what you find in these journals with help keep you up-to-date in this ever-changing medical world.

CLOSING SCENE

We began this chapter with a story about a man teaching his young son about how he could do a better job in less time by using the right tools to cut branches off of a tree (Fig. 1.10). The same is true with rehabilitation, a complex process involving the redevelopment of many performance attributes, each with different goals. It can be facilitated by the judicious use of the right tools—therapeutic modalities.

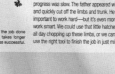

FIGURE 1.10 Just as you would use the right tool for cutting tree limbs, be sure to use the right tool for each stage of rehabilitation.

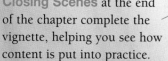

Modality Myths present common misunderstandings, and then set the record straight.

Charts, Tables, and Graphs summarize and serve as a quick reference to key information.

Concept Check Exercises move you beyond rote memorization to deepen your understanding of each chapter.

---

injury has occurred, nor will there be visible signs of the inflammatory process. Nevertheless, each of the inflammation events will occur, even in response to the simplest of injuries.

! Modality Myth

TRAUMA IS FORCE

The word "trauma" is sometimes thought of as the force that causes injuries. This is incorrect. Trauma is the injury that results from physical force, not the force itself.

Ultrastructural Changes

Ultrastructural changes refer to the breaking down and eventual disruption of the cellular membrane and its **organelles**. The cell's contents spill out into the **extracellular spaces** (the spaces between cells) and the cell dies.[7] The cell membrane and contents become debris (waste tissue), which will have to be removed before repair can take place.

With orthopedic or traumatic injuries, ultrastructural changes (and debris) occur from two sources; as a direct result of the initial physical forces, called primary injury, and indirectly as a result of metabolic and/or chemical injury, called secondary injury (discussed in more detail below). Secondary injury occurs in cells adjacent to those that undergo primary injury.

Chemical Mediation

Chemical mediators, such as *histamine, bradykinin,* and *cytokines,* are activated by ultrastructural changes.[6] They signal the rest of the body that cells have been damaged, thereby mobilizing the body's resources to respond. They modify and regulate the rest of the inflammatory response, activities that neutralize the cause of the injury and start to remove the cellular debris so that repair can take place. Chemical mediators are somewhat like police officers; they come to the site of accidents and direct events until the accident is cleaned up.

Hemodynamic Changes

Hemodynamic changes mobilize and transport blood-borne defense components to the injury site and secure their passage through vessel walls into the tissue. These changes occur in blood vessels within the injured area that did not undergo primary injury, and in vessels on the periphery of the injury.

In response to an injury, arteries dilate and blood flow increases. At the same time, many previously inactive capillaries and venules open, thereby expanding the total blood flow to the area. However, the rate of flow through individual vessels is slowed, as shown in Figure 5.3. This slowing of blood flow lets **leukocytes,** white blood cells, fall out of the bloodstream and move to the vessel margins (Fig. 5.4a). After tumbling along the margins for a while, they stick to the **endothelium** (vessel wall) and/or to other leukocytes (Figs. 5.4b and 5.5). Thus the endothelium becomes paved with leukocytes. Eventually, the leukocytes will pass through gaps in the endothelium and move through the tissue to the injury (Fig. 5.4c–g).

Metabolic Changes

Changes in metabolic processes are a cause of injury, as mentioned above. They are discussed in more detail here because they play a major role following acute injuries. Primary injury and the body's response to it, cause additional ultrastructural damage in the tissue. This additional insult is called secondary injury because it occurs as a result of the primary injury. Thus the total injury includes tissue debris from both primary and secondary injury.

Normal cellular functioning (specifically the cell membrane and organelles within the cell) requires energy in the form of **ATP (adenosine triphosphate),** which is usually supplied by aerobic (oxygen-using) metabolism.[9] When a cell is deprived of oxygen, a state known as **hypoxia,** it switches to anaerobic metabolism, or glycolysis, to satisfy its energy requirements. Glycolysis generates ATP by converting glucose to lactic acid when insufficient oxygen is available. It is not long lasting, however, and continued hypoxia leads to a steady decrease in energy production. Cell membrane functions slow down as the

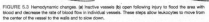
(a)   (b)

FIGURE 5.3 Hemodynamic changes. (a) Inactive vessels (b) open following injury to flood the area with blood and decrease the rate of blood flow in individual vessels. These steps allow leukocytes to move from the center of the vessel to the walls and to slow down.

Many clinicians believe that their hands and exe[...] best tools for treating orthopedic injuries. The[...] only tools, however, and integrating therapeuti[...] as part of a treatment regime often facilitates t[...] treatment. For example, cryokinetics involves [...] joint with cold, followed by active exercise. If th[...] not ice the ankle prior to exercise, pain and inhi[...] compromise the exercise, thereby making it less[...] this case, ice is the tool that causes numbing, s[...] can perform a higher level of exercise. The exer[...] good, but numbing and exercise together are sm[...]

In **physical medicine,** a therapeutic moda[...] for bringing about a desired therapeutic respo[...] book, you learn why, how, and when to use sev[...] your treatment regimens.

Defining and Classifyin[g] Therapeutic Modalities

A **therapeutic modality** is a device or appl[...] delivers a physical agent to the body for thera[...] poses. The most common **physical agents** use[d in] orthopedic injuries are:

- Heat
- Cold
- Light
- Electricity
- Exercise

TABLE 1.1	GENERAL CLASSIFICATIONS OF THERAPEUTIC MODALITIES	
CLASSIFICATION	DESCRIPTION	EXAMPLES
Cryotherapy	Use of cold (usually between 32°F and 70°F; 0°C and 21°C).	Ice massage, ice packs, *ice slush/ice immersion*, part of contrast therapy, cold *whirlpool*, and vapocoolant sprays.
Thermotherapy	Use of superficial and deep heat (usually between 98.6°F and 109.4°F; 37°C and 43°C)	moist heat packs, warm whirlpool, paraffin wax baths, ultrasound, *pulsed shortwave diathermy*, and ultraviolet
Hydrotherapy	Application of water	*Whirlpool* and aquatic therapy pools, and *ice slush/ice immersion*
Electrotherapy	Use of electricity	EMS, iontophoresis, TENS, and *diathermy*
Light therapy	Use of electromagnetic radiation	Laser, light therapy, *infrared*
Mechanotherapy	Use of motion, force, or pressure	Massage, mobilization, intermittent compression, continuous passive motion, traction, *whirlpool*, and *ultrasound*
Exercise	Activities the patient performs to bring about a desired response	Various

Modalities in italics are classified in more then one category.

[...]ss each of the four erroneous concepts of reha-
[...]tion. What effect do these misconceptions have
[...]erapeutic modality users?
[...]ibe the 12 principles of rehabilitation.
[...]ibe the 10 core goals of rehabilitation.

therapeutic purpose.
- Describe the relationship between the theory and the application of therapeutic modalities.
- Identify the various therapeutic modality classification systems.
- Discuss the roles of physicians and ATs in determining which therapeutic modality is used, and the selection criteria.
- Define rehabilitation, and the relationship between therapeutic modalities and rehabilitation.

2. Write three to five questions for discussion with your class instructor, clinical instructor, classmates, and clinical colleagues.
3. Get together with classmates and quiz each other on the concepts of this chapter. Use the points in reflection no. 1 and questions you wrote for reflection no. 2 as a beginning. Explaining concepts out loud to others requires a deeper grasp of the material than feeling you understand it as you read.

Concept Check Responses

CONCEPT CHECK 1.1

Knobologists can harm the health professions in several ways:
1. They lack the theory and scientific background to be able to modify or modulate the treatments to cater to the specific needs of their patients.
2. Their patients' health concerns are not resolved as fully or as quickly.
3. They may not be able to fully answer questions asked by their patients.
4. They do not stay current with changes and updates to their profession.
5. They give their profession a bad name or poor image because they are perceived as technicians rather than professions.

CONCEPT CHECK 1.2

When performance is evaluated and the performer is given specific feedback regarding that performance, she is able to make corrections. For example, in the number guessing game, if your friend chose 55 and was told it was wrong, her next choice would be any one of 99 numbers. In the second example, however, telling her that the number was lower would reduce the choices to one of 54 numbers. With each choice and feedback, she gets closer to the right answer. The same is true when you give performance goals and feedback on how the patient performed.

REFERENCES

1. Merriam-Webster's Online Dictionary. Accessed via OneLook Dictionary Search, OneLook.com [website]. Available at: http://www.merriam-webster.com/dictionary/rehabilitation. Accessed November, 2011.
2. MedFriendly Glossary. Accessed via OneLook Dictionary Search, OneLook.com [website]. Available at: http://www.medfriendly.com/letterr.php3. Accessed November, 2011.
3. Knight KL. Quadriceps strengthening with the DAPRE technique: case studies with neurological implications. Med Sci Sports Exerc. 1985;17:646-650.
4. Knight KL. Guidelines for rehabilitation of sports injuries. Clin Sports Med. 1985;4:405-416.
5. Knight KL. Total injury rehabilitation. Phys Sports Med. 1979;7(8):111.
6. DePalma MT, DePalma B. The use of instruction and the behavioral approach to facilitate injury rehabilitation. J Athl Train. 1989;24:217-222.
7. Kegerreis S. The construction and implementation of functional progressions as a component of athletic rehabilitation. J Orthop Sports Phys Ther. 1983;5(1):14-19.
8. Delorme TL, Watkins AL. Technics of progressive resistance exercise. Arch Phys Med. 1948;29(5):263-273.
9. Kvist H, Jarvinen M, Sorvari T. Effect of mobilization and immobilization on the healing of contusion injury in muscle. A preliminary report of a histological study in rats. Scand J Rehabil Med. 1974;6(3):134-140.

Application Tips give you tips for practice and understanding.

Original Photographs taken specifically for this text demonstrate how to perform many of the techniques.

Five-Step Application Procedure Templates streamline how you organize the information needed to apply a modality, helping you quickly learn new modalities.

Special Topic Boxes cover a range of interesting topics such as anecdotes about great pioneers and interactions with patients that illustrate key principles.

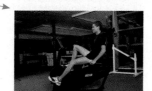

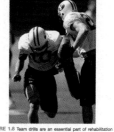

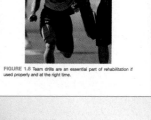

---

266   Part IV • Therapeutic Heat and Cold

gel is applied to the treatment area in sufficient amounts to maintain good contact and lubrication between the soundhead and the skin, but not so much that air pockets form from movement of the soundhead. A direct technique of exposure may be used as long as the surface being treated is larger than the diameter of the soundhead. If a smaller surface area is being treated, use a soundhead with a smaller surface so that direct application can still be performed. In the absence of a smaller soundhead, use the immersion technique.

THE IMMERSION TECHNIQUE

Water is a great coupling medium, but it is not suited for surface application because it will not stay in one place, like gel. There are, however, some instances where you might want to use the underwater technique. The immersion technique is recommended if the area to be treated is smaller than the diameter of the available soundhead, or if the treatment area is irregular with bony prominences (Fig. 14.16).

Use a plastic, ceramic, or rubber basin; a metal basin or whirlpool will reflect some of the ultrasound, thereby increasing the intensity near the basin walls. Tap water seems to be just as effective as degassed water as a coupling medium for the immersion technique and less likely to produce surface heating than mineral oil or glycerin. The soundhead should be moved parallel to the surface being treated at a distance of 0.5–1 cm. If air bubbles accumulate on the soundhead or over the treatment area, wipe them

APPLICATION TIP

CONSIDER THESE POINTS WHEN ADMINISTERING UNDERWATER ULTRASOUND

• If thermal effects are desired, don't use room temperature water; use a water bath at least as warm as body core temperature 98.6°F (37°C).
• Ask yourself if the condition would be better served by using an ultrasound gel pad.

THE GEL PAD TECHNIQUE

If the treatment area is irregular but cannot be immersed in water, you can use a gel pad as a medium. Companies have recently been manufacturing ultrasound gel packs, which consist of gel housed in a thin plastic envelope, or gel pads, which resemble gel-filled clear hockey pucks.

A few studies have been performed on the efficacy of gel pads. Two studies suggest that ultrasound gel pads are as effective as ultrasound gel.[34,35] When the gel pad is used over bony prominences, such as the lateral malleolus of the ankle or the knuckles of the hand, you need to apply a thin layer of ultrasound gel on both sides of the gel pad.[35] The bottom layer ensures that no air is trapped between the bony prominences and the gel pad, and the top layer helps the soundhead glide smoothly on the gel pad (Fig. 14.17).

In another study, two thicknesses of gel pads were

Goal 6: Muscular Speed

Muscular speed is the speed at which a muscle contracts. A good way to develop muscular speed is participation in team drills at half speed, then three-fourths speed, and finally at full speed, focusing on explosive-type activities (short duration, maximal power). Isokinetic exercise also

FIGURE 1.7 A stationary bike is a versatile tool that can be used for developing range of motion, endurance, and power.

FIGURE 1.8 Team drills are an essential part of rehabilitation if used properly and at the right time.

Chapter 14 • Therapeutic Ultrasound   277

Application of Therapeutic Ultrasound

STEP 1: FOUNDATION

A. Definition. Therapeutic ultrasound is inaudible, acoustic vibrations of high frequency that produce either thermal or nonthermal physiologic effects in tissues.
B. Effects
  1. Thermal effects include:
    a. Diminished pain perception
    b. Increased metabolism
    c. Increased blood flow
  2. Nonthermal effects include:
    a. Tissue regeneration
    b. Wound healing
    c. Cell membrane alteration
C. Advantages
  1. Can heat deep tissues without overheating the surface
  2. Heats the deepest of all modalities (except

  6. Pelvis immediately following menstruation
  7. Pregnancy
  8. Pacemaker
  9. Malignancy
  10. Infection
G. Precautions
  1. Epiphyseal areas in young children
  2. Metal implants
  3. Areas of decreased temperature sensation
  4. Areas of decreased circulation
  5. Total joint replacements

STEP 2: PREAPPLICATION TASKS

A. Make sure ultrasound is the proper modality for this situation.
  1. Reevaluate the injury/problem. Make sure you understand the patient's condition.
  2. If ultrasound was applied previously, review the patient's response to the previous treatment.
  3. Confirm that the objectives of therapy are compatible with ultrasound.
  4. Make sure ultrasound is not contraindicated in this situation.

---

188   Part IV • Therapeutic Heat and Cold

BOX 10.2 METRIC SYSTEM ABBREVIATIONS

ABBREVIATIONS	MEANING	VALUE
K	kilo	10^3 or 1000
M	mega	10^6 or 1,000,000
c	centa	10^{-2} or 1/100
m	milli	10^{-3} or 1/1000
u	micro	10^{-6} or 1/1,000,000
um	millimicro	10^{-9} or 1/1,000,000,000
n	nano	10^{-9} or 1/1,000,000,000
A	angstrom	10^{-10} or 1/10,000,000,000

SIMILARITIES AND DIFFERENCES AMONG FORMS OF RADIATION

As mentioned earlier, radiation propagates energy through empty space as **electromagnetic waves**, which take many forms, including heat, light, electricity, x-rays, and cosmic rays (Fig. 10.2). Forms of radiation have the following in common:

The various forms of radiation have these main differences:

• Some forms are visible (such as light).
• Some forms are audible (such as radio waves).
• Some forms you can feel (such as electricity and infrared).
• Some forms can pass through you (such as x-rays).
• Each form has different energy.
• Each form has a unique wavelength and a unique frequency.

The differences between various forms of radiation result from their different energy levels, which result from their specific wavelengths and frequencies (see Fig. 10.2).

ELECTROMAGNETIC WAVES

Electromagnetic waves consist of oscillating electric and magnetic fields at right angles to one another and at right angles to the propagation direction (Fig. 10.3). Individual electromagnetic waves, although dual in nature, behave as a single wave and are often represented as such. Each has a unique wavelength and frequency.

Wavelength is the distance, expressed in meters or centimeters, of one repetition of the wave (Fig. 10.4).

Special Study Tools

These special study tools enhance your learning and your success of applying therapeutic modalities in the future.

Reflections are open-ended questions and tasks at the end of each chapter that help you apply your skills dealing with real-world issues.

Review Questions at the end of each part (with answers in the appendix) help you assess your knowledge as you progress through the text.

Case Studies in the final chapter ask you to apply what you've learned by choosing specific modalities to meet particular patient needs.

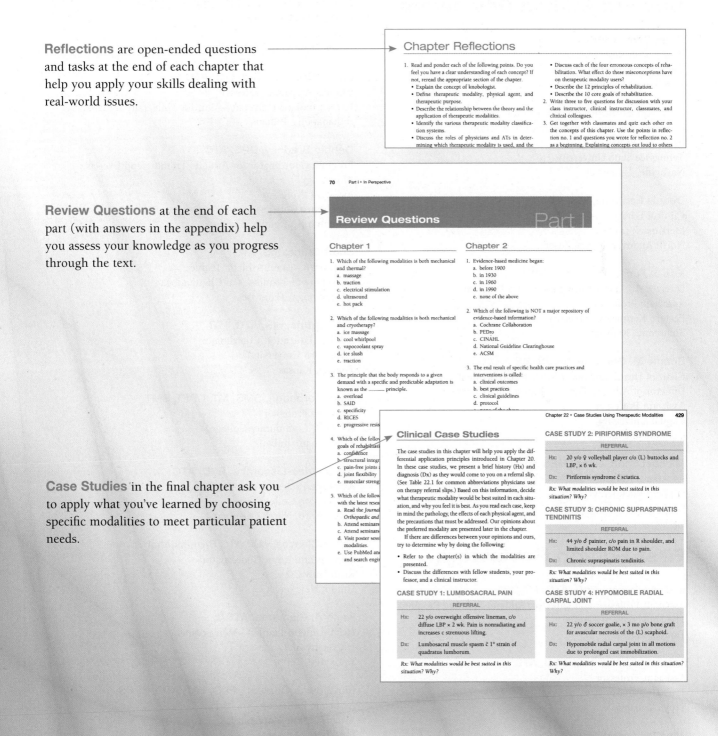

Reviewers

Second Edition Reviewers

Brian Czajka, MS
Assistant Professor
The University of Michigan
Ann Arbor, Michigan

Deborah Edmondson, PT, EdD, CWcHP
Academic Coordinator of Clinical Education
Associate Professor
Tennessee State University
Nashville, Tennessee

Dennis Fontaine, MS, ATC
Clinical Education Coordinator
Merrimack College
North Andover, Massachusetts

Eric J. Fuchs, DA, ATC, EMT
Director Athletic Training Education Program
Associate Professor
Eastern Kentucky University
Richmond, Kentucky

Bonnie M. Goodwin, MESS, BS
Chair of Health and Sport Sciences Department
Director of Athletic Training Education Program
Assistant Professor
Capital University
Columbus, Ohio

Michael Scott Zema, MEd, ATC
Assistant Professor
Slippery Rock University
Slippery Rock, Pennsylvania

First Edition Reviewers

J. C. Andersen, PhD, ATC, PT, SCS
Assistant Professor and Director, Athletic Training Program
The University of Tampa
Tampa, Florida

Amanda K. Andrews, PhD, ATC
Assistant Professor
Troy University
Troy, Alabama

Jennifer Austin, PhD, ATC
Assistant Professor
Colby-Sawyer College
New London, New Hampshire

Barbara Belyea, PT, MS, CSCS
Clinical Associate Professor
Ithaca College
Ithaca, New York

Jay A. Bradley, MEd, LAT, ATC
Clinical Assistant Professor
IUPUI: Indiana University—Purdue University Indianapolis
Indianapolis, Indiana

Debbie Bradney, DPE, ATC
Program Coordinator for Athletic Training and Exercise Physiology
Assistant Professor
Lynchburg College
Lynchburg, Virginia

Scott Bruce, MS, ATC
Lecturer/Assistant Athletic Trainer
University of Tennessee at Chattanooga
Chattanooga, Tennessee

John Burns, MS, ATC, LAT
Clinical Education Coordinator
Washburn University
Topeka, Kansas

Mary Carbaugh, SMS, MT, CPFT, SMT
Assistant Professor
Ivy Tech Community College
Fort Wayne, Indiana

BC Charles-Liscombe, EdD, ATC
Associate Professor
Greensboro College
Greensboro, North Carolina

Gwen Cleaves, MA, ATC Professional
Clinical Education Coordinator
Kean University
Union, New Jersey

Keith A. Clements, ATC/L
Head Athletic Trainer—Men's Athletics
University of Tennessee
Knoxville, Tennessee

Matthew J. Comeau, PhD, LAT, ATC, CSCS
Associate Professor
Arkansas State University
Jonesboro, Arkansas

Shawna Jordan, PhD, ATC, LAT
Assistant Professor
Athletic Training Education Program Director
Kansas State University
Manhattan, Kansas

Owen Keller, ATC
Associate Professor
Athletic Trainer
Ohio Northern University
Ada, Ohio

Robin E. Kennel, MS, LAT, ATC, CSCS
ATEP Director/Assistant Athletic Trainer
Mars Hill College
Mars Hill, North Carolina

Casey Kohr, MS, PT, ATC, LAT
Instructor of Athletic Training
Clarke College
Dubuque, Iowa

Mark Lafave, PhD (ABD), MSc, CAT(C)
Department Chair and Instructor
Mount Royal College
Calgary, Alberta

Rifat Latifi, MD, FACS
Professor of Clinical Surgery
The University of Arizona College of Medicine
Tucson, Arizona

Christine A. Lauber, EdD, LAT, ATC
Associate Professor
University of Indianapolis
Indianapolis, Indiana

Barbara H. Long, MS, VATL, ATC
Chair, Health and Exercise Science
Bridgewater College
Bridgewater, Virginia

Susan Lowe, PT, DPT, MS, GCS
Associate Clinical Professor
Northeastern University
Boston, Massachusetts

William T. Lyons, MS, ATC
Director of Athletic Training Education
University of Wyoming
Laramie, Wyoming

Brendon P. McDermott, MS, ATC
Laboratory Instructor/Research Assistant
University of Connecticut
Storrs, Connecticut

Tsega A. Mehreteab, PT, MS, DPT
Clinical Professor
New York University
New York, New York

Mark A. Merrick, PhD, ATC
Associate Professor and Director
Division of Athletic Training
The Ohio State University
Columbus, Ohio

Angela Mickle, PhD, ATC
Associate Professor
Radford University
Radford, Virginia

Charles Miller, MS, ATC, CSCS, PES
Athletic Trainer
West Liberty State College
West Liberty, West Virginia

Matthew Miltenberger, MS, ATC, CSCS
Instructor
East Stroudsburg University
East Stroudsburg, Pennsylvania

Kyle Momsen, MA, ATC
ATEP Clinical Education Coordinator
Gustavus Adolphus College
St. Peter, Minnesota

Brad Montgomery, MAT, ATC
Head Athletic Trainer/Instructor
The University of West Alabama
Livingston, Alabama

Patricia Morganroth, MSN, RN, CDE
Program Chair—Health and Fitness
Cincinnati State Technical and Community College
Cincinnati, Ohio

Christopher W. O'Brien, MS, ATC
Athletic Training Education Program Director
Assistant Professor of Health and Physical Education
Marywood University
Scranton, Pennsylvania

Matthew S. O'Brien, PhD, ATC
Assistant Professor
Oklahoma State University
Stillwater, Oklahoma

Kim O'Connell-Brock, MS, ATC/L
Assistant Director, ATEP
New Mexico State University
Las Cruces, New Mexico

Gretchen D. Oliver, PhD, ATC
Assistant Professor
University of Arkansas
Fayetteville, Arizona

Robert W. Pettitt, PhD, ATC, CSCS
Program Director, Athletic Training
California State University, Fresno
Fresno, California

Roberta L. Pohlman, PhD
Associate Professor
Wright State University
Dayton, Ohio

Kristyn Powell-Holmes, MS
Department Head
Utah Career College
West Jordan, Utah

Kris Ring, MS, ATC, LAT
Head Athletic Trainer/Lecturer
Texas Woman's University
Denton, Texas

Jeffrey J. Roberts, MS, ATC, NASM-PES
Clinical Coordinator of Athletic Training
San Jose State University
San Jose, California

Mack D. Rubley, PhD, ATC, CSCS
Associate Professor
Director, Athletic Training Education Program
University of Nevada, Las Vegas
Las Vegas, Nevada

Chris Schmidt, PhD, ATC
Assistant Professor
Azusa Pacific University
Azusa, California

Lisa Schniepp, MA, ATC
Athletic Trainer/Instructor
University of Nebraska at Omaha
Omaha, Nebraska

Chris Schommer, MEd, ATC
Program Coordinator Athletic Training
Bowling Green State University
Bowling Green, Ohio

Kent Scriber, EdD, ATC, PT
Professor
Department of Exercise and Sport Sciences
Ithaca College
Ithaca, New York

Carlyn Sikes, MFA, E-RYT
Faculty
Scottsdale Community College
Scottsdale, Arizona

Veronica Southard, PT, DHSc, GCS
Associate Professor
New York Institute of Technology
Old Westbury, New York

Robert Stow, PhD, ATC, CSCS
Assistant Professor, Director—Athletic Training Education
University of Wisconsin—Eau Claire
Eau Claire, Wisconsin

Lorna R. Strong, MS, ATC, LAT
Instructor
West Texas A&M University
Canyon, Texas

Jeff Sullivan, PhD, ATC
Associate Professor/Director of Rehabilitation
Point Loma Nazarene University
San Diego, California

Scott Sunderland, MS, ATC
Head Certified Athletic Trainer/Assistant Adjunct Professor
Knox College
Galesburg, Illinois

Derek Suranie, MEd, ATC
Assistant Professor
North Georgia College & State University
Dahlonega, Georgia

Erik E. Swartz, PhD, ATC
Associate Professor and Clinical Coordinator
Athletic Training Education Program, Department of Kinesiology
University of New Hampshire
Durham, New Hampshire

LesLee Taylor, PhD, ATC, LAT
Assistant Professor
Texas Tech University Health Sciences Center
Lubbock, Texas

Adam J. Thompson, PhD, ATC, LAT
Associate Professor
Indiana Wesleyan University
Marion, Indiana

Brian Udermann, PhD, ATC, FACSM
Associate Professor
University of Wisconsin—La Crosse
La Crosse, Wisconsin

Heather L. VanOpdorp, MSEd, ATC
Instructor/Athletic Training Room Coordinator
University of Tampa
Tampa, Florida

Ben Velasquez, DA, ATC, LAT
Associate Professor
University of Southern Mississippi
Hattiesburg, Mississippi

Gary Ward, MS, ATC, PT
Assistant Professor and Program Director
Department of Sports Medicine and Athletic Training
Missouri State University
Springfield, Missouri

Scot A. Ward, MS, ATC
Clinical Coordinator/Athletic Trainer
Keene State College
Keene, New Hampshire

Tony Ward, MS, ATC, LAT
Assistant Professor
Director
Athletic Training Education Program
Shawnee State University
Portsmouth, Ohio

Susie Wehring, MS, ATC, LAT
Associate Professor
Loras College
Dubuque, Iowa

Chuck Whedon, MS, ATC, CSCS
Coordinator of Athletic Training Services
Instructor, Health and Exercise Science
Rowan University
Glassboro, New Jersey

Jackie Williams, PhD, LAT, ATC
Director of Athletic Training Education
University of Idaho
Moscow, Idaho

Scott Woken, MA, ATC
Director of Sports Medicine
North Dakota State University
Fargo, North Dakota

Michael Scott Zema, MEd, ATC
Assistant Professor/Football Athletic Trainer
Slippery Rock University of Pennsylvania
Slippery Rock, Pennsylvania

Contents

PART III: PAIN AND ORTHOPEDIC INJURIES

PART IV: THERAPEUTIC HEAT AND COLD

PART V: ELECTROTHERAPY

PART VI: OTHER MODALITIES

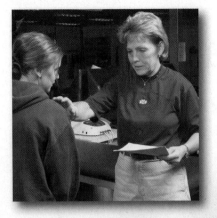

In Perspective

What are therapeutic modalities? Why are they used? How do they relate to therapeutic exercise? How do you know what therapeutic modality to use and when to use it? What is evidence-based practice? The objective of Part I is to answer these questions and thus establish an overall perspective for therapeutic modality use. We define therapeutic modalities and help you understand their place in orthopedic injury management and explain how they relate to total rehabilitation. We discuss the concept of medical practice, why it must be based on the best scientific evidence available, and how to acquire such evidence. We then present a rationale for using a standardized systems approach to therapeutic modality application. Finally, we present a case for proper record keeping, indicating how doing so can strengthen both the efficacy of your treatments and the quality of your health care. Thus Part I is a foundation for the rest of the book.

The material in chapter 2, Evidence-Based Practice, is much more in-depth than will be covered in a typical therapeutic modalities class. There is, however, no other source in the athletic training literature with an extensive, over-all treatment of evidence-based medicine and practice. As a result, many have a confused and/or incomplete understanding of the concept. We feel this comprehensive treatment of the topic will help reduce that confusion.

Evidence-based medicine should be part of most, if not every, every athletic training curriculum class. We recommend that the history and basic concepts be introduced early in the curriculum and additional aspects be taught in subsequent classes, using this chapter as the text for the units in those additional classes.

Therapeutic Modalities:
What They Are and Why They Are Used

Chapter Outline

OPENING SCENE

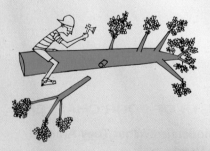

FIGURE 1.1 You can get the job done with the wrong tool, but it takes longer and the result might not be as successful.

A father enlisted his young son to help remove a small dead tree from their yard. The eager boy got a small hatchet from the garage and began feverishly chopping away at tree limbs (Fig. 1.1). Although he worked very hard, his progress was slow. The father appeared with a power saw and quickly cut off the limbs and trunk. He said, "Son, it's important to work hard—but it's even more important to work smart. We could use that little hatchet and work hard all day chopping up these limbs, or we can work smart and use the right tool to finish the job in just minutes."

Many clinicians believe that their hands and exercise are the best tools for treating orthopedic injuries. These aren't the only tools, however, and integrating therapeutic modalities as part of a treatment regime often facilitates the hands-on treatment. For example, cryokinetics involves numbing a joint with cold, followed by active exercise. If the patient did not ice the ankle prior to exercise, pain and inhibition would compromise the exercise, thereby making it less effective. In this case, ice is the tool that causes numbing, so the patient can perform a higher level of exercise. The exercise alone is good, but numbing and exercise together are smart.

In **physical medicine**, a therapeutic modality is a tool for bringing about a desired therapeutic response. In this book, you learn why, how, and when to use several tools in your treatment regimens.

Defining and Classifying Therapeutic Modalities

A **therapeutic modality** is a device or application that delivers a physical agent to the body for therapeutic purposes. The most common **physical agents** used in treating orthopedic injuries are:

- Heat
- Cold
- Light
- Electricity
- Exercise

The **therapeutic purposes** of these agents are to promote or improve:

1. Wound healing
2. Pain relief
3. Flexibility and range of motion
4. Muscular strength
5. Muscular endurance
6. Muscular speed
7. Muscular coordination or skill
8. Muscular power
9. Agility
10. Cardiorespiratory endurance

There are several systems of classifying therapeutic modalities. They can be classified according to the physical agent used, such as hydrotherapy, thermotherapy, and electrotherapy. They can be classified according to tissue responses, such as deep heating, superficial heating, and cooling. However, these categories are not exclusive, and many therapeutic modalities fit into different categories. For example, ultrasound can be classified as thermotherapy, mechanical, or deep heating. Contrast therapy is both cryotherapy and thermotherapy. General classifications are shown in Table 1.1. Modalities in italics are classified in more than one category.

Which of the classification systems is preferred? None of them. Because so many modalities fit into multiple categories, trying to force one particular classification system is an exercise in futility.

TABLE 1.1	GENERAL CLASSIFICATIONS OF THERAPEUTIC MODALITIES	
CLASSIFICATION	**DESCRIPTION**	**EXAMPLES**
Cryotherapy	Use of cold (usually between 32°F and 70°F; 0°C and 21°C).	Ice massage, ice packs, *ice slush/ice immersion*, part of contrast therapy, cold *whirlpool*, and vapocoolant sprays.
Thermotherapy	Use of superficial and deep heat (usually between 98.6°F and 109.4°F; 37°C and 43°C)	moist heat packs, warm whirlpool, paraffin wax baths, ultrasound, *pulsed shortwave diathermy*, and ultraviolet
Hydrotherapy	Application of water	*Whirlpool* and aquatic therapy pools, and *ice slush/ice immersion*
Electrotherapy	Use of electricity	EMS, iontophoresis, TENS, and *diathermy*
Light therapy	Use of electromagnetic radiation	Laser, light therapy, *infrared*
Mechanotherapy	Use of motion, force, or pressure	Massage, mobilization, intermittent compression, continuous passive motion, traction, *whirlpool*, and *ultrasound*
Exercise	Activities the patient performs to bring about a desired response	Various

Modalities in italics are classified in more than one category.

Maximizing the Effectiveness of Therapeutic Modalities

Therapeutic modalities can be powerful tools for caring for and rehabilitating orthopedic injuries, or they can contribute little to the process. They are effective only when the proper modality is applied in the proper way to injured tissue. There is little value in using the wrong modality properly or in using the right modality improperly. Consider the following ideas as you develop your personal philosophical basis for using therapeutic modalities.

ART AND SCIENCE

The use of therapeutic modalities, like all practices in the health professions, is an art—an art influenced by experience and tradition and by science and theory (Fig. 1.2). It would be ideal if the use of therapeutic modalities were based entirely on scientific fact. But this is unrealistic for two reasons. First, the human body is very complex, and there has not been enough research to fully explain its response to either injury or the application of therapeutic modalities. Second, many clinicians are not current with the modality research that has been done, and therefore their use of modalities is outdated.

Your initial use of therapeutic modalities will be influenced heavily by the traditions and theories of your clinical instructors. These may or may not agree with the concepts presented in this text. We have heard horror stories over the years of clinics where most patients were treated the same way regardless of their injury. For example, in one clinic 95% of patients were "HUM'd," treated with hot packs, ultrasound, and mobilization. Regardless of the approach of your initial clinical instructors, strive to gradually increase the scientific and theoretical influence on your own clinical practice.

KNOBOLOGY

Knobology is a tongue-in-cheek term for the study of application without theory. One of our colleagues uses the term "knobologist" for students and clinicians who want to know only which knobs on a therapeutic modality to turn but are uninterested in why they are doing so (Fig. 1.3). Not only would there be little advancement in medicine if all clinicians were knobologists, but patients would suffer from inadequate treatment. Don't be a knobologist!

 CONCEPT CHECK 1.1. List some ways that "knobologists" can harm the health professions.

APPLICATION: EVIDENCE VERSUS OPINION, RUMOR VERSUS REALITY, FACT VERSUS FICTION

The ideal is that all application is based on scientifically derived evidence and theory. Yet this is not possible, because application almost always precedes theory, and there is a lack of valid research. A clinician, frustrated with a particular case, or group of similar cases, tries something new to help her patients. It seems to work, so she modifies the approach, talks to colleagues, talks to patients, fine-tunes some more, and shares the approach with others. As the popularity and acceptance of the technique grow, people begin trying to explain why the application works. These explanations become a theory. In time, scientists test the theory with research. The research either strengthens or alters the

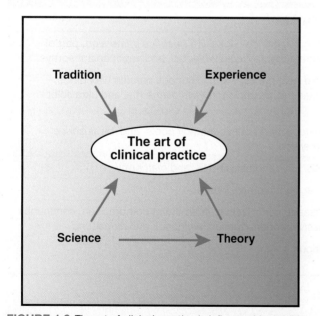

FIGURE 1.2 The art of clinical practice is influenced by tradition, experience, science, and theory.

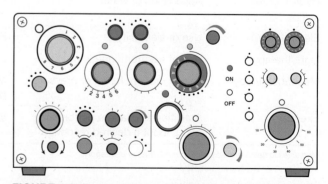

FIGURE 1.3 Knobologists know the knobs but not why they use the knobs.

theory and often results in adjustments to the application. Thus, application, theory, and research are intertwined, each stimulating the other.

It is critical for a clinician to learn both application and theory. She must adjust the application and its theoretical basis as new knowledge becomes available. This practice may even provide opportunities for participating in the discovery of new approaches.

CLINICAL DECISION MAKING

Clinical decision making is the process of determining how to treat patients. It is an ongoing, dynamic process that should occur before every therapeutic modality application. It requires critical thinking and evaluation of the evidence available for the specific injury, patient, availability of therapeutic modalities, and other therapeutic interventions, such as drugs and therapeutic exercise. The process begins with a thorough evaluation of the patient and the specific injury or condition. Analysis of the subjective and objective data leads to a tentative diagnosis. A plan of action is then outlined, which prescribes how the patient will be treated, which includes the role of therapeutic modalities.

Following are the four main sources of information that clinicians draw upon when formulating plans of action. They are:

1. *Tradition*. How it has always been done. Techniques and procedures that have been handed down from one clinician to the next to the next, etc.
2. *Experience*. The result of successes and failures with similar patients and similar conditions in the past.
3. *Research*. The result of scientific investigation. This evidence will range from general to specific (see Chapter 2).
4. *Theory*. The best guess of what is going on, based on a logician evaluation of evidence. The strength of a theory is determined by the strength of the evidence upon which it is based and the care with which the evidence is tied together.

In Chapter 2, we discuss the essential role of research in selecting and using therapeutic modalities and the roles and relative value of various types of research evidence. The concepts of "best practices" and "evidence-based practice" are also discussed.

Selecting a Therapeutic Modality

Who selects the modality to treat patient X? On what criteria is that decision based? In this section, we discuss the philosophy and general principles of modality selection.

WHOSE DECISION?

Who selects which therapeutic modality to use in treating a patient? The athletic trainer (AT)? A physical therapist (PT)? The team physician? The patient's family physician? The decision depends on your specific state practice act, which usually stipulates that ATs apply therapeutic modalities under the direction of a physician. This can be problematic, however, when physicians do not provide specific guidelines and leave clinicians to determine the treatment. For instance, if a physician prescribes "therapy for _____ due to pain and swelling of the left ankle," the clinician must choose the specific modality to use.

PTs and ATs sometimes work under the direction of a **physiatrist**, an MD who is a specialist in **physical medicine and rehabilitation**, the medical subspecialty relating to the treatment and rehabilitation of physical conditions. Physiatrists usually provide clear prescriptions, so the clinician knows exactly what modality to use. But most PTs and ATs receive prescriptions from physicians who either have not been trained in the use of therapeutic modalities or are not up-to-date concerning their use. What then? Does the AT make his own decision and ignore the physician? This is not only against the law, but it is unethical. Instead, you must help the physician understand why and when to use various therapeutic modalities so that he can adequately direct their use.

SELECTION CRITERIA

To responsibly decide which modality to use, you should:

1. Have a correct diagnosis, which results from analysis of the subjective and objective data obtained during a thorough evaluation of the patient and the specific injury or condition
2. Have a definite concept of the pathological and physiological changes associated with the injury
3. Outline an overall treatment plan which includes long range, medium range, and short range therapeutic goals
4. Understand the modality's effects, indications, and contraindications, including the type and strength of evidence supporting this information (see Chapter 2)
5. Match your therapeutic goal with a modality that will help you achieve that goal

Rehabilitation and Therapeutic Modalities

Many will question having a section on rehabilitation in a therapeutic modality text. A proper understanding of the role of therapeutic modalities depends, however, on understanding the overall orthopedic injury rehabilitation process. The definition of rehabilitation (given in the next subsection) will help you appreciate how therapeutic modalities fit into the rehabilitation process. You must begin now to understand that therapeutic modality use is part of rehabilitation, not something that precedes it.

In this and subsequent sections, we discuss some erroneous concepts about rehabilitation, present some basic principles to guide rehabilitation, develop a rationale for a systems approach to rehabilitation, and discuss some of the psychological factors that can optimize rehabilitation.

REHABILITATION DEFINED

Rehabilitation means restoring to a former capacity by providing training or therapy.[1] (The term is derived from the Latin *rehabilitate*, "to make fit again.")[2] The entire process of returning an injured patient to her pre-injury status, including the use of therapeutic modalities, is rehabilitation.

FOUR ERRONEOUS CONCEPTS ABOUT REHABILITATION

There are many erroneous concepts about rehabilitation, which, if applied, might compromise proper and complete rehabilitation. Four are discussed here. Clinicians should try to avoid letting these ideas become part of their thinking about rehabilitation.

Misconception 1: Treating Injuries, Then Rehabilitating Them

Some clinicians think treating injuries is separate from rehabilitation. They "treat" their patients with modalities and then "rehabilitate" them with exercise. This is inconsistent with the definition of rehabilitation. Rehabilitation is the entire process of returning an injured person to her normal habits. So treatment with modalities is part of rehabilitation, not something that precedes it.

Does it matter how you define these processes? Yes. If you define treatment and rehabilitation as separate processes, you would be inclined to use therapeutic modalities and therapeutic exercise sequentially, rather than together. As you will see throughout this text, therapeutic modalities and therapeutic exercise complement each other and in many cases must be used together.

The following two erroneous concepts are part of the reason that some think treatment and rehabilitation are separate. Tie each of these concepts back to this one as you read them.

Misconception 2: Rehabilitation is Reconditioning

Injury rehabilitation is often called **reconditioning**, meaning conditioning again. The two processes do share some common principles, but there are also some fundamental differences. Rehabilitation includes conditioning, but it also involves the promotion of healing and pain relief. For instance, a patient who has torn a tendon cannot begin a reconditioning program until the tendon has healed. Pain relief is also part of rehabilitation. Because pain activates neural mechanisms that inhibit strength, flexibility, and so on, pain must be addressed before reconditioning can begin.

Another difference is that the speed at which physical attributes redevelop during rehabilitation can be much faster than during original conditioning.[3] Thus, rehabilitation can be much more aggressive than conditioning.

Misconception 3: Working with Weights

Although the "rehab area" of many athletic training and sports medicine clinics is the area that contains the weight-training equipment, the terms *rehab, working with weights,* and *strength training* are not synonymous. Rehabilitation is not complete if the patient works only with weights, regardless of how creative and intense the work.

Misconception 4: The Cookbook Approach

In the **cookbook approach to rehabilitation,** the clinician follows a specific recipe or protocol for treating each injury. The protocol includes phases with specific time periods and therapeutic interventions. For instance, phase 2 might last from 2 to 6 weeks post-injury and include thermotherapy, isokinetic exercises, isotonic exercises, StairMaster, cycling, swimming, and light running. The appeal of the cookbook approach is that it is easy to follow because there is a specific protocol for each injury. Its limitation is that all patients with the same or similar injury are treated the same, without regard for individual differences. Variables that are disregarded in the cookbook approach include:

- The patient's genetic makeup, general health, pre-injury state of conditioning, psychological profile, and work ethic
- The severity of the injury and associated problems
- The rate of progress (patients respond differently to the same interventions)
- The difference in demands placed on the injured body part during sport participation (a runner must spend more time developing muscular endurance than a golfer; a football player must develop more muscular speed than a distance runner)
- The time of the season (demands on a patient are greater during the sport season than during the off-season)

Every patient and every injury is different, so rehabilitation programs must be individualized. Optimal rehabilitation is not planned by the calendar and not achieved by specific exercises.

This erroneous concept developed because application techniques generally precede theory; clinicians tend to use treatments or rehabilitation techniques before they know why they are effective. As a result, many professionals have a bag of tricks, an assortment of techniques, that have not been brought together under an overall theoretical umbrella. This is changing, however; professionals are more often looking at the entire process and taking a systems approach to rehabilitation.[4,5]

A Systems Approach to Rehabilitation

The guiding philosophy of the **systems approach to rehabilitation** is that each patient and each injury is unique and therefore treatment must be individualized, dynamic, and interactive. Therapeutic intervention is based on the patient's initial signs and symptoms, customized to the patient's needs, and adjusted according to patient progress. The systems approach is based on 12 principles of rehabilitation and directed by 10 core goals related to the independent but interrelated physical **performance attributes**, such as pain-free movement, muscular strength, and motor control. Since injury disrupts one or more of the performance attributes, rehabilitation consists of systematically reestablishing the attributes. The principles and core goals are discussed in the next two sections.

TWELVE PRINCIPLES OF ORTHOPEDIC INJURY REHABILITATION

This section covers 12 essential principles of rehabilitation. All of them apply, regardless of the type of injury being rehabilitated. These principles provide the theoretical framework for decision making during rehabilitation. They are discussed below in random order.

The SAID Principle
Rehabilitation is dominated by the **SAID principle**, an acronym for "specific adaptation to imposed demands." Stated another way, the body responds to a given demand with a specific and predictable adaptation. For a specific adaptation to occur, a specific demand must be imposed. For example, if you want to develop endurance in a particular muscle group (the specific adaptation), you must require that particular muscle group to repeatedly contract over a longer time (the imposed demand).

An AT (or other clinician) must identify and use training to specifically address each performance attribute to be redeveloped (or developed if the patient was not properly conditioned prior to the injury). A patient can only achieve total rehabilitation if the AT works with him to redevelop each aspect of conditioning through individual specific imposed demands.

Therapeutic Goals
Therapeutic goals establish your aim or desired result. To put the SAID principle into practice, you must establish therapeutic goals and then select a therapeutic regimen that elicits the physiological and psychological responses required for achieving those goals. Goals help you determine the specific demand to impose on the patient. Plan your work and then work the plan.

Plan specific goals for a variety of time frames. Daily goals should lead to short-range goals, which in turn should progressively lead to helping the patient attain long-range goals. Be flexible in adjusting or adding goals as the rehabilitation progresses and the needs of the patient change.

Another advantage of goal-oriented rehabilitation is that by directing the rehabilitation using numerous specific goals, patients can see regular progress as they achieve these goals.[6] The satisfaction in achieving the goals gives patients a psychological boost. Use goals liberally during rehabilitation.

Continual Evaluation
Proper application of the SAID principle does not end at determining a specific adaptation and planning goals after the initial diagnosis of the nature and severity of the injury. Reevaluation is necessarily almost daily to determine the patient's response to the therapeutic regimen and progress toward her goals (Fig. 1.4).

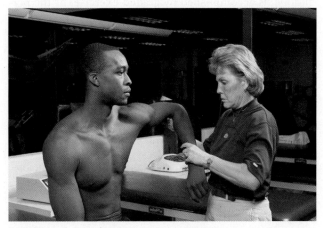

FIGURE 1.4 Evaluation of the anatomical and pathological changes induced by the injury is essential to establishing therapeutic goals and selecting the appropriate modality. Also periodic reevaluation is essential in determining the success of the treatment regimen and in altering the course of treatment.

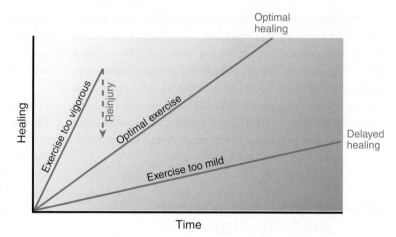

FIGURE 1.5 Therapeutic exercise is essential to healing an injury. Optimal healing requires a balance between exercise that is so vigorous that it might cause further injury and exercise that is so mild that healing is delayed. Reinjury (*vertical dashed line*) can result from exercise that is too vigorous.

Overload and Progression

Overload is the concept of challenging the body to greater function by pushing it beyond its comfort zone to near its limits. The body likes to have a reserve, so when you demand near-total functioning by a system, the body attempts to develop a reserve. Of course, if your demands are too great, you will injure the system (Fig. 1.5). Once the body adapts to the overload, you increase the challenge (load) and thus require additional adaptation.

Weight training is a good example of this concept. If a muscle's maximal strength is 50 lb and a person trains by lifting 40 lb for a few sessions, the muscle will adapt so that it can lift 55 lb. Increasing the training weight to 45 lb will result in an additional strength increase. Continuing the process with incremental increases once the body has adapted is known as **progression**.

Functional Progression

Functional progression, also known as *progressive reorientation*, is accomplished by **graded exercise**, or the performance of functional activities in an ordered sequence, beginning with simple, easy activity and progressing to full sport or work activity.[7] It is based on the concept of progressive resistive exercise (PRE) to regain strength during rehabilitation, developed by Delorme and Watkins.[8] Functional progression facilitates the acquisition or reacquisition of skills required for the safe and effective performance of complex skills.[7] Patients usually progress from:

- unloaded activities to
- loaded activities to
- overloaded activities

And from:

- single-plane activities to
- multiple-plane activities

Both of which progress from:

- slow speed to
- normal speed to
- high speed

And with:

- slow transition to
- normal transition to
- very quick transition

The Absence of Pain

All therapeutic exercise should be relatively pain free. If the activity is more than mildly uncomfortable, this is a signal from the body that something is wrong. The rehabilitation exercise or activity should not evoke pain. If it does, the activity is too vigorous and should be simplified.

✔ APPLICATION TIP

REHABILITATION MUST BE PAIN-FREE

"No pain no gain" does not apply to rehabilitation, but "Ignore the pain equals no brain" does.

Biofeedback

Biofeedback is a process of measuring a biological mechanism using some objective means and then telling the patient his scores. The feedback stimulates more rapid patient progress. Although there are commercial biofeedback devices that measure variables such as electrical activity in a muscle or the temperature in a finger, biofeedback does not require these devices. The concept is much greater in scope and simpler to use than a machine. For instance, when you are trying to develop elbow flexibility, you could tell the patient to "move your arm so that your fingers touch the wall during extension and my hand during flexion." Tell the patient to perform a specific number of repetitions, say 10. Count each repetition out loud so the patient hears you. If a repetition is incomplete (does not reach both the wall and your hand), tell the patient the repetition does not count. You can provide further biofeedback by timing the patient's performance: "Let's see how long it takes you to perform 10 complete repetitions." Tell the patient the time and then ask "do you think you can perform 10 more repetitions faster than before?" The second set of repetitions will almost always be faster than the first.

Do you think Rodger Bannister would have broken the 4-minute mile if he just went out and ran without keeping track of his time? Of course not. Performance improves when the patient or athlete is given specific feedback concerning his performance.

Use your imagination to determine specific performance goals for every therapeutic exercise you have the patient do. Then measure the performance and report the results to the patient. The combination of specific performance goals and feedback concerning how the patient performed relative to the goals has a powerful effect on performance.

 CONCEPT CHECK 1.2. Try the following biofeedback exercise. Think of a number between 1 and 100. Ask a friend to guess the number. Unless she is very lucky, she will guess wrong. Say, "Wrong, try again." Continue this process until she eventually gets lucky and guesses the number. Repeat the process, perhaps with someone else, but this time give more effective feedback; say, "lower [or higher]" after each guess. The specific feedback should cause the friend to guess the number much more quickly. Why?

Early Exercise

Early exercise is essential to rehabilitation. Not only does the proper use of exercise speed the healing process,[9–13] but a lack of exercise during the early stages of rehabilitation can result in permanent disability.[14] Caution is essential, however, because exercise that is too vigorous can also result in permanent disability.[14] The optimal conditions for healing depend on a fine balance between protection from too much stress and a return to normal functioning at the earliest possible time[12] (see Fig. 1.5).

A classic series of studies by Jarvinen and associates[9–13] supports this theory. Immediate mobilization following contusions to the legs of rats led to a more pronounced macrophage reaction, quicker hematoma resolution, an increased vascular ingrowth, quicker regeneration of muscle and scar tissue, and increased tensile strength of the

healed muscle. Immobilization for only 2 or 5 days, on the other hand, delayed contraction and maturation of the scar when measured 42 days later. Exercise during rehabilitation also results in stronger ligaments and tendons.

Relatively Rapid Rate of Reconditioning

As mentioned, many physical attributes can be redeveloped much more quickly than they were developed originally. Much of the loss of performance with injury is the result of pain-induced neural inhibition. Rehabilitation involves systematically removing the inhibitions rather than developing the attribute from the beginning.

Timelines

Rehabilitation should begin immediately after the injury occurs and end only when the patient can fully participate in her sport, with no limitations imposed by the injury. Obviously the complexity of rehabilitation will depend on the magnitude and type of injury sustained, as well as the requirements of the sport. A runner with a sprained finger usually will not have to worry about it as much as a quarterback would. But even for a quarterback, rehabilitation of a sprained finger would not be as complicated, or take as long, as rehabilitation of a sprained ankle. Whether the process is simple or complex, it should follow the same general process to ensure complete rehabilitation.

It is important to accomplish the rehabilitation process as quickly as possible. Many negative consequences result from prolonged absence from participation. Inactivity can lead to atrophy of specific muscle groups, loss of overall conditioning, skills becoming rusty, loss of the patient's sixth sense, and emotional trauma. Often an injury is accompanied by feelings of frustration, discouragement, and self-doubt that become greater the longer the patient is unable to participate.

Prioritizing

The return of the patient to full performance is the priority, and the motivating force, of early rehabilitation. No matter how valuable an athlete is to the team, the interests of neither the team nor the coach should take precedence over the health of the patient.

Maintain Conditioning

It is important to maintain conditioning of uninjured body segments and systems while the injury is being rehabilitated. If you allow the whole body to decondition while the injury is rehabilitating, you have additional problems to resolve before the patient can return to full activity. It is relatively easy for an active person to maintain conditioning; she just has to alter her physical activities. For example, a patient with an upper extremity injury can run or peddle an exercise bike. Or a person with a lower extremity injury can swim, peddle an exercise bike with a single leg, or run in chest high water in a swimming pool.

THE 10 CORE GOALS OF ORTHOPEDIC INJURY REHABILITATION

The fundamental goal of orthopedic injury rehabilitation is to return the patient to full, unhindered activity. For an athlete, this means the ability to fully perform his sport. Injury results in torn tissue and/or pain, both of which cause **neural inhibition** (decreasing or stopping) of performance attributes. Thus during rehabilitation you must be concerned with healing damaged tissue, removing pain, and reestablishing each of the performance attributes.

The 10 core goals of rehabilitation are listed in Table 1.2. Goals 3–10 are performance attributes necessary for an athlete to be successful. Goals 1 and 2 are prerequisites for the last 8. When a healthy athlete develops these attributes, she is conditioning; when a patient redevelops them following injury, she is being rehabilitated. Think of these 10 core goals as long-term goals.

The 10 core goals are somewhat sequential. With two exceptions, each attribute builds upon the previous attributes. For example, since muscle power is a combination of strength and speed, both muscular strength and speed must be redeveloped before muscle power. Goals 1–4 must be developed in sequence. Goals 5–7 can be developed in any order or at the same time, but before goals 8–10. Goals 8–10 can be developed in any order or at the same time.

A thorough evaluation of the patient's injury and the limitations imposed on the patient by the injury must precede rehabilitation. Functional activities are often part of the evaluation. Not all injuries involve torn tissue, and pain is sometimes not present until the patient exceeds a specific level of performance. You then select the appropriate core goal to begin working on, establishing specific short-range goals to guide the patient in meeting the core goal. You then select specific therapeutic modalities and techniques that will help the patient progressively meet the core goal. Once the patient achieves the core goal, you repeat the process for the next core goal.

Goal 1: Structural Integrity

Structural integrity refers to the health of a patient's anatomical structures, such as bones, muscles, ligaments, and tendons. Any disrupted structure has to be repaired before its function can be rehabilitated. In general, both surgery and immobilization are necessary for repairing a severely injured musculoskeletal structure. Immobilization and/or rest are used to protect less seriously injured structures during the healing process.

Although immobilization is often necessary, it can also cause problems.[15,16] It often increases neural inhibitions, thereby resulting in decreased neuromuscular function. Exercising the immobilized part helps minimize neural inhibition, but it must not be so vigorous that it disturbs the structure that is healing.

Thermotherapy is often used during healing. It increases circulation and metabolism, thus speeding the healing process (see Chapter 6).

Goal 2: Pain-Free Joints and Muscles

Immobilization, therapeutic modalities, cryotherapy, and exercise are all used to reduce pain. Graded exercise (functional progression) is especially important in pain reduction, by helping the patient overcome neural inhibitions and by gradually readjusting or reorienting the body part to full pain-free activity.

It is important to monitor pain throughout the rehabilitation process. Pain accompanying an activity indicates the activity is too difficult, and the patient should revert to a lower level of activity. **Residual pain**, or pain the next day, is a signal that the previous day's activity was too demanding and the current day's activity needs to be decreased accordingly. Activities that cause pain during rehabilitation will compromise the rehabilitation by invoking neural inhibition.

Goal 3: Joint Flexibility

The ability of a joint to move through its full range of motion is known as **joint flexibility**. Impaired joint flexibility is the result of muscle spasm, pain, and/or neural inhibition secondary to acute injury, or from connective tissue adhesions and contractures secondary to surgery

TABLE 1.2   THE 10 CORE GOALS OF REHABILITATION*

GOAL OR PERFORMANCE ATTRIBUTE	
1	Structural integrity
2	Pain-free joints and muscles
3	Joint flexibility
4	Muscular strength
5	Muscular endurance
6	Muscular speed
7	Motor skill
8	Muscular power (strength and speed)
9	Agility (speed and skill)
10	Cardiorespiratory endurance

*Goals 1–4 should be developed sequentially, followed by goals 5–7 and then goals 8–10. Goals 5–7 and 8–10 can be developed in any order or at the same time with others in their groups.

and/or immobilization. Therapeutic exercise is essential to restoring flexibility, and its effects are enhanced by applications of hot packs and cold packs. Cold packs are generally more effective in treating muscular conditions, and hot packs are preferred when connective tissue is involved.[17]

During periods of immobilization, limited motion can help limit the loss of joint flexibility. After an appropriate period of immobilization, static stretch and **proprioceptive neuromuscular facilitation (PNF)** techniques, such as hold-relax (static stretch interspersed with isometric contraction of the involved muscle) and contract-relax (static stretch interspersed with isometric contraction of the antagonistic muscle), are effective. Flexion and extension exercises to range-of-motion limits and riding a stationary bike are other good ways to restore flexibility.

For acute muscle spasm, the two most effective modalities are the cryostretch technique (see Chapter 13), which combines cold applications with hold-relax, and electrical muscle stimulation (EMS), if applied in order to cause successive maximal tetanic contractions (see Chapter 17). For restoring range of motion to stiff, frozen joints, heat the joint capsule with pulsed shortwave diathermy and then follow with joint mobilization (see Chapter 15).

Goal 4: Muscular Strength

Muscular strength is a measure of the ability of a muscle to exert force. Some type of PRE must be performed on a regular basis by the involved muscles if an increase in strength is desired (Fig. 1.6). Elastic tubing exercises

TABLE 1.3	THE DAPRE TECHNIQUE	
SET	**PORTION OF WORKING WEIGHT USED**	**NUMBER OF REPETITIONS**
1	½	10
2	¾	6
3	Full	Maximum*
4	Adjusted	Maximum†

*The number of repetitions performed during the third set is used to determine the adjusted working weight for the fourth set according to the guidelines in Table 1.4.

†The number of repetitions performed during the fourth set is used to determine the adjusted working weight for the next day according to the guidelines in Table 1.4.

Source: Adapted from Knight.[20]

will help some, but weight training is more effective. Manufacturers of strength equipment constantly assert the merits of their products, but the strengthening program used is more important than the equipment.

The **daily adjustable progressive resistive exercise (DAPRE) technique** is a four-set, isotonic muscle strengthening technique that leads to rapid strength gains during rehabilitation (Tables 1.3 and 1.4).[3,18,19] An individual's strength can be redeveloped more quickly than it was originally developed. The DAPRE technique maximizes this because patients are required to perform maximal repetitions during their third and fourth sets, and the number of repetitions is used as a basis for adjusting the resistance during the fourth set and on the next day, respectively.

It is essential to exercise both sides of the body independently, which prevents the injured side from depending on the uninjured side. You must also establish a strength development goal for the injured side. The uninjured limb will lose strength following the injury, so if its strength is not reestablished, it is not a proper goal.

Once the strength of the injured side reaches 90–95% of the strength in the noninjured side, the program is changed from strength development to strength maintenance, and the rehabilitation goal changes to developing muscular endurance. Muscular strength can usually be maintained with one or two workouts per week at near maximal resistance.

Goal 5: Muscular Endurance

Muscular endurance refers to the ability of a muscle to contract repeatedly without becoming fatigued. Some ATs use a stationary bike to redevelop muscular endurance (Fig. 1.7). Although this is effective, running (or an equivalent upper body exercise for upper extremity injuries) is more specific to most sports and is therefore preferred. For

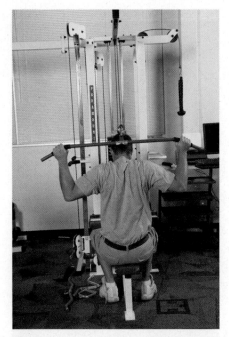

FIGURE 1.6 Muscular strength development is important early in the rehabilitation process to establish a basis for developing performance attributes such as endurance, speed, skill, agility, and power.

TABLE 1.4   GENERAL GUIDELINES FOR ADJUSTMENT OF WEIGHT WHEN USING THE DAPRE TECHNIQUE

NUMBER OF REPETITIONS PERFORMED DURING SET	ADJUSTMENT FOR THE FOURTH SET*	WORKING WEIGHT FOR THE NEXT DAY†
0–2	Decrease 2–5 kg and repeat the set	
3–4	Decrease 0–2 kg	Keep the same
2–7	Keep the same	Increase 2–5 kg
8–12	Increase 2–5 kg	Increase 2–7 kg
13+	Increase 5–7 kg	Increase 5–10 kg

*The number of repetitions performed during the third set is used to determine the adjusted working weight for the fourth set according to the guidelines in column 2.

†The number of repetitions performed during the fourth set is used to determine the adjusted working weight for the next day according to the guidelines in column 3.

Source: Adapted from Knight.[20]

example, the patient should jog 400 m the first couple of days and increase this distance 200–400 m each day as tolerance increases. Pain or soreness indicates the previous day's activity was too much and the distance should be decreased for a few days. After the patient can run a distance appropriate for his sport, (say 1600 m for a football player), start working toward other goals. But distance running should continue, reaching a level proportionate to the needs of the patient's sport.

Weight lifting is not recommended for developing muscular endurance. Repetitions of more than 100–300 would be necessary for reaching significant endurance levels, and this is impractical.

Goal 6: Muscular Speed

Muscular speed is the speed at which a muscle contracts. A good way to develop muscular speed is participation in team drills at half speed, then three-fourths speed, and finally at full speed, focusing on explosive-type activities (short duration, maximal power). Isokinetic exercise also

successfully develops muscular speed, but it is not needed if the patient develops near maximal strength and then progresses through team drills at increasing speed.

Goal 7: Motor Skill

Motor skill is the integration and coordination of many muscles acting together to produce a desired movement. Practicing sport-specific skill patterns, such as increasingly complex team drills will develop both motor skills and muscular speed (Fig. 1.8). Observe the patient closely to ensure the correct performance of the activities.

It is often necessary to isolate a particular part of the skill pattern and work on it individually. This involves reverting to earlier rehabilitation goals. Focus first on

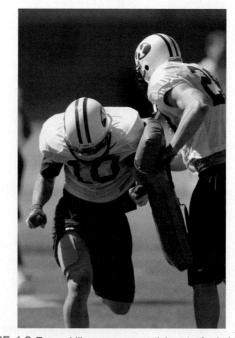

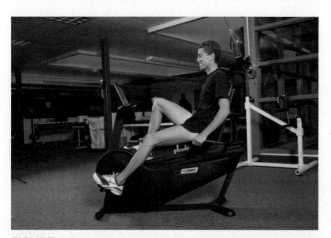

FIGURE 1.7 A stationary bike is a versatile tool that can be used for developing range of motion, endurance, and power.

FIGURE 1.8 Team drills are an essential part of rehabilitation if used properly and at the right time.

flexibility development while performing the specific part of the skill pattern, then progress through strength, endurance, and speed development with the particular muscles involved in the isolated part of the skill pattern.

Goal 8: Muscular Power

Power is a measure of the rate of doing work. **Muscular power** is a combination of strength and speed of movement, so it must be developed after those attributes. It can be developed with an isokinetic device, or with high-speed resistive exercises with traditional weights. Traditional weights, or weight machines, are recommended because they are less expensive and more accessible.

Goal 9: Agility

Agility is a combination of muscular speed and coordination, and it is developed in the course of performing skill patterns quickly. As with redeveloping motor skill, sport-specific team drills are used to redevelop agility.

Goal 10: Cardiorespiratory Endurance

Cardiorespiratory endurance is the ability of the heart and lungs to supply exercising muscles with adequate oxygen to produce the energy needed to maintain the activity. The exercises used to develop muscular endurance may stimulate some cardiorespiratory endurance development. Other sport-specific conditioning drills should be used, gradually at first and then increasing in difficulty.

If it looks like it will take more than 2 weeks to complete the total rehabilitation program, you should try to minimize the patient's loss of cardiovascular endurance. The method depends on the body part injured. If the injury does not compromise the patient's ability to perform normal conditioning activities, it's fine to continue with them. For instance, a football player with an arm injury can still run. If the injury prevents running, a substitute activity should be used. A football player with a thigh injury, for example, can run in a swimming pool in chest-high water or ride a stationary bike.

Modality Effectiveness in Achieving the Core Goals

When using a systems approach in rehabilitation, you must have some basis for choosing certain therapeutic modalities when working toward specific goals. The correct therapeutic modality must be matched with the therapeutic goal. For instance, a whirlpool treatment is clearly not the best choice for improving cardiorespiratory endurance.

Table 1.5 presents various therapeutic modalities rated according to their effectiveness in achieving each of the 10 core goals of rehabilitation. The most commonly used modalities are given one of three ratings for each of the core goals on which they have some effect. Here are the three ratings:

1. The modality has a direct effect and is a good choice for this rehabilitation goal.
2. The modality can be effective if used in a specific way. For example, performing several hundred isotonic resistive exercises three times per week would be effective in developing muscular endurance, but performing 10–15 repetitions would not develop significant muscular endurance.
3. The modality is somewhat effective but not the best choice for this rehabilitation goal.

As you look at Table 1.5, notice the general shape of the body of the table forms an L shape. What does this tell you about the use of therapeutic modalities during rehabilitation? They are most effective during the earlier stages of rehabilitation, when trying to promote healing, relieve pain, and restore full range of motion and flexibility. Achieving the core goals of strength and beyond requires mostly therapeutic exercise; therapeutic modalities have little effect here.

Teaching Versus Applying Therapeutic Modalities

Teaching therapeutic modalities is exactly opposite of the way we use them. Through most of the text, we talk about a specific modality and its **indications**. In the real world, however, you start with a problem (an injury), not with the modality. The scenario is "Here is a problem, here are my therapeutic goals, so which of the myriad modalities should I use?" You must understand the capabilities of each modality before you can choose from among them for treating a specific condition.

In Chapter 21, we reverse the process of the bulk of the book and begin with specific injuries and phases of injury/healing and discuss the best modality choices for treating them. In essence, we expand the information given in Table 1.5. And in the process, we help you change your orientation from learning about therapeutic modalities, to the real-world approach of using therapeutic modalities.

The Psychology of Rehabilitation

Rehabilitation is usually discussed in terms of physiological aspects, but the psychological side is important as well. In fact, some say that rehabilitation is 75% psychological and 25% physiological. Some patients seem to give

TABLE 1.5 THE EFFICACY OF VARIOUS THERAPEUTIC MODALITIES WHEN USED TO ACHIEVE EACH OF THE 10 CORE GOALS*

MODALITY	Structural Integrity	Pain-Free Joints and Muscles	Joint Flexibility	Muscular Strength	Muscular Endurance	Muscular Speed	Motor Skill	Muscular Power	Agility	Cardiorespiratory Endurance
Cold packs		1	2							
Ice massage		1	2							
Whirlpool, cold		1	2							
Whirlpool, hot	1	1	2							
Hot packs	1	1	2							
Paraffin baths	1	1	2							
Contrast baths	1	1	2							
Infrared	1	1	2							
Laser	1	1	2							
Ultrasound	1	1	2							
Diathermy	1	1	2							
LV muscle Stimulation	?	1	3	2						
HV muscle Stimulation	2	1								
TENS		1								
Traction		1	2							
Massage		1	2							
Joint mobilization		1	1							
Exercise										
Passive		2	1							
Assistive		2	3	?						
Active										
Range of motion	2	2	3							
Jogging (or EUBA)†		2		3	1					1
Running (or EUBA)†		2		3	2	1				1
Agility drills		2		3	2	1		1		2
Team drills		2		3	2	2		1		2
Team practice		2		3	2	2		1		2
Restive										
Manual				2						
Isometric				2						
Isotonic										
Free weights				1	2	2		3		3
Machine, weight				1	2	2				3
Machine, cam			2	1	2	2				3
Isokinetic				1	2	2				3

*1 = good choice, 2 = effective under certain conditions, 3 = somewhat effective—not the best choice.
†EUBA, equivalent upper body activity.

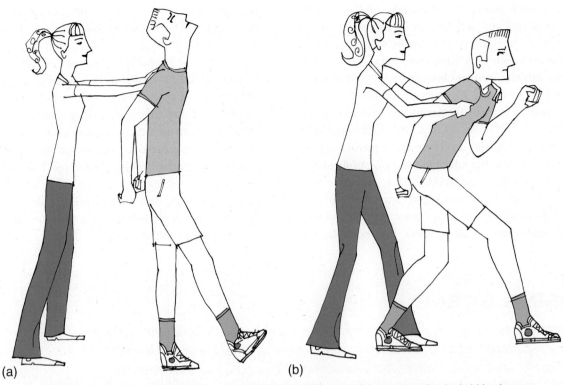

(a)   (b)

FIGURE 1.9 (a) Some patients must be prodded and cajoled, and **(b)** others need to be held back so as to prevent reinjury.

up after being injured, and must be encouraged regularly to reach their rehabilitation goals (Fig. 1.9a). The clinician has to constantly check on them to make sure they comply. Other patients can be overly aggressive and must be held back to avoid overworking and possible reinjury (Fig. 1.9b). Both types of patients require the same amount of time and effort during rehabilitation.

Another psychological aspect of rehabilitation is the direct connection that exists between the mind and the body's physiological functioning. The way a person thinks is manifested in the way her body performs. There is power in positive thinking. During rehabilitation, the clinician needs to make every effort to ensure that the patient doesn't give up on herself or her ability to recover from the injury and perform again. Pointing out even the smallest sign of progress can help.

Preparation for Using Therapeutic Modalities

Ideally, anyone who is properly trained in the correct theory and application and remains up-to-date with current research is qualified to use therapeutic modalities. However, many clinicians do not find the time to stay current with research. Regardless, state regulations determine who can legally administer therapeutic modality

treatments, so you need to be aware of the laws in the state in which you are employed.

To prepare yourself to use therapeutic modalities, keep the following in mind:

1. *Be an active learner.* This is not a spectator sport. You will not learn therapeutic modalities simply by reading the text, listening to classroom lectures, cramming for exams, and spitting out the answers. You must do these things, but also you must make this information part of yourself. How do you do that? You interact with the information by:

   - Writing questions as you read and then discussing the questions with classmates, other students, professors, clinical instructors, and even patients
   - Writing reflectively about the material
   - Experimenting with various forms of application

2. *Aside from classroom experiences, try to use the various modalities every day.* A model of education that combines academics in the morning and clinical work in the afternoon or evening is powerful. During your clinical experiences, question, consider, and reflect on what you have been taught in the classroom. Experiment on yourself. For example, put your foot in a container of ice water and record how many minutes it takes for your foot to go numb. When treating patients, think about whether there is a better way to do something, and discuss it with both your clinical instructor and your classroom teacher.

3. *Once you finish your formal education, take the opportunity to attend and actively participate in continuing education seminars.* Some professions will require you to maintain continuing education units (CEUs). The National Athletic Trainers' Association (NATA) requires its members to obtain 75 hours of additional learning every 3 years. Currently the American Physical Therapy Association (APTA) does not require this, but some individual state regulations do. There are numerous opportunities for continuing education at many professional meetings, including the NATA, APTA, and American College of Sports Medicine (ACSM) annual meetings.

4. *Most professional organizations sponsor a peer-reviewed journal that is sent to all members.* For example, the keystone journal for ATs is the *Journal of Athletic Training*; for PTs, *Physical Therapy*; and for physiatrists, the *Archives of Physical Medicine* and *Rehabilitation* (APM&R). The *Journal of Orthopaedic & Sports Physical Therapy (JOSPT)* serves as a crossover journal for orthopedic and sports PTs, and generally has more therapeutic modality information than *Physical Therapy*. Make it a habit to study the journal of your primary professional organization, and periodically peruse the journals of related health professions. They represent the most current science and clinical practice in your specialty. Reading and implementing what you find in these journals with help keep you up-to-date in this ever-changing medical world.

CLOSING SCENE

We began this chapter with a story about a man teaching his young son about how he could do a better job in less time by using the right tools to cut branches off a tree (Fig. 1.10). The same is true with rehabilitation, a complex process involving the redevelopment of many performance attributes, each with different goals. It can be facilitated by the judicious use of the right tools—therapeutic modalities.

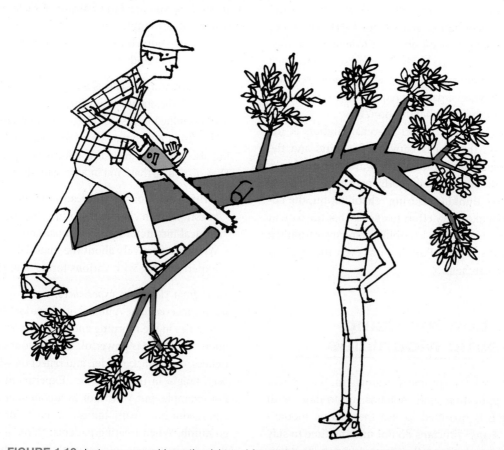

FIGURE 1.10 Just as you would use the right tool for cutting tree limbs, be sure to use the right tool for each stage of rehabilitation.

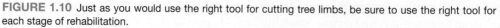

Chapter Reflections

1. Read and ponder each of the following points. Do you feel you have a clear understanding of each concept? If not, reread the appropriate section of the chapter.
   - Explain the concept of knobologist.
   - Define therapeutic modality, physical agent, and therapeutic purpose.
   - Describe the relationship between the theory and the application of therapeutic modalities.
   - Identify the various therapeutic modality classification systems.
   - Discuss the roles of physicians and ATs in determining which therapeutic modality is used, and the selection criteria.
   - Define rehabilitation, and the relationship between therapeutic modalities and rehabilitation.
   - Discuss each of the four erroneous concepts of rehabilitation. What effect do these misconceptions have on therapeutic modality users?
   - Describe the 12 principles of rehabilitation.
   - Describe the 10 core goals of rehabilitation.
2. Write three to five questions for discussion with your class instructor, clinical instructor, classmates, and clinical colleagues.
3. Get together with classmates and quiz each other on the concepts of this chapter. Use the points in reflection no. 1 and questions you wrote for reflection no. 2 as a beginning. Explaining concepts out loud to others requires a deeper grasp of the material than feeling you understand it as you read.

Concept Check Responses

CONCEPT CHECK 1.1

Knobologists can harm the health professions in several ways:
1. They lack the theory and scientific background to be able to modify or modulate the treatments to cater to the specific needs of their patients.
2. Their patients' health concerns are not resolved as fully or as quickly.
3. They may not be able to fully answer questions asked by their patients.
4. They do not stay current with changes and updates to their profession.
5. They give their profession a bad name or poor image because they are perceived as technicians rather than professions.

CONCEPT CHECK 1.2

When performance is evaluated and the performer is given specific feedback regarding that performance, she is able to make corrections. For example, in the number guessing game, if your friend chose 55 and was told it was wrong, her next choice would be any one of 99 numbers. In the second example, however, telling her that the number was lower would reduce the choices to one of 54 numbers. With each choice and feedback, she gets closer to the right answer. The same is true when you give performance goals and feedback on how the patient performed.

REFERENCES

1. Merriam-Webster's Online Dictionary. Accessed via OneLook Dictionary Search, OneLook.com [website]. Available at: http://www.merriam-webster.com/dictionary/rehabilitation. Accessed November, 2011.
2. MedFriendly Glossary. *Accessed via OneLook Dictionary Search, OneLook.com* [website]. Available at: http://www.medfriendly.com/letterr.php5. Accessed November, 2011.
3. Knight KL. Quadriceps strengthening with the DAPRE technique: case studies with neurological implications. *Med Sci Sports Exerc.* 1985;17:646–650.
4. Knight KL. Guidelines for rehabilitation of sports injuries. *Clin Sports Med.* 1985;4:405–416.
5. Knight KL. Total injury rehabilitation. *Phys Sports Med.* 1979;7(8):111.
6. DePalma MT, DePalma B. The use of instruction and the behavioral approach to facilitate injury rehabilitation. *J Athl Train.* 1989;24:217–222.
7. Kegerreis S. The construction and implementation of functional progressions as a component of athletic rehabilitation. *J Orthop Sports Phys Ther.* 1983;5(1):14–19.
8. Delorme TL, Watkins AL. Technics of progressive resistance exercise. *Arch Phys Med.* 1948;29(5):263–273.
9. Kvist H, Jarvinen M, Sorvari T. Effect of mobilization and immobilization on the healing of contusion injury in muscle. A preliminary report of a histological study in rats. *Scand J Rehabil Med.* 1974;6(3):134–140.

10. Jarvinen M. Immobilization effect on the tensile properties of striated muscle: an experimental study in the rat. *Arch Phys Med Rehabil.* 1977;58(3):123–127.

11. Jarvinen M. Healing of a crush injury in rat striated muscle. 3. A micro-angiographical study of the effect of early mobilization and immobilization on capillary ingrowth. *Acta Pathol Microbiol Scand A.* 1976;84(1):85–94.

12. Jarvinen M. Healing of a crush injury in rat striated muscle. 4. Effect of early mobilization and immobilization on the tensile properties of gastrocnemius muscle. *Acta Chir Scand.* 1976;142(1):47–56.

13. Jarvinen M. Healing of a crush injury in rat striated muscle. 2. A histological study of the effect of early mobilization and immobilization on the repair processes. *Acta Pathol Microbiol Scand A.* 1975;83(3):269–282.

14. Dehne E, Torp RP. Treatment of joint injuries by immediate mobilization. Based upon the spinal adaptation concept. *Clin Orthop.* 1971;77:218–232.

15. Enwemeka CS. Inflammation, cellularity, and fibrillogenesis in regenerating tendon: implications for tendon rehabilitation. *Phys Ther.* 1989;69(10):816–825.

16. Morrissey MC. Reflex inhibition of thigh muscles in knee injury causes and treatment. *Sports Med.* 1989;7:263–276.

17. Sapega AA, Quedenfeld TC, Moyer RA, Butler RA. Biophysical factors in range-of-motion exercise. *Phys Sports Med.* 1981;9(12).

18. Wadey VM, Knight KL. Four week training of quadriceps strength with electrical muscle stimulation and the isotonic DAPRE technique. *J Can Athl Ther Assoc.* 1989;16(2):14–20.

19. Knight KL, Ingersoll C, Bartholomew J. Isotonic contractions may be more effective that isokinetic contractions in developing muscle strength. *J Sport Rehabil* 2001;10:124–131.

20. Knight KL. Knee rehabilitation using a adjustable progressive resistive exercise technique. *Am J Sports Med.* 1979;7:336–337.

2

Evidence-Based Practice

OPENING SCENE

Kate is in her second clinical rotation. She noticed that Eric, her clinical instructor, approaches some situations differently than Jane, her first clinical instructor, did. When questioned about the differences, Eric replied, "There is more than one way to skin a cat. This is the way I was taught, and it has worked fine for me." She then sought out Jane, concerning the disparity. Jane gave her a similar answer. "How can that be?" she thought. "Are the two approaches really equivalent? Is there evidence that proves or suggests that one approach is better than the other?"

The Philosophy of Evidence-Based Medicine

Evidence-based medicine (EBM) and its cousin evidence-based practice (EBP) have become buzzwords throughout medicine. Indeed, EBP has "taken health care by storm,"[1] and "is almost at the level of a cult or fashion."[2] Some speak of EBM as if it is a new phenomenon, or the latest advancement in medicine. In 1998, Sweeney et al.[3] wrote that it was a "new deity in clinical medicine: physicians worship it, managers demand it, and policy makers aspire towards it." Don't be misled, however. Although the recent popularity of the phrase "evidence-based" implies that medical practitioners did not use evidence as a basis for their medical decisions until recently, that is not true. Every clinical decision is based on evidence of some sort.

BOX 2.1 • FALSE EVIDENCE LEADS TO WRONG CLINICAL DECISIONS

It was once thought, and taught, that isolated anterior cruciate ligament (ACL) tears did not occur in isolation.[4] ACL tears were thought to occur only with injury to other structures, usually in conjunction with medial collateral ligament and medical meniscus tears (the "Terrible Triad"). It wasn't until orthopedic surgeons began to use the arthroscope to actually look inside the knee and the Lachman test was devised[5] that clinicians concluded they had been misdiagnosing patients with torn ACLs. In retrospect, clinicians concluded that the *anterior drawer test* is inadequate because it returns too many false-negative results; that is, the test indicates the ligament is not torn when in fact it is. Thus, the evidence upon which clinicians were basing their decision that the ACL was intact (a negative anterior drawer test) was false, thereby leading to wrong decisions.

The problem has been that some of the evidence used was/is false or inadequate for the situation. *Inaccurate evidence may lead to inaccurate decisions.* Box 2.1 outlines an example of how an inaccurate decision can be made when using incomplete or inadequate evidence.

Inaccurate evidence in any phase of injury or illness care can compromise the resolution of the injury or illness. This includes making the diagnosis, choosing the clinical intervention, administering the intervention, and patient compliance. There is a direct correlation, therefore, between the quality of evidence and the quality of health care.[6]

EVIDENCE-BASED MEDICINE OR EVIDENCE-BASED PRACTICE?

EBM and EBP are closely related, and yet they are different concepts. The following definitions will help clarify the similarities and differences:

- Medicine is a learned profession devoted to preventing, alleviating, or curing diseases and injuries.
- Practice is the exercise of a profession, meaning the customary way that a professional behaves or performs his/her duties.
- **Evidence-based medicine (EBM)** is medicine based on the latest and most rigorous scientific evidence,[7,8] integrated with clinical experience and patient preferences and circumstances.[9,10]
- **Evidence-based practice (EBP)** is the application of the principles of EBM to patient care; health care that is based on scientific evidence; and patient preferences. Its goal is to improve the quality and effectiveness of health care.[11,12]

The phrase "evidence-based practice" is actually a misnomer—an incorrect or unsuitable name. Literally, EBP is practicing medicine under the influence of evidence—any evidence. As used in the medical literature, though, the term refers to practicing medicine under the influence of the best possible evidence.[7] Since the phrase "best possible evidence-based practice" is a bit cumbersome, we accept the shorter, but technically incorrect, version of the term.

The original concepts of EBP were both new and important. They emphasized the need for medical practitioners to learn to identify the strength of evidence for their diagnoses and interventions, and then use only the best evidence to guide their medical decisions. Generally, the best evidence comes from the latest and most rigorous science.[8]

THE HISTORY OF EVIDENCE-BASED MEDICINE AND PRACTICE

EBM grew from two seeds, although its philosophical origins extend back to the middle of the nineteenth century. The first seed was a concept advocated by the British epidemiologist Archie Cochrane[13] in a 1972 book. He stated that health care decisions should be based on randomized clinical trials (RCTs) because they provide more reliable information than other sources of evidence.[13] There is much more to consider than just RCTs, however. Also, RCTs do not always provide reliable evidence. We'll discuss these concepts later in the chapter.

The second seed was planted by faculty members at McMaster University Medical School in Canada in the 1970s and 1980s, as they incorporated more clinical learning in their medical education[9,14–16] requirements. They coined the term "evidence based medicine" (no hyphen) in the 1980s to label their clinical learning strategy,[17] the essence of which was that every aspect of medical care should be based on the best available scientific evidence.[9]

Cochrane's work led to setting up the Cochrane Collaboration.[18] This entity developed into what is now a worldwide endeavor to collect, evaluate, synthesize, and maintain a database of RCTs in all areas of medicine (Box 2.2).

EBP quickly became a major initiative of the U.S. Department of Health and Human Services, the American Medical Association, and America's Health Insurance Plans (see Box 2.2).[19] Twelve Evidence-Based Practice Centers, housed in major medical schools, have been established to conduct systematic reviews of the scientific literature related to specific diseases or health problems. The goal is to determine whether specific **interventions** (treatments) for specific conditions work. Guidelines are then written for treating the problem, including statements concerning the strength of clinical evidence for the intervention. The guidelines from these reviews are housed in a national database for use by medical and health-related personnel. The database[19] is not limited to reports from the Evidence-Based Practice Centers. Reports from many other professional and private organizations are also referenced. This is a great source of information for the clinician who wants to provide the best care possible to his/her patients.

BOX 2.2   EVIDENCE-BASED MEDICINE REPOSITORIES

The five most important repositories of evidence-based information are:

- Cochrane Database of Systematic Reviews (COCH) <http://www.ovid.com/site/products/ovid-guide/cochdb.htm>or The Cochrane Collaboration <http://www.cochrane.org>
- Pubmed or Medline, U.S. National Library of Medicine, National Institutes of Health. <http:/// www.pubmed.gov>
- National Guideline Clearinghouse, U.S. Department of Health & Human Services <http:// www.guideline.gov/>
- PEDro Physiotherapy Evidence Database <http:// www.pedro.org.au/> or Center for Evidence-Based Physiotherapy <https://www.cebp.nl/>
- CINAHL, the Cumulative Indices to Nursing and Allied Health Literature http://www.ebscohost. com/cinahl/

In addition to the National Guideline Clearinghouse, the U.S. National Library of Medicine publishes Medline, also known as PubMed. It is the largest collection of journal citations and abstracts for biomedical literature in the world. Its collection includes literature from around the world.

The Australian Physiotherapy Association has led the charge to incorporate EBM in orthopedic injury care. They established the Physiotherapy Evidence Database, or PEDro[20] (see Box 2.2), and developed the PEDro Scale, to help evaluate the quality of published clinical trials and thereby help determine the validity of the data.

Nurses have also become advocates of EBP.[21] Like many medical specialty organizations, nursing organizations in many countries have established Centers for Evidence-Based Nursing to promote EBP through research, education, and the dissemination of research findings to nurses.

EVIDENCE-BASED VERSUS PATIENT-CENTERED MEDICINE

Two very powerful, but different and somewhat contradictory, general belief systems have driven medical care: "evidence-based medicine" and "patient-centered medicine."[1,22] Both concepts are generally accepted as important in clinical decision making, even though they developed independently (at about the same time), and philosophically were totally different. They existed in separate worlds and had little in common because they focused on different aspects of medical care.[1] For example, a Medline search reported in 2000 produced 1023 hits from "evidence-based medicine," 317 hits from "patient-centered medicine," but only 12 from a combination of the two terms, 10 of which were in the previous year.

How are they different? EBM approaches patient care from a biomedical perspective, based solely on scientific facts[1]; it is referred to as a cognitive-rational enterprise. It is a doctor-oriented,[3] disease-centered model[23] that focuses on gathering, synthesizing, and providing clinicians with the best available scientific evidence for how to treat specific diseases.[1,3] The goal of EBM is to improve quality by standardizing medical care, through clinical guidelines and best practices.[22] Patients' major signs and symptoms classify them as part of a group, and the science specifies the best way to treat patients who fit within that group. Patient uniqueness, needs, preferences, and emotional status become irrelevant.[3]

Patient-centered medicine, on the other hand, is a humanistic, biopsychosocial approach. Its focus is on patient participation in clinical decision making, using in-depth patient communication to understand patients' complaints, unique needs in the context of their lives, preferences, culture, beliefs, backgrounds, behaviors, and emotional status—in essence, who the patient is.[22,23] It moves care from clinician control to patient empowerment.[23,24] One author describes it as allowing patients to use the clinician as a tool to manage their own illness.[25] The concepts are different enough that they require different medical records.[26] A patient-centered medical record must address the person and perspective of the patient as competently as it addresses the patient's disease. For example, it must include a more in-depth patient profile and a section for "chief concerns," rather than "chief complaints."

Many physicians feel that patient centeredness is a requirement for maintaining the high standards and good quality of medical and health care, for the following reasons[24]:

1. Patients are experts in the experience of their symptoms.
2. Patients are different in their preferences in health care, even patients with the same objective diseases and the same symptom patterns. Diversity is more common than uniformity.
3. Much of health care depends on the patient's own adaptation and coping capabilities. A clinician can facilitate the patient more by acting as a "teacher" or "consultant" than as an "expert" or "guardian."

Not Either-Or, but Both
In a paper published in 2000, Bensing,[24] an authority in medical communications, challenged the medical profession to increase efforts to bring these separate worlds

together. Interchanging ideas and principles, she wrote, would benefit both approaches and therefore lead to enhanced medical care. The science is absolutely necessary, but clinicians must interpret the clinical science *not just* in terms of mathematical/statistical terms, but also with, and in the context of, the individual patient,[3] as well as in the context of their own (the clinician's) clinical experience.[22] Personal significance is the key.

One of the most ardent early advocates of EBM opposed the notion that EBM would cause a physician to approach patients with a "cookbook" reliance on scientific evidence. Sackett et al.[27] stated: "It requires a bottom up approach that integrates the best external evidence with individual clinical expertise and patient choice.... External clinical evidence can inform, but can never replace, individual clinical expertise, and it is this expertise that decides whether the external evidence applies to the individual patient at all, and if so, how it should be integrated into the clinical decision."

It is important to remember, however, that the science cannot be ignored under the guise of being patient centered; both approaches must be integrated.[27]

Cultural Diversity
Part of patient-centered health care is understanding, acknowledging, and respecting the health beliefs, values, and behaviors of individuals. This philosophy started with rather simplistic attempts to teach doctors about population groups, their cultural norms, and especially cultural peculiarities regarding health and health care.[22] Clinicians must seek to understand the patient's stories and integrate what is important to the individual into decisions about his/her care.[22]

BECOMING AN EVIDENCE-BASED PRACTITIONER

Becoming an evidence-based practitioner is not an easy task; in fact, it is not even a task that can be completed. Rather, it is a complex philosophy that evolves and develops over time; a philosophy of systematically searching for and evaluating contemporary research findings, and incorporating them into your medical practice.[9] Becoming an evidence-based practitioner does not happen in a week, a month, or a year. Fully understanding, and practicing, EBM requires a lifelong commitment. It begins with understanding the vocabulary, philosophy, and complexity of EBP (as discussed in this chapter), expanding your use and application of that philosophy during future educational and clinical classes and experiences, and then following that philosophy and critically questioning your practice throughout your health care career.

Don't be discouraged by the complexity of the matter. Resolve to begin your understanding of the philosophy and to develop some ability to access, and use, EBM clinical tools during this class. Periodically review the concepts and techniques introduced here and progressively apply them throughout all classes in your AT curriculum. Constantly question the validity of the evidence for the individual skills and techniques you learn. Make referencing the EBM repositories a regular and frequent habit during your clinical experiences (see Box 2.2). With a commitment to the task, you can become an accomplished evidence-based practitioner over time.

Clinical Decision Making

The bottom line of EBP is to use the best evidence possible when making clinical decisions. You must understand clinical decision making to fully understand and become an evidence-based practitioner.

Clinical decision making has traditionally been defined as the process of physicians making a diagnosis,[28] but it also includes determining how to treat patients.[29] It begins with collecting evidence from a variety of sources, ends with a specific plan for treating the patient, and involves careful analysis of, and critical thinking about, the collected data and treatment options.

All clinical decision making is an educated guess, and can range from totally accurate to totally wrong. The ideal, obviously, is that decisions are accurate and lead to full, speedy resolution of patient's disability or disease. Unfortunately, this does not always happen. Why?

Clinical decisions are based on interpreting and integrating four elements, as shown in Figure 2.1: (1) clinical data, (2) patient preferences and actions, (3) research evidence, and (4) the clinician's expertise and experience.[30,31] The fourth element overrides the other three. Failure to collect the proper data, failure to correctly interpret the data, or a lack of critical thinking during the process can lead to inaccurate conclusions.

The specific process of clinical decision making involves the following steps:

1. Evaluate the patient's injury/illness, in order to understand his clinical state and circumstances. This involves a thorough physical and mental evaluation of him and his specific injury or condition, and his response to previous interventions, if available. Consider the latest research concerning diagnostic tests for the possible injury or disease.
2. Analyze the subjective and objective data, to establish a tentative diagnosis or a list of possible causes of the disorder; this is known as the *differential diagnosis*. Determine what tests to order to help refine the list or identify the specific injury or disease responsible for the disability.[28] Critical thinking is especially important here.
3. Determine a final diagnosis.
4. Establish therapeutic goals, taking into account patient preferences and actions.
5. Develop a *plan of action*, which prescribes how the patient is to be treated to reach the established therapeutic goals. Consider the patient's preferences and actions, the availability of therapeutic modalities and other therapeutic interventions, such as drugs and therapeutic exercise, and available research evidence.
6. Administer therapeutic interventions as prescribed by the plan of action.
7. Periodically repeat steps 1–6, adjusting as necessary for changing conditions, such as healing.
8. Continue until the condition is resolved.

CLINICAL OUTCOMES

Clinical outcomes are the end results of specific health care practices and interventions.[32] They include the pathophysiological, social, and psychological results of the intervention—for example, how an athletic injury healed as measured by laboratory tests, such as x-rays, and clinical functional tests, such as strength and endurance; the patient's self-confidence in his ability to perform, his perception about his coach's confidence in his ability to perform, his relationships with teammates; and related quality-of-life issues.

BEST PRACTICES

Best practice is both a philosophy of action and specific techniques, methods, activities, or processes.[33] It refers to dealing with specific conditions or circumstances in a

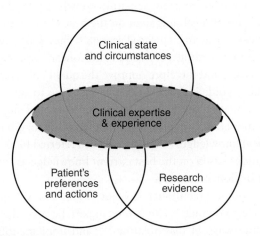

FIGURE 2.1 A model for evidence-based clinical decisions, integrating the four key elements of evidence-based medicine. (From Haynes et al.[10])

way that experts believe will result in the best outcome, meaning the most effective and/or with the least amount of effort. "Best practices" is sometimes used incorrectly to refer to standard operating procedures, which, in business or manufacturing, are procedures designed to give a consistent result. For example, your favorite burger from a specific restaurant chain will be the same in any city you visit. Also, the floor plan of a specific chain of big box stores is the same at all locations, so you always know where specific items are. In these cases, best practices are merely a standard way of doing things, a set of rules for accomplishing specific tasks.[33]

In medicine, best practices refers to treating a specific patient's specific condition in the way that will lead to resolution of the condition in the most complete and expedient manner possible (Box 2.3). It is also known as *standard of care* and *standard therapy*, and is treatment that experts agree is appropriate, accepted, widely used, and reproducible.[16,34] Best practices involve the appropriate use of the current best evidence in making clinical decisions.[16]

Developing best practices is difficult in some areas of health care because of differences of opinion and an ever-evolving knowledge base.[35] Nevertheless, societies and interdisciplinary teams should constantly strive to improve the quality of their care by studying issues and updating best practices.[36,37] The evolution of technology,

increasing knowledge about diseases and treatments, and ongoing research all contribute to improved therapeutics, which in turn lead to updating best practices.

Health care providers have a moral obligation to provide patients with the best practice available[34]; it "must happen for every patient every time."[38] Providing patients with the best practice is not always possible, however, and here are some of the reasons:

- There is no practice that is best for everyone or in every situation.[39]
- It is estimated that good guidelines apply to only 80% of patients.[40]
- A given best practice is only applicable to a specific condition or circumstance and may have to be modified or adapted for similar circumstances.[39]

Despite the limitations, however, every effort should be made to use, and update, best practices.[41]

The best practice concept is operationalized (put into practice) though protocols[42] and Clinical Practice Guidelines.[31,42] When followed, they are expected to produce a benchmark outcome.

PROTOCOLS

A *protocol* is a plan or a set of specific steps to be followed in an investigation or intervention; it provides a strict process for monitoring and taking care of a patient with a disease.[42] In many instances, protocols provide a practical, step-by-step framework for implementing guidelines.

CLINICAL PRACTICE GUIDELINES

Clinical Practice Guidelines, also known as *Best Practice Statements*,[43] *Recommendation Statements*,[44] or *Health Care Guidelines*,[45] are systematically developed statements that describe best and achievable practice in specific areas of care; they reflect current scientific knowledge of practices and expert clinical judgment on the best ways to prevent, diagnose, treat, or manage diseases.[42] They guide practitioners in providing a consistent and cohesive approach to health care, and therefore improve the quality of care.[31,42,43]

These guidelines are a positive response to the reality that clinicians need "help in assimilating and applying the exponentially expanding, often contradictory, body of medical knowledge."[46] They have been referred to as "how to" guides based on the best current knowledge as synthesized by domain experts.

Too often, practitioners are not aware of pertinent best practice guidelines.[47] This is due, in part, because there are multiple ways of dissimilating[48–51] and implementing[47,52] them. Development of these guidelines is explained later in the chapter.

BOX 2.3   AN EXAMPLE OF A BEST PRACTICE IN ATHLETIC TRAINING

Joint mobilization is often used to treat a frozen shoulder. Properly applied, it will result in increasing the range of motion (mobility) of the shoulder. Application of therapeutic heat to the shoulder before mobilization will increase its effectiveness, if applied properly. Some use a hot pack, which will help to a certain extent, but a hot pack does not heat the deeper tissues. Others use ultrasound, which is limited to heating a smaller area. The best choice is pulsed shortwave diathermy, which heats a large area and penetrates deeply. None of the heating is effective, however, unless it is applied for at least 15 minutes and the mobilization is applied immediately (seconds, not minutes) after heating. Therefore, the best practice for a frozen shoulder is to apply shortwave diathermy for 15–20 minutes followed immediately by joint mobilization (see Chapter 15). Although there are other approaches to treating a frozen shoulder, according to current research, other methods would not be as effective.

Principles of Evidence-Based Medicine

Since EBP is the application of the principles of EBM to patient care, it is necessary to identify these principles. These are the conscientious, explicit, and judicious application of the best available scientific facts to medical/clinical decision making concerning the care of individual patients.[7,27]

The efforts of two groups of professionals are essential to EBM: (1) the medical-scientific community, in seeking new knowledge through research, and (2) individual clinicians, in developing a personal philosophy of patient care that includes the use of evidence-based principles, and becoming aware of the latest research in their specialty. Following are the major aspects of seeking new EBP knowledge on the part of the medical and scientific communities:

- Classify those parts of medical practice that are, in principle, subject to scientific methods.[7]
- Promote the collection, interpretation, and integration of valid, important, and applicable patient-reported, clinician-observed, and research-derived evidence.
- Assess the quality of evidence about the risks and benefits of diagnostic tests and treatments, or lack of treatment.[7]
- Apply the best available evidence, moderated by patient circumstances and preferences, to ensure the best prediction of outcomes in medical treatment,[7] improve the quality of clinical judgments, and facilitate cost-effective care.

The philosophy of patient care for individual clinicians practicing EBM includes the following six steps for each individual patient[16,53]:

1. Convert the need for information about a specific patient/case into a specific, structured, and answerable question.
2. Find the best evidence to answer the question.
3. Critically evaluate the evidence for validity, impact, and applicability.
4. Integrate the critical evaluation with your clinical expertise and with the patient's biology, values, and life circumstances.
5. Reevaluate the previous four steps to determine if you can improve the effectiveness and efficiency of the process.
6. Execute the plan.

Evidence

Evidence is anything used to establish a fact, or to give a reason to believe something. Both parts of this definition are essential to understanding EBP, and to providing quality health care. The first is about seeking indisputable scientific facts. For example, ultrasound applied to an area about twice the size of the soundhead will heat the underlying tissue, whereas if applied to an area larger that about six times the size of the soundhead will not heat the underlying tissue (see Chapter 14). The second part of the definition has a much broader application. It can mean the same thing as the first; we believe something because of scientific fact. But it also means that we may believe false ideas and concepts because either they are unproven or we are unaware of the evidence that proves the concepts wrong. For example, many people continue to believe the disproved concept that ice application to acute injuries is effective because it constricts blood vessels, thereby decreasing blood flow, and thus limits swelling (see Chapter 6).

In the past, many areas of professional practice were based on loose bodies of knowledge, much of which had no scientific basis. Myths, based on generations of clinical experience, were used to justify various medical theories and procedures. This allowed quackery by uneducated and unscrupulous individuals. Unfortunately these practices still exist, resulting in ineffective medical care and the waste of large sums of money.

SOURCES OF MEDICAL EVIDENCE

Following are the four main sources of evidence upon which clinicians base their clinical beliefs:

1. Tradition: How it has always been done. These are theories, techniques, and procedures that have been handed down from one clinician to the next. This evidence ranges from solid factual reality to unfounded opinion, rumor, and fiction. Be cautious, even if the opinion is popular. As Russell[54] observed, "The fact that an opinion has been widely held is no evidence whatever that it is not utterly absurd; indeed in view of the silliness of the majority of mankind, a widespread belief is more likely to be foolish than sensible."
2. Experience: The result of successes and failures in treating similar patients and similar conditions in the past. This evidence also ranges from solid factual reality to unfounded opinion, rumor, and fiction. Be cautious about rejecting alternative options, just because something may have worked in the past. But also don't jump on every new idea that comes along, unless it is based on solid scientific fact.
3. Research: The result of scientific investigation. This evidence will range from general to specific, as explained below.
4. Theory: The best guess of what is going on, based on a logical evaluation of evidence (solid, false, and everything in between). The strength of a theory lies in the strength of the evidence upon which it is based, and the care with which the evidence is tied together.

RESEARCH EVIDENCE

There are many types of research evidence, each of which has a role in clinical decision making. Although their relative value varies, each is essential, if used properly. Research evidence has been classified into three broad categories, based on the location and nature of the research: laboratory, observational, and clinical trials.

Laboratory research, which is conducted in a laboratory, is the least expensive and easiest type of research to do, and allows the greatest control over interventions. Its key elements are detailed, written explanations of the following:

- A prospectus, or research design, written prior to data collection, in which all elements of the research are described
- A control group and one or more treatment groups (interventions)
- How the treatment interventions will be applied
- How the subjects will be selected
- The method of randomly assigning subjects to treatment groups

Laboratory research typically assesses:

- Physiological responses of healthy, uninjured humans to specific interventions. It allows comparisons of various interventions, and levels of specific interventions. This research provides good, but limited, information. The greatest limitation is that healthy, uninjured tissue often does not respond to specific interventions the same as injured tissue does.
- Pathophysiological responses of injured animals to specific interventions. Injury or diseased states can be modeled with this research, but the value of the results depends on how closely the animal's responses mimic human responses.

Observational research is carried out within a particular context. The observations occur as people go about routine activities in their natural environment. In medical research, observational research involves a wide range of study designs, including prospective (designed before data are collected) and retrospective (designed to study existing data) studies.[55] The dependent (or measurement) variable of these studies is determined by clinical practice rather than a scientific protocol. Here are some common observational study designs:

- *Case study*: The details of specific interventions in a single patient, or preferably, in multiple patients with the same injury/illness, are carefully recorded. The latter is called a case series or cohort study. Case studies identify patient responses to a specific intervention for a specific injury/illness. They are limited because they lack control subjects, and because they give no indication of their relative value compared to other interventions.
- *Cohort study*: A group of patients is followed over time. Outcomes of interest are measured prior to an intervention (baseline), and periodically following an intervention. Differences from baseline indicate the effects of the intervention.[56]
- *Cross-sectional study*: A group of patients is examined at a single time during, or following, an intervention concerning their current and past history regarding the effects of an intervention on the outcomes of interest.[56]
- *Case-control study*: Two groups of patients are selected based on the presence or absence of an outcome, and examined concerning their involvement with the intervention of interest.[56]

Clinical trials research is a cross between observational and laboratory research. They are observational in that patients are studied while receiving normal clinical treatment. They are like laboratory studies in that they are prospective, they usually include a control group, treatment groups (interventions) are more closely standardized, and subjects may be randomly assigned to treatment groups. These are by far the most expensive to conduct. Here are the common types of clinical trials:

- *Clinical or controlled trials (CTs)*: Controlled research of a specific medical intervention on patients with a specific injury or disease. Clinical trials may be randomized or nonrandomized, meaning patients may be randomly assigned to one of the treatment groups, or not. Generally, CT refers to nonrandomized trials, while randomized trials are referred to as RCTs.
- *Randomized clinical trials (RCTs)*: Quantitative scientific experiments conducted to test the effectiveness of medical interventions, services, or technologies.[57,58] Participants with a specific injury, disease, or disorder are assigned randomly to one of two or several treatment groups, or clinical interventions, one of which is a control or standard of comparison.[57] The control may be a standard practice, a placebo ("sugar pill"), or no intervention at all. Patient outcomes (responses to the intervention) are measured and compared between groups.[59]

The RCT is one of the simplest and most powerful tools in clinical research.[57] As such, it was the basis for the concept of EBP. As mentioned earlier, in 1972 Cochrane[13] emphasized the importance of basing health care decisions on evidence from RCTs because these were likely to provide much more reliable information than other sources of evidence. Be aware, however, that RCTs are not the "do all-be all" of medical evidence. RCTs are discussed in detail later in the chapter.

QUALITY OF EVIDENCE

The core of EBM is quality of evidence.[60] The higher the quality of evidence upon which a clinical decision is based, the better that decision[6] will be. Obviously, it is important for clinicians to know the relative quality of evidence. A few of the many systems of classifying levels of evidence are presented later in the chapter.

ADVANCING THEORY

When reviewing any research, it is important to recognize the difference between two concepts: that something "proves the theory" and "is consistent with the theory." Only RCTs are capable of providing definitive proof of a specific treatment. Other types of research evidence, however, can get us closer to the truth. And in some cases, other types of evidence provide evidence that RCTs cannot. Also, remember this important point: *The absence of evidence is not evidence of absence.*[61] Just because evidence has not been established for a clinical technique or practice does not mean it is false. But most clinical techniques have an underlying theory. Careful examination of the theory to make sure all its elements are consistent with known scientific facts, and with each other, is critical.

Generating Evidence for Evidence-Based Practice

EBM has broad support within the medical community because clinicians who base their clinical decisions on evidence derived from rigorous scientific research are most likely to provide optimal patient care.[8] This discipline requires interaction of knowledge creation and knowledge application (Fig. 2.2). Knowledge is of little value until it is applied; and as knowledge is applied, deficiencies, or holes, are identified that lead to additional research questions and additional knowledge creation (sometimes called knowledge refinement). Neither is optimized without the other.

Both laboratory (human- and animal-centered) and clinical (patient-centered) research provide information to enhance clinical decision making and patient care. All types of research are necessary. However, RCTs, if conducted and interpreted correctly, provide the most rigorous scientific research. Thus, RCTs are considered the highest grade of research evidence[62]—the gold standard for determining the efficacy of therapeutic agents.[63]

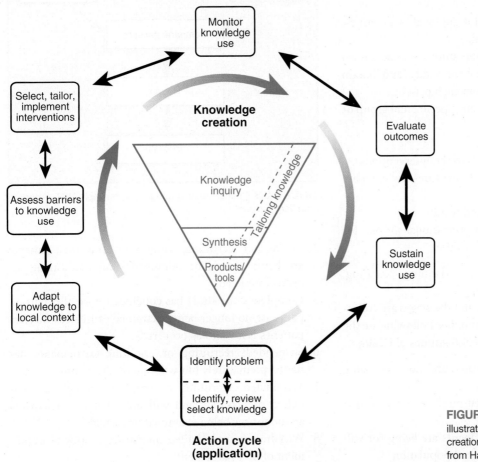

FIGURE 2.2 The knowledge-to-action cycle illustrates the interdependence of knowledge creation and knowledge application. (Adapted from Harrison et al.[31])

RANDOMIZED CLINICAL (CONTROLLED) TRIALS

A **randomized clinical trial** (RCT),[63–65] also known as a *randomized controlled trial*,[66–70] is a scientific study of a specific medical intervention on patients with a specific injury or disease. Both forms of the term are used interchangeably, and they refer to a specific type of controlled, clinical research.

In an RCT, a group of participants are randomly assigned to one of two or more treatment groups, called *arms*, one of which may be a control group.[58] These groups are followed up for the variables/outcomes of interest.[59] The trial is "blind" if the participants or the investigator is unaware of who is in which arm or group. If both are blinded, the experiment is called "double blind." Blinding helps eliminate bias (prejudice) for or against the treatment.[65]
Here are the major steps of the process, summarized in Figure 2.3:

1. Conceive of a clinical problem that needs to be researched.
2. Translate the problem into one or more specific research questions.
3. Develop a study plan (or methods) that clearly identifies subject characteristics and detailed intervention protocols.
4. Submit the proposed study for approval by an ethics, or institutional, review board.
5. Recruit patients that meet the study criteria, inform them of pertinent details of the study, and obtain informed written consent from each patient.
6. Randomly assign patients to an experimental group or a control group.
7. Implement the intervention.
8. Measure outcomes (responses to the interventions).
9. Apply appropriate statistical measures to compare outcomes between groups.
10. Write a report of the study and results.
11. Submit the manuscript to a professional journal for peer review and possible publication.

Tables and checklists usually help in planning, executing, and reporting the results of trials.[71]

RCTs are conducted in stages, and the stages are collectively referred to as the *recruitment status*. Following are the stages outlined by the U.S. National Institutes of Health:

1. Not yet recruiting: participants are not yet being recruited or enrolled
2. Recruiting: participants are currently being recruited and enrolled
3. Enrolling by invitation: participants are being (or will be) selected from a predetermined population

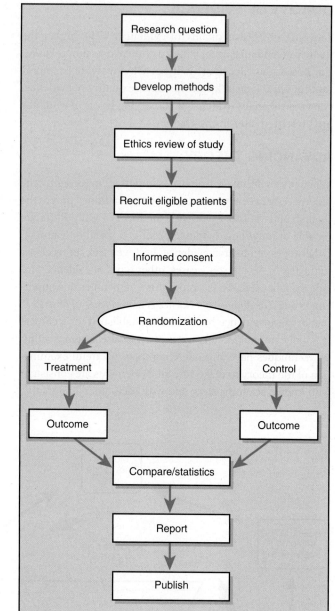

FIGURE 2.3 Critical steps in conducting a simple RCT. (Adapted from Torpy et al.[65])

4. Active, not recruiting: study is ongoing (i.e., patients are being treated or examined), but enrollment has been completed
5. Completed: the study has concluded normally; participants are no longer being examined or treated (i.e., last patient's last visit has occurred)
6. Suspended: recruiting or enrolling participants has halted prematurely but will potentially resume
7. Terminated: recruiting or enrolling participants has halted prematurely and will not resume; participants are no longer being examined or treated
8. Withdrawn: study halted prematurely, prior to enrollment of first participant

Concerns About RCTs

RCTs are the most rigorous type of scientific research,[62,63] if performed properly, meaning they are well designed, properly executed, and the design, conduct, and analysis of the study are thoroughly and accurately described in the report.[62,63,72] Not all RCTs are performed and/or reported properly, however, and therefore clinical decisions based on this evidence may be faulty. Following are factors that lead to faulty RCTs:

- Meta-analyses of studies with a small number of trials are not always as reliable as those with a larger number of trials.[73,74]
- Although RCTs are considered the highest grade of research evidence, properly conducted trials investigating the same association often yield conflicting results. These conflicting results may represent a spectrum of "real" outcomes for specific treatments. Such trials are best evaluated by considering concurrently both the validity of study design and the generalizability of patients and interventions involved.[62]
- Inappropriate measurements and statistical analysis of data.[75]
- Poor-quality intervention, or variation in applying interventions, represents a failure to deliver the intended care, so the trial becomes a measure of deliverability rather than the efficacy of the treatment.[76]
- Blinding is not always possible, such as a study comparing the effectiveness of applying various therapeutic modalities.[8]
- Ethical limitations exist about the types of comparisons that can be undertaken; that is, a conflict between established best practices for an individual and trial protocols of the RCT.[8,76]
- Positive clinical trials are published more often than negative trials, leading to publication bias.[66] Thus, a review of the literature concerning a specific intervention is biased in favor of the effectiveness of the intervention.
- There is inadequate reporting of RCTs.[72]

Many of the above problems can be avoided by including an epidemiologist and statisticians in the design of trials,[76] and by following the CONSORT (Consolidated Standards of Reporting Trials-discussed below) statement when publishing the results of the RCT.[72]

Assessing and Reporting the Quality of RCTs

There is overwhelming evidence that the quality of reporting of RCTs is not always optimal.[72] Thus, readers can neither judge the reliability and validity of a particular RCT nor extract valid information for systematic reviews. It appears that inadequate reporting and design are associated with biased estimates of treatment effects, which

negates one of the primary advantages of RCTs—the ability to minimize or avoid bias.[72] The results of such studies should not be trusted. Assessing the quality of RCTs is relatively new.[77] It is important because it gives an estimate of the likelihood that the results are a valid supposition of the truth. Numerous scales and checklists have been developed to assess quality, some of which are discussed in an annotated bibliography.[77]

Checklists are most useful to scientists. They provide guidelines for what information should be included in reporting RCTs. Scales, on the other hand, were developed for clinicians and other consumers of research. They give readers a quantitative index of the likelihood that the reported methods and results are free of bias.[77]

Even the highest quality of RCT research is of little value to clinicians if the published reports of the research are incomplete and inaccurate, which many have been.[72] To improve the quality of RCT reports, and thus the quality of RCTs, a group of scientists and editors developed the CONSORT (Consolidated Standards of Reporting Trials) statement in 1996.[78] Many leading medical journals and major international editorial groups have endorsed this set of standards,[72] although not all strictly enforce it.[79] The standards were updated in 2001[80–83] and again in 2010.[72,84] It appears that reports are improving,[85] in spite of some lax application.[79]

The initial CONSORT statement consisted of a checklist and flow diagram that facilitated critical appraisal and interpretation of RCTs.[78] The revisions consisted of updates to the checklist and a greater explanation of the meaning and rationale for each new and updated checklist item. They also provided examples of good reporting and references to relevant empirical studies.[72,83,84] Minor additions and updates continue to be added.[84] (See the CONSORT website for the latest information.)

RCT: Gold or Fools' Gold?

RCTs are considered the highest grade of research evidence,[62] the gold standard for determining the efficacy of therapeutic agents.[63] This is true in theory, but not always true in reality. Many clinical trials are badly flawed,[76] as discussed above. Resist the tyranny of the RCT; don't accept all RCTs as being completely accurate. And recognize that the conclusions of RCTs are, at best, only guidelines and at worst the result of a flawed trial rather than of a flawed intervention.[75] Use their data judiciously.

Research Other Than RCTs—Useful and Necessary

Some have misinterpreted Cochrane's plea as meaning that other forms of evidence were of limited value, and that all research should be RCTs. Not true. Positive clinical trials provide the best evidence, but the only conclusion that can be made from negative clinical trials is that the treatment was of no value as it was applied. For example, an RCT of the use of 10-minute applications of ice packs for acute sprained ankles would probably be negative. Does this mean that ankle sprains should not be treated with ice packs? No. It only means that 10-minute applications are ineffective. If the clinical trial had been done with 30-minute applications, the results would have probably been overwhelmingly positive.

RCTs are extremely difficult and expensive to conduct (e.g., millions of dollars for a multicenter surgical RCT[76]). The greatest difficulty is finding enough patients who meet the specific criteria for participation. Selection criteria are rigid. Therefore, the geographical area from which patients are selected must be enlarged. Also, many qualified patients are unwilling to participate because they may be assigned to a control or a less than optimal treatment group and thereby not get the best care.[8] This is especially true of athletes. Can you imagine an athlete, AT, or coach who would consent to the athlete *not* being treated so the effectiveness of the treatment could be proven? The difficulty in obtaining qualified patients means that those who are qualified and will volunteer must be compensated for their time and travel, which makes the research quite expensive.

The limited number of eligible patients limits the number of research questions that can be studied. How much time and money would it take to test every possible way of treating every possible injury in every possible type of patient? Laboratory and lower-level observational research is conducted to eliminate way-out ideas, develop theory, and establish treatment parameters with some degree of potential for success.

In addition, answers to some clinical questions can come from observational studies.[8] Some interventions are so powerful that their efficacy is obvious from case series. And they may be the best methods if researchers are studying the outcomes of uncommon treatments or diseases, if funding is scarce, or if there is only one acceptable intervention and the physician is ethically obligated to provide it.[8] Remember, however, that observational studies can only demonstrate associations between intervention and outcomes and therefore are inferior to RCTs, which can show causality.[56]

The data from large, prospective observational studies provide information about the safety and effectiveness of interventions used in daily clinical practice.[55] These studies are limited because of their susceptibility to bias and confounding, so their data should not be used to determine the cause and effect of interventions. They may, however, provide clinically relevant information that RCTs do not provide, if a more heterogeneous patient population and more heterogenous medical interventions are involved. The value of such information can be strengthened if the studies are designed to maximize their validity by identifying and measuring potential causes of bias and confounding.[55]

So although properly conducted RCTs provide the best clinical research evidence,[57,62,63] they cannot stand alone. Answers to clinical questions come from both observational studies and RCTs.[8]

HEALTH-RELATED QUALITY OF LIFE RESEARCH

Quality of life has become an important concept in health. Patients and clinicians realize that there is more to life than just breathing. It is a broad, multidimensional, patient-centered concept that measures a person's general feeling of personal well-being or satisfaction with life[86,87] (Fig. 2.4). It helps identify the effects of individual experiences, beliefs, values, expectations, and perceptions on physical and psychosocial dimensions of life.[86]

Health-Related Quality of Life (HRQoL) research is an emerging field of rehabilitation evidence generation. It supplements physical and performance evidence (the traditional basis of EBM) with psycho-social evidence. Thus it is an excellent tool for incorporating more patient-centered medicine into health care.

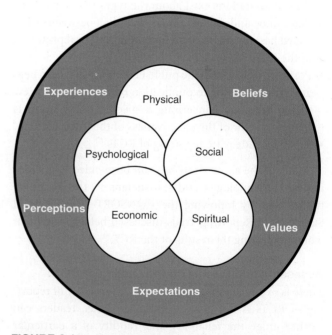

FIGURE 2.4 Health-related quality-of-life research encompasses the effects of beliefs, values, expectations, perceptions, and experiences on the physical and psychosocial aspects of an individual's life. (Adapted from Parsons and Snyder.[86])

The term "quality of life" appeared in the 1960s in the United States.[88] It is used with and without "health-related" and is abbreviated numerous ways: QOL,[89,90] QoL,[91] HRQL,[92] HEQoL,[93] and HRQOL.[86]

Numerous generic and disease/population/cultural-specific HRQoL assessment instruments have been developed,[88,94] and validated for many uses. As with any research, however, the validity and reliability must be established before using a specific instrument for a specific project.[89,92]

The HRQoL assessment instruments can be:

- Self-administered or interviewer-administered,[92] simple or complex[95]
- Used for patient management and policy decisions[92]
- Used to measure cross-sectional differences in HRQoL between patients at a point in time (discriminative instruments) or within individual patients over a period of time (evaluative instruments)[92]
- Used to detect trivial, small, moderate, and large differences[92]

Quality of life has become an important measure of patient responses to illness[92,94] and injury. It has not yet, however, become routine in sports rehabilitation clinical research and patient care.[86] Parsons and Snyder[86] make a strong argument for using HRQoL measurement as a primary outcome in rehabilitation of sports injuries.[86] Their published research paper is the most comprehensive primer on the definition, scientific validity, and use of HRQoL in sports rehabilitation. We recommend it as the first source you turn to for additional information on the subject.

JUDICIOUS USE OF EVIDENCE

Medical practice is an art as well as a science. EBP should not become robotic, prescriptive, or cookbookish. Even the best evidence available should not replace the clinician's experience and judgment.[76,96] The RCT has an important but limited role to play. As Cooper[76] stated, "Invest the RCT with dogma that it is the only valid method for confirming the value of new procedures is to disguise it with the emperor's new clothes." This does not justify a casual attitude toward continually seeking evidence, including RCTs. It means that you critically think about all research, as well as practical and acceptable alternatives to standard interventions. Recognize that there is no "average" patient.

Synthesizing Evidence-Based Medical Data

Data synthesis is the process of combining and summarizing results and opinions from many related individual studies and commentary. It serves two major purposes:

1. Pulling together many studies gives a clearer picture than individual studies, and thus saves clinicians and scientists from being overly influenced by studies that are extremely positive or extremely negative.
2. It gives readers more information in a shorter time; they don't have to read all the individual studies.

The multiple forms of data synthesis of medical literature are presented in the sections that follow. These include narrative review, meta-analysis, systematic review, clinical practice guidelines, clinical practice statements, and critically appraised topics (CATs).

NARRATIVE REVIEW

A **narrative review**, or literature review, of health care research is an approach that has existed for many decades; however, they are often not systematic. Narrative reviews may have been written by a recognized expert, but it is not realistic for one person to identify and bring together all relevant studies. Of more concern, an individual or company might actively seek to discuss and combine only the research that supports their opinions, prejudices, or commercial interests. In contrast, systematic reviews aim to circumvent this bias by using a predefined, rigorous, and explicit methodology (described in more detail below).

META-ANALYSIS

Meta-analysis, also known as *data synthesis* or *quantitative overview*,[97] is a technique that uses statistical tools to systematically combine and summarize the results of several individual/independent primary studies on a specific topic[97-101] (such as RCTs). Meta-analysis contrasts and compares results from related studies in an attempt to identify consistent patterns and sources of disagreements, thereby providing a stronger conclusion than individual studies alone.[102] This method is essentially an observational study of evidence,[98] the primary tool of systematic reviews (see below).

Well-conducted meta-analyses are valuable for a variety of reasons:

- They are considered to be the highest level of evidence, if the individual studies are high-quality RCTs.[103-108]
- They have greater statistical power than most individual studies because they pool the results of multiple smaller studies.[105,109] Thus, a clinician can have greater confidence in the study.
- They allow a more objective appraisal of the evidence than traditional narrative reviews.[110]
- They allow for a more objective appraisal of the evidence, which may lead to a resolution of uncertainty and disagreement.[110]

- They provide a more precise estimate of a treatment effect.[98]
- They identify conclusions that cannot be made from examining individual studies.[99]
- They may explain heterogeneity (differences) between the results of individual studies.[98,100]
- They may reduce the probability of false-negative results (Type II error) and thus prevent undue delays in the use of effective treatments in clinical practice,[110] especially when small studies show no treatment effect.[111]
- They optimize time spent by clinicians trying to remain current in their field of medicine.[105,112,113] Reading one meta-analysis takes less time than reading each of the individual studies, which can number in the hundreds.
- They provide preliminary data for calculating sample size for a definitive large trial.
- They provide preliminary data for selecting hypotheses to be tested in, and for calculating sample size for, a definitive large trial.[111]

Poorly conducted meta-analyses may be biased because of methodological factors and random error.[107] Bias can be introduced by the exclusion of relevant studies or the inclusion of inadequate studies.[104,112,114,115] The quality is only as good as the original studies included in the meta-analysis.[105,106] An insufficient number of cases and limited controls also can cause invalid[73,114,116–118] or questionable results.[98,104,119–122] Meta-analysis of nonrandomized studies has considerable limitations.[115] Even the tool recommended by the Cochrane Musculoskeletal Group, which assesses the quality of non-randomized studies[121,123] has been challenged.[124] Therefore, the methods of each individual study included in the meta-analysis review, the number of subjects in the individual studies,[73] and the methods of the review itself should be scrutinized before accepting the results.[105,118,125,126]

The characteristics of a high-quality meta-analysis include:[98]

- Carefully planned methods, with a detailed written protocol prepared in advance
- An *a priori* (based on theory) definition of eligibility criteria for studies to be included
- A comprehensive search of the literature
- An intermediate step of a graphical display of results from individual studies on a common scale, which allows a visual examination of the degree of heterogeneity among all the studies
- Appropriate statistical methods. There is no single "correct" method; one of many can be used to combine the data.
- A thorough sensitivity analysis to assess the robustness of combined estimates to different assumptions and inclusion criteria

Although meta-analysis is an important tool in understanding medical interventions and clinical decision making, it is not the sole tool, and not always the best tool.[127] As already mentioned, you must carefully consider the methods and studies included in a meta-analysis before accepting the conclusions.[99,118]

Meta-analysis is not statistical alchemy that makes life easier by distilling one magic number from confounded data; it is a scientific discipline that aims to quantify evidence and to explore bias and diversity in research systematically. We should keep trying to improve clinical trials and meta-analyses, not undermine them.[128]

Remember that meta-analysis is a method for studying studies rather than a shortcut for conducting large, randomized trials.[129] A meta-analysis of a number of RCTs with small numbers of subjects does not equal a single large-subject RCT.[73] For example, LeLorier et al.[73] compared 12 large RCTs and 19 meta-analyses of small sample-sized studies that had addressed the same questions, and included 40 primary and secondary outcomes. The meta-analyses, which were conducted prior to the large RCTs, did not accurately predict 35% of the 40 primary and secondary outcomes of the RCTs.

Comprehensive Literature Search

An exhaustive literature search is of utmost importance to a meta-analysis.[99] This type of synthesis should include searches of a multitude of databases, such as Medline/PubMed, Cochrane, National Clearing House, PEDro, and CINAHL (see Box 2.2). Limiting the search to a single database, such as PubMed, will probably result in a less than optimal search,[99,130] such as missing articles that should be included and returning articles that do not fit the search criteria.

Presenting Meta-Analysis Results

Results must be presented in formats that facilitate their integration into the health care decisions of clinicians and consumers.[131] The Cochrane Musculoskeletal Group (CMSG) developed specific guidelines to help scientists and authors convert the pooled estimates of meta-analyses to user-friendly numbers (Figs. 2.5 and 2.6). Doing so, they felt, would improve the impact and usability of systematic reviews. They recommended three methods for aiding knowledge translation (KT) from the laboratory to the clinic, and for facilitating the exchange between clinicians and patients:

- Produce clinical relevance tables of absolute and relative benefits or harms, and the numbers needed to treat (NNT) (Table 2.1).
- Create graphical displays using face figures (Fig. 2.6). The faces represent a group of 100 people and are shaded according to how many people out of 100 benefited or were harmed by the interventions.

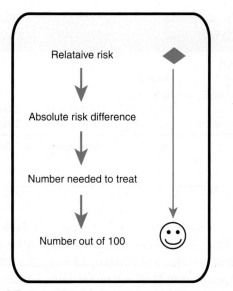

FIGURE 2.5 Translating numbers from systematic reviews into user-friendly graphs facilitates application of the results by clinicians and patients. The relative risk, represented as a diamond on a blobbogram, is converted to an absolute number needed to treat, and then to the number of patients out of 100 who benefit from the intervention. Compare with Figure 2.6. (Reproduced with permission from Santesso et al.[131])

• Write short consumer summaries (such as clinical practice statements and CATs, see below) for clinicians and to facilitate discussions between patients and their clinicians.

STATISTICS OF EBM

Interpreting RCTs, meta-analysis, and other evidence requires an understanding of some basic statistical concepts. These are presented in this section; however, an introductory statistics class is highly recommended. We also recommend a paper on how to read systematic reviews and meta-analysis results.[101]

Validity and Reliability

Validity is a measure of how well a test or intervention does what it is supposed to do; it is a property of the meaning of the test, not of the test itself.[132,133] For example, using the *Lachman test* for diagnosing anterior cruciate deficiency returns more correct answers than the *anterior drawer test* (see Box 2.1), and therefore is more valid. **Reliability** is a measure of how reproducible, or consistent, a test or intervention is. When it is administered numerous times in the same situation, it gives similar results. Box 2.4 presents an example of validity and reliability in sports performance.[132]

Sensitivity and Specificity of Diagnostic Tests

Diagnostic tests are used to determine the presence (or absence) of an injury or condition of interest. A test is considered positive if it indicates the structure is damaged or the condition is present, whether or not it actually is.

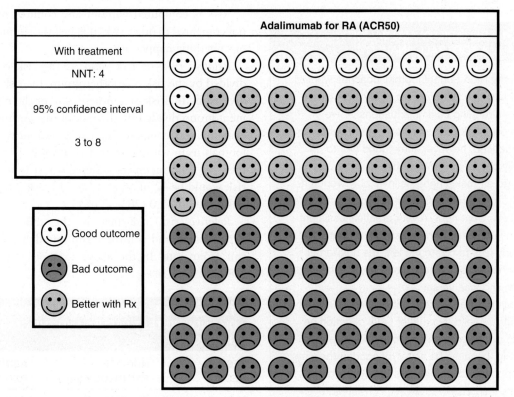

FIGURE 2.6 A face figure graph is another example of a user-friendly presentation recommended by the Cochrane Collaboration. Compare with Figure 2.5 for alternative graphical format, and to Table 2.1, which presents the same data. (Reproduced with permission from Santesso et al.[131])

TABLE 2.1   A CLINICAL RELEVANCE TABLE BASED ON META-ANALYSIS IN THE COCHRANE SYSTEMATIC REVIEW FOR ADALIMUMAB FOR RHEUMATOID ARTHRITIS

OUTCOME	NUMBER OF PATIENTS (NUMBER OF TRIALS)	EVENT RATE IN CONTROL GROUP, %	WEIGHTED ABSOLUTE RISK DIFFERENCE, %	WEIGHTED RELATIVE PERCENTAGE CHANGE (IMPROVEMENT)	NUMBER NEEDED TO TREAT (BENEFIT)	STATISTICAL SIGNIFICANCE	QUALITY OF EVIDENCE
ACR 50	1067 (3)	10.5	30 (30 more people out of 100)	273	4	Significant	Gold

A test is considered negative if it indicates the structure is intact or the condition is not present. So there are four possible results/interpretations of any test: two that are correct and two that are false or incorrect (Table 2.2). The incorrect interpretations are known as either *false positive*, meaning the test is interpreted as positive (injured/diseased) but the structure is normal (uninjured), or *false negative*, meaning the test is interpreted as negative (uninjured/nondiseased) but the structure is abnormal (injured).

The degree of correctness of diagnostic tests is captured by the terms sensitivity and specificity. **Sensitivity** is the proportion of true positives that are correctly identified by the test.[134] **Specificity** is the proportion of true negatives

that are correctly identified by the test.[134] In Table 2.3 (fictional data), sensitivity is 17/20 = 0.85, so if the structure is normal, the test will correctly identify this 85% of the time. Specificity is 31/47 = 0.66 for Table 2.3 data. Thus if the structure is abnormal, the test will only identify it as such 66% of the time.

Risk, Relative Risk, Risk Ratio, and Relative Risk Reduction[98]

Risk is the number of patients who fulfill the criteria for a given end point, divided by the total number of patients, reported as *x* of *x*, or as a percentage. For example, if 25 of the 90 members of your football team had a lost time injury during the first week of spring football, the risk would be 25 of 90, or 28%.

Risk is computed without any context, meaning it is not compared to other risk. It is just the simple probability of something happening.

Relative risk, or *risk ratio*, is the risk of one group divided by the risk of another group, the risk of one team divided by the risk of another team, or the risk of a treatment group divided by the risk of the control group. For example, let's compare the first week injury rates of your football team with your arch rival football team. If 12 of their 86 team members suffered a lost time injury, their risk would be 12 of 86 or 14%. The risk ratio, or relative risk, would be 2.0 (28% ÷14%).

Relative risk reduction is the difference between experimental and control group rate divided by the control group rate. In the above example it would be 1.0 (28% − 14% ÷ 14%).

BOX 2.4   RELIABILITY AND VALIDITY: A FOOTBALL ANALOGY

Grand County High School football coaches wanted to occasionally use Bobby, a big strong offensive lineman, as a running back in situations where they needed to pick up a small amount of yardage. As they practiced, however, they found him to be directionally challenged. When they called a play for him to go off tackle right, he invariably went left. Conversely, when they called for him to go off tackle left, he always went right. A very practical assistant coach came up with a commonsense solution. When Bobby was to run to the left, the quarterback instructed the rest of the team to block as if he were going right, and vice versa.

The statistical application: Bobby was 100% reliable, but 0% valid. No matter what direction he was told to go, he went the opposite way. He was totally invalid, because he never responded the way he was supposed to. But he was totally reliable, because his response was always consistent, even though it was wrong.

TABLE 2.2   THE RELATIONSHIP BETWEEN A DIAGNOSTIC TEST RESULT AND THE CORRECT DIAGNOSIS

TEST RESULT	NORMAL PATHOLOGY (−)	ABNORMAL PATHOLOGY (+)
Normal (−)	Correct	False positive
Abnormal (+)	False negative	Correct

TABLE 2.3 THE RELATIONSHIP BETWEEN A DIAGNOSTIC TEST RESULT AND THE CORRECT DIAGNOSIS, WITH SAMPLE DATA

TEST RESULT	NORMAL PATHOLOGY (–)	ABNORMAL PATHOLOGY (+)	TOTAL
Normal (–)	17	16	24
Abnormal (+)	3	31	34
Total	20	47	58

Odds and Odds Ratio

Odds is the probability of an event occurring versus the probability of it not occurring. In the example of your football team above, it would be 25 to 65 (or 25:65, or 25/65, or 0.38); since 25 of the 90 were injured, leaving 65 of 90 uninjured. Your rival team's odds would be 12:74, or 0.16.

The *odds ratio* represents the odds of an event occurring in one group versus the odds of it occurring in another group. Thus, the odds ratio of injury between the above two football teams would be 2.38 (0.38 ÷ 0.16). Using the same data we got a relative risk of 2.0, but an odds ratio of 2.38, very different numbers. Let's investigate that.

The odds ratio is a measure of effect size, or the strength of association or nonindependence between two values. It is a descriptive statistic that relates to the substantive, rather than the statistical, significance of a research result.[135] It is a difficult concept to grasp, in part because it can be confused with relative risk, which it is not.[136] The odds ratio is a ratio of odds, not percentages, as in the case of relative risk. It also is not the probability (or chance, or likelihood) of something happening, as odds are typically defined. As the probability gets smaller, there is less difference between relative risk and the odds ratio. At higher probabilities, however, the difference between them grows much greater. Consider a control group in which 8 of 10 subjects respond positively and a treatment group in which 9 of 10 respond positively. The relative risk would be 1.25 (9 ÷ 10 and 8 ÷ 10; 0.9 ÷ 0.8), and the odds ratio would be 2.25 (9 ÷ 1 and 8 ÷ 2; 9 ÷ 4). Using an odds ratio in this case would distort reality.

In medical research, the odds ratio is favored for case-control studies and retrospective studies. Relative risk is used in RCTs and cohort studies.[135]

Risk-Benefit Analysis

Risk-benefit analysis is the comparison of the risk of a situation to its related benefits. Two examples will help clarify this concept. An infrared lamp provides very low-cost ($25–$50) superficial heating (see Chapter 11). However, it is very easy to burn a patient with this modality, and a burn injury can take 1–2 weeks to heal. On the other hand, hydrocollator packs, which cost about $300 for a 4-pack unit, have little incidence of burning. The difference of a few hundred dollars is not worth the risk of using an infrared lamp.

The second example is rehabilitating a 2° ankle sprain with cryokinetics 3–6 days as opposed to 10–15 days with traditional thermotherapy (see Chapter 13). The initial cooling with cryokinetics is quite painful, but tolerable. And the body quickly adapts to the cooling, so that little pain is felt after a day or so. Most patients feel the benefits of quicker rehabilitation far outweighs the initial pain from cooling.

Numbers Needed to Treat

Numbers needed to treat (NNT) represents the number of patients who would be required to receive a particular intervention in order for one of them to benefit from the intervention.[137] NNT is popular because it combines an estimate of the relative benefit of a particular treatment with the background risk of patients. It is the inverse of the absolute risk reduction.

Calculating NNT from meta-analysis data is more complex than from individual trials.[131] There are various methods for making these calculations, and each method yields different results. Therefore, the method used to compute NNT should be clearly identified.[131]

Inference, Bayesian Inference, and Confidence Intervals

Research rarely measures an entire population having the characteristic of interest (e.g., people with ankle sprains). Not only is measuring an entire population much too time-consuming and costly, it is usually impossible to even identify the entire population. Scientists, therefore, measure or sample a small subset of the population and estimate the population characteristic from the subset, a process known as inference.

Inference, the process of forming an opinion about something based on partial information, allows us to expand knowledge in the face of uncertainty.[138] Often the bridge between evidence and clinical decisions,[139] inference uses statistical methods of calculating the probability that a hypothesis may be true.[138–140] It does not prove the hypothesis; it just infers the probability that the hypothesis is true.

There are two statistical approaches to inference: frequentist inference and Bayesian inference. *Frequentist inference* is the classical approach, using techniques such as the *t*-test and analysis of variance (ANOVA). *Bayesian inference* uses Bayes' theorem (named after Thomas Bayes) in its calculation.[139,141] The frequentist approach uses a sampling distribution and the Bayesian approach uses prior probability to test a hypothesis.[142] Fully exploring the differences in approaches requires a course in statistics.

The conclusion of probability testing is the chance, or probability (most often expressed as $p < 0.05$), that the mean of subjects in one group is different than the mean of one or more other groups of subjects. The p value simply states that the groups are different; it tells nothing about the magnitude of the difference between the groups.

A *confidence interval (CI)* is a statistical measure that indicates the reliability of the sample mean[143]; a range of values that tries to quantify the uncertainty of the inference. Consider it as a range of plausible values. The interval is always associated with a percentage. For example, the 95% CI indicates that if you take multiple samples, 95% of the time the true mean will lie within the upper and lower ranges of the CI.

SYSTEMATIC REVIEW

A **systematic review** is a structured literature review that addresses a specific clinical question.[97] It provides an overview of primary research studies[101] by summarizing evidence for the end user in an easily understandable format that is appropriate to the needs of a wide audience of people, especially clinicians, patients, and health care policy makers.[131] Systematic reviews address two needs: (1) minimize the chances of making an incorrect decision because of basing it on a few studies that may not have been conducted properly and therefore might have incorrect conclusions, and (2) help clinicians manage information overload.

Medical research is exploding. Over 12,000 new published articles (including more than 300 RCTs) are added to the Medline database each week.[144] To keep current with their field, it is estimated that health care professionals would have to average reading 17–20 original articles every day.[145] Increasingly, systematic reviews are being advocated as a way to keep up with current medical literature.[146]

The goal of systematic reviews is to determine whether specific interventions (treatments) work for a specific condition. They summarize the research, give direction for treating the problem, and include statements concerning the strength of clinical evidence for the intervention.

A systematic review involves systematically searching, analyzing, and summarizing evidence from numerous research studies.[113,147] It often includes a meta-analysis to quantitatively synthesize the results of the individual studies, thereby providing a numerical summary of the combined effect.[147] A systematic review has many of the same goals as a meta-analysis: helping clinicians stay up-to-date with the rapidly growing health care literature, minimizing the influence of flawed individual studies, and managing conflicting conclusions, thus making relevant evidence more accessible to decision makers.[113] A systematic review also helps expose areas where evidence about particular interventions is lacking.[113]

Systematic reviews are very different than narrative reviews (standard literature reviews) that have been part of medical literature for years (Tables 2.4 and 2.5). The major difference is that a systematic review includes strategies to avoid bias in selecting studies to review.[110] This necessitates that it includes a material and methods section. Systematic reviews may include formal meta-analyses,[110,113] although this is not a requirement. Other statistical methods can be used to analyze the data.

Systematic reviews are based on the idea that only rarely will a single research study of a treatment or test yield sufficiently strong evidence for using it.[113,148] Evidence from individual tests must be interpreted in the context of evidence from multiple tests. Systematic reviews provide such context.

A systematic review is conducted like any other type of research study, by following these steps[148]:

1. Formulating a specific research question
2. Outlining rigorous, objective methods of searching the literature and specific criteria for deciding which studies to include and exclude (Fig. 2.7)
3. Collecting the relevant data
4. Critically analyzing and synthesizing the data, using a variety of methods, including meta-analysis
5. Drawing conclusions and formulating clinical applications
6. Preparing a structured report

TABLE 2.4 FEATURES OF NARRATIVE REVIEWS AND SYSTEMATIC REVIEWS

FEATURE	NARRATIVE REVIEW	SYSTEMATIC REVIEW
Question	Broad	Focused
Sources/Search	Usually unspecified; possibly biased	Comprehensive; explicit
Selection	Unspecified; biased?	Criterion-based; uniformly applied
Appraisal	Variable	Rigorous
Synthesis	Usually qualitative	Quantitative
Inference	Sometimes evidence-based	Usually evidence-based

TABLE 2.5   CHARACTERISTICS OF THREE TYPES OF REVIEWS

CHARACTERISTIC	NARRATIVE REVIEW	SYSTEMATIC REVIEW	SHORTCUT REVIEW
Intent	Reviews current knowledge and practice in a clinical topic area	Reviews all available evidence on a focused question for the purpose of deriving a single best estimate of the true result	Selects the best or most applicable studies to maximize the role of evidence from research in clinical decision making
Topic	Clinical topic area	Focused clinical research question	Question arising from a practitioner's patient care
Author	An established expert or researcher on the topic	A team including methodologic and clinical expertise	Busy clinicians (either academic or nonacademic)
Searching	Frequently extensive, aimed at gathering literature on the topic area in question	Extensive, aimed at locating all primary studies relevant to a single research question	Limited search aimed at locating the strongest evidence addressing the question
Level of rigor	Criteria not uniform because of the relatively broad scope of the review	Follows established published criteria for research investigations of this type	Follows the methods of systematic reviews often with substantial limitations
Advantages	Provides an overview of a defined clinical topic area for practitioners needing primary information or an update	Provides an estimate of the "true answer" based on available clinical research pertaining to a focused research question	Provides an estimate of the "true answer" but with a weaker inference than a systematic review
Disadvantages	Does not provide the definitive answers to specific focused questions	Requires specialized expertise and a formal research protocol to prepare; results relevant to a single question only	Article search and selection may miss key evidence; methods of integrating discordant studies not rigorously addressed; results relevant to a single question only

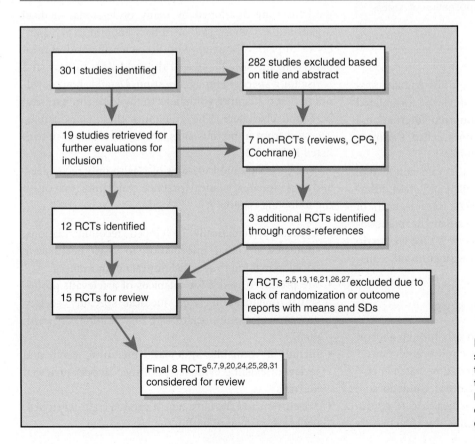

FIGURE 2.7 Study selection for a systematic review. CPG, clinical practice guideline; RCT, randomized clinical trial; SD, standard deviation.[131] (Note: References in the figure are from the original paper; they do not refer to this chapter.) (Source: Kim et al.[64])

BOX 2.5 CONCLUSION OF A SYSTEMATIC REVIEW BY KIM, ET AL.[64]

The present review supports the use of NMES in conjunction with exercise during the first 4 weeks following ACL reconstruction to improve quadriceps strength. The effectiveness of NMES on quadriceps strength was observed with lower treatment volumes and fewer sessions, an observation that should warrant further study into the cost-effectiveness of NMES treatment. Conclusions regarding self-reported outcomes cannot definitively be made, but the limited existing data suggest that there may be at least a trivial effect to, at best, a clinically meaningful benefit on patient-oriented outcomes on the Knee Outcome Survey. The effect of NMES upon functional performance is unconvincing, and the imprecision in the limited reported results suggest that a clinically meaningful benefit may or may not exist based upon both the ES point estimates and the width of 95% CIs. Moreover, methodological flaws and suboptimal parameter selection is likely to have impacted the results of the RCTs included in this review. Recommendations are given for future clinical trials to improve methodological quality and NMES treatment parameter consistency. Further recommendations are made for development of clinical practice guidelines in the application of NMES following ACL reconstruction.

Many groups prepare, maintain, and disseminate systematic reviews of treatments.[148] Reviews formulated by one of the 50 groups of the nonprofit international Cochrane Collaboration are sometimes called *Cochrane Reviews*.[30,149] Box 2.5 presents an example.

In spite of the care with which they are conducted, systematic reviews may differ in quality, and yield different answers to the same question.[150] As a result, users of systematic reviews should critically evaluate the methodological quality of the available reviews.[125,151] One way to do this is with the 11-item AMSTAR assessment tool[152] (discussed later).

CLINICAL PRACTICE GUIDELINES

The best practice concept is put into use through clinical practice guidelines,[31] also known as clinical guidelines,[44] best practice statements,[43] recommendation statements,[31] CMSG (Cochrane Musculoskeletal Group) Guidelines,[131] nursing best practice statements,[44] or health care guidelines.[45] These describe best and achievable practice in specific areas of care, in a clinician-friendly format, ready to be assist in forming health care decisions.[131] They guide practitioners in providing a consistent and cohesive approach to health care, and therefore improve the quality of care.[31] For example, see the *Ottawa Panel Evidence-Based Clinical Practice Guidelines for Electrotherapy and Thermotherapy Interventions in the Management of Rheumatoid Arthritis in Adults*.

Clinical practice guidelines are systematically developed statements that help clinicians and patients make appropriate decisions for specific clinical circumstances by doing the following[153–155]:

- Describing a range of specific, generally accepted approaches for diagnosing, managing, or preventing specific diseases or conditions
- Defining specific practices that meet the needs of most patients in most circumstances
- Identifying gaps in the research. This often leads to further research in order to fill the gap.

The statements contain recommendations based on evidence from a rigorous systematic review and synthesis of the published medical literature.[45,131] They do not contain fixed protocols that must be followed; rather, they encourage clinicians to use responsible judgment to develop individual treatment, tailored to an individual patient's specific needs and circumstances.[154] Clinical practice guidelines are developed by many professional medical organizations, whose staff members appoint expert panels of unpaid volunteers who are scientific and clinical experts in the specific area of the guideline, to draft and revise for a specific clinical question. Details about developing[154] and adapting guidelines to the local context[31] can be found elsewhere. The guidelines themselves can be accessed from numerous sites, including the repositories listed in Box 2.2.

The U.S. National Institutes of Health only recognizes, and disseminates, clinical practice guidelines that meet the following criteria[156]:

- Contain systematically developed recommendations, strategies, or other information to assist health care decision making in specific clinical circumstances
- Are produced under the auspices of a relevant professional organization (e.g., medical specialty society, government agency, health care organization, or health plan)
- Include a verifiable, systematic literature search and review of existing evidence published in peer-reviewed journals
- Are current and the most recent version (i.e., developed, reviewed, or revised within the last 5 years)

CLINICAL PRACTICE STATEMENTS

Some medical groups, such as the American College of Physicians, also publish clinical practice statements, which are reviews and critiques of available clinical practice guidelines.[155] They are digest versions of specific clinical practice guidelines.

CRITICALLY APPRAISED TOPICS: CATS AND CAPS

A **critically appraised topic (CAT)** is a short summary of evidence on a topic of interest, usually focused on a clinical question. A CAT is a shorter and less rigorous version of a systematic review, summarizing the best available research evidence on a topic. Usually more than one study is referenced in a CAT.

A **critically appraised paper (CAP)** is similar to a CAT, differing only in that it summarizes a single study, as opposed to multiple studies.[157] CATs and CAPs are one way for busy clinicians to collate and share their appraisals.

A CAT involves the following steps [157]:

1. Identify a common clinical problem.
2. Capture the essence of the problem into a written, focused clinical question.
3. Conduct a literature search for the best available evidence to answer the question, especially studies on the effectiveness of an intervention. The aim is to locate current best evidence, such as systematic reviews and RCTs. However, in the absence of such research, lower-level studies may be used.
4. Appraise and summarize the evidence.
5. Write a report.

Increasingly, CATs are being used as a university assignment to assess student skill and knowledge, and many of the more recent topics were completed by Australian undergraduate occupational therapy students in their final year of study.[157] There are multiple sites on the Internet containing CATs or CAPs, and some professional journals publish them—for example, the *Journal of Sport Rehabilitation* (*http://journals.humankinetics.com/jsr*) and the *Journal of Athletic Training* (*http://www.nata.org/journal-of-athletic-training*), which puts them under a heading of *Evidence-Based Medicine*. Some CATs and CAPs are peer-reviewed (such as those published in professional journals); some are not, especially those on some Websites, such as the Australian Occupational Therapy site (*http://www.otcats.com/intro.html*). Keep this fact in mind if using these CATs or CAPs to guide your practice.

Laboratory to the Bedside: Using Evidence

Medical knowledge is of little benefit to patient care if it remains in the realm of science; obviously, clinicians have to be aware of it. Regardless of the clinician's skill and compassion, her ability to help patients is limited by her knowledge of current information about how to treat the patient's specific problem.[6] One of the many initiatives of EBM is the emergence of a new medical discipline, clinical and translational science, to facilitate getting evidence into the hands of medical practitioners.[158]

KNOWLEDGE TRANSLATION

Knowledge translation (KT), also known as *knowledge exchange, knowledge transfer, knowledge mobilization, knowledge brokering,*[159] *knowledge diffusion,*[160] *research utilization, knowledge utilization, implementation science,*[161] and over 85 other terms,[162] is the process of translating science from the research lab to the clinician[163]—in other words, putting knowledge into action.[164] It is the link between knowledge developers and knowledge users.[165] Laboratory discoveries are of little value to the clinician until they are translated, transformed, and ultimately applied to current practice conditions.[166]

Not all research is clinically relevant, and that which is relevant is too massive for individual practitioners to keep abreast of.[113,144,167] There is simply too much information in too many places.[168] Thus, the task of those involved in KT is to sift thorough the masses of uncensored and nonprioritized information and synthesize it into a form clinicians can use in patient care,[159] and that patients and health care policy makers can use to evaluate clinical care.

Science does not benefit patients until the clinician understands the results of scientific investigations, decides the information is relevant and useful,[169] and then uses the knowledge in decision making.[159,162]

KT involves the synthesis, dissemination, exchange, and ethically sound application of knowledge to improve health care, provide more effective health care services and products, and strengthen the health care system.[162] It includes all the topics discussed in this chapter in the context of EBP, plus the many educational interventions that promote incorporating best evidence into health care practices.[170]

Despite the great explosion of medical knowledge, acting on that knowledge is lagging.[30,161,163,171] There are gaps between evidence and decision making at all levels of health care, including those of patients, health care professionals, and policy makers.[162] Many clinicians have a favorable impression of EBP, but they rely more on their clinical experience, colleagues, and informal continuing education experiences to guide their practice.[30,161,171] Transforming research into practice is a demanding task, requiring intellectual rigor and discipline, as well as creativity, skill, and organizational savvy and endurance.[163] Even so, the integration of new knowledge into best practices must be accelerated, and the best practices must be observed by more practicing clinicians.[166,172]

Implementation of evidence into practice requires much more than a practitioner's ability to critically appraise evidence and make rational decisions.[173] It is a multifaceted, complex process.[173]

Here are strategies to make KT more effective in universities[173]:

1. Defining and setting up a system to assess the KT cycle
2. Implementation and use of information technology
3. Identification and encouragement of face-to-face interactions between researchers and decision makers
4. Exchanging knowledgeable individuals among centers
5. Creating mutual trust, a common language, and a common culture for the creation of organizational knowledge
6. Using important motivational tools in the university
7. Using multidimensional methods for knowledge transfer. Universities depend primarily on the passive dissemination of knowledge, such as through publications and changing of individual behavior. Such passive diffusion of knowledge, however, is not sufficient to guarantee its adoption into practice.[163]

Knowledge Brokers

Knowledge brokers facilitate KT, the transfer of research and other evidence between researchers and practitioners.[174] Their activities include initial and ongoing needs assessments; scanning the horizon; knowledge management; knowledge translation and exchange; network development, maintenance, and facilitation; facilitation of individual capacity development in evidence-informed decision making; and facilitation of and support for organizational change.[175] The Canadian Institute of Health Research[176] maintains a repository of resources for individuals who want to learn about the science and practice of KT, and access tools that facilitate their own KT research and practices.

Bidirectional Knowledge Translation: Clinician Responsibility

The idea of KT is often thought of as the movement of information from the laboratory to the clinic, from the scientist to the clinician. However, this gives the impression that new knowledge is discovered only by the scientist,

and therefore the information that drives clinical practice comes primarily from the laboratory.[166] Such is not true, for two reasons: (1) There must be real-world verification of laboratory research.[166] (2) Aggressive, curious, and critical-thinking clinicians often try innovative approaches on patients who do not respond to traditional interventions. Many of these interventions are discarded, but others prove to be effective (see, for example, the discussion of cryokinetics in Chapter 12). The clinical success of the technique leads to scientific investigation, which results in verification and refinement of the technique.

As important as RCTs and systematic reviews are, they look only at the effectiveness of current interventions; as such, they are important, but limited, pieces of the health care puzzle. In addition, clinicians must help shape future research by sharing their clinical questions and observations.[6] The foundation of all research is the *research question*, and clinicians must help shape those questions.

There must be a bidirectional flow of discovery from the clinic to the laboratory and vice versa.[166] Best practices development requires the continual, active interaction of scientists and clinicians.

Bedside is the Sports Rehabilitation Laboratory

Sports rehabilitation defines the traditional medical model of research flowing from the laboratory to the bedside.[177] In sports, rehabilitation is driven by the calendar; athletic competition marches forward with or without the injured athlete. As a result, patients, and clinicians working with them, are more highly motivated to rehabilitate so the patient-athlete can return to participation. Consequently, new therapies often stem from innovative clinicians.[177] Sauers and Snyder[177] used accelerated ACL rehabilitation as an example of how "innovation at the point of care sparked research at every level of the clinical continuum."[177] "Only those who provide care, can improve care" (Slutsky,[178] quoted by Sauers and Snyder[177]).

Although the process is reversed, all elements are necessary for optimal clinical improvements. Intraprofessional teams of clinicians, scholars, and educators must be involved.[177] They must work together to select and refine clinical outcomes with which to monitor rehabilitation, teach clinicians how to use measure these outcomes, and motivate them to do so. The routine assessment of clinical outcomes in sports rehabilitation lags behind other professions,[179] in part due to a lack of understanding of basic concepts.[180] An excellent introduction to clinical outcomes assessment are papers by Mattacola,[181,182] Herrimann and Ragan,[181,182] Evans and Lam,[180] and Michener.[183] All six of these papers are necessary, as they address different aspects.

LEVEL, QUALITY, AND STRENGTH OF EVIDENCE

The core of EBM is quality of evidence.[6,60] Understanding the relative quality of evidence is necessary for clinicians to make the most informed decisions during injury diagnosis and treatment. Unfortunately, there is no uniformity in the use of terms or in classification systems. Despite the variations, however, their purposes are the same: to assist users of clinical research information to determine, through careful critical appraisal, the studies that are likely to be most valid.[7]

Level of Evidence: Individual Studies

Level of evidence is based on the type of research design used to generate the evidence[184]—in other words, the degree to which it maximizes the validity of the results by minimizing opportunities for the results to be influenced by bias and other confounding factors. There are differences of opinion about evidence hierarchies—differing in the number of levels, the types of research designs included, the relative order of some designs, and whether expert opinion, consensus panels, and unsystematic observations are included.[60,149,184–187]

The first quality of evidence grading systems were developed by the United Kingdom National Health Service[188] and the U.S. Preventive Services Task Force[189] to rate the quality of individual research studies. They consisted of four and five levels, respectively, and one used letters to designate the levels, while the other used roman numerals. Despite the differences between systems, in general, levels of evidence are graded 1 through 5 in decreasing order of quality.[190] Types of studies at each level vary somewhat with the clinical question (e.g., of diagnosis, treatment, or economic analysis), but typically follow this general organization:

- Level 1 evidence (the highest quality) consists of systematic reviews or meta-analyses of multiple RCTs and high-quality, single RCTs.
- Level 2 evidence is from well-designed cohort studies.
- Level 3 evidence is from case-control studies.
- Level 4 evidence is from case series and poor-quality cohort and case-control studies.
- Level 5 evidence is from expert opinion, based not on critical appraisal, but on reasoning from physiology, bench research, or underlying principles.

Level of Evidence: Synthesized Studies

As scientists began synthesizing groups of related research (such as meta-analysis and systematic reviews), additional classifications were needed. Table 2.6 is an example of additional grading.[45] Note that reports are assigned a

TABLE 2.6	EVIDENCE GRADING BY TYPE OF REPORT
CLASS	**DESCRIPTION**
Primary Reports of New Data Collections	
A	Randomized, controlled trial
B	Cohort study
C	Nonrandomized trial with concurrent or historical controls Case-control study Study of sensitivity and specificity of a diagnostic test Population-based descriptive study
D	Cross-sectional study Case series Case report
Reports That Synthesize or Reflect upon Collections of Primary Reports	
M	Meta-analysis Systematic review Decision analysis Cost-effectiveness analysis
R	Consensus statement Consensus report Narrative review
X	Medical opinion

Reports are assigned a letter indicating the class of report based on design type for individual, primary research (A, B, C, D) or by method used to synthesize collections of individual primary reports (M, R, X).[45]

letter to indicate the method used to compile the report. Letters A–D are for individual primary research, and the letters M, R, and X indicate reports that synthesize primary reports.

Level of evidence does not give clinicians a clear picture of how much faith to have in various clinical tests and interventions. Unfortunately, there is no top level of evidence to answer many clinical questions. It became clear that additional grading was necessary, thereby leading to the concepts of quality and strength of evidence.[184]

Be aware that some refer to *level of evidence* and *quality of evidence* as the same. We prefer the practice of defining them as separate characteristics.

Quality of Evidence

Quality of evidence relates to the credibility, clinical significance, and applicability of evidence.[191–193] How confident are you that it represents the "truth"?[193] Can you trust the results of the research (are they valid); will the procedure make a difference when applied clinically (results are both statistically and clinically significant); and to what patient population and setting do the results apply?[184]

TABLE 2.7 EXAMPLES OF CRITERIA FOR THE CRITICAL APPRAISAL OF VARIOUS STUDY DESIGNS

STUDY DESIGN	SELECTED CRITERIA
Systematic reviews	Were all relevant studies identified? Was the process by which reviewers assessed the quality of included studies described? Was the rationale for excluding studies provided?
RCTs	Is sample size based on power analysis? Were patient, clinicians, and study personnel blind to treatment group assignment? Were subjects analyzed in groups to which they were randomized (intent-to-treat)?
Cohort studies	Was follow-up sufficiently long and complete? Were dropout rates reported and reasons given? Was subgroup analysis performed?
Case-control studies	Were the controls appropriate for the study? Were potential confounding factors identified and handled properly? Was an estimate of effect given?
Qualitative studies	Were methods used for data collection described adequately? Were negative or discrepant results fully addressed? Are the explanations of results presented in a plausible and coherent manner?
Descriptive studies	Is the sample representative of the patient population under study? Are all critical outcomes being measured? Are the results influenced by temporal or secular trends?

Source: Jones[184]

Answering these questions requires an in-depth structured critical appraisal of the research. Checklists, such as those in Table 2.7,[184] or presented by the AGREE Collaboration,[194] may help in the analysis.

Strength of Evidence and Strength of Recommendation

Strength of evidence and strength of recommendation are intertwined. **Strength of evidence** is a combination of level of evidence and quality of evidence.[184] **Strength of recommendation** refers to the confidence in the belief that adherence to a particular recommended intervention (which is based on the evidence) will do more good than harm.[193]

The GRADE (grading quality of evidence and strength of recommendations) system is based on the fact that there is a difference between quality of evidence and strength of recommendation.[185,193,195] Thus, it integrates the two. It has four grades (ranks) of evidence (high quality, moderate, low, and very low)[195] and corresponding strength of recommendation (strong, weak, or conditional) to an intervention (pro or con) for the top three grades (Table 2.8). There appears to be a direct relationship between the strength

TABLE 2.8 QUALITY OF EVIDENCE AND AN EXPLANATION OF THE CATEGORIES IN THE GRADE SYSTEM

RANK	EXPLANATION	EXAMPLES*
High	Further research is very unlikely to change our confidence in the estimate of effect.	Randomized trials without serious limitations Well-performed observational studies with very large effects (or other qualifying factors)
Moderate	Further research is likely to have an important impact on our studies confidence in the estimate of effect and may change the estimate.	Randomized trials with serious limitations Well-performed observational yielding large effects
Low	Further research is very likely to have an important impact on our confidence in the estimate of effect and is likely to change the estimate.	Randomized trials wit very serious limitations Observational studies without special strengths or important limitations
Very low	Any estimate of effect is very uncertain.	Randomized trials with very serious limitations and inconsistent results. Observational studies with serious limitations. Unsystematic clinical observations (e.g., case reports)

*The examples are not comprehensive. See text[195] for criteria for upgrading or downgrading the quality of evidence.

of recommendations made in clinical practice guidelines and the quality of evidence as measured by the GRADE system.[193]

SORT: Strength of Recommendation Taxonomy[187,196]

Certain journals are beginning to rate the strength of the clinical recommendations made in some of the narrative review and clinical technique articles they publish (see Salata et al.[197]). They base the article recommendations on the types of evidence on which the authors base their recommendations. The three levels of recommendations are:

A: Consistent, good-quality patient-oriented evidence
B: Inconsistent or limited quality patient-oriented evidence
C: Consensus, disease-oriented evidence, usual practice, expert opinion, or case series

Strength of Recommendations of Preventive Measures

The U.S. Preventive Services Task Force (USPSTF) is responsible for conducting scientific evidence reviews of a broad range of clinical preventive health care services

(such as screening, counseling, and preventive medications) and developing recommendations for primary care clinicians and health systems.[198] It is a two-part evaluation, with grades for both the strength of its recommendations and the quality of the evidence upon which the recommendations are based[199] (Table 2.9). The classifications (A, B, C, D, I) reflect the USPSTF's opinion of the strength of evidence and magnitude of net benefit (benefits minus harms). The quality of the overall evidence for a service is graded on a 3-point scale (good, fair, poor).

EVIDENCE REPOSITORIES AND DATABASES

The five most important repositories for evidence-based information are in Box 2.2. Become familiar with each of them. Most university and hospital libraries have access to these. Visit the reference desk of your favorite library to learn how to use them, how to access them remotely, and how to obtain copies via interlibrary loan if your library does not subscribe to the journals referenced. In the process of writing this chapter, I (KK) have browsed over 500 articles, and obtained pdf copies of over 300, all from my home office. (See Box 2.2 for online references to each of these databases.)

TABLE 2.9 STRENGTH OF RECOMMENDATIONS OF PREVENTIVE MEASURES

STRENGTH OF RECOMMENDATIONS

A.	The USPSTF strongly recommends that clinicians provide [the service] to eligible patients. The USPSTF found good evidence that [the service] improves important health outcomes and concludes that benefits substantially outweigh harms.
B.	The USPSTF recommends that clinicians provide [this service] to eligible patients. The USPSTF found at least fair evidence that [the service] improves important health outcomes and concludes that benefits outweigh harms.
C.	The USPSTF makes no recommendation for or against routine provision of [the service]. The USPSTF found at least fair evidence that [the service] can improve health outcomes but concludes that the balance of benefits and harms is too close to justify a general recommendation.
D.	The USPSTF recommends against routinely providing [the service] to asymptomatic patients. The USPSTF found at least fair evidence that [the service] is ineffective or that harms outweigh benefits.
I.	The USPSTF concludes that the evidence is insufficient to recommend for or against routinely providing [the service]. Evidence that the [service] is effective is lacking, of poor quality, or conflicting and the balance of benefits and harms cannot be determined.

QUALITY OF EVIDENCE

Good:	Evidence includes consistent results from well-designed, well-conducted studies in representative populations that directly assess effects on health outcomes.
Fair:	Evidence is sufficient to determine effects on health outcomes, but the strength of the evidence is limited by the number, quality, or consistency of the individual studies, generalizability to routine practice, or indirect nature of the evidence on health outcomes.
Poor:	Evidence is insufficient to assess the effects on health outcomes because of limited number or power of studies, important flaws in their design or conduct, gaps in the chain of evidence, or lack of information on important health outcomes.

Note that this is a two-part evaluation. Reproduced with permission from the U.S. Preventive Services Task Force (USPSTF).[198]

? CONCEPT CHECK 2.1. Log on to one of the evidence-based databases (see Box 2.2) and enter a topic related to sports medicine. Read one of the guideline summaries returned. If by chance there are no hits, try another condition. How could accessing this, or similar, sites in the future contribute to your education?

Application of Evidence-Based Medicine

EBM uses techniques from medicine and science to help practitioners make conscientious decisions about the current and best use of tasks in their everyday practice. Its core activities are[2]:

- A questioning approach to practice, leading to scientific experimentation
- Meticulous observation, enumeration, and analysis replacing anecdotal case description
- Recording and cataloguing the evidence for systematic retrieval
- There are three distinct, but interdependent, areas of EBP:
- Treating individual patients with treatments supported in the most scientifically valid medical literature
- Systematically reviewing medical literature to evaluate the best studies on specific topics
- Advocating and popularizing the methods and usefulness of EBP to the public, patient communities, educational institutions, and continuing educators

Impediments to Evidence-Based Practice

Despite its obvious benefits, many health care professionals do not observe or practice EBM. There are a variety of reasons.

CULTURAL STAGNATION

One major hindrance to KT is that the movement requires a cultural shift in professional practice.[161,200] Implementing new evidence requires changing behavior, which is not easy for either individuals or groups.[165] Surveys of occupational therapists, for example, indicate that even though they have access to relevant research evidence, they often lack the confidence and skills to interpret and apply the research to clinical practice.[30,180] Greater efforts must be made to get clinicians to regard EBP as a clinical attitude, a mind-set—an approach to making health care decisions based on the best available evidence, the practitioner's

clinical expertise, and the patient's values.[180] Patients deserve nothing less than the best efforts of clinicians who are working on their behalf.

CONSTANTLY EVOLVING KNOWLEDGE

Keeping up to date is difficult, and keeping totally up to date is impossible. It's like shooting at a moving target—the evidence is constantly evolving. For instance, 10 years after the publication of a meta-analysis showing that a specific stroke treatment reduced the likelihood of death and disability by up to 30%, less than one third of acute stroke patients in Canadian hospitals received that specialized care.[167]

Here is a concrete example of the pace of knowledge evolution: The American College of Physicians state that their guidelines are automatically withdrawn or invalidated after 5 years, if they have not been updated.[155]

OBSTACLES TO BEST PRACTICES

The quality of care a patient receives can be limited by many factors, including the following:

- Clinician indifference to keeping current
- Lack of available facilities and resources[201]
- Policies of the payer[47,201]
- The absence of "high-level" research evidence.[16] The quality of relevant research evidence to answer many of the questions of clinicians and patients is still not available.[2,202,203]
- Delays in translating evidence into practice[16,202]
- Lack of acceptance of guidelines by some educators[47]
- Lack of time to keep up with the latest information[16]
- Too much information in too many places[168]
- The fact that good guidelines apply to only an estimated 80% of patients[40]
- A given best practice is only applicable to a specific condition or circumstance and may have to be modified or adapted for similar circumstances.
- Best practices don't remain best for very long, as people continually find better ways of doing things.[38]
- There is no single practice that is best for everyone or in every situation.[38,202]
- It is probably impossible for any individual practitioner to be fully versed in best practices. Indeed, at one health authority, there are 955 best practice guidelines for their practioners.[2]

ATHLETIC INJURY-SPECIFIC RESEARCH IS LACKING

A major impediment to fully using EBP in sports medicine is the lack of evidence about treatments on athletes. Most of the available evidence was collected from patients who were not athletes. One example is the increasing reporting of the sensitivity and specificity of diagnostic tests[134] in orthopedic evaluation texts.[204] However, these data come from patients rarely seen within minutes following the injury. And although a ligament tear in an athlete and a nonathlete are similar, the evaluation of a ligament tear 10 minutes after it happened often reveals different information than the same tear evaluated an hour later, and different still when evaluated a day or two later. This is not to say that these results should be ignored, rather that they should be interpreted with caution.

Another example is the lack of definitive data for some interventions, such as the application of cryotherapy for immediate care of acute injuries. These data are almost nonexistent.[205,206] Why? Although clinical experience and laboratory research (Level 5) indicate that immediate care cryotherapy is essential, there are no RCTs of immediate care (within 15 minutes of injury) of acutely injured competitive athletes. And such a study probably will never be done. What AT (or coach) would allow active athletes to participate in a study that required 50% of the subjects to be randomly assigned to a control (nontreatment) group? And what athlete would comply if assigned to a no-treatment group? Most athletes would self-treat with ice packs, thus invalidating the results.

APPLICATION PRECEDES THEORY AND EVIDENCE

Another impediment to EBM, especially with orthopedic injury intervention (including therapeutic modality application), is that application almost always precedes theory, and theory usually precedes research. A clinician, frustrated with a particular case, or group of similar cases, tries something new to help her patients. It seems to work, so she might fine-tune the approach, talk to colleagues about it, and share the approach with others. As the acceptance and popularity of the technique grow, people begin trying to explain why the application works. These explanations become a theory, but without any direct research evidence. In time, scientists test the theory with research, which may support or challenge the theory, and result in adjustments to the application.

The lack of research evidence should not deter you from using interventions based on clinical evidence, as long as you strive to understand and develop the theoretical basis of the technique. We do not condone the practice, however, of the continuous use of techniques based only on tradition, with the empty explanation of "I get good results."

It is critical that you learn both application and theory, and are aware of the strength of the theory—that is, what level of evidence the theory is based on. Then you can, and should, adjust the application and its theoretical basis as new knowledge becomes available. This approach may even lead to the discovery of new approaches.

POOR COMMUNICATION SKILLS

Communication is the "royal pathway to patient-centered medicine."[24] Training programs for enhancing communication skills for health care practitioners have been described by many authors.[207-210]

A Patient-Doctor Depth-of-Relationship Scale[211] has recently been developed to help clinicians understand how well they are relating to their patients. This is a conceptually grounded questionnaire that is easy for patients to complete, and it is psychometrically robust.[211] Its validity, and whether or not it correlates to the patient's quality of care, are questions for future research.

Becoming an Evidence-Based Practitioner, Revisited

Despite the concerns and problems with EBP, health care providers must provide patients with the best practice available.[34,38] This is a lofty goal that will never be met, yet educators, leaders of professional organizations (such as the National Athletic Trainers Association), and truly dedicated practitioners must persist in increasing the influence of EBM in patient care.[212] The discussions that follow are suggestions for accomplishing that goal.

TEACHING WITH, AND ABOUT, SYSTEMATIC REVIEWS

Becoming an evidence-based practitioner takes considerable effort, starting with a change in educational approach.[213] Critical appraisal of studies through the traditional use of journal clubs appears to not significantly increase the amount of medical research read by professionals-in-training. Teaching with systematic reviews, on the other hand, links learning to the numerous medical questions that physicians generate while providing patient care, because they model the rational and effective use of information. Systematic reviews should be made available at clinical sites for use during "teachable moments."

Students must also be taught early in their training how to read scientific literature, especially systematic reviews and meta-analyses,[101] and how to evaluate their quality before accepting their results.[125] Many systematic reviews are not valid. For example, Lundt et al.[125] reviewed the quality of 117 pediatric oncology systematic reviews

(99 published in regular journals and 18 in Cochrane Reviews) using a 10-item quality assessment tool.[214] The average methodological quality of these reviews was low, scoring only 1 (range 1–7) on those published in regular journals, compared to 6 (range 3–7) in Cochrane systematic reviews ($p < 0.001$).

The point that systematic reviews are meant to assist, not replace, clinical decision making, must also be emphasized.[213] They are a tool, not the law.

EVIDENCE IS NOT THE BASE OF MEDICINE

There is a growing sentiment that evidence cannot be the base for medicine; rather, it is one of multiple perspectives upon which medical practice is based.[215–217] An analogy is that medical practice should not be seen as a chain (outcomes evidence), but as a cable with multiple, intertwined threads, including traditional EBM outcomes evidence, basic and clinical sciences, clinician experiences, patient and family experiences and preferences, and societal values and perspectives.[216]

This does not justify an indifferent attitude toward continually seeking EBM evidence, such as RCTs.[76] It means you must critically think about all research, as well as practical and acceptable alternatives to standard interventions. Clinical judgment depends on both a fund of information and extensive experience.[218]

MULTIFACTORIAL CLINICAL DECISION MAKING

EBM can improve a clinician's negotiation between general medical knowledge and the patient's particulars, but it cannot replace patient input.[218] Patients should be involved as active partners with clinicians in making medical decisions, in clarifying acceptable medical options, and in choosing the preferred course of clinical care.[219] The major factor, however, in most patients' decisions is their doctor's opinion on the matter.[220,221]

NO AVERAGE PATIENT

There is no "average" patient[76]; each one is an individual. It is crucial to remember this when making any clinical decision. Research is usually reported as a mean ± a SD—that is, the "average" patient. This is relevant in the clinic because the majority of your individual patients will respond similar to the mean, but some will deviate from that mean throughout the continuum. And there is no way to know, as you sit eyeball to eyeball with an individual, where he/she fits. Begin with the assumption that your patient will fit the norm, but be ready to adjust care if that is not the case.

CRITICAL THINKING: ESSENTIAL TO EBP

Practicing EBM is impossible without critical thinking.[222–227] We have mentioned critical thinking throughout this chapter. Why? Why is it essential to EBP? What is it? How do you become a critical thinker?

Thinking Versus Critical Thinking

"Everyone thinks. It is our nature to do so. But much of our thinking, left to itself, is biased, distorted, partial, uninformed, or downright prejudiced. Yet the quality of our life and that of what we produce, make, or build depends precisely on the quality of our thought. Shoddy thinking is costly, both in money and in quality of life."[228] It leads to inadequate health care.

Some feel there is a crisis in medicine due to clinicians' decreasing critical thinking skills.[224–226] One physician-educator claims physicians are graduating from medical school as "hyposkilliac" (with deficient skills).[225] Another physician-educator questioned how (or if) physicians were taught to think.[226] Members of other health professions are concerned as well.[222–224,229]

Critical thinking is a complex subject that has stimulated thousands of volumes of written work. There were over 1850 articles in the CINAHL database from 1980 to 2005, and over 300 articles from 2004 to 2007.[227] This represents only nursing and allied health. Think how many tens of thousands of critical thinking articles there must be in the rest of medicine and other professional literature, such as philosophy, education, and engineering. It is impossible to present a complete or exhaustive review of critical thinking here.

It is essential, however, for ATs to cultivate critical thinking skills. We will introduce the topic here, and strongly encourage further study. We recommend the books by Brookfield[230] and by Paul and Elder[228] as a beginning for additional study.

Defining and Explaining Critical Thinking

Critical thinking is a process that requires explanation rather than a definition.[227] Related terms include critical decision making, critical analysis, critical awareness, critical reflection, and clinical reasoning; however, the process is more complex than those names imply. Brookfield[230] identified five characteristics and four key components of the process (Box 2.6). Paul and Elder[228] summarized five attributes of a critical thinker (Box 2.7).

Thinking Outside the Box

Critical thinking is often inappropriately defined as "thinking outside the box." While there is a basis for this concept, the phrase is so overused without context that it lacks significance. In short, it has become a cliché. What does this mean? What is "the box"?

BOX 2.6   CHARACTERISTICS AND COMPONENTS OF CRITICAL THINKING

Characteristics of Critical Thinking

1. Critical thinking is a productive and positive activity.
2. Critical thinking is a process, not an outcome.
3. Manifestations of critical thinking vary according to the contexts in which it occurs.
4. Critical thinking is triggered by positive as well as negative events.
5. Critical thinking is emotive as well as rational.

Components of Critical Thinking

1. Identify and challenge assumptions that underlie the ideas, beliefs, values, and actions that we (and others) take for granted. Asking (sometimes awkward) questions concerning our workplaces, interpersonal relationships, and all the realities of our lives helps us to understand who we are, why we do things, and how we might change our lives and actions for the better.
2. Challenge the importance of the context (framework, background, circumstance) of our life and activities. Actions result from context, and context is based on assumptions, often hidden and sometimes false.
3. Try to imagine and explore alternatives to existing ways of thinking and living. Exploring alternatives may lead to ideas and concepts that when integrated into our lives results in enhanced performance and living.
4. Become a reflective skeptic. Don't blindly accept claims to universal truth or ultimate explanations. But also don't be cynical.

BOX 2.7   ATTRIBUTES OF A CRITICAL THINKER

A well-cultured critical thinker:

- Raises vital questions and problems, formulating them clearly and precisely
- Gathers and assesses relevant information, and can effectively interpret it
- Comes to well-reasoned conclusions and solutions, testing them against relevant criteria and standards
- Thinks open-mindedly within alternative systems of thought, recognizing and assessing as need be, their assumptions, implication, and practical consequences
- Communicates effectively with others in figuring out solutions to complex problems

Critical thinking is, in short, self-directed, self-disciplined, self-monitored, and self-corrective thinking. It presupposes assent to rigorous standards of excellence and mindful command of their use. It entails effective communication and problem-solving abilities

Adapted from Paul and Elder.[228]

With context, however, the phrase can be helpful. If you think of "thinking within the box" as rigid, constrained, or unimaginative, then "thinking outside the box" would be open, unrestricted, unrestrained[231]—thinking differently, unconventionally, or from a new perspective, looking beyond the obvious.[232] The "nine dots" puzzle illustrates this concept (Box 2.8).

Developing Critical Thinking Skills

Critical thinking is a process that must be cultivated, rather than learned.[228] It requires adopting the attributes of a critical thinker, summarized in Box 2.7. Here are some suggestions for enhancing your critical thinking skills.

- Follow the advice of Sir Francis Bacon (1561–1626), who, although he did not use the phrase "critical thinking," expressed the concept in the early 1600s as follows:

Read not to contradict and refute
Nor to accept and take for granted
But to weigh and consider.

- Question, question, question. Why? Why? Why? Get beyond the surface. Dig deep. Why is a certain idea or technique being advocated? Is it based on assumptions, solid evidence, or most likely, a combination of both?
- Evaluate the evidence upon which theories, concepts, procedures, and techniques are based. Determine the validity and strength of that evidence.
- Identify and evaluate the validity of the assumptions underling theories, concepts, procedures, and techniques. (An assumption is something taken for granted, a supposition, without proof.) This involves probing, reflecting on, and questioning usual ways of thinking, as well as the morals, beliefs, values, and stereotypical notions of the author of the papers you read.[230] This process helps demonstrate the importance of the context wherein one's assumptions are formed.
- Practice "reflective skepticism" that is not cynicism, but rather the belief that ideas and practices must be subjected to careful testing against experiences.[230] (This is basically what Bacon advocated.)
- Differentiate between assumptions, theories, and reproducible scientific data.
- Ask "What evidence is needed to solidify this concept?" Then, "Where can I get that evidence?"

BOX 2.8   THE NINE DOTS PUZZLE

Connect all nine dots with four or fewer straight lines, without lifting your pencil from the paper and without passing through any dot more than once.

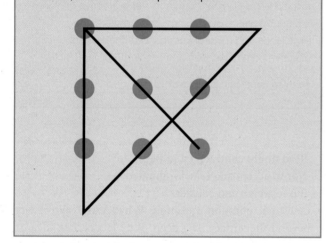

The solution is impossible if you stay within the box containing the nine dots. If you go outside the box, however, the solution is quite simple.

- Don't reject any evidence; rather, try to pull it all together. You can't sweep inconvenient information under the rug. Truth is often revealed as we resolve apparent inconsistencies and contradictions between our thoughts and observations and those of others.
- Consider and imagine alternatives to your own thoughts, ideas, and ways of acting, including your policies and procedures of patient care and management.

Critical Thinking Requires an Extensive Knowledge Base

Practicing EBM requires critical thinking *and* a storehouse of knowledge to think about.[233] One cannot exist without the other. You must memorize facts and figures, as well as theories and concepts. This must occur during your formal training (schooling) as well as throughout your career (Box 2.9). Continually add to your knowledge base. You must learn about and engage in critical thinking until it becomes second nature.

You need to study long and hard, memorize key concepts, and review material previously learned for updates and additional developments. Best practices are going to evolve and change as research advances knowledge about the condition.[38] Therefore, a commitment to using best practices requires a commitment to stay current with evolving knowledge. Plan a specific time to study; don't make it discretionary time. Schedule it, don't put it on a "to do list" that you will get to when you have time. And critically evaluate what you read.

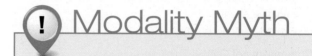

Modality Myth

Rote Memory has no Place in Higher Education. There is a naive notion that rote learning has no place in higher education, that students should engage in "higher-order" educational activities requiring critical thinking. A corollary is that rote learning is a waste of time. It is true that rote learning without higher-order thinking is of limited value. However, critical thinking cannot occur without a knowledge base upon which to think.

BOX 2.9   KEEPING UP WITH THE JONESES (ALLSEN AND NUTTALL)

Being an evidence-based practitioner requires keeping current with developing research and theories of sports injury care. Two of our colleagues at BYU are great examples of professional dedication to staying current with knowledge development. We offer them as models to emulate.

Phil Allsen, an exercise physiologist and strength and conditioning consultant, has read a professional book every month for the past 45 years. No wonder he is respected as one of the top strength and conditioning experts in the world.

Ron Nuttall, AT, has spent time reading for a half-hour every day for the past 30 years. He is known as one of the top overuse injury clinicians in the world. It is easy to see why US Track and Field and the BYU world championship dance troupes want him to travel with them.

When asked how many times they failed in reaching their reading goals, both gentlemen stated they could probably count on one hand the number of times they missed. What an example of dedication to continuing education and keeping up with professional advances. And what a gift to their clients and patients.

CLOSING SCENE

After reading this chapter, Kate still cannot resolve her dilemma about the differences in approaches between her two clinical instructors. If there is evidence that favors one approach over the other, she has an idea of how to find it. There is still much about the application of evidence to clinical decision making that she does not understand, but she is convinced that the principles of EBM will lead to better health care for her patients. She is committed to becoming an evidence-based practitioner, who seeks the best evidence possible and critical thinking to guide her clinical decisions.

Chapter Reflections

1. Read and ponder each of the following points. Do you feel you have a clear understanding of each concept? If not, reread the appropriate section of the chapter.
   - Discuss the philosophy and history of EBM.
   - Differentiate between evidence-based and patient-centered medicine. Which is most important? Why?
   - How will you become an evidence-based practitioner?
   - Discuss clinical decision making.
   - Explain, and differentiate between, clinical outcomes, best practices, protocols, clinical practice guidelines.
   - Define evidence and discuss sources of medical evidence, research evidence, and quality of evidence.
   - What is meant by advancing theory?
   - Discuss the process of generating evidence for EBP.
   - What are randomized controlled trials? How do they differ from randomized clinical trials?
   - Discuss the concerns the scientific/medical community has about RCTs.
   - Describe assessing and reporting the quality of RCTs.
   - What is meant by the phrase "RCT: gold or fool's gold"?
   - Explain how research other than RCTs is useful and necessary.
   - What is meant by health-related quality of life?
   - What is meant by judicious use of evidence? How to use evidence judiciously?
   - Explain how evidence-based medical data are synthesized.
   - Define, and differentiate between, narrative reviews, meta-analysis, systematic review, clinical practice guidelines, clinical practice statements, and critically appraised topics and papers (CATs and CAPs). Briefly explain how each is done and presented.
   - Discuss the following statistical concepts used with EBM: validity, reliability, sensitivity, and specificity of diagnostic tests; risk, relative risk, risk ratio, and relative risk reduction; odds and odds ratio;

   risk-benefit analysis; NNT; inference, Bayesian inference, and CIs.
   - What is meant by laboratory to the bedside?
   - Discuss KT.
   - What is the role of knowledge brokers?
   - Describe bidirectional KT. What are the roles and responsibilities of scientists and clinicians in this process?
   - Describe the concepts of level, quality, and strength of evidence, and identify how each one applies to individual and synthesized studies.
   - Describe quality of evidence, strength of evidence, and strength of recommendation, strength of recommendation taxonomy, and strength of recommendations of preventive measures.
   - What are evidence repositories and databases? Name the five most prominent ones for EBP.
   - Describe the following impediments to EBP: cultural stagnation, constantly evolving knowledge, obstacles to best practices, lack of athletic injury-specific research, application precedes theory and evidence, poor communication skills.
   - Discuss the following concepts as they relate to EBM: multifactorial clinical decision making, evidence is not the base of medicine, no average patient.
   - Describe what critical thinking is, how it differs from regular thinking, how to develop it, its role in EBP, and the role of knowledge in EBP.

2. Write three to five questions for discussion with your class instructor, clinical instructor, classmates, and clinical colleagues.

3. Get together with classmates and quiz each other on the concepts of this chapter. Use the points in reflection no. 1 and questions you wrote for reflection no. 2 as a beginning. Explaining concepts out loud to others requires a deeper grasp of the material than feeling you understand it as you read.

REFERENCES

1. Bensing J. Bridging the gap. The separate worlds of evidence-based medicine and patient-centered medicine. *Patient Educ Counsel.* 2000;39:17–25.

2. Peile E. Reflections from medical practice: balancing evidence-based practice with practice based evidence. In: Thomas G, Pring R, eds. *Evidence-Based Practice in Education.* Maidenhead, Berkshire, UK: McGraw-Hill Education. Open University Press, 2004:102–115.

3. Sweeney K, MacAuley D, Gray D. Personal significance: the third dimension. *Lancet.* 1998;351(9096):134–136.

4. Klafs C, Arnheim D. *Modern Principles of Athletic Training.* 4th ed. St. Louis, MO: CV Mosby Co., 1977.

5. Torg JS, Conrad W, Kalen V. Clinical diagnosis of anterior cruciate ligament instability in the athlete. *Am J Sports Med.* 1976;4:84–92.

6. Merrick MA, Dolan MG. Introduction to this special issue on clinical and translational science. *J Sport Rehab.* 2010;19(1):357–358.

7. Evidence-based medicine. *Wikipedia, The Free Encyclopedia.* Available at: http://en.wikipedia.org/wiki/Evidence-based_medicine. Accessed September, 2010.

8. Campbell A, Bagley A, Van Heest A, James M. Challenges of randomized controlled surgical trials. *Orthop Clin North Am.* 2010;41(2):145–155.

9. Maternal and newborn health: Republic of Moldova: evidence-based medicine— a new approach to childbirth. *World Health Organization Europe.* Available at: http://www.euro.who.int/en/what-we-do/health-topics/Life-stages/maternal-and-newborn-health/activities/evidence-based-care/republic-of-moldova-evidence-based-medicine-a-new-approach-to-childbirth. Accessed January, 2011.

10. Haynes RB, Devereaux PJ, Guyatt GH. Clinical expertise in the era of evidence-based medicine and patient choice. *Evid Based Med.* 2002;7:36–38.

11. Hootman JM. New Section in JAT: evidence-based practice. *J Athl Train.* 2004;39(1):9.

12. Steves R, Hootman JM. Evidence-based medicine: what is it and how does it apply to athletic training? *J Athl Train.* 2004;39(1):83–87.

13. Cochrane AL. *Effectiveness and Efficiency. Random Reflections on Health Services.* London: Nuffield Provincial Hospitals Trust, 1972 (reprinted in 1999 by the Royal Society of Medicine Press, London).

14. Haynes R. What kind of evidence is it that Evidence-Based Medicine advocates want health care providers and consumers to pay attention to? *BMC Health Serv Res.* 2002;2:3.

15. Guyatt G. Evidence-based medicine [editorial]. *ACP J Club.* 1991;114:A-16.

16. Groah S, Libin A, Lauderdale M, et al. Beyond the evidence-based practice paradigm to achieve best practice in rehabilitation medicine: a clinical review. *J Inj Func Rehabil.* 2009;1(10):941–950.

17. Rosenberg W, Donald A. Evidence based medicine: an approach to clinical problem solving. *Br Med J.* 1995;310(6987):1122–1126.

18. The Cochrane Database of Systematic Reviews. Available at: www.cochrane.org. Accessed August, 2010.

19. Agency for Healthcare Research and Quality (AHRQ) USDoHaHS. National Guideline Clearinghouse [web page]. Available at: http://www.guideline.gov/. Accessed August, 2005.

20. Association AP. PEDro Physiotherapy Evidence Database. *Centre for Evidence-Based Physiotherapy (CEBP).* [web page]. Available at: www.pedro.fhs.usyd.edu.au. Accessed August 2010.

21. Introduction to evidence-based nursing. Available at: http://ktclearinghouse.ca/cebm/syllabi/nursing/intro. Accessed January, 2011.

22. Hasnain-Wynia R. Is evidence-based medicine patient-centered and Is patient-centered care evidence-based? *Health Serv Res.* 2006;41(1):1–8.

23. Yeheskel A, Biderman A, Borkan JM, Herman J. A course for teaching patient-centered medicine to family medicine residents. *Acad Med.* 2000;75:494–497.

24. Bensing JM, Verhaak PF, van Dulmen AM, Visser AP. Communication: the royal pathway to patient-centered medicine. *Patient Educ Couns.* 2000;39:1–3.

25. Balint E. The possibilities of patient-centered medicine. *J R Coll Gen Pract.* 1969;17:269–276.

26. Donnelly WJ. Patient-centered medical care requires a patient-centered medical record. *Acad Med.* 2005;80:33–38.

27. Sackett DL, Rosenberg WMC, Gray JAM, Haynes RB, Richardson WS. Evidence based medicine: what it is and what it isn't. *Br Med J.* 1996;312:71.

28. Clinical decision making. *Encyclopaedia Britannica Online.* Available at: http://www.britannica.com/EBchecked/topic/121745/clinical-decision-making. Accessed October, 2010.

29. McGee D. Clinical decision making. *Merck Manuals Online Medical Library.* Available at: http://www.merck.com/mmpe/sec22/ch328/ch328a.html. Accessed October, 2010.

30. Menon A, Korner-Bitensky N, Kastner M, McKibbon K, Straus S. Strategies for rehabilitation professionals to move evidence-based knowledge into practice: a systematic review. *J Rehabil Med.* 2009;41(13):1024–1032.

31. Harrison M, Légaré F, Graham I, Fervers F. Adapting clinical practice guidelines to local context and assessing barriers to their use. *Can Med Assoc J.* 2010;182(2):E78–E84.

32. Agency for Healthcare Research and Quality. Outcomes research fact sheet. *US Department of Health & Human Services.* Available at: http://www.ahrq.gov/clinic/outfact.htm. Accessed September 2010.

33. Best Practice. *Wikipedia.* Available at: http://en.wikipedia.org/wiki/Best_practice. Accessed September, 2010.

34. National Cancer Institute. Dictionary of Cancer Terms: Best practice. *National Cancer Institute, US National Institutes of Health.* Available at: http://www.cancer.gov/Templates/db_alpha.aspx?CdrID=346526. Accessed August, 2010.

35. Cook D. Quality improvement: best evidence in clinical practice and clinical evidence of best practice. *Crit Care Med.* 2006;34(1):261–262.

36. Curtis J, Cook D, Wall R, et al. Intensive care unit quality improvement: a "how-to" guide for the interdisciplinary team. *Crit Care Med.* 2006;34(1):211–218.

37. Droller M. Peer review of guidelines, best practice statements and new documents: what this means for how we use them. *J Urol.* 2008;180(6):2297–2298.

38. Sturgeon N. Best practice must happen for every patient every time. *Nurs Times.* 2010;106(24):43.

39. Best Practices. *BusinessDictionary.com.* Available at: http://www.businessdictionary.com/definition/best-practice.html. Accessed September, 2010.

40. Carlisle D. How do we deliver best practice. *Nurs Times.* 2010;106(18):22–27.

41. Lautz D, Jiser M, Kelly J, et al. An update on best practice guidelines for specialized facilities and resources necessary for weight loss surgical programs. *Obesity.* 2009;17(5):911–917.

42. Scalise D. Evidence-based medicine. *Hosp Health Netw.* 2004/12//2004;78(12):32.

43. Ring N, Malcolm C, Coull A, Murphy-Black T, Watterson A. Nursing best practice statements: an exploration of their implementation in clinical practice. *J Clin Nurs.* 2005;14(9):1048–1058.

44. US Preventative Services Task Force. Aspirin for the prevention of cardiovascular disease: U.S. preventive services task force recommendation statement. *Ann Intern Med.* 2009;150:396–404.

45. Vinz C, Foreman J, Cummings K. An integrated approach to developing health care guidelines and measures. *Agency for Health Care Reserach and Quality.* May 17, 2010. Available at: http://www.guideline.gov/expert/expert-commentary.aspx?id=23793. Accessed November, 2010.

46. Manchikanti L, Datta S, Gupta S, et al. A critical review of the American Pain Society Clinical practice guidelines for interventional techniques: part 2. Therapeutic interventions. *Pain Physician.* 2010;13(4):E215–E264.

47. Lawrence D, Polipnick J, Colby E. Barriers to and opportunities for the implementation of best practice recommendations in chiropractic: report of a focus group. *J Allied Health.* 2008;37(2):82–89.

48. Price P. Disseminating best practice at conferences. *Nurs Stand.* 2010;24(25):35–41.

49. Price P. Disseminating best practice through publication in journals. *Nurs Stand.* 2010;24(26):35–41.

50. Price P. Disseminating best practice through education. *Nurs Stand.* 2010;24(27):35–41.

51. Price P. Disseminating best practice through workshops. *Nurs Stand.* 2010;24(28):35–41.

52. Marchionni C, Ritchie J. Organizational factors that support the implementation of a nursing best practice guideline. *J Nurs Manag.* 2008;16(3):266–274.

53. Sackett D, Straus S, Richardson W, Rosenberg W, Haynes R. *Evidence-Based Medicine: How to Practise and Teach EBM.* Edinburg: Churchill Livingstone, 2000.

54. Russell B. Marriage and Morals, Ch 5. (British author, mathematician, & philosopher; 1872–1970). *The Quotations Page.* Available at: http://www.quotationspage.com/quote/30147.html. Accessed November, 2010.

55. Yang W, Zilov A, Soewondo P, et al. Observational studies: going beyond the boundaries of randomized controlled trials. *Diabetes Res Clin Pract.* 2010;88(Suppl 1):S3–S9.

56. Hulley SB, Cummings SR, Browner WS, Grady DG, Newman TB. *Designing Clinical Research.* 3rd ed. Philadelphia, PA: Lippincott Williams & Wilkins, 2007.

57. Randomized controlled trial. *MedicineNet.com.* Available at: http://www.medterms.com/script/main/art.asp?articlekey=39532. Accessed November, 2010.

58. Glossary of Clinical Trials Terms. *ClinicalTrials.gov, US National Institutes of Health.* Available at: http://clinicaltrials.gov/ct2/info/glossary. Accessed November, 2010.

59. CEBM Glossary. *Centre for Evidence Based Medicine.* Available at: http://www.cebm.net/index.aspx?o=1116. Accessed November, 2010.

60. Hujoel P. Grading the evidence: the core of EBD. *J Evid Based Dent Pract.* 2008;8(3):116–118.

61. Sagan C. Carl Sagan quotes (American astronomer, writer and scientist, 1934–1996). *Think exist.com.* Available at: http://thinkexist.com/quotation/absence_of_evidence_is_not_evidence_of_absence/154055.html. Accessed November, 2010.

62. Jane-Wit D, Horwitz R, Concato J. Variation in results from randomized, controlled trials: stochastic or systematic? *J Clin Epidemiol.* 2010;63(1):56–63.

63. Floriani I, Garattini S, Torri V. Looking for efficiency rather than efficacy in randomized controlled trials in oncology. *Ann Oncol.* 2010;21:1391–1396.

64. Kim K-M, Croy T, Hertel J, Saliba S. Effects of neuromuscular electrical stimulation after anterior cruciate ligament reconstruction on quadriceps strength, function, and patient-oriented outcomes: a systematic review. *J Orthop Sports Phys Ther.* 2010;40(7):383–391.

65. Torpy J, Lynm C, Glass R. Randomized controlled trials. *JAMA.* 2010;303(12):1216.

66. Dickerson K, Rennie D. Registering clinical trials. *JAMA.* 2003;290:516–523.

67. Beckerman H, de Bie R, Bouter L, De Cuyper H, Oostendorp R. The efficacy of laser therapy for musculoskeletal and skin disorders: a criteria-based meta-analysis of randomized clinical trials. *Phys Ther.* 1992;72:483–491.

68. Kokoszka A, Scheinfeld N. Evidence-based review of the use of cryosurgery in treatment of basal cell carcinoma. *Dermatol Surg.* 2003;29(6):566–571.

69. Peto R, Pike M, Armitage P, et al. Design and analysis of randomized clinical trials requiring prolonged observation of each patient. I. Introduction and design. *Br J Cancer.* 1976;34(6):585–612.

70. Peto R, Pike M, Armitage P, et al. Design and analysis of randomized clinical trials requiring prolonged observation of each patient. II. analysis and examples. *Br J Cancer.* 1977;35(1):1–39.

71. Hanson BP. Designing, conducting and reporting clinical research. A step by step approach. *Injury, Int J Care Injured.* 2006;37:583–594.

72. Moher D, Hopewell S, Schulz K, et al. CONSORT 2010 Explanation and Elaboration: updated guidelines for reporting parallel group randomised trials. *BMJ.* 2010;340:c869.

73. LeLorier J, Grégoire G, Benhaddad A, Lapierre J, Derderian F. Discrepancies between meta-analyses and subsequent large randomized, controlled trials. *N Engl J Med.* 1997;337(8):536–542.

74. Rerkasem K, Rothwell P. Meta-analysis of small randomized controlled trials in surgery may be unreliable. *Br J Surg.* 2010;97(4):466–469.

75. Senn S, Julious S. Measurement in clinical trials: a neglected issue for statisticians? *Stat Med.* 2009;28:3189–3209.

76. Cooper J. Randomized clinical trials for new surgical operations: Square peg in a round hole? *J Thorac Cardiovasc Surg.* 2010;140(4):743–746.

77. Moher D, Jadad A, Nichol G, et al. Assessing the quality of randomized controlled trials: an annotated bibliography of scales and checklists. *Control Clin Trials.* 1995;16:62–73.

78. Begg C, Cho M, Eastwood S, et al. Improving the quality of reporting of randomized controlled trials: the CONSORT statement. *JAMA.* 1996;276:637–639.

79. Plint A, Moher D, Morrison A, et al. Does the CONSORT checklist improve the quality of reports of randomised controlled trials? A systematic review. *Med J Aust.* 2006;185(5):263–267.

80. The Consort Group. Consort Statement 2001. Available at: http://www.consort-statement.org/about-consort/history/consort-statement-2001/. Accessed June, 2011.

81. Moher D, Schulz K, Altman D, CONSORT Group. The CONSORT statement: revised recommendations for improving the quality of reports of parallel group randomized trials. *JAMA.* 2001;285(15):1987–1991.

82. Rennie D. CONSORT revised—improving the reporting of randomized trials. *JAMA.* 2001;285(15):2006–2007.

83. Altman D, Schulz K, Moher D, et al. The revised CONSORT statement for reporting randomized trials: explanation and elaboration. *Ann Intern Med.* 2001;134(8):663–694.

84. The Consort Group. Consort Statement 2010. Available at: http://www.consort-statement.org/consort-statement/. Accessed June, 2011.

85. Moher D, Jones A, Lepage L. Use of the CONSORT statement and quality of reports of randomized trials: a comparative before-and-after evaluation. *JAMA.* 2001;285(15):1992–1995.

86. Parsons JT, Snyder AR. Health-related quality of life as a primary clinical outcome in sport rehabilitation. *J Sport Rehabil.* 2011;20(1):17–36.

87. Spilker B. Introduction. In: Spilker B, ed. *Quality of Life and Pharmacoeconomics in Clinical Trials.* 2nd ed. Philadelphia, PA: Lippincott-Raven, 1996:1–10.

88. Wood-Dauphinee S. Assessing Quality of Life in Clinical Research: from where have we come and where are we going? *J Clin Epidemiol.* 1999;52(4):355–363.

89. Rey de Castro J, Rosales-Mayor E, Ferreyra-Pereyra J. Using a generic measure of quality of life in patients with obstructive sleep apnea. *Sleep Breath*. 2011;15(4):792–735.

90. Olestad B, Holm I, Engebretsen L, Risberg M. The association between radiographic knee osteoarthritis and knee symptoms, function and quality of life 10–15 years after anterior cruciate ligament reconstruction. *Br J Sports Med*. 2011;45(7):583–588.

91. Anneken V, Hanssen-Doose A, Hirschfeld S, Scheuer T, Thietje R. Influence of physical exercise on quality of life in individuals with spinal cord injury. *Spinal Cord*. 2010;48(5):393–399.

92. Guyatt GH, Feeny DH, Patrick DL. Measuring health-related quality of life. *Ann Int Med*. 1993;118(8):622–629.

93. Vainiola T, Roine R, Pettilä V, et al. Effect of health-related quality-of-life instrument and quality-adjusted life year calculation method on the number of life years gained in the critical care setting. *Value Health*. 2011;14(8):1130–1134.

94. Wells GA, Russell AS, Haraoui B, Bissonnette R, Ware CF. Validity of quality of life measurement tools—from generic to disease-specific. *J Rheumatol*. 2011;88(Suppl 1):2–6.

95. Grunnesjö M, Bogefeldt J, Blomberg S, Strender L, Svärdsudd K. A randomized controlled trial of the effects of muscle stretching, manual therapy and steroid injections in addition to 'stay active' care on health-related quality of life in acute or subacute low back pain. *Clin Rehabil*. 2011;25(11):999–1010.

96. Timmermans S, Mauck A. The promises and pitfalls of evidence-based medicine. *Health Affairs*. 2010;24(1):18–28.

97. National Information Center on Health Services Research and Health Care Technology (NICHSR). HTA 101: Glossary. *National Library of Medicine, United States National Institutes of Health*. Accessed October, 2010.

98. Egger M, Smith G, Phillips A. Meta-analysis: principles and procedures. *BMJ*. 1997;315(7121):1533–1537.

99. Winchester D, Bavry A. Limitations of the MEDLINE database in constructing meta-analyses. *Ann Int Med*. 2010;153(5):347–348.

100. Tak L, Meijer A, Manoharan A, de Jonge P, Rosmalen J. More than the sum of its parts: meta-analysis and its potential to discover sources of heterogeneity in psychosomatic medicine. *Psychosom Med*. 2010;72(3):253–265.

101. Greenhalgh T. Papers that summarise other papers (systematic reviews and meta-analyses). *BMJ*. 1997;315(7109):672–975.

102. Nestoriuc Y, Kriston L, Rief W. Meta-analysis as the core of evidence-based behavioral medicine: tools and pitfalls of a statistical approach. *Curr Opin Psychiatry*. 2010;23(2):145–150.

103. Wallace B, Schmid C, Lau J, Trikalinos T. Meta-Analyst: software for meta-analysis of binary, continuous and diagnostic data. *BMC Med Res Methodol*. 2009;9. Available at: http://www.biomedcentral.com/1471-2288/1479/1480

104. Moayyedi P. Meta-analysis: can we mix apples and oranges? *Am J Gastroenterol*. 2004;99(12):2297–2301.

105. Temple C. A primer in meta-analysis for the plastic surgeon. *Ann Plast Surg*. 2010;64(4):506–509.

106. Suebnukarn S, Ngamboonsirisingh S, Rattanabanlang A. A systematic evaluation of the quality of meta-analyses in endodontics. *J Endod*. 2010;36(4):602–608.

107. Brok J, Thorlund K, Wetterslev J, Gluud C. Apparently conclusive meta-analyses may be inconclusive—trial sequential analysis adjustment of random error risk due to repetitive testing of accumulating data in apparently conclusive neonatal meta-analyses. *Int J Epidemiol*. 2009;38(1):287–298.

108. van der Tweel I, Bollen C. Sequential meta-analysis: an efficient decision-making tool. *Clin Trials*. 2010;7:136–146.

109. Rosenthal L, Schisterman E. Meta-analysis: drawing conclusions when study results vary. *Methods Mol Biol*. 2010;594:427–434.

110. Egger M, Smith G. Meta-analysis: potentials and promise. *BMJ*. 1997;315(7119):1371–1374.

111. Borzak S, Ridker P. Discordance between meta-analyses and large-scale randomized, controlled trials. *Ann Intern Med*. 1995;123:873–877.

112. Dijkman B, Abouali J, Kooistra B, et al. Twenty years of meta-analyses in orthopaedic surgery: has quality kept up with quantity? *J Bone Joint Surg Am*. 2010;92(1):48–57.

113. *Systematic Reviews: CRD's Guidance for Undertaking Reviews in Health Care*. Heslington, York, UK: Centre for Reviews and Dissemination, University of York, 2008.

114. Athanasiou T, Rao C, Buxton B. Meta-analysis covers the horizon when the literature search is undertaken through a keyhole. *J Thorac Cardiovasc Surg*. 2010;139(6):1667–1670.

115. Jonker F, Trimarchi S, Verhagen H, et al. Meta-analysis of open versus endovascular repair for ruptured descending thoracic aortic aneurysm. *J Vasc Surg*. 2010;51(4):1026–1032.

116. Juni P, Altman D, Egger M. Systematic reviews in health care: assessing the quality of controlled clinical trials. *BMJ*. 2001;323(7303):42–46.

117. Nuesch E, Juni P. Commentary: which meta-analyses are conclusive? *Int J Epidemiol*. 2009;38:298–303.

118. Coyne J, Thombs B, Hagedoorn M. Ain't necessarily so: review and critique of recent meta-analyses of behavioral medicine interventions in health psychology. *Health Psychol*. 2010;29(2):107–116.

119. Steptoe A, Chida Y, Hamer M, Wardle J. Author reply: meta-analysis of stress-related factors in cancer. *Nat Rev Clin Oncol*. 2010;7(5):1.

120. Cremieux P. Methodological issues in a meta-analysis. *Hepatology*. 2010;52(1):395–397.

121. Navarese E, Buffon A, De Luca G, De Servi S. Regarding "a closer look at meta-analysis of observational data." *J Vasc Surg*. 2010;52(3):819.

122. Ingham R, Bothe AK. Letter to the editor. Thomas and Howell (2001): yet another "exercise in mega-silliness"? *J Fluency Disord*. 2002;27:169–174.

123. Wells G, Shea B, O'Connell D, et al. The Newcastle-Ottawa Scale (NOS) for assessing the quality of nonrandomized studies in meta-analyses. Available at: http://www.ohri.ca/programs/clinical_epidemiology/oxford.htm. Accessed October, 2010.

124. Stang A. Critical evaluation of the Newcastle-Ottawa scale for the assessment of the quality of nonrandomized studies in meta-analyses. *Eur J Epidemiol*. 2010;25(9):603–605.

125. Lundh A, Knijnenburg S, Jørgensen A, van Dalen E, Kremer L. Quality of systematic reviews in pediatric oncology—a systematic review. *Cancer Treat Rev*. 2009;35(8):645–652.

126. Katz RT, Campagnolo DI, Goldberg G, et al. Critical evaluation of clinical research. *Arch Phys Med Rehabil*. 1995;76(1):82–93.

127. Mak A, Cheung M, Fu E, Ho R. Meta-analysis in medicine: an introduction. *Int J Rheum Dis*. 2010;13(2):101–104.

128. Ioannidis JP, Cappelleri JC, Lau J. Meta-analyses and large randomized, controlled trials; letter. *N Engl J Med*. 1998;338:59–62.

129. Sim I, Lavori P. Meta-analyses and large randomized, controlled trials; letter. *N Engl J Med*. 1998;338:59–62.

130. Wilczynski N, Haynes R. Consistency and accuracy of indexing systematic review articles and meta-analyses in medline. *Health Info Libr J*. 2009;26:203–210.

131. Santesso N, Maxwell L, Tugwell P, et al. Knowledge transfer to clinicians and consumers by the cochrane musculoskeletal group. *J Rheumatol*. 2006;33:2312–2318.

132. Denegar C, Fraser M. How useful are physical examination procedures? Understanding and applying likelihood ratios. *J Athl Train*. 2006;41(1):201–206.

133. Messick S. Validity of psychological assessment: validation of inferences from person's response to performances as inquiry into score meaning. *Am Psychol*. 1995;20:741–749.

134. Altman DG, Bland JM. Diagnostic tests 1: sensitivity and specificity. *Br Med J*. 1994;308:1554.

135. Odds ratio, effect size, relative risk. *Wikipedia*. Available at: http://en.wikipedia.org/wiki/Odds_ratio. Accessed January, 2011.

136. Goldin R. Odds Ratios. *George Mason University*. Available at: http://stats.org/stories/2008/odds_ratios_april4_2008.html. Accessed January, 2011.

137. Cates C. What is NNT? *Dr Chris Cates' EBM Web Site*. Available at: http://www.nntonline.net/. Accessed November, 2010.

138. Holyoak K, Lee H, Lu H. Analogical and category-based inference: a theoretical integration with Bayesian causal models. *J Exp Psychol Gen*. 2010;139(4):702–727.

139. Lilford R, Braunholtz D. Who's afraid of Thomas Bayes? *J Epidemiol Community Health*. 2000;54(10):731–739.

140. Fong Y, Rue H, Wakefield J. Bayesian inference for generalized linear mixed models. *Biostatistics*. 2020;11(3):397–412.

141. Bowalekar S. Adaptive designs in clinical trials. *Perspect Clin Res*. 2011;2(1):23–27.

142. Johnson SR. Bayesian inference: statistical gimmik or added value? *J Rheumatol*. 2011;38(5):794–795.

143. Dorey FJ. In brief: statistics in brief: confidence intervals: what is the real result in the target population? *Clin Orthop Relat Res*. 2010;468(11):3137–3138.

144. Glasziou PP. Information overload: what's behind it, whats beyond it? *Med J Aust*. 2008;189:84–85.

145. Davidoff F, Haynes B, Sackett D, Smith R. Evidence based medicine. *BMJ*. 1995;310(6987):1085–1086.

146. Lau J, Ioannidis J, Schmid C. Summing up evidence: one answer is not always enough. *Lancet*. 1998;351(9096):123–127.

147. Sutton AJ, Abrams KR. Bayesian methods in meta-analysis and evidence synthesis. *Stat Methods Med Res*. 2001;10(4):277–303.

148. Editorial commentary (2007). Systematic reviews of all the relevant evidence. *The James Lind Library*. Available at: www.jameslindlibrary.org. Accessed June, 2011.

149. Maxwell L, Santesso N, Tugwell P, et al. Method guidelines for cochrane musculoskeletal group systematic reviews. *J Rheumatol*. 2006;33:2304–2311.

150. Moher D, Soeken K, Sampson M, et al. Assessing the quality of reports of systematic reviews in pediatric complementary and alternative medicine. *BMC Pediatr*. 2002;2(2):3.

151. Jadad A, Moher M, Browman G, et al. Systematic reviews and meta-analyses on treatment of asthma: critical evaluation. *BMC Pediatr*. 2000;320:537–540.

152. Shea B, Grimshaw J, Wells G, et al. Development of AMSTAR: a measurement tool to assess the methodological quality of systematic reviews. *BMC Med Res Methodol*. 2007;7:10. http://www.biomedcentral.com/1471-2288/7/10

153. Ottawa Panel Evidence-Based Clinical Practice Guidelines for Electrotherapy and Thermotherapy Interventions in the Management of Rheumatoid Arthritis in Adults. *Phys Ther*. 2004;84:1016–1043.

154. National Heart and Blood Institute. About clinical practice guidelines. *US National Institutes of Health*. Available at: http://www.nhlbi.nih.gov/guidelines/about.htm. Accessed September.

155. Qaseem A, Snow V, Owens D, Shekelle P. The development of clinical practice guidelines and guidance statements of the American college of physicians: summary of methods. *Ann Int Med*. 2010;153:94–199.

156. Agency for Healthcare Research and Quality (AHRQ). The National Guideline Clearinghouse Fact Sheet. *U.S. Department of Health and Human Services* [website]. Available at: http://www.ahrq.gov/clinic/ngcfact.htm. Accessed September, 2010.

157. McCluskey A. CATS: Occupational therapy critically appraised topics. *University of Western Sydney*. Available at: http://www.otcats.com/intro.html. Accessed October, 2010.

158. Balke CW, Umberger GH, Mattacola CG. "Oh, the Places You'll Go" 1: Transformation of the Nation's Biomedical Research Enterprise in the 21st Century. *J Sport Rehabil*. 2010;19(4):359–368.

159. Reimer-Kirkham S, Varcoe C, Browne A, et al. Critical inquiry and knowledge translation: exploring compatibilities and tension-snup_405. *Nurs Philos*. 2009;10(3):156–166.

160. Thompson G, Estabrooks C, Degner L. Clarifying the concepts in knowledge transfer: a literature review. *Adv Nurs*. 2006;53(6):691–701.

161. Kent B, Hutchinson A, Fineout-Overholt E. Getting evidence into practice–understanding knowledge translation to achieve practice change. *Worldviews Evid Based Nurs*. 2009;6(3):183–185.

162. Straus S, Tetroe J, Graham I. Defining knowledge translation. *Can Med Assoc J*. 2009;181(3–4):165–168.

163. Majdzadeh R, Sadighi J, Nejat S, Mahani A, Gholami J. Knowledge translation for research utilization: Design of a knowledge translation model at Tehran university of medical sciences. *J Contin Educ Health Prof*. 2008;28(4):270–277.

164. Graham I, Logan J, Harrison M, et al. Lost in knowledge translation: time for a map? *J Contin Educ Health Prof*. 2006;26(1):13–24.

165. MacDermid J, Graham I. Knowledge translation: putting the "practice" in evidence-based practice. *Hand Clin*. 2009;25(1):125–143.

166. Mattacola C. Sport rehabilitation and the clinical and translational science initiative. *J Sport Rehabil*. 2010;19(6):355–356.

167. Bayley M, Lindsay P, Hellings C, Woodbury E, Phillips S. Balancing evidence and opinion in stroke care: the 2008 best practice recommendations. *CMAJ*. 2008;179(2):1247–1249.

168. Leng G, Thomason C. NHS evidence—promoting efficiency and quality through evidence-based decisions. *Ann R Coll Surg Engl*. 2010;92(6):527–528.

169. Bucknall T. A gaze through the lens of decision theory toward knowledge translation science. *Nurs Res*. 2007;56(4 Suppl):S60–S66.

170. Davis D, Davis N. Selecting educational interventions for knowledge translation. *CMAJ*. 2010;182(2):E89–E93.

171. Gross D, Lowe A. Evaluation of a knowledge translation initiative for physical therapists treating patients with work disability. *Disabil Rehabil*. 2009;31(11):871–879.

172. Zerhouni E. Translational research: moving discovery to practice. *Clin Pharmacol Ther*. 2007;81(1):126–158.

173. Rycroft-Malone J, Bucknall T. Using theory and frameworks to facilitate the implementation of evidence into practice. *Worldviews Evid Based Nurs*. 2010;7(2):57–58.

174. Ward VL, House AO, Hamer S. Knowledge brokering: Exploring the process of transferring knowledge into action. *BMC Health Serv Res*. 2009;9:12.

175. Dobbins M, Robeson P, Ciliska D, et al. A description of a knowledge broker role implemented as part of a randomized controlled trial evaluating three knowledge translation strategies. *Implement Sci*. 2009;4:23.

176. Joint Program in Knowledge Translation. KT Clearinghouse. *Canadian Institute of Health Research*. Available at: http://ktclearinghouse.ca/. Accessed January, 2011.

177. Sauers EL, Snyder AR. A team approach: demonstrating sport rehabilitation's effectiveness and enhancing patient care through clinical outcomes assessment. *J Sport Rehabil*. 2011;20(1):3–7.

178. Slutsky J. Patient-Centered Outcomes Research: Closing the Gaps between Research, Practice and Policy. Agency for Healthcare Research and Quality. Paper presented at the Association of Schools of Allied Health Professions Annual Conference, Charlotte, NC. October 20, 2010.

179. Mattacola CG. Outcomes assessment in sport rehabilitation. *J Sport Rehabil*. 2011;20(1):1–2.

180. Evans TA, Lam KC. Clinical outcomes assessment in sport rehabilitation. *J Sport Rehabil*. 2011;20(1):8–16.

181. Herrmann S, Ragan BG. Outcome assessment part 1: measurement of physical activity. *Athl Ther Today*. 2008,13(2):25–28.

182. Herrmann S, Ragan BG. Outcome assessment part 2: measurement of person-environment interaction. *Athl Ther Today*. 2008;13(2):29–33.

183. Michener LA, Snyder AR, Leggin BG. Responsiveness of the numeric pain rating scale in patients with shoulder pain and the effect of surgical status. *J Sport Rehabil*. 2011;20(1):115–128.

184. Jones K. Rating the level, quality, and strength of the research evidence. *J Nurs Care Qual*. 2010;25(4):304–312.

185. Terracciano L, Brozek J, Compalati E, Schünemann H. GRADE system: new paradigm. *Curr Opin Allergy Clin Immunol*. 2010;10(4):377–383.

186. Gagiu P, Gugiu M. A critical appraisal of standard guidelines for grading levels of evidence. *Eval Health Prof*. 2010;33(3):233–255.

187. Ebell M, Siwek J, Weiss B, et al. Strength of recommendation taxonomy (SORT): a patient-centered approach to grading evidence in the medical literature. *J Fam Pract*. 2004;69(3):548–556.

188. Ranking the quality of evidence, National Health Service. *Wikipedia*. Available at: http://en.wikipedia.org/wiki/Evidence-based_medicine#National_Health_Service. Accessed November, 2010.

189. US Preventive Services Task Force. *Guide to Clinical Preventive Services*. 2nd ed. Washington, DC: Office of Disease Prevention and Health Promotion, 1996.

190. McGee D. Evidence-based medicine and clinical guidelines. *Merck Manuals Online Medical Library*. Available at: http://www.merck.com/mmpe/sec22/ch328/ch328b.html. Accessed October, 2010.

191. Brown S. *Evidence-Based Nursing: The Research-Practice Connection*. Sudbury, MA: Jones & Barlett, 2009.

192. Johnson L, Fomepit-Overholt E. Teaching EBP: the critical step of critically appraising the literature. *Worldviews Evid Based Nurs*. 2006;3(1):44–46.

193. Djulbegovic B, Trikalinos T, Roback J, Chen R, Guyatt G. Impact of quality of evidence on the strength of recommendations: an empirical study. *BMC Health Serv Res*. 2009;9:120.

194. AGREE Collaboration. Appraisal of guidelines research and evaluation (AGREE) instrument. Available at: http://www.agreecollaboration.org/pdf/agreeinstrumentfinal.pdf. Accessed November, 2010.

195. Brozek J, Akl E, Alonso-Coello P, et al. Grading quality of evidence and strength of recommendations in clinical practice guidelines. Part 1 of 3. An overview of the GRADE approach and grading quality of evidence about interventions. *Allergy*. 2009;64(4):669–677.

196. Ebell M, Siwek J, Weiss B, et al. Simplifying the language of evidence to improve patient care: Strength of recommendation taxonomy (SORT): a patient-centered approach to grading evidence in medical literature. *J Fam Pract*. 2004;53(2):111–120.

197. Salata M, Gibbs A, Seklya J. The effectiveness of prophylactic knee bracing in americal football: a systematic review. *Sports Health*. 2010;2(5):375–379.

198. U.S. Preventive Services Task Force. About the USPSTF. Available at: http://www.uspreventiveservicestaskforce.org/index.html. Accessed June, 2011.

199. U.S. Preventive Services Task Force. Grade Definitions. Available at: http://www.uspreventiveservicestaskforce.org/3rduspstf/ratings.htm. Accessed June, 2011.

200. Rycroft-Malone J. The politics of evidence-based practice. *Worldviews Evid Based Nurs*. 2005;2(4):169–171.

201. Fink-Samnick E, Muller L. Case management across the life continuum: ethical obligations versus best practice. *Prof Case Manag*. 2010;15(3):153–156.

202. Newnham E, Page A. Bridging the gap between best evidence and best practice in mental health. *Clin Psychol Rev*. 2010;30(1):127–142.

203. Tunis SRR, Stryer DB, Clancy CM. Practical clinical trials increasing the value of clinical research for decision making in clinical and health policy. *JAMA*. 2003;290(12):1624–1632.

204. Starkey C, Brown SD, Ryan JL. *Evaluation of Orthopedic and Athletic Injuries*. 3rd ed. Philadelphia, PA: FA Davis Company, 2009.

205. Bleakley C, McDonough S, MacAuley D, Bjordal J. Cryotherapy for acute ankle sprains: a randomised controlled study of two different icing protocols. *Br J Sports Med*. 2006;40(8):700–705.

206. Hubbard TJ, Aronson SL, Denegar CR. Does cryotherapy hasten return to participation? A systematic review. *J Athl Train*. Mar 2004;39(1):88–94.

207. Roter D. The enduring and evolving nature of the patient-physician relationship. *Patient Educ Couns*. 2000;39(1):5–15.

208. Mead N, Bower P. Measuring patient-centredness: a comparison of three observation-based instruments. *Patient Educ Couns*. 2000;39(1):71–80.

209. Hargie O, Morrow N, Woodman C. Pharmacists' evaluation of key communication skills in practice. *Patient Educ Couns*. 2000;39:61–70.

210. Smith R, Marshall-Dorsey A, Osborn G, et al. Evidence-based guidelines for teaching patient-centered interviewing. *Patient Educ Couns*. 2000;39(1):27–36.

211. Ridd M, Lewis G, Peters T, Salisbury C. Patient-doctor depth-of-relationship scale: development and validation. *Ann Fam Med*. 2011;9(6):538–545.

212. Rosenberg WMC, Sackett DL. On the need for evidence-based medicine. *Therapie*. 1996;51:212–217.

213. Oxman A, Guyatt G. Validation of an index of the quality of review articles. *J Clin Epidemiol*. 1991;44(11):1271–1278.

214. Badgett R, O'Keefe M, Henderson M. Using systematic reviews in clinical education. *Ann Intern Med*. 1997;126:886–891.

215. Buysse V, Wesley PW. Evidence-based practice: How did it emerge and what does it really mean for the early childhood field? In: Buysse V, Wesley PW, eds. *Evidence-Based Practice in the Early Childhood Field*. Washington, DC: Zero to Three Press, 2006:1–34.

216. Upshur REG. If not evidence, then what? Or does medicine really need a base? *J Eval Clin Pract*. 2002;8(2):113–119.

217. Assael L. Evidence-based practice: what does it really mean? *J Oral Maxillofac Surg*. 2008;66(10):1979–1980.

218. Montgomery K. Thinking about thinking: implications for patient safety. *Healthc Q*. 2009;12:e191–e194.

219. Sheridan S, Harris R, Woolf S. Shared decision-making workgroup of the U.S. Preventive Services Task Force. *Am J Prev Med*. 2004;26:56–66.

220. Mazur D, Hickam D, Mazur M, Mazur M. The role of doctor's opinion in shared decision making: what does shared decision making really mean when considering invasive medical procedures? *Health Expect*. 2005;8(2):97–102.

221. Bowling A, Culliford L, Smith D, Rowe G, Reeves B. What do patients really want? Patients' preferences for treatment for angina. *Health Expect*. 2008;11(2):137–147.

222. Finn P. Critical thinking: knowledge and skills for evidence-based practice. *Lang Speech Hear Serv Sch*. 2011;42(1):69–72.

223. Profetto-McGrath J. Critical thinking and evidence-based practice. *J Prof Nurs*. 2005;21(6):364–371.

224. Knight KL. Hyposkillia & critical thinking: What's the connection. *Ath Train Ed J*. 2008;3(3):79–81.

225. Fred. Hyposkillia—deficiency of clinical skills. *Tex Heart Inst J*. 2005;32(3):255–257.

226. Groopman J. *How Doctors Think*. Boston, MA: Houghton Mifflin Co., 2007.

227. Riddell T. Critical assumptions: thinking critically about critical thinking. *J Nurs Educ*. 2007;46(3):121–126.

228. Paul R, Elder L. *Critical Thinking: Tools for Taking Charge of Your Learning and Your Life*. Upper Saddle River, NJ: Prentice Hall, 2001.

229. Jones S, Crookes P, Johnson K. Teaching critical appraisal skills for nursing research. *Nurse Educ Pract*. 2011;11(5):327–332.

230. Brookfield SD. *Developing Critical Thinkers: Challenging Adults to Explore Alternative Ways of Thinking and Acting*. Reprint ed. San Francisco, CA: Jossey-Bass, 1991.

231. Finder TP. Think outside the box. Available at: http://www.phrases.org.uk/meanings/think-outside-the-box.html. Accessed April, 2012.

232. Wikipedia. Thinking outside the box. Available at: http://en.wikipedia.org/wiki/Thinking_outside_the_box. Accessed April, 2012.

233. Knight K, Draper D. Critical thinking and therapeutic modalities. *Athl Ther Today*. 2004;9(6):28–29.

General Application Procedures

OPENING SCENE

Jennie, a new student, is in her 5th day of clinical observation/experience. She has noticed that patients with similar injuries are treated the same, with little regard to how they respond to the treatment. She reflects on the three times she sprained her ankle during her high school athletic career. Even though she was told with each one that it was a lateral sprain, her response to the injuries was different in each instance. With one, her ankle hurt constantly for the 1st week; with another, she had pain only when she tried jumping or running. As she talked to the patients, she learned they were responding differently to the treatments. Then why were they all being treated the same way?

Jennie is also amazed at the number of different therapeutic modalities and the variety of their knobs, switches, and applicators. And the clinic has three machines called "electrical muscle simulators" that appear to be quite different modalities. She asks, "How long will it take me to master the use of all of these machines? What if I get mixed up and use the procedures of one modality when applying another modality?"

Jennie's two concerns are the basis of this chapter. How do you modify treatment to the specific needs of the patient? How do you learn the application of so many different modalities and keep them straight?

Application Approaches

Therapeutic modalities can be either powerful rehabilitation tools or a waste of time. What makes the difference? Using the right tool in the right way. Successful application requires more than knowing which knob to turn or what button to push (being a knobologist). You must know how to apply the modality, but you must also know:

- What your specific goals are
- That the modality you have chosen is the proper modality for achieving those goals
- What other therapy, such as therapeutic exercise, is beneficial and should be applied in combination with the modality

The application must be part of a carefully thought-out, goal-driven rehabilitation plan. This is sometimes called the rifle approach, as contrasted to the shotgun approach. The following analogy helps explain these contrasting approaches.

When a hunter fires a shotgun, hundreds of small round pellets are emitted from the gun. If a few of these pellets hit the target, they might kill a small animal, even though many pellets missed. On the other hand, when a hunter shoots a rifle, only one bullet comes out of the barrel. The hunter must take careful aim or else the target will be missed. With the shotgun approach, the patient is treated with every possible modality, with the hope that one will be effective. The rifle approach is more focused; the patient is treated with one or two specific modalities, targeted to achieve a particular goal (Fig. 3.1).

In Chapter 1, we discouraged the use of a cookbook approach to rehabilitation, and we repeat that advice here. The cookbook approach is rigid; it follows a specific recipe. In contrast, the critical thinker approach is more flexible. Just as some clinicians fall into the habit of using the same rehabilitation protocol for every injury, some also use the same modalities (and settings) when treating several different types of injuries. Although the one-recipe-fits-all

approach to modality application is easier to learn and use, it is not in the best interest of patients. No two patients or injuries are alike, and not everyone responds the same way to all treatments. With the cookbook approach, clinicians often treat the symptoms rather than the cause of the injury.

 CONCEPT CHECK 3.1. Can you think of some ways that you might be a better clinician by applying the rifle approach when you use therapeutic modalities? List several, then turn to the end of the chapter and compare your responses with ours.

THE CRITICAL THINKER APPROACH

The **critical thinker approach to rehabilitation** uses an organized procedural outline that includes fairly broad guidelines to help the clinician choose the most appropriate modality and mode of applying that modality.[1] It is patient driven, rather than specific modality driven. The modality is not the focus; it is part of an overall rehabilitation plan.

This approach begins with a thorough evaluation of the injury, establishing long-, medium-, and short-term goals and then selecting modalities and application parameters that will accomplish the specific goals. As the patient progresses, the application is altered to reflect the changing patient needs. Because no two patients or conditions are identical, the skilled clinician can use several tools (modalities) to reach certain treatment goals. The clinician who understands and employs critical thinking adapts to various situations. He alters the application parameters to best meet patient needs and to address the cause of the injury or condition. The critical thinker approach is more flexible than the cookbook approach because it empowers the clinician to adjust the rehabilitation approach to the specific patient and injury. For example, a critical thinking clinician might speculate and ask questions such as, "I wonder what might happen if I try this modality in this situation?" or "What if I adjust the application parameters to …?" (Fig. 3.2).

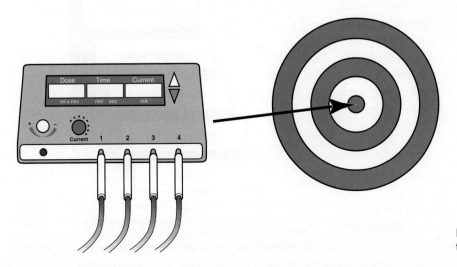

FIGURE 3.1 Use modalities that target the specific needs of the patient.

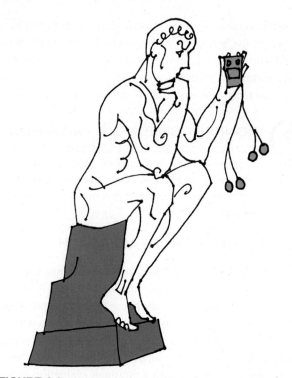

FIGURE 3.2 A critically thinking clinician is always seeking more efficient ways of treating patients.

STANDARD YET FLEXIBLE OPERATING PROCEDURES

Standard operating procedures (SOPs) are specific guidelines and protocols for performing a specific task. Having SOPs is a form of quality control. A knowledgeable person, or team of people, develops SOPs for all to follow when performing the task. For example, your favorite fast food will be the same in Moab, Utah, as it is in New York City, because it was prepared by people using the same SOPs. Having SOPs for complex tasks promotes consistency. They help you remember the specific steps and ensure that all essential elements are performed.

Using SOPs for therapeutic modality operation can have some disadvantages, however. They may lead to cookbook applications, and the task of learning SOPs for each of the dozens of modalities can be daunting and confusing, especially for those that you use infrequently.

The five-step approach outlined below is a framework for therapeutic modality application.[1] It is not as rigid as typical SOPs because it does not dictate all the specifics of each modality application—it is not a cookbook. We call it a *framework* because it contains all the essential elements. A clinician thinks critically and then adds the specifics of each modality to the general framework. Using the same framework for each modality is a quality control measure because it ensures that all essential elements are included. Using the same five-step procedure for all modalities minimizes the amount of information you need to learn for each modality, thus adding another element of quality control. Remember that the following is a general outline. Specific information will be presented in subsequent chapters for a variety of modalities.

 The Five-Step Application Procedure

The application of all therapeutic modalities should follow a standard procedure to ensure that all essential elements occur and to prevent rogue applications (Fig. 3.3). Although there is a wide range of therapeutic modalities, each one can follow a general application process. The **five-step application procedure** below eliminates the need to learn SOPs for each modality.[1] After learning the five-step framework, you can plug in specifics for each therapeutic modality. By learning and applying this system, you will be more organized and effective in delivering therapeutic modality treatments.

STEP 1: FOUNDATION

A. Definition. A description of the modality and the basics of how it operates (Fig. 3.4).
B. Effects. The physiological and/or pathological changes the modality evokes, both locally and systemically (throughout the body).

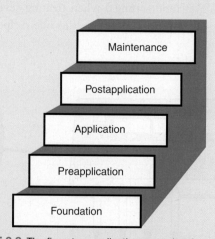

FIGURE 3.3 The five-step application procedure is a standardized framework for applying any therapeutic modality. It is rigid enough for quality control, yet flexible enough to allow the clinician to use modalities in the context of a critical thinking approach to rehabilitation.

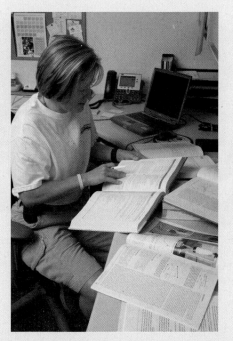

FIGURE 3.4 Before a therapeutic modality can be properly applied, you must have foundational knowledge about the modality and how specific types of injuries respond to the various ways of applying it.

C. Advantages. The benefits of the modality that make it more effective in treating injuries than other modalities.

D. Disadvantages. The possible negative effects the modality might cause as well as the benefits that might be lost from using this modality over another.

E. Indications. Situations in which the modality should be used or for which it is a suitable treatment or remedy for the condition.

F. Contraindications. Situations in which the modality should not be used—that is, situations in which it may do more harm than good.

G. Precautions. Situations that could cause harm if the clinician is not careful—for example, failure to move the soundhead during ultrasound treatment could damage tissue or cause extreme pain.

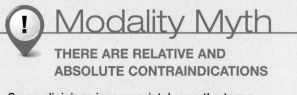

! Modality Myth

THERE ARE RELATIVE AND ABSOLUTE CONTRAINDICATIONS

Some clinicians inappropriately use the terms absolute and relative contraindications to refer to contraindications and precautions, respectively. The term "absolute contraindication" is redundant. Contraindication means "do not use," so it is already *absolute*. The term "relative contraindication" contradicts itself. It is impossible to *relatively* not use a modality. Use the more precise terms contraindications and precautions.

▣ STEP 2: PREAPPLICATION TASKS

A. Selecting the proper modality
   1. Determine the pathological and physiological changes associated with the injury by doing the following:
      a. Evaluate (or reevaluate) the injury or problem.
      b. Review the patient's response to any previous treatment (Fig. 3.5).
   2. Establish the objectives (goals) of the therapy.
   3. Match your therapeutic goal with a modality that will help you achieve that goal; consider effects, advantages, disadvantages, indications, contraindications, and precautions of all the possible modalities you could use to reach your goals.
   4. Make sure the modality is not contraindicated for the injury/condition.

B. Preparing the patient psychologically. This step entails more than just good bedside manners. As we will discuss in Chapter 8, there is a strong connection between emotions and physiological responses. The patient's psychological state modifies tissue responses to the therapy.
   1. Explain the purpose and expected outcome of the procedure.
   2. Describe the body's basic physiological response to the treatment, if the patient is interested.
   3. Explain what the patient should expect to feel—for example, tingling, pins and needles, or gentle warmth.
   4. Demonstrate the procedure on yourself if the patient is apprehensive.
   5. Warn the patient about precautions.

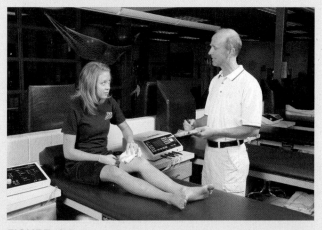

FIGURE 3.5 Patient interaction is an essential preapplication task. Detailed questions about how the patient responded to previous treatments help you decide whether to continue with the present modality or select another one. Explaining the purpose, the expected outcome, the body's physiological response, and what the patient should feel help prepare the patient psychologically for the treatment.

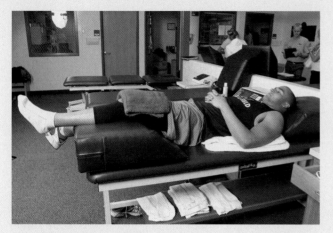

FIGURE 3.6 Pillows and bolsters are helpful in positioning a patient for treatment. You can never have too many pillows and bolsters in an athletic training clinic.

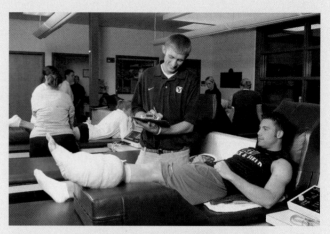

FIGURE 3.7 Properly recording specifics of the therapeutic modality application, patient response, and postapplication instructions to the patient is an essential part of modality application. Do not neglect these tasks.

C. Preparing the patient physically
   1. Remove clothing as necessary.
   2. Remove bandages, braces, and so on, as necessary.
   3. Position the patient in a manner that will be comfortable, yet allow accessibility to the modality. Have an ample supply of pillows or bolsters (supports) to use in positioning the patient (Fig. 3.6).
D. Equipment preparation
   1. Set up the equipment.
   2. Check the equipment operation.
   3. Perform a safety check.

3 STEP 3: APPLICATION PARAMETERS

A. Procedures
   1. Turn on the unit (if necessary).
   2. Adjust the output parameters as needed.
   3. Check the patient's response, and readjust the output as needed.
B. Dosage
C. Length of application
D. Frequency of application
E. Duration of therapy

4 STEP 4: POSTAPPLICATION TASKS

A. Equipment removal; patient cleanup
B. Equipment replacement; area cleanup
C. Instructions to the patient. *Note:* These should be written if they are extensive or complicated.
   1. Schedule the next treatment.
   2. Instruct the patient about the level of activity and/or self-treatment she should administer prior to the next formal treatment.
   3. Instruct the patient about what she should feel following treatment.
D. Record of treatment, including unique patient responses (Fig. 3.7).

5 STEP 5: MAINTENANCE

A. Regular equipment cleaning
B. Routine maintenance
C. Simple repairs

CLOSING SCENE

Recall from the opening scene, Jennie, a new student, seemed a bit confused that patients with similar injuries were treated with the same method, even though they responded differently to the treatments. She was also overwhelmed by all of the different kinds of therapeutic modalities housed in the clinic. She wondered about the purpose of each modality and the function of each of the knobs, switches, and lights on the devices. She wondered how long it would take her to master the correct use of all of those machines.

Jennie was fortunate to be assigned to work under the direction of a clinical instructor who understood when and why to use specific modalities. This instructor cautioned her about the flaws of the cookbook approach to treatment. He encouraged her to be a critical thinker. This included looking at each patient individually and then determining the appropriate modality to use for the patient's condition. He also taught her the five-step procedure to use when applying modalities. Under his watchful eye, he allowed her to experience what each modality treatment felt like. Within a few months, Jennie understood the functions of each modality and felt confident in using them. As Jennie became more confident, her clinical instructor turned the treatment of some patients over to her. Much to her surprise, the patients got better! Jennie succeeded where others had failed, because she became a clinician skilled in the art of critical thinking.

Chapter Reflections

1. Read and ponder each of the following points. Do you feel you have a clear understanding of each concept? If not, reread the appropriate section of the chapter.
   - Define a standard operating procedure.
   - Explain the cookbook and critical thinker approaches to therapeutic modality application.
   - Discuss the similarities and differences between SOPs and the five-step application procedure.
   - Describe the five-step application procedure, including the subelements of each step.
   - Identify the differences between indication, contraindication, and precaution with respect to therapeutic modalities.
   - Explain the importance of each of the following elements in selecting a therapeutic modality: evaluating the patient/injury, therapeutic goals, the physiological effects of the modality on the body, and its advantages over another modality.
2. Write three to five questions for discussion with your class instructor, clinical instructor, classmates, and clinical colleagues.
3. Get together with classmates and quiz each other on the concepts of this chapter. Use the points in reflection no. 1 and questions you wrote for reflection no. 2 as a beginning. Explaining concepts out loud to others requires a deeper grasp of the material than feeling you understand it as you read.

Concept Check Response

CONCEPT CHECK 3.1

There are several possible answers:

1. You treat the cause of the injury instead of the symptoms.
2. Your patients get better faster.
3. You know which modality/treatment regimen worked, because you tried one or two at a time and there is a cause-and-effect relationship to the outcome.
4. Your patients develop confidence in you.
5. You are able to establish which regimens work and which ones don't.

REFERENCE

1. Knight K, Draper D. Critical thinking and therapeutic modalities. *Athl Ther Today.* 2004;9(6):28–29.

4

Injury Record Keeping

OPENING SCENE

Both of us have served as witnesses and consultants in legal cases dealing with the alleged improper use of therapeutic modalities. One such case involved a podiatrist who treated an elderly woman with ultrasound during an office visit following a bunionectomy. The patient complained that the treatment hurt and asked him to stop. He informed her that she should not feel anything and that the treatment would last for only 10 minutes. The patient thought the pain and swelling intensified in the days following the treatment. After several weeks of pain, she hired an attorney, who claimed her pain and scarring were excessive, and the result of the ultrasound treatment. Were the pain and scarring due to the surgery or the ultrasound? The patient's treatment records were inadequate to answer this question, describing the treatment simply as "ultrasound for 10 minutes." The records included only the treatment duration, while omitting several important parameters such as frequency, intensity, treatment size, and duty cycle. If the clinician had kept detailed records in this case, he might not be in such a predicament.

Record Keeping

You may think a textbook on health care administration[1,2] is a more appropriate place for a chapter on record keeping. However, maintaining injury and treatment records is essential for all rehabilitation professionals. You must understand, early in your career, the absolute necessity of keeping accurate records, so we introduce the basics here. You must make record keeping a part of your clinical education from the beginning.

STANDARDS OF PROFESSIONAL PRACTICE

Accurate and detailed **record keeping** is a mandatory part of any health care program. Standard 7 of the *Board of Certification's (BOC) Standards of Professional Practice* states: "All services are documented in writing by the Athletic Trainer and are part of the patient's permanent records. The Athletic Trainer accepts responsibility for recording details of the patient's health status."[3] Failure to comply with this standard is unethical. It also could lead to loss of certification and licensure.

The Purpose of Keeping Records

Injury records are necessary for the following reasons, in order of importance:
1. *Communication and quality control*: Communicating with other clinicians, the patient, and yourself to increase the quality of care provided to patients.
2. *Legal protection*: Protecting the clinician in the event of a lawsuit.
3. *Research*: Documenting treatment details to help establish evidence of the effectiveness of the treatment, and/or find newer approaches.
4. *History*: Tracking a patient's injury history.
5. *Traffic patterns*: Monitoring injury and modality use frequency, as well as clinic workflow.

COMMUNICATION AND QUALITY CONTROL

By far the most important reason for keeping records is communication with yourself, with others involved in the treatment, and with the patient. Records enhance the quality of care by preserving details that otherwise might be forgotten or known only to a single person.

It is impossible for a busy clinician to remember all the details of numerous patients without written records. Periodic review of the records helps a clinician see what progress a patient has made, and may stimulate ideas for improved treatment.

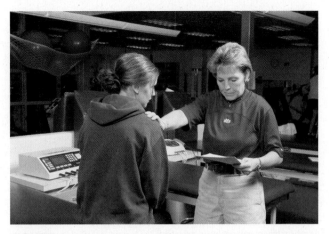

FIGURE 4.1 Clear, concise, and numerous entries on treatment notes help clinicians communicate with each other and thereby provide better care.

Written records help various treatment team members understand and discuss the approach, thereby adding continuity to the rehabilitation program (Fig. 4.1). Treatments are often administered by different people, and if the details are not recorded, no one will know what the others are doing. The efforts of each clinician will be isolated rather than part of a coordinated whole. This often leads to patient confusion, especially if each clinician is giving different advice about self-treatment to supplement the formal regimen. Moreover, the efforts of physicians involved in the rehabilitation program can often be more effective if detailed information about each treatment is communicated to them.

 CONCEPT CHECK 4.1. It is 10 P.M., and the end of a very busy day. You just finished caring for some softball players following a double-header. You want to go home and jump into bed. Unfortunately, you have injury and treatment forms to fill out. You hate to leave them until next morning because you might forget some important information. What can you do?

Another way that records help communication is with the patient. Patients frequently express frustration at not recovering from an injury as quickly as expected, and they want to know what else can be done. Although the patient might claim to be following the prescribed rehabilitation program, the treatment records reveal another story. When confronted with the records, the patient admits to missing some treatments. The problem becomes evident—it is not the program that is wrong; the patient is not following the program. At other times, the program is inadequate and needs to be adjusted. But the adjustments must also be recorded to verify that the patient has faithfully followed the revised program.

LEGAL PROTECTION

An injury record is a legal document. Conflicts concerning the quality of medical care often become legal issues, whether or not they end up in court. One of the first actions of plaintiffs' attorneys is to request copies of injury records. The value of these documents depends on their accuracy and detail.

Written records also help witnesses if the conflict progresses to a lawsuit. Most lawsuits occur years after the event, usually after any clinician would have forgotten the specific details of any treatment. Written records are obviously necessary for providing the details of how a particular patient's injury was treated.

An actual court case, in 1986 in Illinois, illustrates the need for detailed records (Ken Knight was a witness). A former high school athlete sued a coach, the school district, and a cold pack manufacturer for a thermal burn and scarring he claimed resulted from applying a cold pack to his knee overnight. During cross examination by the defense attorney in the case, the young man was asked a series of questions similar to the following:

- "Coach Jones testified that he told you to apply the cold pack for only 30 minutes. Do you contest that?"
- "Yes."
- "Are you sure he didn't tell you to only apply it for 30 minutes?"
- "Yes, I am sure, he never told me how long to apply it."
- "Have you ever doubted whether or not he told you how long to apply it?"
- "No, I have never doubted it—he did not tell me."
- "Did you give a deposition [pretrial testimony] on [date 3 years previous]?"
- "Yes."
- "Will you read the following statement you made during that deposition?"

Three years previously, the patient had testified that he did not think the coach told him how long to apply the cold pack, but he was not sure. Thus, his testimony at trial contradicted his earlier testimony. The jury sided with the coach. Written records help you be consistent in your testimony concerning a lawsuit.

✔ APPLICATION TIP

What did you eat for dinner on February 23rd 4 years ago? Did it include a salad? If so, what vegetables did it include? This illustrates the task you might face in a lawsuit, which typically includes testimony months or years after the fact.

RESEARCH

Research is accomplished by documentation: precise and accurate record keeping. Most clinicians are researchers, whether they realize it or not. Consider the following scenario: A clinician, frustrated with the lack of progress of a patient, tries something new. It seems to work, so he tries it again with other patients, and is again satisfied with the results. He then shares the idea with colleagues, who express interest in the concept and ask specific detailed questions about the cases. The clinician goes back to his treatment records for the details of the case and decides to write a case report. The clinician just conducted a research project. Therapeutic modality use and rehabilitation programs can be improved if clinicians record what they do, and then periodically evaluate the records.

HISTORY

The history of an injury is important to all members of the treatment team, as well as others. Since the need for this information sometimes arises months after the injury occurred, accurate and detailed records are critical. Specific details are essential to an insurance company. Claim settlement is often delayed while companies research details. Records also help a patient verify information concerning past injuries. College and professional team recruiters, the military, and some civic and corporate employers often want a patient to report significant sports injuries they have suffered and the extent of their rehabilitation.

TRAFFIC PATTERNS

Injury records provide the only means of establishing daily, weekly, monthly, and yearly traffic patterns in an athletic training clinic. Records can serve as evidence for verifying to the administration the need for additional budget, facilities, and/or staff, or the disadvantages of proposed cuts in the clinic's program. Records can also demonstrate increases or decreases in the volume of work handled in the athletic training clinic. If, for example, records show that the use of a particular modality has drastically increased, additional modalities might be authorized.

Using Records and Forms

Several components of athletic training and sports medicine clinics require record keeping. Five types of records are listed in Table 4.1, along with the names of the forms that are used at one university for recording that

TABLE 4.1 FORMS TYPICALLY USED IN AN ATHLETIC TRAINING CLINIC

PURPOSE OR TYPE OF RECORD	SPECIFIC FORM
Evaluation of injuries	• Athletic injury report form • SOAP notes
Treatment of injuries	• Daily treatment log • Individual treatment sheet • SOAP note progress • Daily weight recording form
Referrals to/from others	• Medical referral • Rehabilitation referral
Medical information	• Incoming student athlete • Returning student athlete
Equipment upkeep	• Ultrasound calibration • Electrical stimulator maintenance • GFI check (ground-fault interrupter) • Weight equipment maintenance

information. (Most clinics have similar forms but probably name them differently). One of the first things you should do when beginning to work in a new clinic is to familiarize yourself with the various forms and records used in that clinic.

ENTRY DETAIL

A medical record should be complete enough that in 2 days, 2 months, or 2 years from now, you or another clinician could read it and know the complete situation.[4] Language must be objective, specific, and concise but complete. Only standard English and universally recognized medical abbreviations should be included (Table 4.2).

INITIALING AND DATING ENTRIES ON FORMS

It is important that every entry on recording forms be initialed and dated by the person making the entry. Often one clinician needs more information about a patient than what is on the form. The initials tell the clinician who to go to for additional information. The date establishes when the entry was created.

ELECTRONIC RECORD KEEPING

Not all records need to be kept in paper form. Injury tracking and record keeping software programs allow records to be computerized (Fig. 4.2). Two popular ones are the Sports Injury Monitoring System (SIMS)[5] and the SportsWare Injury Tracking System.[5] They are designed to document injury and treatment parameters, and to improve communication between members of the clinic staff.[1] Two key features of these programs with respect to modality use are daily progress and treatment notes.

TABLE 4.2 COMMONLY USED MEDICAL ABBREVIATIONS

ABBREVIATION	DEFINITION	ABBREVIATION	DEFINITION
c/o	complains of	MM	muscle
c̄	with	OA	osteoarthritis
s̄	without	RA	rheumatoid arthritis
Hx	history	LBP	low-back pain
Dx	diagnosis	p̄	post
Rx	prescription	fx	fracture
♀ or F	female	s/p fx	status post-fracture
♂ or M	male	× 6 mo	for 6 months (or 6 months' duration)
y/o	year-old	AA	active assistive
EXER.	exercise	ROM	range of motion
L-S	lumbosacral	MMT	manual muscle test
pt.	patient	Bil	bilateral
ER	emergency room	LLE	left lower extremity
NN	nerve	RUE	right upper extremity
Tx	treatment	p/o	postoperation

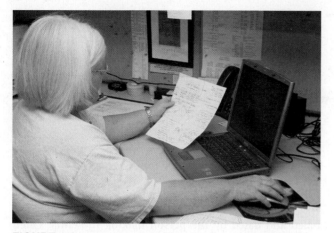

FIGURE 4.2 Computerized record keeping can simplify summary reports.

Computerized record keeping programs must be easy to use. They must allow entry on the fly, meaning treatments can be entered as quickly as, or immediately after, they are given. Systems that require the clinicians to sit down at the computer at the end of the day to enter the day's treatment details will result in records that are inaccurate and incomplete.

SOAP NOTES

The **SOAP note** format is a type of problem-oriented medical record.[7,8] SOAP is an acronym, each letter representing a section of the record: subjective evaluation, objective evaluation, assessment, and plan.[7]

- S = *Subjective*. The subjective evaluation contains information gathered primarily from questioning the patient on her present condition. Patient history and symptoms make up the majority of this information. For example, if a patient presents with ankle pain, saying "I twisted my ankle and it hurts right here," the subjective evaluation would read "Lateral ankle pain from twisting ankle."
- O = *Objective*. The objective evaluation consists of reproducible information the clinician gathers through tests or evaluative measures. Measurable factors, such as laxity during a stress test, girth, volumetric measurements of swelling following a sprained ankle, and joint range of motion as measured with a goniometer, appear in this portion of the record. The objective evaluation of the patient above might read "Pain over ATF during palpation and plantar flexion/inversion. Neg maleolar compression test."
- A = *Assessment*. The assessment is the clinician's professional judgment or impression of the injury. Using the above example, this section would read "Moderate inversion ankle sprain."
- P = *Plan*. The course of action that the clinician and the patient will follow to treat and rehabilitate the injury.

Depending on the extent of the injury, this may include an immediate treatment plan and short-term and long-term goals. An immediate treatment plan for the patient with the sprained ankle would read, "Application of an ice pack with an elastic wrap for 30 minute repeated every 2 hours." A short-term goal might be "Cryokinetics to gain back full, pain-free ROM and decrease swelling," while a long-term goal might be "Hot pack to heat the tissues prior to sport-specific skills and return to competition."

There are three types of SOAP notes[5]:

1. **Initial note**, written after the initial assessment (Fig. 4.3)
2. **Progress note**, or **interim note**, periodic documentation of the results of the treatment plan
3. **Discharge note**, written when treatment is discontinued

 CONCEPT CHECK 4.2. In which of the three types of SOAP notes will most therapeutic modality treatments be recorded?

INITIAL NOTES

Initial SOAP notes are the foundation for care. They establish what the injury is, how the diagnosis was arrived at, and what the initial care plan is/was. They also meet all the requirements of good medical records.

- They provide important information that can be used to determine whether or not a certain modality intervention is working.
- They are a good way to communicate with others. If a clinician is absent from work or busy treating other patients, his protocol can be easily followed by another practitioner.
- In cases where reimbursement might be warranted, clear, concise SOAP notes might make the difference between being paid for modality use or not.
- They are legal documents that protect both the clinician and the patient.

PROGRESS NOTES

Progress notes include updates or additional information regarding the patient's status since the most recent note was written (Fig. 4.3).[5] Below is an example of how progress notes could be written with respect to therapeutic modality use using the ankle sprain patient in the previous example.

- S = *Subjective*. The progress note after 3 days might read, "The pain has decreased by 50%."
- O = *Objective*. Tests and measures are updated or added to the information reported in the last progress note. "Ankle girth has decreased by 1 cm and plantar flexion

Blackfoot State University
Injury Evaluation

Patient: _Likialiki, Moafua_   Date: _19 Oct. 2013_   Status: (new) ongoing recurring

AT: _D. Draper_   Sport: _football_

Subjective: _Stepped in hole on practice field, can't walk_

Objective: _2+ pain over ATF on palpation & wt bearing_
80% ROM-PF & inv, normal ROM ever & DF

Assessment: _2° ATF Sp_

Plan of treatment: _RICES today, cryokinetics tomorrow_
X-ray

FIGURE 4.3 A typical progress SOAP note form.

has increased by 5°" is an example of the objective portion of a progress note.

- A = *Assessment*. This is typically only included in the progress note if the diagnosis has changed.
- P = *Plan*. This includes progress toward short-term or long-term goals and addresses why or why not these goals have been met. The progress note after 1 week might read, "Cryokinetics has resulted in pain free range of motion and decreased swelling."

Progress notes do not substitute for daily treatment logs. Every treatment should be recorded in both the facility's daily treatment log and in the individual patient's injury record. Progress notes are not intended to be used for every treatment.

Discharge Notes

A discharge SOAP note is written at the time the therapy is discontinued, after a final examination and evaluation are performed. A discharge note addresses the results of the final examination and evaluation, the outcomes and goals achieved, a summary of the interventions, and the final disposition of the patient.[6]

Record Use and Abuse

Medical records are essential to providing proper health care, as explained earlier in this chapter. They must be available to those administering health care, but protected from anyone not involved in administering care. In some instances, failure to adequately maintain records is a violation of federal and/or state laws, and thereby an ethics violation.

The three major state and federal regulations concerning medical records are:

- the Health Insurance Portability and Accountability Act (HIPAA)[9]
- the Family Educational Rights and Privacy Act (FERPA)[10]
- Statute of Limitations

PATIENT CONFIDENTIALITY

Two federal laws protect the privacy of an individual's medical records, and information. The HIPAA regulates the dissemination of personal medical information by anyone (including athletic trainers (ATs), physicians, coaches, and other members of the sports medicine team).[9] It guarantees that individual athletes have full access to any information about themselves and gives them control over disclosure of that information to anyone else. Individuals must provide written authorization before any of their personal information is released to third parties, whether the dissemination is written or verbal.

A second federal law also protects the privacy of student educational records, which includes any record created and/or maintained by an educational institution. Parents control dissemination of the records for students under 18 years of age.[10] At age 18, the rights are transferred to the student. Like HIPAA, it requires that you have written permission prior to releasing information.

Written authorization should include at least the following[8]:

- Description of information to be disclosed
- Identification of who is authorized to share the information
- Description of each purpose for which the information will be used
- Expiration date or event for the authorization
- Signature of the individual authorizing the disclosure
- If the person signing the disclosure is some one other than the patient, she must describe her authority to act for the individual.

STATUTE OF LIMITATIONS

A statute of limitations sets the maximum time after an event that a person can initiate legal proceedings related to that event. They vary by state but generally range from 1 to 3 years.

The clock begins at the time an injury is discovered following an alleged negligent act.

Minors generally have an extension.

RECORDS STORAGE

There are two types of record storage: active patient records and inactive patient storage. In a traditional medical facility, or if records are computerized, these will not differ, and records are generally secure from unauthorized persons. In a traditional athletic facility, however, numerous clinicians and many patients intermingle in one large open clinic. And there typically is no traffic cop (receptionist) to direct patients to specific clinicians. And patients usually interact with numerous clinicians. Thus, records of active patients must be readily accessible to all clinicians, yet be secured from unauthorized persons. For example, a central storage area such as a file cabinet or desk, where patients pull their own records could lead to a breach of confidentiality. Any person could look at any patient's records.

Inactive patient records are easier to secure because they do not have to be readily available. How long should these records be kept? Until past the statute of limitations. We recommend 2 to 4 years past the statute of limitations, just to be sure.

CLOSING SCENE

We opened this chapter with an example of how improper record keeping leaves a clinician vulnerable to lawsuits. We could have related the details of any of seven cases when attorneys representing one of our former patients requested our treatment records to review as part of their investigation of a potential lawsuit. No lawsuit was filed, in part because we had good records.

Far more important than protecting us from a few potential lawsuits, our injury records have increased the quality of our care. We have always worked in very busy athletic training clinics, with huge patient loads and numerous clinicians. Our records have been indispensable, as we have treated patients using a critical thinking approach.

Chapter Reflections

1. Read and ponder each of the following points. Do you feel you have a clear understanding of each concept? If not, reread the appropriate section of the chapter.
   - Name the five reasons for keeping treatment records, and discuss why each one is important.
   - Discuss the five specific types of records that each athletic training clinic should maintain, and name specific records at your institution that are examples of each type.
   - Explain why it is important to initial each entry in an injury record.
   - Describe the elements of a SOAP note, and discuss the type of information that is contained in each section.
   - Explain the similarity and differences between initial, progress, interim, and discharge SOAP notes.
   - Discuss the following: HIPPA, FERPA, and Statute of Limitations.
   - Discuss records storage and how this relates to patient confidentiality and length of storage.
2. Write three to five questions for discussion with your class instructor, clinical instructor, classmates, and clinical colleagues.
3. Get together with classmates and quiz each other on the concepts of this chapter. Use the points in reflection no. 1 and questions you wrote for reflection no. 2 as a beginning. Explaining concepts out loud to others requires a deeper grasp of the material than feeling you understand it as you read.

Concept Check Responses

CONCEPT CHECK 4.1

It is the end of a very busy day, but accurate injury and treatment notes are needed. Sure you have the basics jotted down on a notepad or electronic device. But if you wait until morning to fill in the blanks, you might forget something important. Simply use a small tape recorder to record the important details.

CONCEPT CHECK 4.2

Most therapeutic modality treatments are recorded in a progress (interim) note.

REFERENCES

1. Ray RR, Konin J. *Management Strategies in Athletic Training*. 4th ed. Champaign, IL: Human Kinetics, 2011.
2. Rankin JM, Ingersoll CD. *Athletic Training Management: Concepts and Application*. 3rd ed. New York: McGraw Hill Higher Education, 2006.
3. Board of Certification. *BOC Standards of Professional Practice*. [Web page]. Available at: http://www.bocatc.org/images/stories/multiple_references/standardsprofessionalpractice.pdf. Accessed August 2010.
4. Mathewson C. Documentation for athletic trainers: What should we document? How do we document? *Presented at the Rocky Mountain Athletic Trainers' Association 26th Annual District 7 Meeting*, Denver, CO, April 2010.
5. SIMS (Sports Injury Monitoring System). *Flantech Computer Services* [Web page]. Available at: http://www.flantech.net/sims_features.html. Accessed August 2010.
6. CSMI. SportsWare Injury Tracking System. *Computer Sports Medicine Inc.* [Web Page]. Available at: http://www.csmisolutions.com/products/sportsware_online/sportsware_online_overview.shtml. Accessed August 2010.
7. Kettenbach G. *Writing S.O.A.P. notes*. 3rd ed. Philadelphia, PA: FA Davis, 2004.
8. Anderson MK, Parr GP, Hall SJ. *Foundations of Athletic Training*. 4th ed. Baltimore, MD: Lippincott Williams & Wilkins, 2009.
9. US Department of Health & Human Services. *Understanding Health Information Privacy*. Available at: http://www.hhs.gov/ocr/privacy/hipaa/understanding/index.html. Accessed July 2010.
10. US Department of Education. *Family Educational Rights and Privacy Act (FERPA)*. Available at: http://www2.ed.gov/policy/gen/guid/fpco/ferpa/index.html. Accessed July 2010.

Review Questions

Chapter 1

1. Which of the following modalities is both mechanical and thermal?
   a. massage
   b. traction
   c. electrical stimulation
   d. ultrasound
   e. hot pack

2. Which of the following modalities is both mechanical and cryotherapy?
   a. ice massage
   b. cool whirlpool
   c. vapocoolant spray
   d. ice slush
   e. traction

3. The principle that the body responds to a given demand with a specific and predictable adaptation is known as the _____ principle.
   a. overload
   b. SAID
   c. specificity
   d. RICES
   e. progressive resistive

4. Which of the following is not among the 10 core goals of rehabilitation?
   a. confidence
   b. structural integrity
   c. pain-free joints and muscles
   d. joint flexibility
   e. muscular strength

5. Which of the following is not a good way to stay current with the latest research in therapeutic modalities?
   a. Read the *Journal of Athletic Training* and *Journal of Orthopaedic and Sports Physical Therapy*.
   b. Attend seminars that deal with topics on modalities.
   c. Attend seminars for emergency medical technicians.
   d. Visit poster sessions at seminars geared toward modalities.
   e. Use PubMed and explore other online databases and search engines.

Chapter 2

1. Evidence-based medicine began:
   a. before 1900
   b. in 1930
   c. in 1960
   d. in 1990
   e. none of the above

2. Which of the following is NOT a major repository of evidence-based information?
   a. Cochrane Collaboration
   b. PEDro
   c. CINAHL
   d. National Guideline Clearinghouse
   e. ACSM

3. The end result of specific health care practices and interventions is called:
   a. clinical outcomes
   b. best practices
   c. clinical guidelines
   d. protocol
   e. none of the above

4. Which of the following is a source of evidence that medical practitioners use for making medical decisions?
   a. experience
   b. research
   c. theory
   d. tradition
   e. all of the above

5. Which of the following is not a term used to help you determine if you should use a specific test?
   a. specificity
   b. sensitivity
   c. false positive
   d. ratio percent
   e. odds ratio

6. What is the relationship between evidence-based medicine and evidence-based practice?
   a. They are the same.
   b. One is the application of the other.
   c. One is used primarily by health care students and the other by only licensed clinicians.
   d. It depends on what part of the world you live in.
   e. none of the above

7. Which of the following is a source of evidence that medical practitioners use for making medical decisions.
   a. experience
   b. research
   c. theory
   d. tradition
   e. all of the above

8. Following are the five levels of quality of research evidence upon which to make medical decisions, ranked highest to lowest quality. Which of the following is out of place, meaning it is ranked higher than it should be?
   a. systematic reviews or meta-analyses of randomized controlled trials and high-quality, single, randomized controlled trials
   b. well-designed cohort studies
   c. case-control studies
   d. expert opinion, based on reasoning from physiology, bench research, or underlying principles
   e. case series and poor-quality cohort and case-control studies.

9. What is the relationship between evidence-based medicine and patient-based medicine?
   a. They are the same.
   b. One is based on science, the other on tradition.
   c. One is the application of the other.
   d. It depends on what part of the world you live in.
   e. none of the above

Chapter 3

1. What is the main weakness of a clinician who follows the cookbook approach when using therapeutic modalities?
   a. He is a technician.
   b. He is not a critical thinker.
   c. He treats the symptoms of the injury, not the cause.
   d. He doesn't build trust with his patient.
   e. He takes too many shortcuts.

2. What is the main strength of a clinician who follows the critical thinker approach when using therapeutic modalities?
   a. She is not a technician.
   b. She is guided by standard operating procedures.
   c. She builds trust with her patients.
   d. She treats the cause of the injury, not just the symptoms.
   e. She gets results.

3. The five-step framework for applying therapeutic modalities accomplishes all the following except _____.
   a. ensuring that all essential elements occur during application
   b. helping prevent rogue applications
   c. ensuring that each therapeutic modality is applied the same each time
   d. assisting in the use of standard operating procedures (SOP)s
   e. eliminating the need to learn separate SOPs for each modality

4. Which of the following is not one of the five steps of the five-step application procedure?
   a. application parameters
   b. recording treatments
   c. preapplication tasks
   d. postapplication tasks
   e. foundation

Chapter 4

1. What is the most important reason for keeping records?
   a. preventing lawsuits
   b. research
   c. establishing traffic patterns for future modality use
   d. knowing injury history
   e. keeping communication lines open

2. Which of the following contributes to quality control?
   a. preventing lawsuits
   b. research
   c. establishing traffic patterns for future modality use
   d. knowing injury history
   e. keeping communication lines open

3. Information gathered primarily by questioning the patient is what part of the SOAP note?
   a. history
   b. subjective
   c. objective
   d. assessment
   e. plan

4. The clinician's professional judgment or impression of the injury is what part of the SOAP note?
   a. subjective
   b. diagnosis
   c. objective
   d. assessment
   e. plan

5. The choice to use thermotherapy or cryotherapy would be recorded in what part of the SOAP note?
   a. subjective
   b. objective
   c. analysis
   d. plan
   e. none of the above

6. Which of the following is not a type of SOAP note?
   a. progress note
   b. permanent note
   c. interim note
   d. initial note
   e. discharge note

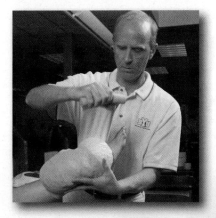

Orthopedic Injury, Immediate Care, and Healing

The basis of using therapeutic modalities is understanding the injury you are trying to treat, and the body's response to that injury. The first topic of Part II is an in-depth look at inflammation, the pathophysiological changes that occur following injury. The second topic, Immediate care—how you respond right away to the injury—involves the use of modalities that are often more important than anything you do in the subsequent weeks to resolve the problem. The third topic is the healing process and how you influence it.

Many professionals will think our ordering of these chapters is odd. Indeed, every other text we have seen places healing immediately after inflammation, and often in the same chapter. For most of our careers, we taught inflammation and healing sequentially. We experimented with the current order a few years ago in an effort to strengthen our presentation of immediate care. It worked so well we haven't even considered going back to our former ordering.

The present sequence is true to the time course of events. Immediate care procedures should be initiated long before healing begins, and indeed, the earlier they are begun, the more effective they are and the quicker healing can begin. Some have argued that since healing follows inflammation (pathophysiologically) they should be presented sequentially. However, since immediate care procedures aim to modify the inflammatory process, they should be discussed immediately following inflammation. And from a chronological and injury management standpoint, healing follows immediate care. Therefore, our immediate care chapter belongs where it is.

Most of Part II is foundational material. The exception is the last part of Chapter 6, where we included specific application parameters for immediate care, including cryotherapy. Our treatment of cryotherapy in Chapter 6, however, is deliberately incomplete. In this part of the book, we are only concerned with immediate care. Chapters 12 and 13 deal with additional uses of cryotherapy during later stages of rehabilitation.

You will find extensive cryotherapy content in Chapter 6. Indeed some may feel it is excessive. We think not. To get the most from cryotherapy you must understand what it is and what it is not. There is a vast amount of misinformation about cryotherapy that much of the medical community accepts as true. In order to debunk this information, we chose to acknowledge the existence of these erroneous ideas and to discuss why they are wrong, rather than to ignore them. We hope to reduce their influence on how clinicians manage acute orthopedic injury, and thereby improve patient care.

PART II CONSISTS OF THREE CHAPTERS:

5

Tissue Response to Injury: Inflammation, Swelling, and Edema

OPENING SCENE

A basketball player grabs a rebound and lands on another player's foot, twisting her ankle and falling to the floor. Rachel, an athletic trainer, rushes to her aid, performs a quick evaluation, and assists her off the court. After a thorough evaluation, Rachel determines that the player has a second-degree inversion ankle sprain. The game is over for her. Rachel applies an ice pack, a compression wrap, and a splint and then sets her on the bench and elevates her ankle. Is all of that necessary? Why?

The Inflammatory Response

Injury to the body results in anatomical, physiological, pathological, and psychological changes. Such changes must be addressed in the course of caring for and rehabilitating a patient following an injury. This chapter focuses primarily on the pathological and physiological changes that are part of the inflammatory response. Psychological factors are discussed in Chapters 8 and 9.

Inflammation, also known as the *inflammatory response*, is the local response of the body to an injury or irritant. It occurs at the tissue level, and has a dual function (Fig. 5.1):

1. To defend the body against foreign substances
2. To dispose of dead and dying tissue so that repair, the regeneration of viable tissue, can take place

Some consider repair part of the inflammatory response,[1] while others consider it to be separate processes.[2,3] Still others divide the two processes into three phases.[4,5] Regardless, inflammation and repair are defined by a series of overlapping but sequential events. We treat them as two separate processes (inflammation and repair), in order to explain them more clearly. Inflammation is the subject of this chapter and repair is the subject of Chapter 7. Thinking of them as one, two, or three process, however, has no bearing on understanding the events that occur from the time of the injury until it is healed.

CARDINAL SIGNS

There are five cardinal, or primary, signs of inflammation, often referred to by their Latin names:

- *Rubor*—redness
- *Calor*—heat
- *Edema*—swelling
- *Dolor*—pain
- *Funca laesa*—functional loss

Each of these signs will occur to some degree when tissue is injured and the body responds with inflammation. Some may argue that a splinter in the finger will not cause loss of function. True if you are thinking of the entire body, but false when you consider the local tissue. It will not prevent the patient from running, but cells in the finger have been damaged, will die, and must be replaced. So there is some loss of function. Also, a splinter in the finger may prevent a baseball pitcher from throwing his best curve ball.

The primary signs of inflammation always occur in response to an injury, but their magnitude and impact on a person's activity depend on the extent of the injury, where it occurred, and the nature of the activity.

COMMON MISCONCEPTIONS

There are many misconceptions about inflammation and injury care. Following are three prominent ones:

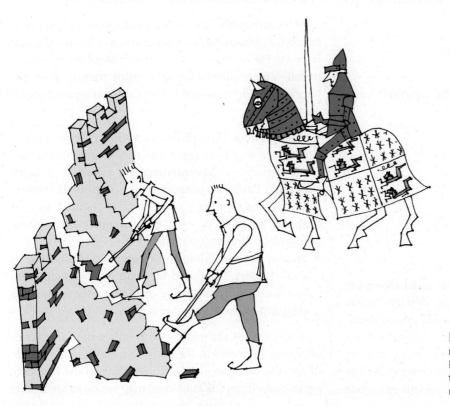

FIGURE 5.1 The dual function of inflammation is illustrated by a soldier (actually a Knight, in shining armor) defending against foreign invaders and two laborers cleaning up debris so that a wall can be rebuilt.

FIGURE 5.2 Swelling, edema, and inflammation are very different events.

- Inflammation is bad and should be eliminated. Just the opposite, inflammation is, in fact, good and necessary. Without inflammation there would be no healing.[6] This misconception persists, in part because the signs of inflammation are often mistaken for the inflammatory response itself. Minimizing the *signs* of inflammation, such as swelling and pain, is beneficial, whereas eliminating inflammation will actually prolong the process of healing instead of shortening it.
- Swelling, edema, and inflammation are synonyms for the same phenomenon. Not true; they are entirely different processes (Fig. 5.2). Swelling and edema occur during inflammation, but inflammation is a much more complex process that prepares the injury for repair. Edema causes swelling, but swelling occurs from other sources as well, so they are not the same. All edema causes swelling, but not all swelling is caused by edema.
- The purpose of ice application to acute injuries is to decrease inflammation. No; as mentioned above, inflammation is a necessary prerequisite to repair. Without inflammation there would be no repair. This misconception stems from the fact that swelling needs to be minimized and the misconception that inflammation and swelling are the same thing.

SEQUENTIAL, INTERRELATED, OVERLAPPING EVENTS

Inflammation consists of a series of eight sequential, interrelated, and overlapping events:

1. Injury
2. Ultrastructural changes
3. Chemical mediation
4. Hemodynamic changes
5. Metabolic changes
6. Permeability changes
7. Leukocyte migration
8. Phagocytosis

These eight events occur in the order listed above, but they can also occur simultaneously at different places within the injured tissue, because they progress at different rates in different parts of the tissue. A helpful analogy is the construction of a highway. The area is first surveyed; then bridges and culverts are built, hills are leveled, depressions are filled, the roadbed is graded, cement or asphalt

is laid, shoulders are graded, lines are painted, and signs are put up. Bulldozers would not begin their work before the area is surveyed, nor would lines be painted before the cement/asphalt is laid. If the project is many miles long, however, as asphalt is being laid at the beginning of the road, bridges could be being built toward the end. Thus the road is built in sequential events at each point, but in overlapping events throughout the entire project, just as in the inflammatory response.

Those who consider inflammation and repair as one process with three phases divide the eight inflammatory events into one phase and repair into two phases, which we discuss in Chapter 6.

Injury

Inflammation is initiated by an injury, an occurrence that impairs the structure or function of tissue and thereby alters the cell's ability to carry out its normal homeostatic mechanisms.[2] There are many types of injury, each of which results in the same basic inflammatory response. Causes of injury include the following:

- Physical agents (physical force, burns, radiation)
- Metabolic processes (ischemia and hypoxia)
- Biologic agents (bacteria, viruses, parasites)
- Chemical agents (acids, gases, organic solvents, endogenous chemicals). Endogenous chemicals are normal secretions in abnormal locations (such as those that cause gout), or in increased quantity in a normal location (such as those that cause stomach ulcers).

Most **orthopedic injuries**, such as sprains, strains, contusions, and fractures, are caused when excessive physical force (stress or strain) causes musculoskeletal structures to fail. These injuries are also called **trauma**, from the Greek word for "a wound." There are two types of physical trauma:

- **Macrotrauma**, also called *impact injury* or *contact injury*, is caused by a large insult and results in immediate tissue disruption. Macrotrauma are classified as *acute injuries*. The terms **primary injury** (or primary trauma) and **secondary injury** (or secondary trauma) are also applied to acute injuries, to differentiate between the causes of ultrastructural changes.
- **Microtrauma**, also known as *overuse, cyclic loading,* or *friction injury*,[2] is caused by small or low-grade stress that wears away the tissue over time. Microtrauma is classified as *chronic injury*.

Regardless of the cause of the injury, the same series of responses occurs in the body, although the magnitude of specific reactions will vary according to the causative agent. Sometimes the individual may not be aware that an injury has occurred, nor will there be visible signs of the inflammatory process. Nevertheless, each of the inflammation events will occur, even in response to the simplest of injuries.

! Modality Myth

TRAUMA IS FORCE

The word "trauma" is sometimes thought of as the force that causes injuries. This is incorrect. Trauma is the injury that results from physical force, not the force itself.

Ultrastructural Changes

Ultrastructural changes refer to the breaking down and eventual disruption of the cellular membrane and its **organelles**. The cell's contents spill out into the **extracellular spaces** (the spaces between cells) and the cell dies.[7] The cell membrane and contents become debris (waste tissue), which will have to be removed before repair can take place.

With orthopedic or traumatic injuries, ultrastructural changes (and debris) occur from two sources; as a direct result of the initial physical forces, called primary injury, and indirectly as a result of metabolic and/or chemical injury, called secondary injury (discussed in more detail below). Secondary injury occurs in cells adjacent to those that undergo primary injury.

Chemical Mediation

Chemical mediators, such as *histamine, bradykinin,* and *cytokines,* are activated by ultrastructural changes.[6] They signal the rest of the body that cells have been damaged, thereby mobilizing the body's resources to respond. They modify and regulate the rest of the inflammatory response, activities that neutralize the cause of the injury and start to remove the cellular debris so that repair can take place. Chemical mediators are somewhat like police officers; they come to the site of accidents and direct events until the accident is cleaned up.

Hemodynamic Changes

Hemodynamic changes mobilize and transport blood-borne defense components to the injury site and secure their passage through vessel walls into the tissue. These changes occur in blood vessels within the injured area that did not undergo primary injury, and in vessels on the periphery of the injury.

In response to an injury, arteries dilate and blood flow increases. At the same time, many previously inactive capillaries and venules open, thereby expanding the total blood flow to the area. However, the rate of flow through individual vessels is slowed, as shown in Figure 5.3. This slowing of blood flow lets **leukocytes**, white blood cells, fall out of the bloodstream and move to the vessel margins (Fig. 5.4a). After tumbling along the margins for a while, they stick to the **endothelium** (vessel wall) and/or to other leukocytes (Figs. 5.4b and 5.5). Thus the endothelium becomes paved with leukocytes. Eventually, the leukocytes will pass through gaps in the endothelium and move through the tissue to the injury (Fig. 5.4c–g).

Metabolic Changes

Changes in metabolic processes are a cause of injury, as mentioned above. They are discussed in more detail here because they play a major role following acute injuries. Primary injury and the body's response to it, cause additional ultrastructural damage in the tissue. This additional insult is called secondary injury because it occurs as a result of the primary injury. Thus the total injury includes tissue debris from both primary and secondary injury.

Normal cellular functioning (specifically the cell membrane and organelles within the cell) requires energy in the form of **ATP (adenosine triphosphate)**, which is usually supplied by aerobic (oxygen-using) metabolism.[9] When a cell is deprived of oxygen, a state known as **hypoxia**, it switches to anaerobic metabolism, or glycolysis, to satisfy its energy requirements. Glycolysis generates ATP by converting glucose to lactic acid when insufficient oxygen is available. It is not long lasting, however, and continued hypoxia leads to a steady decrease in energy production. Cell membrane functions slow down as the

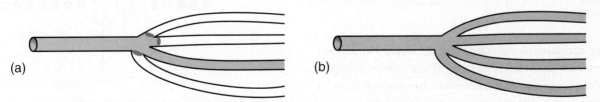

FIGURE 5.3 Hemodynamic changes. **(a)** Inactive vessels **(b)** open following injury to flood the area with blood and decrease the rate of blood flow in individual vessels. These steps allow leukocytes to move from the center of the vessel to the walls and to slow down.

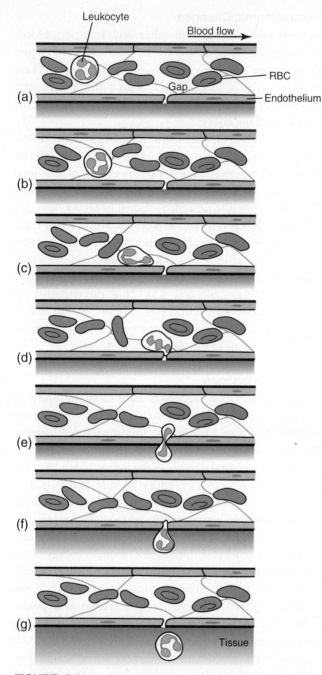

FIGURE 5.4 Hemodynamic changes and leukocyte migration. (a) The leukocyte moves to the margin of the blood vessel. It then (b) sticks to the endothelium (pavementing), (c) moves over the endothelium surface, (d) finds an endothelial gap, (e) passes through the gap, and (f) leaves the vessel. (g) The leukocyte moves about in the tissue. Note, RBC are red blood cells. (Source: Adapted from McLeod.[8])

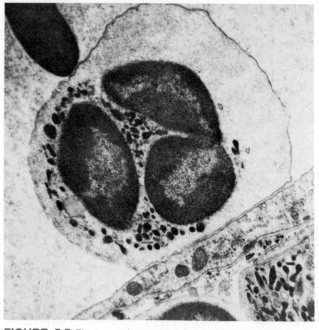

FIGURE 5.5 Electron micrograph of a leukocyte sticking to a blood vessel wall. It will move until it finds a gap in the vessel wall through which it can pass. (Source: Adapted from McLeod.[8])

energy necessary to maintain them decreases. Particularly important is the reduced activity of the sodium pump, a membrane process that maintains the concentration of intracellular sodium at very low levels (Fig. 5.6).

The cell membrane is porous to sodium ions (Na^+); so sodium passively diffuses across the membrane if the concentration of sodium between the inside and outside of the cell is unequal. The cell needs a low internal sodium content to function properly, so the sodium pump actively moves sodium out of the cell. Because this is an active process, it requires energy to function. If sufficient energy is not available, the sodium pump's activity slows or stops and the sodium concentration within the cell and/or its organelles increases. This causes increased amounts of water to pass into the cell, and the cell begins to swell. Excessive swelling causes the cell to burst and die.

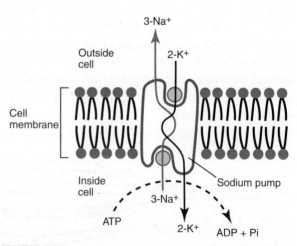

FIGURE 5.6 The sodium pump actively moves sodium (Na^+) out of the cell and lesser amounts of potassium (K^+) into the cell. The energy necessary to drive this process is supplied by breaking down adenosine tri-phosphate (ATP) into adenosine di-phosphate (ADP) and free phosphate (Pi).

Prolonged anaerobic metabolism also leads to intracellular acidosis, and the buildup of acid within the cell further impairs membrane integrity. Cellular organelles called **lysosomes** contain enzymes that digest foreign matter trapped within the cell. If lysosome membranes rupture from acidosis (caused by a failure of the sodium pump), their contents will begin attacking and digesting other cellular components, including the cell membrane, thus increasing the total amount of tissue destruction.

Metabolic changes are an exception to the primary purpose of the inflammatory response to prepare the injured tissue for repair. Metabolic changes are an unfortunate consequence of the primary injury and the body's response through the inflammatory response to repair the damage.

Permeability Changes

Both histamine and bradykinin increase the permeability of small blood vessels (the same ones involved in hemodynamic changes). The endothelial cells contract or round up, thereby pulling away from each other, creating sizable gaps through which leukocytes move out of the blood vessel into the extracellular spaces (see Fig. 5.4e and f). Even though the gaps are large compared to their normal state, the cells have to work to escape (Fig. 5.7; see also Fig. 5.4f).

Although the purpose of increased permeability is to let leukocytes move to the injury site, it also allows great amounts of protein-rich fluid to escape. This results in two concerns:

- As a result of the decreased fluid in the blood vessels, the viscosity of the blood increases, sometimes to the extent that enough cells are packed in the vessel to block circulation.
- The protein molecules are too large to be reabsorbed into the circulation, so they add to the hematoma, and increase tissue oncotic pressure, the major cause of edema. More about that later in the chapter.

Leukocyte Migration

Once the leukocytes have passed to the outside of the vascular wall, **leukocyte migration** to the injury site occurs (see Fig. 5.4g). Leukocyte migration occurs in a concentration-limited fashion, meaning that the number of leukocytes is highest at sites where the greatest tissue damage has occurred and is lowest where there is little or no tissue damage. Concentration-limited leukocyte migration is a response to the concentration of chemical mediators in the area; the stronger concentration is at the site of the most damage.

Two types of leukocytes play primary roles in trauma-induced inflammation; neutrophils and macrophages (Fig. 5.8). **Neutrophils**:

- Are smaller, faster, and more numerous than macrophages
- Arrive at the injury site first and provide a temporary first line of defense
- Are short-lived (~7 hour) and do not reproduce as macrophages do

The main function of neutrophils is to form a first line of defense against bacterial infections.[10] They contain highly toxic substances that destroy microorganisms, and in the process may destroy neutrophils and/or cause

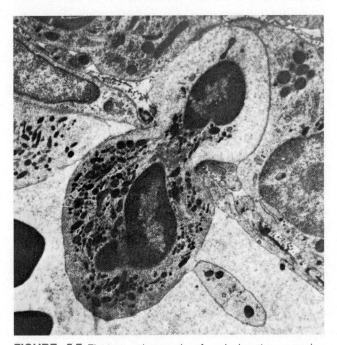

FIGURE 5.7 Electron micrograph of a leukocyte squeezing through an endothelial gap from the vessel into the tissue. Note the platelet (**lower right**) and a portion of another leukocyte (**upper left**) adhering to it. (Source: Adapted from McLeod.[8])

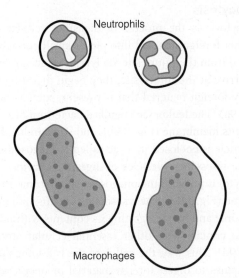

FIGURE 5.8 Neutrophils (**top**) and macrophages (**bottom**) are the most common leukocytes. Because neutrophils are smaller, they migrate out of the blood vessels first. But they soon die and add to the cellular debris that is cleaned up by the macrophages.

collateral damage to adjacent healthy cells and tissues.[3,10,11] Regulatory mechanisms, however, reduce or prevent the neutrophils from damaging healthy cells,[11,12,13,14] although the extent of their regulation is uncertain.

Most sports-related injuries are *closed*, meaning the skin is not broached. So there are no bacteria involved. What, then, is the role of neutrophils in these injuries? First, as they struggle to pass out of the circulation, the neutrophils widen the endothelial gaps, thus making it easier for the larger macrophages to pass through later. Second, when they die, they release chemical mediators that attract additional macrophages to clean up the cellular debris, thus increasing the concentration of chemical mediators in the injured area.

Macrophages live for months and can reproduce, thereby providing a long-lasting second line of defense. But their main function is cleaning up the cellular debris, a perquisite to repair. Through **phagocytosis** they break down cellular debris into much smaller units of free protein. In addition, they release chemical mediators that prolong the inflammatory response and thereby aid in healing. Some types of macrophages also aid tissue repair and regeneration by releasing various essential growth factors into the injury site.[3]

There are two types of macrophages, with different roles.[3] One enters necrotic tissue and is most active in the early stages of tissue clean up and repair. They produce and release more than 100 substances. The other is activated during the later inflammatory stages and congregates in the extracellular matrix. Thus their primary role appears to be in tissue repair through producing cytokines (chemical mediators) and cell signaling.[3]

Phagocytosis

Phagocytosis is the process of digesting cellular debris and other foreign material into pieces small enough to be removed from the injury site via lymph vessels. As leukocytes arrive at the injury site, they begin digesting debris and any foreign material that is present, such as bacteria (Fig. 5.9a). The leukocyte engulfs a bacterium or cell particle in its membrane (Fig. 5.9b), and surrounds it so that the particle is enclosed in a sac called a **phagosome**. One or more lysosomes (vesicles of digestive enzymes in the leukocyte) unite with the phagosome, to become a **phagolysosome** (Fig. 5.9c). The lysosomal contents spill into the phagosome and begin digesting its contents without coming into contact with other essential cellular structures (Fig. 5.9d). This way, the cell uses the lysosome's powerful enzymes to digest foreign material or debris without causing its own destruction. The digested contents of the phagolysosome are expelled from the cell as free protein (not part of a structure).

CHRONIC AND RECURRING INFLAMMATION

The phrase *chronic inflammation* is confusing because it is used to describe events following two very different processes: microtrauma and recurring acute inflammation. **Recurring inflammation** refers to reinitiated acute inflammation before the previous episode of acute inflammation has finished. This occurs when a patient becomes overly aggressive and returns to vigorous activity too quickly. Each time acute inflammation is reinitiated before the previous episode is completed, it takes less of an insult to initiate the inflammatory response. Recurring inflammation is usually initiated by an insult that normally would not cause an injury or inflammation. Avoid using the term "chronic inflammation" to refer to recurring acute inflammation.

Chronic inflammation begins in a slow, often unnoticed manner; it tends to persist for several weeks, months, or years, and has a vague and indefinite termination. It occurs when the inflammatory response is unable to eliminate the cause of the injury (such as with repeated overuse) and restore normal function.[1] The specific mechanisms, however, that cause this condition to become chronic are not known.[2] Most of the phases of acute inflammation are absent. Macrophages proliferate and release chemical mediators that attract additional macrophages. As more macrophages accumulate, it takes less stress or overuse to keep the process going. Thus, activity that normally is nonstressful becomes a chronic inflammatory stimulus.

The suffix *-itis* designates chronic inflammation conditions, such as *bursitis* (inflammation of bursae) and tendinitis (inflammation of a tendon). While these conditions result from microtrauma, not all of them involve an inflammatory response.[16] Cases of clinically diagnosed Achilles tendinitis[16,17] and patellar tendinitis have been reported in which there was no evidence of inflammation. One explanation is that microtrauma can cause significant structural disruption, and microvascular damage can occur, causing pain and other clinical symptoms, before the classic inflammatory response is activated.[2]

An Acute Orthopedic Injury Model

What happens when a muscle is pulled or an ankle is sprained? Although it is correct to answer that the injury evokes the inflammatory response, such a view is somewhat simplistic, and does not explain related peripheral events that impact on immediate care of the injury. It is also overly simplistic to apply ice to every injury without understanding the overall bodily response. Technique must be based on sound theory if it is to be developed and improved. With

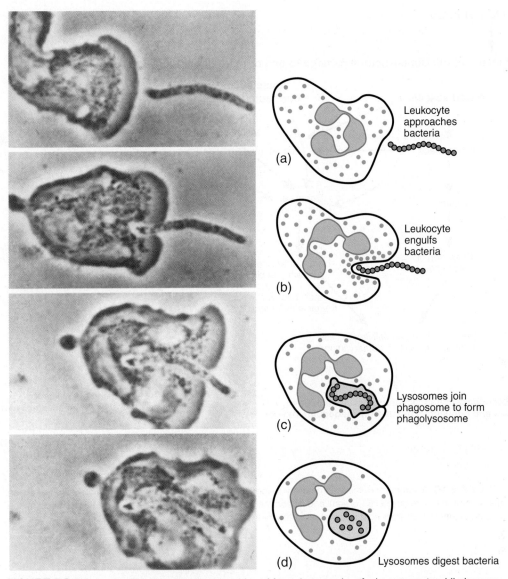

FIGURE 5.9 Phagocytosis is illustrated in this series of four photographs of a human neutrophil phagocytosing a strand of bacteria (**on the left**) and an artist's rendering on the events (**on the right**). Tissue debris is broken down by the same process. (Source: Adapted from Ryan and Majno.[15])

this model, we consider inflammation in context with other events involved in the body's response to injury.

 CONCEPT CHECK 5.1. What is a model, and why are models useful?

The generalized model of the processes that occur after an acute injury is summarized in Figure 5.10. Note that a portion of the inflammatory response path from injury to repair is in green, while the associated responses are in black. Details of individual components of the model are explained and illustrated in following paragraphs.

This model includes an area of tissue composed of cells, blood vessels, and nerves. Figure 5.11 shows the normal pre-injury tissue. When an injury occurs, whether it is a sprain or strain caused by a stretching force or a contusion caused by direct compression, immediate ultrastructural changes take place in the muscle and/or connective tissue. Nerves and blood vessels might be broken at this time as well. All this damage is directly caused by the physical force, and is called primary injury (Fig. 5.12). The damaged tissue becomes debris, which must be removed from the tissue before new cells can replace the damaged ones.

The cellular debris releases chemical mediators that signal the body that an injury has occurred. The torn nerves send impulses to the brain that are interpreted as pain. The broken blood vessels allow extravascular hemorrhaging, resulting in swelling (Fig. 5.13). This hemorrhaging (bleeding) is usually short-lived, however, owing to the clotting mechanism.

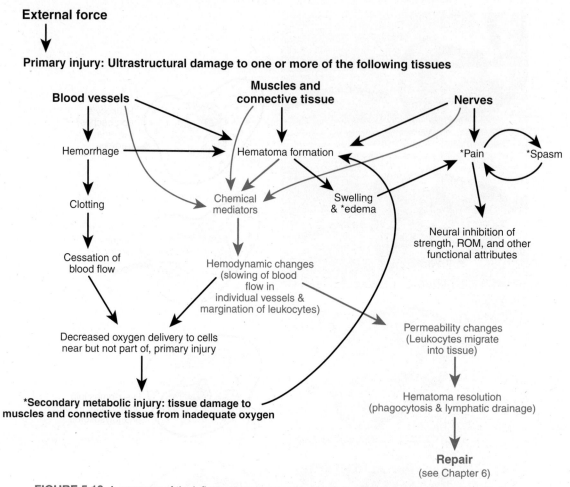

FIGURE 5.10 A summary of the inflammatory response to acute trauma. Note the differentiation between the inflammatory response (in *green*) and associated events (in *black*). *Asterisks* identify phases of the response that benefit from cold application to the injury. (See text and Chapter 6 for details.)

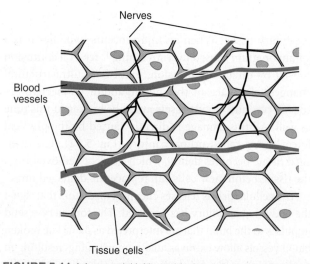

FIGURE 5.11 Injury model I. Normal (uninjured) tissue cells, blood vessels, and nerves.

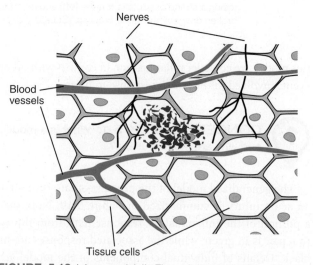

FIGURE 5.12 Injury model II. The primary traumatic damage; trauma, such as a contusion, causes ultrastructural changes to tissue cells, blood vessels, and nerves. All tissues damaged by the trauma have suffered primary injury. Damage to nerves causes pain.

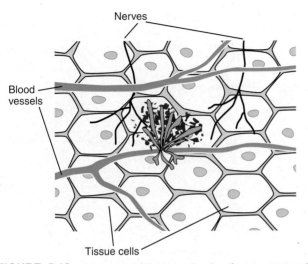

FIGURE 5.13 Injury model III. Hemorrhaging from a ruptured blood vessel into the tissue.

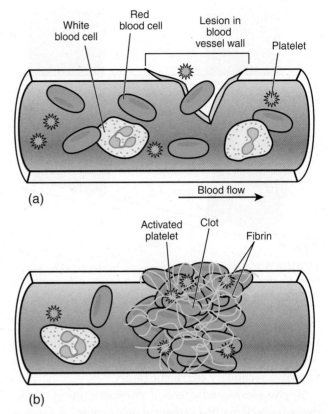

FIGURE 5.14 Injury model IV. Clotting begins immediately after the injury (**a, b**) as strands of fibrin begin forming in the vessel, in the vicinity of the injury, eventually becoming a mesh over the lesion. Platelets, and later red cells, become entrapped in the mesh to form the clot and seal the lesion. As the clot grows, it often plugs the entire vessel.

Clotting is a multistage process that results in *fibrin* and *platelets*, both of which are blood components, closing a damaged blood vessel.[18] The fibrin forms into strands, which in turn create a network. The fibrin net captures circulating platelets, thereby forming a plug that seals the damaged vessel (Fig. 5.14), but also often fills the entire vessel, which completely blocks circulation in the injured vessel, thus depriving distal tissues from oxygen.

The hemorrhaged blood and cellular debris from the primary injury are collectively known as a **hematoma**. As the hematoma forms, it exerts pressure on undamaged nerve fibers in the area, causing more pain. In addition to outward responses to pain, such as discomfort and nausea, the body responds internally with muscle spasm and inhibition of muscular strength, and range of motion. These responses are the body's effort to protect itself by splinting the area, thereby preventing aggravation of the injury.

The body's response to the hematoma is to remove it, and it does so through four of the last five inflammatory events: hemodynamic changes, permeability changes, leukocyte migration, and phagocytosis. These mechanisms take place in the circulatory vessels on the periphery of the injury. Once macrophages get into the tissue, they break down the hematoma and spew the smaller free protein into the tissue spaces. The free protein is removed from the tissue by the lymphatic system. Once the hematoma is resolved, wound healing—repair—can take place (see Chapter 6).

The effects of the inflammatory response are not all positive, however. The combination of slowed blood flow in the vessels on the injury's periphery and a lack of blood flow distal to the clotted, damaged vasculature results in less oxygen delivered to cells near the primary injury. If the inflammatory response is prolonged, metabolic changes will occur in these cells, and they will undergo secondary metabolic injury. Thus, the total amount of damaged tissue is increased, and more debris accumulates in the hematoma.

Secondary Injury

The body's response to the traumatized tissue (primary injury) leads to further tissue damage, known as **secondary injury**.[19,20,21,22] Many viable cells in the immediate area of, but not damaged by, the primary injury undergo secondary injury as a result of two separate mechanisms: enzymatic action and metabolic deficiency.

SECONDARY ENZYMATIC INJURY

When a cell dies (owing to primary injury), its lysosomes release enzymes that digest cellular debris.[2] If these enzymes come into contact with nearby live cells, which

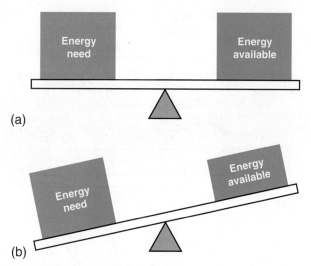

FIGURE 5.15 Injury model V. Secondary metabolic injury results from an imbalance of energy supply and energy consumption in uninjured cells. (**a**) Normal tissues. (**b**) Injured tissue.

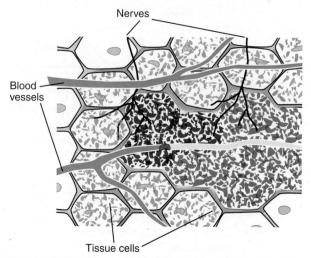

FIGURE 5.16 Injury model VI. A hematoma expands as cellular debris from the secondary injury is added to the debris of the primary injury and hemorrhaging. As the inflammatory process breaks down the cellular debris into free protein, additional secondary injury occurs (see cells at far right).

they often do, they start breaking down the membranes of the live cells, leading to additional cellular death; this is known as **secondary enzymatic injury.**[20, 21, 22]

A possible second cause of enzymatic injury is the excessive presence and activity of neutrophils.[3,22] This is speculation, based on the fact that there are many neutrophils in injured tissue and that in tissues with microorganisms, they have a tendency to cause collateral damage to adjacent healthy cells as they attack the microorganisms.[10,11] The uncertainty of this theory is twofold:

1. We don't know the magnitude of regulatory mechanisms that reduce or prevent the neutrophils from damaging healthy cells.[3,11,12,14]
2. Orthopedic injuries, such as sprains, strains, and contusions, do not involve microorganisms, and the response of neutrophils may be different in the absence of microorganisms. Most of our knowledge of the inflammatory response comes from research involving injury caused by substances that remain in the tissue.[23] With trauma, once the primary injury occurs, the cause of the injury is gone.

SECONDARY METABOLIC INJURY

Secondary metabolic injury, also known as oxidative damage,[24] is caused by three physiological challenges resulting from prolonged local **ischemia**, a deficit of blood to the area. The combination of blood vessel damage by the primary injury and a circulatory slowdown induced by the inflammatory response result in localized ischemia.[24, 25, 26] Ischemia results in: (1) hypoxia, (2) inadequate fuel delivery (glucose, fatty acids, etc.), and (3) inadequate waste removal.[27]

All three challenges lead to a deficiency in ATP production:

- Hypoxia results in cells' switching to anaerobic metabolism.
- Aerobic metabolism is short-lived because the cellular supply of glucose is limited as a result of reduced blood circulation.
- Aerobic metabolism is further reduced because it is inhibited by waste products such as lactic acid, which are normally removed by the circulation.

In areas where metabolic deficiency is severe enough and long enough, the cells die (Fig. 5.15). The resulting debris is added to the hematoma, and the total amount of damaged tissue is increased, causing the hematoma to grow (Fig. 5.16).

! Modality Myth

SECONDARY INJURY IS SECONDARY HYPOXIC INJURY

In 1976, the concept of secondary injury was introduced as secondary hypoxic injury, to describe tissue damage resulting from a metabolic imbalance secondary to acute traumatic sports injuries.[19] In time, however, it became obvious that there was an enzymatic component to secondary injury,[20,21] and that ischemia caused more than just hypoxic challenges to reduced metabolism (as explained in the text).[22] The more inclusive term *secondary metabolic injury* should be used instead of the original term *secondary hypoxic injury*.

Swelling: Hemorrhaging and Edema

Swelling is an increase in tissue volume owing to extra fluid and cellular material in the tissue. Swelling has two sources: direct hemorrhaging into traumatized tissues and edema formation.[28] Initial swelling results from hemorrhaging. Continuing swelling, that which occurs from after about 10 to 15 minutes following the injury is from edema.

Whenever blood vessel walls are damaged from an injury, **hemorrhaging** (bleeding) occurs and continues as long as the vessel walls remain open (see Fig. 5.13). Under normal circumstances, clotting begins within 3 to 5 minutes after the injury occurs,[29,30] thus sealing the vessel walls and stopping the hemorrhaging.

EDEMA FORMATION

Edema is the accumulation of the fluid portion of blood in the tissues.[31] To understand how edema accumulates, it is necessary to first understand normal **fluid dynamics**—the movement of fluid back and forth between capillaries and normal uninjured tissue. Normally, this fluid movement is balanced. If, however, this balanced fluid movement is upset so that more fluid flows into the tissue than is returned to the circulation, the excess fluid accumulates in the tissue. Thus, edema is simply the result of a normal process that is slightly out of balance. The longer it is out of balance, the greater the edema accumulation and the greater the swelling.

NORMAL FLUID EXCHANGE

In normal tissue, fluid constantly passes between the circulatory system and the extracellular spaces.[9,32] Normally, the fluid that moves out of the capillaries is reabsorbed by the body. The vascular system reabsorbs two-thirds of the fluid directly into the venous end of the capillaries. The lymph vessels reabsorb the remaining third and empty it into the venous system.[33] This fluid movement is caused by differences in fluid pressure between the capillary and the tissue. Edema results when the pressures are upset such that more fluid moves out of the capillary than what is reabsorbed. Figure 5.17 illustrates normal fluid exchange.

Two factors make the free movement of fluid possible. First, water molecules diffuse through the capillary walls 80 times more rapidly than blood flows through the capillary.[9] Second, there is a pressure difference between the inside and outside of the vessels. This capillary pressure difference is known as **capillary filtration pressure**; it is the mathematical sum of a number of forces known

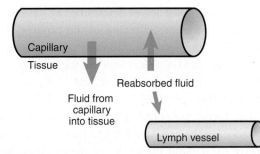

FIGURE 5.17 Normal fluid exchange. Fluid moves constantly between the circulatory system and body tissue. (See text for details.)

as **Starling forces**.[32] Four components influence filtration pressure according to the following equation:

$$\text{Capillary filtration pressure} = (\text{CHP} + \text{TOP}) - (\text{THP} + \text{COP})$$

where, CHP = capillary hydrostatic pressure; TOP = tissue oncotic pressure; COP = capillary oncotic pressure; THP = tissue hydrostatic pressure.

Hydrostatic pressure is pressure exerted by a column of water; the higher the column of water, the greater the pressure. Swimming provides a practical example of hydrostatic pressure. The deeper you go, the higher the column of water is above you, and the greater the pressure. It is the depth of the water, not the amount of water that is important. For example, a person 6 ft under water in a swimming pool will experience the same hydrostatic pressure as a person 6 ft under water in a lake. Hydrostatic pressure is exerted by the water in the blood.

Hydrostatic pressure pushes water. Therefore, **capillary hydrostatic pressure (CHP)** forces fluid out of the capillary and **tissue hydrostatic pressure (THP)** forces fluid back into the capillary (Fig. 5.18).

Oncotic pressure, also called *colloid osmotic pressure*, is pressure resulting from the attraction of fluid by free protein. (It is the similar to osmotic pressure in plants.) Thus, **tissue oncotic pressure (TOP)** tends to pull fluid out of the capillary, and **capillary oncotic pressure (COP)** tends to pull fluid back into the capillary (see Fig. 5.18).

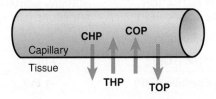

FIGURE 5.18 The influence of the four Starling forces on fluid movement between the capillary and tissue. Arrowheads indicate the direction of fluid movement, and the placement of the labels indicates the action. Hydrostatic forces (CHP and THP) push fluids, while oncotic pressure (COP and TOP) attract fluid.

The net sum of these forces determines which way the fluid travels. At the arteriolar end of the capillary, CHP dominates, and the capillary filtration pressure is positive,[9,32] causing fluid to move out of the capillary and into the tissue. Toward the venular end of the capillary, the pressures that cause fluid to move out decrease and those that cause reabsorption increase, therefore fluid moves back into the capillary. For instance, CHP averages 23 mm Hg throughout the length of the capillary, but it is much higher at the arteriolar end and much lower at the venular end. If all of the pressures along the length of the capillary are summed and averaged, the net (or overall) average capillary filtration pressure is slightly positive. This explains why one-third of the fluid is not reabsorbed directly into the blood vessel—that which is returned to the circulation via the lymphatic system. Table 5.1 summarizes capillary filtration pressure components and their effect on fluid exchange between capillaries and tissues.

FLUID EXCHANGE IN INJURED TISSUE

Following an acute injury, there are alterations in fluid exchange, and more fluid leaves the circulatory system than is reabsorbed. This fluid accumulates in the tissue, causing edema, and the tissue swells. The driving force of edema accumulation is a change in capillary filtration pressure.

Changes in Capillary Filtration Pressure Following Injury

With injury, there is a change in the average capillary filtration pressure, caused primarily by an increase in TOP.[31] The changes in capillary filtration pressure following an injury are presented in Table 5.2 and Figure 5.19. Since TOP pulls fluid into the tissue, and is increased, edema and swelling result.

TOP increases because of increased free protein. As a part of the inflammatory response, tissue debris from primary injury, secondary metabolic injury, and hemorrhaged

TABLE 5.1   NORMAL CAPILLARY FILTRATION PRESSURE

CAPILLARY FILTRATION PRESSURE COMPONENT	NORMAL AVERAGE PRESSURE (MM HG)*
Capillary Hydrostatic (CHP)	+23
Tissue Oncotic (TOP)	+10
Tissue Hydrostatic (THP)	−1 to 4
Capillary Oncotic (COP)	−25
Net (Overall)*	−4 to 7

*If pressure is positive, fluid moves from the capillary into the tissue. If pressure is negative, fluid moves from the tissue into the capillary.

TABLE 5.2   CHANGES IN CAPILLARY FILTRATION PRESSURE COMPONENTS FOLLOWING INJURY

CAPILLARY FILTRATION PRESSURE COMPONENT	NORMAL AVERAGE PRESSURE (MM HG)*	CHANGE IN PRESSURE OWING TO INJURY
Capillary Hydrostatic (CHP)	+23	~
Tissue Oncotic (TOP)	+10	↑↑↑↑↑
Tissue Hydrostatic (THP)	−1 to 4	↑
Capillary Oncotic (COP)	−25	~
Net (overall)*	−4 to 7	↑↑↑↑↑

*If pressure is positive, fluid moves from the capillary into the tissue. If pressure is negative, it moves from the tissue into the capillary.

whole blood is broken down into free protein by macrophages. In addition, some free protein escapes from the circulatory system during the period of hemorrhaging (if a vessel was damaged), or as a result of the increased permeability. The increased tissue free protein upsets the capillary filtration balance, and fluid (edema) builds up in the tissue (see Fig. 5.19b). The greater the injury, the greater the presence of free protein and eventually edema.

 CONCEPT CHECK 5.2. Since the source of most swelling is excess free protein in the tissue, what must happen to remove the swelling? What effect, if any, does ice have on swelling once it has occurred?

This process accounts for the delayed nature of most incidences of swelling following acute injury. Both secondary injury and the breakdown of tissue debris by macrophages occur over an extended period of time. Edema, therefore, begins minutes to hours after the injury and continues to develop over many hours. The swelling that occurs immediately after the injury is caused directly by hemorrhaging.

✔ APPLICATION TIP

USE A COMPRESSION WRAP FOR AN ACUTE INJURY

Always apply a compression wrap for the first day or so following acute injury, even if the injury appears minor and there is no swelling. Swelling is often delayed. Once it occurs, you cannot turn back the clock. And there is no harm in wearing a compression bandage overnight in a situation where swelling would not occur. It is better to be safe than sorry.

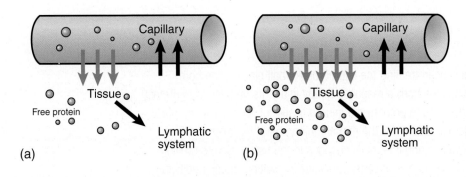

FIGURE 5.19 (**a**) Normal fluid movement. Two-thirds of the fluid exiting the capillary is reabsorbed into the capillary, and one-third returns to the circulation via the lymphatic system. (**b**) Edema results when more fluid moves out of the capillary than is reabsorbed, owing to the progressive buildup of excess free protein during hemorrhaging and phagocytosis.

Secondary injury not only results in increased edema, but increased edema can contribute to increased secondary metabolic injury. Two mechanisms are involved. First, as edema develops, the distance between the blood vessel and tissue cells increases, making it harder for oxygen and other nutrients to diffuse from the circulatory system to the tissue. Second, edema fluid can compress the blood vessel, thus reducing circulation to the area.

If much of the swelling is from edema, why does the area turn black and blue? Isn't this from the breakdown of hemoglobin? Although some discoloration results from oxidized blood, much of the discoloration in muscle may be owing to oxidized **myoglobin**, an oxygen-transporting and storage protein in muscle cells, from damaged musculature.

THE EFFECT OF COLD ON SWELLING

Cold applications to acute injuries can minimize swelling,[34] but cannot decrease it once it has occurred. Cold packs are usually applied after clotting has occurred and therefore have no effect on hemorrhaging. Cold limits edema formation, if applied soon after the injury. The cold reduces secondary metabolic injury,[6,24,26,35] and thus there is less total injury,[25,26] and the amount of free protein in the tissues is decreased. Thus, there will be less TOP (the major factor for edema). This will be covered in more detail in Chapter 6. Remember to act quickly; once edema has developed, cold applications cannot decrease it.

REDUCING SECONDARY INJURY AND EDEMA WITH RICES

Both secondary injury and edema can be reduced if appropriate comprehensive measures are initiated quickly after the injury—within minutes, not hours or days. Although cold is the cornerstone of this treatment, it is only part of the necessary therapy. Appropriate immediate care consists of rest, ice (cold), compression, elevation, and stabilization (RICES). Each of these measures is discussed in detail in Chapter 6, from both a theoretical and a step-by-step application standpoint.

✔ APPLICATION TIP

APPLY COLD PACKS QUICKLY FOLLOWING AN INJURY

The faster you apply the ice, the sooner metabolism will slow down. Thus, you protect more tissue from secondary metabolic injury and have less total tissue damage. Do not, however, forgo a thorough evaluation of the injury in order to apply ice pack.[7] This is the "golden period" for evaluation, the time when you will be able to gain the most information about the injury.

Following injury, the body attempts to protect the inured area by **muscle guarding**, an involuntary process of splinting the injured by inducing low-grade **muscle spasm** of antagonistic muscle groups. The effectiveness of injury evaluation decreases dramatically after muscle guarding has set in.

❗ Modality Myth

ICE IS USED TO REDUCE INFLAMMATION

Many people think the purpose of ice is to decrease inflammation. But inflammation is necessary to prepare the body for healing. Healing cannot take place until much of the cellular debris is removed from the area. So decreasing inflammation is not helpful. This misconception is the result of confusing inflammation with swelling. The purpose of ice is to minimize swelling. The less swelling, the quicker the injury can be healed (see Chapter 6).

Another misconception concerning ice is that it should be used until the swelling is gone. Ice is effective for preventing swelling (i.e., during the 12–24 hours following injury), but not for removing swelling. Swelling reduction occurs as free protein is removed from the area.

CLOSING SCENE

Do you now understand that Rachel's actions in treating the injured basketball player were both appropriate and necessary? Inflammation is the body's response to any injury. Its purpose is to protect the body against invasion by foreign bodies and to prepare the injured tissue for repair. The ice pack Rachel put on the patient's injured ankle did nothing for the primary injury, but it did minimize the secondary injury by decreasing both enzymatic and metabolic changes in the tissue. Some swelling resulted from hemorrhaging, although the bleeding was stopped quickly by clotting. Some additional swelling occurred from an increase in free protein and tissue oncotic pressure. Much more swelling would have occurred if Rachel had not acted quickly to apply ice, compression, and elevation.

Chapter Reflections

1. Read and ponder each of the following points. Do you feel you have a clear understanding of each concept? If not, reread the appropriate section of the chapter.
   - Describe the inflammatory response, its purpose, its cardinal signs, and the eight inflammatory events, and relate each one to a typical orthopedic injury.
   - Define trauma and its relationship to physical force.
   - Differentiate between macrotrauma and microtrauma.
   - Define metabolic changes, ischemia, and hypoxia. What is their relationship to secondary injury?
   - Explain the function of the sodium pump and its role in inflammation.
   - What is chronic inflammation?
   - Differentiate between primary and secondary injury. What are their causes? How should you manage each one?
   - Explain phagocytosis and the role of neutrophils and macrophages in this process.
   - Explain the common misconceptions about recurring inflammation.
   - Define swelling, and differentiate between hemorrhaging and edema.
   - What is capillary filtration pressure? Explain the forces that contribute to capillary filtration pressure and how they are altered following acute orthopedic injury.
   - Describe the difference between preventing and removing swelling. Explain the role of cold in the two processes.
2. Write three to five questions to discuss with your class instructor, clinical instructor, classmates, and clinical colleagues.
3. Get together with classmates and quiz each other on the concepts of this chapter. Use the points in reflection no. 1 and questions you wrote for reflection no. 2 as a beginning. Verbally explaining concepts to others requires a deeper grasp of the material than feeling you understand it as you read.

Concept Check Responses

CONCEPT CHECK 5.1

A model is either a description or an analogy that helps demonstrate or visualize something (such as an atom) that cannot be directly observed, or a simplified description of a complex entity or process. The orthopedic injury model presented in this chapter fits both descriptions because the response to orthopedic injury cannot be directly observed; the physiological and pathological processes are far beyond the scope of this text. By presenting this complexity as a model, you get a general idea of what happens following an orthopedic injury and therefore can understand why and how ice is used to treat injuries.

CONCEPT CHECK 5.2

To reduce or remove swelling, you must remove its source, the free protein. If the fluid is removed without removing the excess free protein, it will just form again. Ice has no effect on removing the free protein; it must be removed by stimulating the lymphatic system.

REFERENCES

1. Ferkel RD, Karzel RP, Del Pizzo W, Friedman MJ, Fischer SP. Arthroscopic treatment of anterolateral impingement of the ankle. *Am J Sports Med.* 1991;19(5):440–446.
2. Leadbetter WB. An introduction to sports-induced soft-tissue inflammation. In: Leadbetter WB, Buckwalter JA, Gordon SL, eds. *Sports-Induced Inflammation.* Chicago, IL: American Academy of Orthopaedic Surgeons, 1990:3–23.
3. Butterfield T, Best T, Merrick MA. The dual roles of neutrophils and macrophages in inflammation: A critical balance between tissue damage and repair. *J Athl Training.* 2006;41(4):457–465.
4. Anderson MK, Hall SJ, Martin M. *Foundations of Athletic Training.* 3rd ed. Baltimore, MD: Lippincott Williams & Wilkins, 2004.
5. Prentice WE. *Arnheim's Principles of Athletic Train.* 12th ed. St Louis, MO: McGraw-Hill, 2006.
6. Järvinen T, Järvinen T, Kääriäinen M, Kalimo H, Järvinen M. Muscle injuries: biology and treatment. *Am J Sports Med.* 2005;33(5):745–764.
7. Fisher BD, Baracos VE, Shnitka TK, Mendryk SW, Reid DC. Ultrastructural events following acute muscle trauma. *Med Sci Sports Exerc.* 1990;22(2):185–193.
8. McLeod I. *Inflammation.* Kalamazoo, MI: Upjohn, 1973.
9. Guyton AC, Hall JE. *Textbook of Medical Physiology.* 10th ed. Philadephia, PA: WB Saunders Company, 2000.
10. Jones P. Multiple Sclerosis Encyclopedia [web page]. Available at: http://www.mult-sclerosis.org/neutrophil.html. Accessed January 2006.
11. Mathison RD, Befus AD, Davison JS, Woodman RC. Modulation of neutrophil function by the tripeptide feG. *BMC Immunol.* 2003;4:3.
12. Nkemdirim M, Kubera M, Mathison R. Modulation of neutrophil activity by submandibular gland peptide-T (SGP-T). *Pol J Pharmacol.* 1998;50:417–424.
13. Fujishima S, Aikawa N. Neutrophil-mediated tissue injury and its modulation. *Intensive Care Med.* 1995;21(3):277–285.
14. Fialho de Araujo A, Oliveira-Filho R, Trezena A, et al. Role of submandibular salivary glands in LPS-induced lung inflammation in rats. *Neuroimmunomodulation.* 2002–2003;10:73–79.
15. Ryan G, Majno G. *Inflammation.* Kalamazoo, MI: The Upjohn Co., 1977.
16. Clancy WGJ. Tendinitis and plantar fasciitis in runners. In: D'Ambrosia R, Drez DJ, eds. *Prevention and Treatment of Running Injuries.* Thorofare, NJ: Charles B. Slack, 1982:77–87.
17. Osterman AL, Heppenstall RB, Sapega AA, et al. Muscle ischemia and hypothermia: a bioenergetic study using 31phosphorus nuclear magnetic resonance spectroscopy. *J Trauma.* 1984;24(9):811–817.
18. Rote N. Inflammation. In: McCance K, Huether S, eds. *Pathophysiology: The Biologic Basis for Disease in Adults and Children.* 4th ed. St Louis, MO: Mosby-Elsevier, 2002:197–226.
19. Knight KL. The effects of hypothermia on inflammation and swelling. *Athl Train.* 1976;11:7–10.
20. Knight KL. *Cryotherapy in Sport Injury Management.* Champaign, IL: Human Kinetics, 1995.
21. Merrick MA, Rankin JM, Andres FA, Hinman CL. A preliminary examination of cryotherapy and secondary injury in skeletal muscle. *Med Sci Sports Exerc.* 1999;31(11):1516–1521.
22. Merrick MA. Secondary injury after musculoskeletal trauma: a review and update. *J Athl Train.* 2002;37(2):209–217.
23. Jutte L. *The Effects of Acute Blunt Trauma Muscle Injury and Local Cryotherapy on Local TNF-a and IL-10 Concentrations.* Provo, UT: Exercise Sciences, Brigham Young University, 2005.
24. Schaser K, Disch A, Stover J, et al. Prolonged superficial local cryotherapy attenuates microcirculatory impairment, regional inflammation, and muscle necrosis after closed soft tissue injury in rats. *Am J Sports Med.* 2007;35(1):93–102.
25. Carvalho N, Puntel G, Correa P, et al. Protective effects of therapeutic cold and heat against the oxidative damage induced by a muscle strain injury in rats. *J Sport Sci.* 2010;28(9):923–935.
26. Oliveira NML, Rainero EP, Salvini TF. Three intermittent sessions of cryotherapy reduce the secondary muscle injury in skeletal muscle of rat. *J Sport Sci Med.* 2006;5:228–234.
27. Majno G, Joris I. *Cells, Tissues, and Disease: Principles of General Pathology.* 2nd ed. New York City: Oxford University Press, 2004.
28. Weisman GB. Introduction. In: Weisman G, ed. *Mediators of Inflammation.* New York: Plenum Press, 1974;1–9.
29. Johnson MG. Potential role of the lymphatic vessel in regulating inflammatory events. *Surv Synth Path Res.* 1983;1:111–119.
30. Mutschler TA, D'Antonio JA, Ferguson GM, Morsch R, Spinola A. Cold therapy reduces blood loss after primary TKA; but pain and swelling are unaffected. *Orthop Today.* 1993;16.
31. Huether S. The cellular environment: Fluids and electrolytes, acids and bases. In: McCance K, Huether S, eds. *Pathophysiology: The Biologic Basis for Disease in Adults and Children.* 4th ed. St Louis, MO: Mosby-Elsevier, 2002:86–113.
32. Porth CM. *Pathophysiology.* 7th ed. Baltimore, MD: Lippincott Williams & Wilkins, 2004.
33. Kaempffe FA. Skin surface temperature reduction after cryotherapy to a casted extremity. *J Orthop Sports Phys Ther.* 1989;10:448–450.
34. Deal DN, Tipton J, Rosencrance E, Curl WW, Smith TL. Ice reduces edema. A study of microvascular permeability in rats. *J Bone Joint Surg Am.* 2002;84-A(9):1573–1578.
35. Prandini MN, Filho AN, Lapa AJ, Stavale JN. Mild hypothermia reduces polymorphonuclear leukocytes infiltration in induced brain inflammation. *Arq Neuropsiquiatr.* 2005;63(3-B):779–784.

6

Immediate Care of Acute Orthopedic Injuries

Chapter Outline

OPENING SCENE

During a first-aid class, the instructor told Sammy that ice is applied almost universally to sprains, strains, cuts, and bruises. This agreed with what Sammy had observed in the athletic training clinic, and it got him thinking. He realized he had many questions regarding ice: Does it matter when you apply ice after an injury? Does it matter what kind of ice you use? Is it okay to apply an ice pack directly to the skin, or should there be a towel between the skin and the ice bag? How long should ice be applied? Is ice used to reduce swelling or pain or both? Is immediate care just about ice? What about compression, elevation, and rest? During a break, Sammy asked his questions but was disappointed with many of the instructor's answers. How could such a basic, simple modality be so confusing, he wondered.

RICES: The Prescription for Immediate Care

In Chapter 5, we discussed the inflammatory response, a series of physiological and pathological changes that occur following an injury. Some of these changes are necessary prerequisites to healing; without them, healing would not occur (see Chapter 7). But some of the changes can lead to further injury and complications that extend the recovery period. Immediate care techniques are designed to limit the unwanted changes, while allowing the necessary changes to occur and thereby facilitate healing and repair.

When applied properly, rest, ice, compression, elevation, and stabilization—known as **RICES**—limit secondary injury, swelling, muscle spasm, pain, and neural inhibition (Fig. 6.1). These efforts result in quicker healing of the injury and thus reduced disability time. Although there seems to be no doubt about using RICES, there is confusion about the pathophysiological response to, and specific protocols for using, these modalities.

MYTHS AND HALF TRUTHS

There is more confusion about the proper use of cryotherapy than any other therapeutic modality. It is a testament to the power of cryotherapy that it is beneficial even when used improperly.

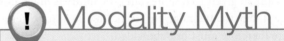

! Modality Myth

Following are modality myths about the immediate care of orthopedic injuries. Immediate care procedures based upon one or more of these myths will result in less than optimal care. Each is discussed in this chapter.

- Acute care and immediate care are the same.
- Ice decreases swelling.
- The goal of injury immediate care is to decrease inflammation.
- The purpose of ice is to decrease hemorrhaging by vasoconstricting blood vessels.
- Inflammation and swelling are the same.
- Water is a better conductor of thermal energy than ice.
- A cold pack composed of a solution of ice and water is more effective than one of all ice.
- A package of frozen peas is as effective as a crushed ice pack for treating acute injuries.
- Ice massage is one of the most effective ways to treat a soft tissue injury.

FIGURE 6.1 The immediate care of all acute injuries includes RICES: rest, ice, compression, elevation, and stabilization.

- All injuries should be treated for the same amount of time, regardless of the body part involved or body composition.
- Icing an injury longer than 20 minutes can cause further damage to the soft tissues, and even result in frostbite damage.

IMMEDIATE CARE VERSUS ACUTE CARE

Injuries are usually classified as acute or chronic. **Acute injuries** are of sudden onset, are caused by high-intensity forces, and are of short duration—for example sprains, strains, and contusions. The term **chronic injury** is used to describe two entirely different types of injuries; those caused by low-intensity forces of long duration, as in tendinitis or bursitis, and recurring acute injuries, such as a chronic sprained ankle.

The care of acute (and recurring acute) injuries is often divided into three stages: acute (0–4 days), subacute (5–14 days), and post-acute (after 14 days). Although this classification is used extensively, there are three problems with it:

- It does not incorporate the concepts of immediate care and emergency care.
- Acute care spans too wide a range of treatments. Treatment given 10 minutes after the injury is much different than treatment given 3 days after the injury. Acute care therefore must be subdivided.
- Injuries heal at different rates, depending on the type and severity of the injury and individual patient differences. Care must be dictated by patient progress, not by specific time frames.

Stages of Acute Injury Care

We suggest the following classification of acute injury care. Consider the time frames as general points of reference rather than specific markers. Actual patient care should be based on patient needs and progress, not on these general time frames.

1. **Acute care**: 0–4 days
   a. **Emergency care**, such as CPR or transportation to a hospital, if needed
   b. Immediate care: 0–12 hours
   c. Transition care: 12 hours to 4 days
2. **Subacute care**: 4–14 days. An injury in this stage is moving beyond acute but is still "somewhat" or "bordering on" acute.
3. **Post–acute care**: after 14 days

ICE, RICE, PRICE, OR RICES?

The acronym ICE was developed to communicate the combined use of ice, compression, and elevation for treating acute injuries. Most clinicians use RICE because part of the standard practice is for the patient to refrain from activity or to rest the injured part. PRICE is used by some because it emphasizes the need to protect the injury from further damage. We prefer to use RICES because stabilizing, or splinting, the injury lessens pain and neural inhibition in addition to protecting the injury.

RICES is applied to protect the injury from further damage and to decrease or minimize the development of:

- Swelling
- Pain
- Muscle spasm
- Neural inhibition
- Secondary injury
- Total injury (because of decreased secondary injury)
- Inflammation? *No!* Review Chapter 5.

Each of these elements is important. The majority of professional and public attention, however, has been on controlling swelling through cold application. This is somewhat shortsighted, as we unfold throughout this chapter.

EVIDENCE FOR THE EFFECTIVENESS OF RICES

Most sports medicine clinicians feel that RICES used immediately post-injury (begun within the first 10–20 minutes) will control swelling and other negative **sequelae**, or aftereffects, of acute musculoskeletal injuries. Not all agree with this opinion, however. Those who disagree generally cite research in which the cold was applied incorrectly, in our opinion.[1,2] Their conclusions should not have been that cold is ineffective, but that *improperly applied* cold is ineffective. Others disagree because there is not enough clinical evidence.[3,4]

The few clinical studies on RICES support the effectiveness of the treatment.[5,6] They involve hospital patients, whose treatment was not initiated as early as typically occurs in athletics. Had treatment been initiated earlier, the results probably would have been even more impressive.

One reason for the lack of clinical studies is that athletic trainers (ATs) are so convinced of the efficacy of RICES that they cannot in good conscience withhold treatment from athletes who would be assigned to a control group. (The scientific method requires that studies have a treatment group and a control group that does not receive treatment.) ATs have seen the consequences of enough cases of athletes who were not treated properly (because the injury occurred away from campus) to know RICES is necessary. In addition, studies based on patients treated in hospitals and physician's offices do not help because RICES is not applied quickly enough following the injury to be considered immediate care. For example, in one study, cold was not applied to some patients in the "early cryotherapy" group for 36 hours after the injury.[6]

TYPES OF INJURIES FOR USING RICES

All acute musculoskeletal injuries should be treated with RICES. In all cases of tissue damage, there is the potential of secondary injury. Failure to properly apply RICES will result in greater soft tissue damage and thus delay the final resolution of the injury.

Some authorities advocate RICES for sprains and dislocations, but only ice packs for strains.[7] There is no logic to this recommendation. All acute orthopedic injuries should be treated with RICES.[8]

The Theoretical Basis for RICES

Each element of RICES contributes to the effectiveness of the treatment. None of the elements should be left out. Understanding how the body responds to each element will help you maximize the use of RICES.

REST LIMITS INJURY AGGRAVATION

Rest during immediate care means moving the injured limb as little as possible. The goal is to not aggravate damaged tissue, which could cause further injury[9] and pain, thereby contributing to the pain-spasm-pain cycle. Some define rest during immediate care as "relative rest," meaning decreased activity rather than inactivity.[10] This philosophy is the result of an inadequate definition of immediate care—that is, the idea that immediate care lasts 4–5 days. According to the stages of acute injury care outlined earlier in this chapter, during immediate care patients should be as inactive as possible. During transition care, they transition to relative rest, which means protecting the injury but using the rest of the body to prevent reconditioning.

The problem of pain following an injury is not only the discomfort, but the body's response to the pain. Pain causes the body to shut things down in an attempt to protect itself. It does so by a process called **neural inhibition**, a decrease or absence of normal neuromuscular functions such as strength and range of motion—thus, an inhibition of most activity. Often these neural inhibitions continue long after the injury itself has healed, thereby preventing the patient from a full return to normal activity. Keeping activity below the level where it causes pain following an injury, avoids the complications of neural inhibition.[1] (See Chapter 9 for further explanation.)

The primary rationale for a patient using crutches following a lower-extremity injury is to remove pain. Limping results from pain. Even though a patient might think she can "hobble along," doing so invokes pain, which invokes neuromuscular inhibition. A patient should always use crutches until she can walk with a normal gait. (See p. 117 for crutch use instructions)

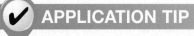 **APPLICATION TIP**

AVOID PAIN LIKE THE PLAGUE

Two rules of thumb for rehabilitation are: "If it hurts, don't do it" and "Work up to the level of pain, but don't go beyond it." The concept of "no pain, no gain" is OK during conditioning exercises, but totally wrong during rehabilitation. Pain causes neural inhibition that prolongs rehabilitation (see Chapter 9). It's not a question of how tough a patient is, but how smart he is in dealing with pain. Tell patients to work around the pain, not force their way through it.

Too little activity might be as detrimental as too much activity (see Fig. 1.5). Too little activity results in:

- Delayed healing
- Adhesions
- Muscular atrophy
- Loss of conditioning
- Skills becoming "rusty"
- Loss of confidence

You must keep patients as active as possible without causing further problems. Usually this means exercising noninvolved body parts to the maximum, and exercising the involved body part to a level just under that which causes pain.

CONCEPT CHECK 6.1. Why is a three-point gait (walking on both legs, but using the crutches to support the injured leg) more effective than a swing gait (no pressure on the injured leg, it just swings) for a patient on crutches 3 days after a moderate ankle sprain?

ICE LIMITS SECONDARY INJURY

Many think controlling swelling is a major goal of immediate care. Controlling swelling is important, but it is only part of immediate care. Limiting secondary injury and neural inhibition are more important than swelling control.

As explained in Chapter 5, swelling is an increase in tissue volume owing to extra fluid and cellular material in the tissue. It results from direct hemorrhaging into traumatized tissues and edema formation. Edema forms when fluid accumulates in the extracellular spaces because of a disruption in the normal fluid exchange between the vascular system and the extracellular spaces; more fluid moves out of the circulatory system than moves back into it. Thus fluid accumulates in the tissues. Cold applications are commonly used to treat swelling.

There are two major theories for why **cryotherapy**, the therapeutic use of cold, is indicated for the immediate care of orthopedic injuries: the decreased blood flow theory (or the circulatory theory) and the decreased secondary injury theory.

The Decreased Blood Flow Theory

The traditional theory for immediate care is that cold limits swelling by decreasing blood flow.[7,11,12] The logic of the theory is as follows:

- Cold causes vasoconstriction, which
- Decreases blood flow, therefore
- Decreases hemorrhaging, and therefore
- There is less swelling.

Cold does decrease blood flow[13] by vasoconstriction and decreased vascular permeability,[14,15] compression decreases underlying blood flow,[16,17] and elevation reduces blood pressure.[18] However:

- Cold is rarely applied sooner than 5–15 minutes following injury. It takes 5–10 minutes to perform even a cursory evaluation of the injury, transport the patient off the court/field, remove equipment, and then apply RICES. Often a more comprehensive evaluation of the injury is performed on the sidelines, so the time is extended even longer.
- Once the cold is finally applied, it takes 5–30 minutes (depending on the depth of the injury) to get significant cooling in the target tissue.
- For most injuries, clotting occurs within minutes after the injury.[19] Thus, hemorrhaging ceases long before the blood vessels at the injury site are constricted.
- Therefore, the beneficial effects of cold on swelling cannot be attributed to decreased circulation.

Despite the illogical basis of this theory, many still believe it.[7,12] It is, however, being replaced by the secondary injury theory.[20]

The Decreased Secondary Injury Theory

An alternative theory, proposed in 1976[21] and refined in 1995[22] and 2002,[21] is that cryotherapy has little effect on hemorrhaging; rather, it limits the amount of secondary injury and edema.[22] The logic of this theory is twofold. First:

- Without cryotherapy, cells within the injured tissue that escaped ultrastructural damage from the physical insult (primary injury), and many cells on the periphery of the primary injury, suffer secondary metabolic injury because of inadequate blood flow and oxygen
- Cryotherapy, however, decreases the metabolic needs of these cells so they require less oxygen. They are put into a state of temporary hibernation
- These cells are therefore more resistant to the ischemic state caused by the compromised circulation[23]
- The result is less secondary metabolic injury, so
  - Less total injury,[14,23,24] which means
  - Less free protein is generated by phagocytosis, and
  - Less edema develops.

Second:
- Damaged cells release chemicals that attack the tissue and uninjured cells in the vicinity, thus causing secondary enzymatic injury.[25]
- Decreased secondary metabolic injury means there are fewer damaged cells to release these chemicals.

The decreased secondary injury theory is modeled in Figure 6.2. Cryotherapy has no effect on primary traumatic injury, or on the hemorrhaging that occurs prior to clotting. Nothing can be done to limit primary injury or

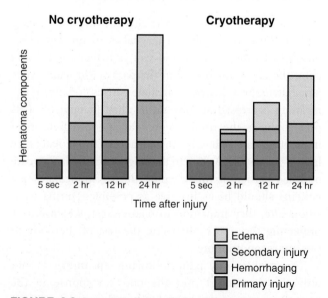

FIGURE 6.2 A model of the effects of immediate cryotherapy on the components of acute orthopedic injury: primary injury, secondary injury, hemorrhaging, and edema. (Source: Adapted from Knight.[22])

hemorrhaging once they have occurred. Early applications of cryotherapy decrease the amount of secondary injury, but they do not totally eliminate it.

The major goal of cryotherapy during immediate care is, therefore, to minimize secondary injury. With less secondary injury, the total injury is decreased, so there is less damaged tissue to repair. The repair process is shorter because with less tissue debris to remove, healing begins more quickly. And, with less total damage, repair runs its course faster.

Cryotherapy and Metabolism

Cryotherapy limits secondary metabolic injury by decreasing tissue metabolism and bringing oxygen demand back into balance with the reduced supply (Fig. 6.3). Damage to blood vessels and the hemodynamic changes of the inflammatory response result in decreased oxygen supply. Cooling reduces cellular energy needs, thereby decreasing the tissue's need for oxygen.[26–29] This same mechanism is used to preserve organs for tissue transplantation; an organ can now be removed at one site, packed in a cooler of ice, transported great distances, and safely implanted into another body.[30,31]

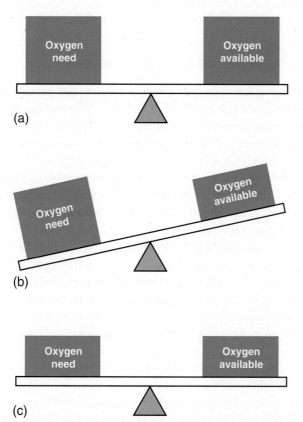

(a)

(b)

(c)

FIGURE 6.3 Cold helps rebalance the oxygen supply and demand that existed prior to injury. **(a)** Before injury, tissue oxygen needs and oxygen available to from the circulation are equal. **(b)** Following injury, circulation is decreased so the availability of oxygen is less than needs. **(c)** Post-injury cryotherapy reduces tissue oxygen demand and thus reestablishes the balance.

There is a direct relationship between tissue temperature and metabolism (Fig. 6.4).[26–28] The greater the cooling, the greater the decrease in metabolism (see Knight[25] Chapter 6 for more detail). And the sooner the cold is applied, the more effective it is. Cryotherapy must be applied within minutes after the injury for maximal results.

Heat applications during this period have just the opposite effect. Heat causes an increase in metabolism, and therefore an increase in tissue oxygen consumption. This causes greater secondary metabolic injury, and thus more total injury.

Cryotherapy and Swelling: Decreased Edema, Not Decreased Hemorrhage

Cryotherapy reduces edema but has little effect on hemorrhaging. With orthopedic injuries, however, most swelling occurs from edema not hemorrhaging, the exceptions being the immediate "goose egg" and hemarthrosis. A goose egg occurs when a moderate to large vessel near a loose skinned surface is ruptured. Hemorrhaging occurs immediately, into the loose skin, creating a mound of blood. **Hemarthrosis**, the presence of blood in a joint, occurs when the injury involves a joint capsule. Synovial fluid within the capsule prevents total clotting, and there is prolonged oozing of blood into the joint.

When Does Edema Occur? When Should Ice Be Applied?

Most edema occurs hours after the injury. The inflammatory process breaks down tissue debris into free protein, which increases tissue oncotic pressure (TOP) and gradually increases capillary filtration pressure (see Chapter 5). Over time, this shift in capillary filtration pressure increases tissue fluid. It is not uncommon for a patient to go to bed a few hours after an acute injury with little swelling and wake up the next morning with significant swelling (edema).

However, it would be misguided to think that the proper time for applying ice is hours after the injury when edema begins to be manifested. Even though it is not apparent, edema begins soon after the injury; initially, however, it fills in spaces within the tissue (see further explanation and Fig. 6.5 in next section). The sooner ice is applied—minutes after the injury—the more effective it is.

How Does Ice Decrease Edema?

Cryotherapy cannot decrease TOP, but it can limit the amount of increase by limiting the amount of tissue debris (Table 6.1). This is done in two ways: by decreasing metabolism, and by decreasing permeability. Decreased metabolism results in decreased secondary metabolic injury, and thus less tissue debris. With less tissue debris, there is less free protein and, therefore, a lower TOP.

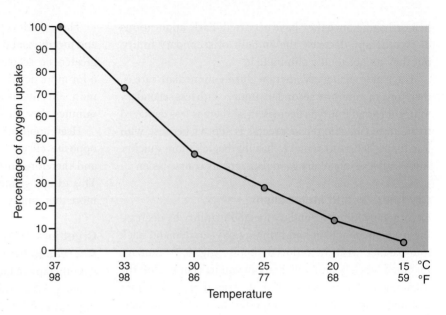

FIGURE 6.4 The relationship between tissue temperature and oxygen consumption is basically linear. The cooler the tissue, the lower is its metabolism. (Source: Adapted from Blair.[27])

Increased permeability of the blood vessel wall is a necessary part of the normal inflammatory response. In addition to allowing leukocytes to pass through the vessel wall and into the extracellular spaces, permeability lets great amounts of protein-rich fluid escape. This

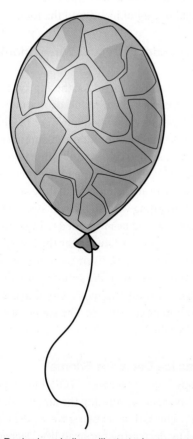

FIGURE 6.5 Rocks in a balloon illustrate how compression on uninjured tissue has no effect on tissue volume. The rocks give the balloon structure (as bones and muscles do for tissue) and therefore prevent it from collapsing under external compression.

additional protein contributes to increased TOP and increased edema.

Thus cryotherapy, when used immediately after the injury, limits not only the extent of the injury but also the amount of edema that develops as a consequence of the injury. But once secondary injury has occurred, cryotherapy will have no effect on edema or swelling.

COMPRESSION CONTROLS EDEMA

Compression increases pressure outside the capillaries, which, although not a Starling force, decreases capillary filtration pressure and thus helps control edema formation (see Table 6.1). External force pressure—compression—is most beneficial once edema begins occurring and will be effective as long as edema is present. Since it is unknown when edema begins developing, compression should be applied within minutes following the injury and continue until edema is resolved.

Compression has no effect on normal fluid exchange. An analogy with a balloon will help explain this concept.[25] When the balloon is filled with water, it expands. If the opening of the balloon is not held tightly, the elasticity in the balloon will force the water out. If, however, the balloon is first filled with rocks, the water will occupy spaces between the rocks (Fig. 6.5). As long as just enough water is added to fill the spaces between the rocks, the water will not be forced from the balloon— the rocks overcome the balloon's elasticity. Squeezing the balloon (or putting an elastic bandage around it) will similarly have no effect on the water. As more water is added, however, and the balloon expands (swells) beyond the rocks, pressure is exerted on the water by the elasticity of the balloon. An elastic bandage around

TABLE 6.1 THE EFFECT OF RICES ON CAPILLARY FILTRATION PRESSURE COMPONENTS FOLLOWING ACUTE INJURY

CAPILLARY FILTRATION PRESSURE COMPONENT	NORMAL AVERAGE PRESSURE (MM HG)*	CHANGE IN PRESSURE FROM			
		Injury	Ice	Compression	Elevation
Capillary hydrostatic (CHP)	+23				↓
Tissue oncotic (TOP)	+10	↑↑↑↑↑	Less ↑		
Tissue hydrostatic (THP)	−1 to 4	↑			
Capillary oncotic (COP)	−25				
External	0			↓	
Net (overall)†	−4 to 7	↑↑↑↑↑	↑↑↑	↑↑	↑

*If pressure is positive, fluid moves into the tissue. If pressure is negative, fluid moves out of the tissue.

†The net change in pressure owing to the application of ice, compression, and elevation illustrates the additive effect as each one is added to the treatment.

Source: Adapted from Knight.[32]

this "swollen" balloon would increase the external force. Also, if the elastic bandage were placed around the balloon before the extra water was added, it would be much harder (i.e., take more force) to add the extra water. The same is true with the human body. An elastic bandage around a normal ankle will have no effect on fluid exchange, but it will tend to retard and/or cause reabsorption of swelling. This explains why compression applied immediately after the injury has little effect on total injury.[24]

Some clinicians have believed that compression is more important than cryotherapy for treating acute injuries.[33,34] Research, however, indicates just the opposite—that compression alone is not as effective as cryotherapy and compression.[24] In fact, compression alone is no better than no treatment. Three bouts of 30-minute treatments were applied, with 1½ hours between them.

Constant or Intermittent Compression?

Constant compression is essential during immediate care when the goal is to prevent edema. Once the swelling fills the interstitial spaces and expands the external skin, constant pressure is needed to minimize it.

Intermittent compression is most effective when the goal is to remove edema (Table 6.2). Intermittent compression stimulates the lymphatic system, which is the route through which tissue debris is removed from the tissue. (Intermittent compression is discussed in more detail later in the chapter.)

Compression also enhances the cooling effect of ice packs, probably by compressing superficial blood vessels and thereby reducing the amount of heat the blood delivers to the tissue (Fig. 6.6).[17]

ELEVATION CONTROLS EDEMA

Elevation decreases capillary hydrostatic pressure (CHP), and therefore decreases the major factor (in a noninjured state) in forcing fluid out of the capillary (see Table 6.1). Elevation also decreases tissue hydrostatic pressure (THP), but this has little consequence since THP is small and thus has a minimal effect on fluid filtration.

As discussed in Chapter 5, hydrostatic pressure is caused by the weight of water.[35] The more water above a particular point, the greater the hydrostatic pressure at that point. CHP is greater when a body part is in a dependent position than when it is elevated because there is more water above.[18,36]

STABILIZATION LIMITS NEURAL INHIBITION

The goal of **stabilization** is to support the injured limb so that surrounding muscles can relax. This reduces both pain and neural inhibition. Stabilization should not be

TABLE 6.2 SWELLING MANAGEMENT WITH COLD AND COMPRESSION

MODALITY	CONTROL/LIMIT SWELLING	REMOVE SWELLING
Cold, intermittent (30–60 min)	x	
Compression, continuous	x	
Compression, intermittent		x

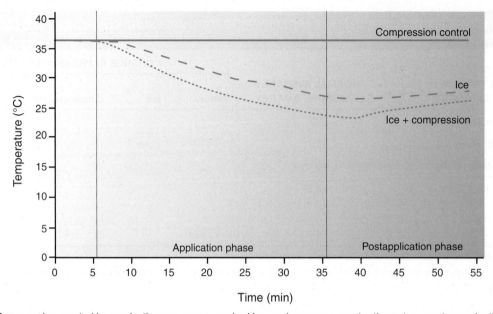

FIGURE 6.6 Compression exerted by an elastic wrap over a crushed ice pack causes a greater tissue temperature reduction than application of the ice pack alone.

confused with compression or rest; its purpose is quite different. It is true that stabilization might provide compression, and might force the injured body part to rest, but these are only secondary effects.

Muscle guarding is an unwanted response to injury. The body attempts to protect the traumatized tissue from further injury by causing muscles to spasm, and thus splint the joints surrounding the injury. But muscle spasm also causes pain, which causes more muscle spasm, which causes more pain, and so on. Thus, a pain-spasm-pain cycle is perpetuated. Early stabilization lets the muscles relax, thereby easing the pain-spasm-cycle. There are numerous braces and splints that can be used for stabilization (Fig. 6.7).

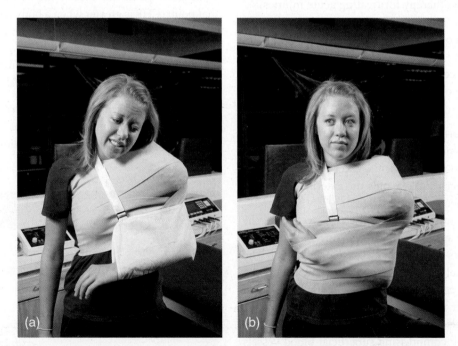

FIGURE 6.7 Stabilization is essential during immediate care. **(a)** Muscles around the injury normally go into spasm in order to splint the injury, resulting in great pain, even when compression or a sling are used. **(b)** Stabilization allows the muscles to relax, thus lessening the pain-spasm-pain cycle.

CONCEPT CHECK 6.2. Early in the chapter, we stated that focusing the majority of attention concerning RICES on controlling swelling through cryotherapy is somewhat shortsighted. Give a reason for agreeing with this statement, and a reason for disagreeing with it.

The Physics and Physiology of Cryotherapy

When ice is applied to the body, it cools the structure it is applied to. Although it sounds simple and straight forward, there are many factors that determine the amount of cooling. First, we must define cold. **Cold** is not a physical substance like heat, which is the kinetic energy of atoms and molecules. Cold is merely the absence of **heat**. The state of being cold is relative. Consider, for example, that in October, after a hot summer, when the temperature gets down to 40°F (4.4°C) you feel cold and want to put on a jacket. In March, however, after a cold winter, when the temperature gets up to 40°F (4.4°C) you feel warm and want to take off your jacket. (Obviously this example doesn't apply to the tropics where there is little change in seasons, and the months would be reversed in the southern hemisphere.)

THE PHYSIOLOGY OF HEAT TRANSFER

During cooling, heat is transferred from the body tissues to the cold modality through a process known as conduction. **Conduction** is the exchange of energy (heat) between two substances of uneven temperatures that are in contact with each other. Heat moves from the body of higher energy to the body of lower energy, causing the warmer body to cool and the cooler body to warm until they reach equilibrium.[37]

Rate of Conduction

The rate of heat conduction, and therefore the rate of tissue temperature decrease, depends on the interaction of many factors, listed below. These same principles apply to superficial heating modalities (discussed in Chapter 10) when heat is added to the body:

- *The temperature differential between the body and the cold modality.*[38,39] Heat will conduct more quickly from 95°F (35°C) tissue into a 34°F (1°C) cold pack than it will into a 50°F (10°C) cold pack.
- *The regeneration of body heat and/or modality cooling.*[39] As the tissue gives up heat to the modality, some lost tissue heat is replaced by circulating blood and conduction from surrounding tissues. Simultaneously, the heat given up to the cold modality either is held by the modality, which therefore increases its temperature, or

is removed from the modality (e.g., as with a cryomatic unit), which maintains its lowered temperature. Both reheating the body and recooling the modality affect the temperature differential.
- *The heat storage capacity of the cold modality* (explained in the next section). Various modalities can accept differing amounts of heat before they begin warming. Thus, a modality that can accept greater amounts of heat will maintain a greater temperature differential between the modality and the tissue. If two cold packs are identical except for their size, the larger one will have a greater heat storage capacity.
- *The size of the cold modality.* The larger the cold pack, the more heat it can accept.
- *The amount of tissue in contact with the cold pack.* The greater the contact area, the more heat that will be extracted from the body and thus more cooling. This is why immersing the forearm in 34°F (1°C) water will cool it to the same degree as a 34°F (10°C) cold pack (Fig. 6.8). If other things are equal, a large cold pack will cool a body part more than a smaller one because it covers a larger area of the body and therefore extracts heat from a larger area.
- *The length of application.*[39] The longer the application of the cold modality, the more time it takes for energy to be exchanged, and thus there will be more heat removal from the body.
- *Individual variability due to adipose tissue between the skin and muscle.*[41] Adipose tissue is an insulator that interferes with, and thus reduces, the transfer of heat between the surface application and deeper tissue.[41,42] The greater the adipose thickness, the longer it takes to cool the underlying tissue.[41] For example, in one study, the time to reduce the temperature 44.6°F (7°C) at 1 cm below the adipose tissue ranged from ~8 minutes in subjects with 0–10 cm skinfold to ~59 minutes in subjects with 30–40 cm skinfold.[41]

The distribution of adipose varies both within and between individuals.[43] Thus sex, body part, fitness level, and individuals' morphology must factor into the time that a cold pack should be applied. This means that you should measure skinfold thickness to determine the appropriate cryotherapy duration.

An analysis of each of the above factors in every type of cold application is beyond the scope of this book. You can evaluate the relative contribution of each factor to the cold modalities of your choice.

Heat Capacity of Modalities

The amount of heat that the same sizes and shapes of various cold modalities can accept depends on their specific heat, their latent heat of fusion, and whether or not they

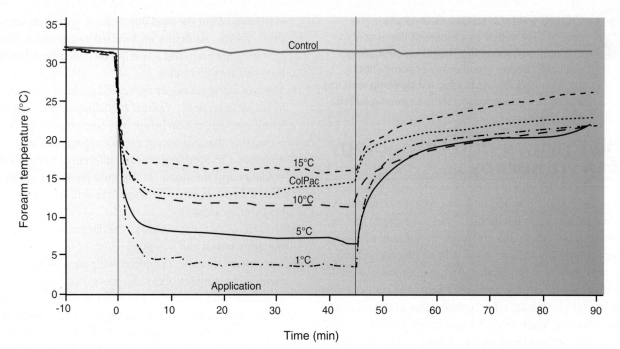

FIGURE 6.8 The influence of the amount of contact between the body and the cold modality on cooling. Note the similarity in tissue temperature during the application of a 32°F (0°C) cold pack and immersion in 50°F (10°C) water. (Source: Data from Knight et al.[40])

undergo a phase change.[37] **Specific heat** is the amount of heat energy required to raise 1 kg of a substance 1°C.[44] Therefore, the greater the specific heat of a substance, the more heat energy it can withdraw. Water has a very large specific heat, greater than most substances, so it is excellent for cold packs.

Phase change refers to the change from one state (solid or liquid or gas) to another without a change in chemical composition or temperature.[37] Of particular interest here is the phase change from ice to water. The **latent**

heat of fusion is the amount of energy needed to convert a substance from its solid state to its liquid state—that is, to undergo a phase change. It takes tremendous amounts of heat energy to change ice at 32°F (0°C) to water at 32°F (0°C).

For example, a 1-kg ice pack would extract 85 kcal of heat from the body if left on until the ice melted and warmed to 41°F (5°C). A gel pack of the same mass would extract only 22 kcal by the time it warmed to the same temperature, about 25% as much (Fig. 6.9; Box 6.1 lists

FIGURE 6.9 Crushed ice packs are more effective than gel packs because they undergo a phase change, which results in more heat being withdrawn from the body. Note the tremendous amount of energy required for ice to change from ice to water at 0°C.

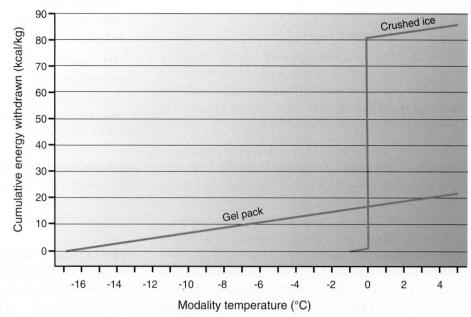

BOX 6.1   LATENT HEAT OF FUSION: COOLING CAPACITY OF AN ICE PACK AND A GEL PACK

The following example illustrates the difference in heat energy extracted from tissue during applications of a crushed ice pack and a cold pack (a fourfold difference in this example). For purposes of the illustration, assume:

- Both packs weigh 1 kg
- Both packs are applied to the same surface
- Both packs are applied until they withdraw enough heat to warm to 41°F (5°C)
- The crushed ice came from a free-standing ice machine, which stored it at 30°F (–1°C)
- The gel pack was stored in a freezer unit at 1°F (–17°C)

Constants required for the equations[44]:

- Heat of fusion of ice (L) = 80 cal/g
- Heating ice (Q) = 0.5 cal/g
- Heating water (Q) = 1 cal/g

Computing the energy associated with the heat withdrawn from the respective modalities requires a single step for the gel pack and three steps for the ice pack (degrees Celsius is the standard convention for these calculations):

Gel pack

1. Heat water 22°C (from –17°C to 5°C)

   Q = 1 kg × 1 cal/g water/°C × 22°C = 22,000 cal or 22 kcal

Ice pack

1. Heat ice 1°C (from –1°C to 0°C)

   Q = 1 kg ice × 0.5 cal/g water/°C × 1°C = 500 cal or 0.5 kcal

2. Heat of fusion (ice to water at 0°C)

   Q = 1 kg ice × 80 cal/g = 80.000 cal or 80 kcal

3. Heat water 5°C (from 0°C to 5°C)

   Q = 1 kg ice × 1 cal/g water/°C × 5°C = 5000 cal or 5 kcal

   Total = 85.5 kcal

- Energy differential 85.5 kcal (for ice pack) vs. 22 kcal (for gel pack)
- 85.5/22 = 3.886

Thus, the total energy available for cooling is 3.9 times greater with an ice pack than a gel pack of equal size and shape.

specific calculations). This is one of the advantages of crushed ice over gel packs for cooling the body. Crushed ice packs freeze solid and therefore undergo a phase change and absorb more heat than gel packs which do not freeze solid.

TEMPERATURE CHANGES RESULTING FROM CRYOTHERAPY

The beneficial effects of cryotherapy are related to tissue temperature changes. The magnitude and rate of these changes, and rewarming after application, vary according to the depth of the tissue and the rate of conduction.

Surface Temperature

Cold applications cause an immediate and rapid decline in the temperature of the surface to which the cold is applied, as heat is conducted from the body to the cold modality (see Fig. 6.8). The rate of cooling steadily slows until the surface temperature eventually plateaus a few degrees above the temperature of the modality.[45–49] Following application, there is an immediate sharp temperature increase, like the initial decrease but of lesser magnitude, followed by a gradual and prolonged return toward preapplication temperature.

The type of cold modality affects the magnitude of the difference between the modality temperature and the plateaued tissue temperature, and whether or not the tissue temperature begins to rise before the modality is removed. For instance, compare the temperature curves for the ColPac to the 34°F (1°C) and 50°F (10°C) water baths in Figure 6.8. Although the ColPac was initially colder than the 34°F (1°C) water bath, it does not have the capacity to cool the forearm as much as the 34°F (1°C) water bath. In fact, it appears much like the 50°F (10°C) water bath during the first 15 or so minutes of application. After 15 minutes, the arm temperature treated with ColPacs began to increase, while those in the 50°F (10°C) water bath continued to decrease slightly.

The degree of cooling, but not the rate of cooling, is affected by previous activity (Fig. 6.10).[49,50] Stationary bike riding at a moderate intensity (enough to increase the heart rate to 60–80% of the subject's heart rate range) resulted in an increase of 3.6°F (2°C) in the ankle[49,50] and thigh[49] before, during, and after ice pack application.

Cooling during repeated applications is not consistent. The degree of cooling during a second application depends on the length of the first application, the time between,[49] and the activity of the patient between the two applications.[49,51] The following are principles based on our research on the intermittent application of cold[49,51]:

- Mild activity, such as walking on crutches and showering, causes more rapid rewarming. Therefore, during

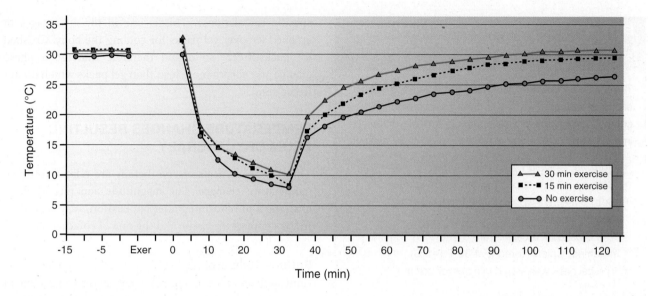

FIGURE 6.10 Exercise prior to cold pack application moderates the temperature decrease during and after application. (Source: Adapted from Mancuso and Knight.[50])

immediate care, cold should be reapplied immediately after these activities.

• Protocols with cooling/rewarming ratios of 1:2 (i.e., 30/60) and less resulted in lower temperatures during the second application-rewarming cycle than the first. If additional reapplication has an additional cooling effect, this might result in tissue damage.

• A compression wrap over an ice pack causes a greater decrease in temperature during application and a compression wrap over the body part following application results in less of an increase following application of an ice pack, in both surface and deep temperatures (see Fig. 6.6).[17]

Tissue Temperature

The response of deep tissue to surface cooling depends on the depth and type of the tissue.[52,53] The reaction of subcutaneous (just below the skin) tissues is the same as that of the skin, but decreased in magnitude[54–56]; temperature initially decreases sharply, followed by a more gradual decrease until it eventually plateaus (Fig. 6.11). Like skin temperature, subcutaneous tissue temperature immediately begins to increase following the application.

Deeper tissue temperatures, on the other hand, do not begin decreasing until minutes after the cold application (see Figs. 6.6 and 6.11).[52,53,58] They then decrease more gradually and to a lesser magnitude than subcutaneous

FIGURE 6.11 Subcutaneous temperature responds much like surface tissue temperature (compare with Fig. 6.8). Deep temperature, on the other hand, decreases much more slowly, continues to decrease following application, and returns to preapplication levels much more slowly. (Source: Adapted from Hartviksen.[57])

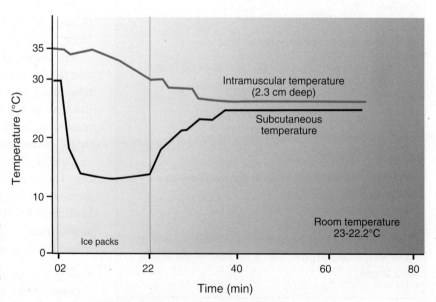

temperature.[52,59,60] Both the delayed response and decreased magnitude of temperature changes in the deeper tissue are the result of the time it takes for heat to exchange between various layers of molecules in the tissue (see Chapter 12).

After cold application, deep tissue temperature continues to decrease (see Figs. 6.6 and 6.10).[53,58,59] The length of the decrease depends on the depth of the tissue[52]; for example, following 5 minutes of ice massage to the calf, temperatures decreased for an additional 2.5 minutes at 1.0 cm deep, 10 minutes at 2.0 cm deep, 30 minutes at 3.0 cm deep, and 50 minutes at 4.0 cm deep.[52]

The magnitude of the temperature change in deep tissues (at all levels) depends on the magnitude of cold application (the amount of heat removed from the body). This relationship can be seen in the data of Waylonis,[52] who reported that skin temperature was basically the same following 5 and 10 minutes of ice massage, but the temperature at 4.0 cm decreased more than twice as much following the 10 minutes ice massage. This difference in deep tissue temperature reflects a greater conduction owing to the longer application of ice. Some researchers have misinterpreted the effects of ice massage by considering tissue temperature change during application rather than following application.[61]

Adipose tissue insulates deeper tissues and thus decreases the effect of cooling on them.[41,62] Changes in deep tissue temperature correlate with the amount of adipose tissue over the biceps brachii muscle[61] and the thigh muscles[63] when cold is applied to the skin over these muscles, and to the percentage of fat of the entire body when application and measurement involve the lower leg.[64]

Intra-articular Temperature

Intra-articular temperature, or temperature within a joint, resembles that in other tissues—the temperature seems to be a function of the magnitude of heat lost. For instance:

- Cold immersion results in a greater temperature decrease than crushed ice packs (~38°F [21°C] vs. 7.2°F [4°C] in 15 minutes) and ethyl chloride spray (4.5°F [2.5°C] in 15–30 minutes).[65]
- Intra-articular temperatures decrease more than adjacent muscle; 4.5°F (2.5°C) vs. 3.6°F (2.0°C), 1.9 cm intramuscularly with 15–30 minutes ethyl chloride spray[58] and 33°F (18.4°C), 31°F (17.4°C), and 30°F (16.4°C) in the knee joint, adjacent muscle and adjacent subcutaneous tissue, respectively, owing to cold packs (43–50°F [6–10°C]) applied for 1 hour.[66]
- Like other deep tissues, the minimum temperature is reached after the ice pack is removed.[65,67]
- The longer the application, the greater is the decrease in temperature.[65] For instance, ice packs applied for 5,

15, and 30 minutes resulted in decreases of 3.6°F (2°C), 7.2°F (4°C), and 11.9°F (6.5°C), respectively.
- Rewarming following cold applications is delayed for hours[67–69]; 215 minutes following a 30-minute application of a frozen gel pack (–23°C) applied over a thin towel to the knees of 10 young healthy bulls,[68] and 150 minutes following a 30-minute crushed ice pack application to 42 human knees, their intra-articular knee temperature was still depressed 8°F (4.5°C).[67]

Rewarming After Cryotherapy

Rewarming after cryotherapy is a function of three factors:

1. The activity level prior to cryotherapy
2. The amount of heat removed from the body during application (i.e., magnitude and duration of cold exposure)
3. The amount of heat available to rewarm the area, which is a function of circulation, environmental temperature, and activity

The fingers rewarm much more quickly than the ankle,[46,48] forearm,[48] calf,[59] and interarticular knee.[67,68] Fingers rewarm in 15–20 minutes, whereas the other body parts take >3 hours (Fig. 6.12). Presumably, this is owing to the increased circulation in the fingers.

Deep tissue rewarming is not as straightforward as is surface temperature rewarming. It varies according to the depth of the tissue. Tissues that are more superficial (up to ~2 cm deep) begin rewarming immediately after the cold is removed.[52,64] Deeper tissues continue to decrease.[52,57,59] The longer the cold is applied, and the deeper the tissue, the slower the rewarming following application.

Activity during rewarming increases the rate of rewarming.[49] Even mild activity, like walking on crutches and standing in a shower for 20 minutes, significantly increases the rate of rewarming.

Rewarming following a second application is generally the same as following the first application, as long at the ratio of application time to interval between applications is >2:1, and the application times and the activity level during rewarming are the same.[49]

Cryotherapy Application Principles

Does it matter how you apply cold? Absolutely! The cold modality chosen and how it is applied result in great differences in tissue cooling. Understanding the factors that affect tissue cooling will help you make proper decisions. There is great confusion on this matter, however.[70,71]

Various protocols have been suggested for applying cold during immediate care. In a review of 45 sports

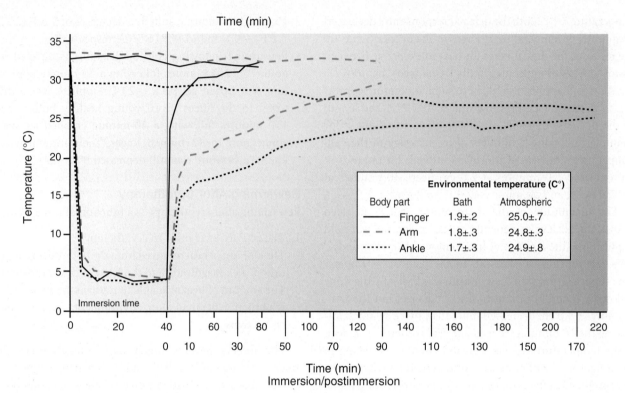

FIGURE 6.12 Fingers rewarm quickly following the removal of a cold pack. Most other body parts take hours to rewarm, as illustrated by the arm and ankle shown here. (Source: Adapted from Knight and Elam.[48])

medicine textbooks, 17 gave no specific guidance and 28 that did varied greatly.[70] In another review of the recommended length, frequency of application, and duration of therapy of >30 published protocols, there were only two instances in which the two recommendations were the same.[71] The following few pages will help solve some of the confusion.

FACTORS THAT AFFECT TISSUE COOLING

Numerous factors influence tissue cooling during cold pack application. Some of these were discussed above, including:

- The temperature differential between the body and the cold modality
- The regeneration of body heat and/or modality cooling
- The heat storage capacity of the cold modality
- The size of the cold modality; the larger the cold pack, the more cooling
- The amount of tissue in contact with the cold pack. The greater the area of contact with the cold modality, the more is the cooling
- The length of application; the longer the application, the more is the cooling and the slower the rewarming
- Individual variability
- Heat capacity of modalities
- Amount of adipose tissue at the site of application

Other factors that influence tissue cooling are:

- Types of cold packs
- Application directly to the skin rather than over a towel or elastic wrap
- Length of application
- Rate of intermittent application
- The duration of therapy (number of treatments)

These factors, and their implications on application guidelines, are discussed below.

TYPES OF COLD PACKS

The four main types of **cold packs** are crushed ice packs, gel packs, artificial ice packs, and crushable chemical packs (Fig. 6.13). Each are discussed in this section, along with frozen peas and ice massage.

Crushed Ice Pack

A **crushed ice pack** is crushed ice, typically from an ice machine, in a plastic or cloth bag (Fig. 6.13a). Ice packs are typically 30°F (–1°C) to 32°F (0°C) when applied to the body. They are the most effective type of cold modality because they undergo a phase change and therefore extract great amounts of heat from the body (see Fig. 6.9). Yet, they are not so cold that they cause frostbite, unless applied for hours.

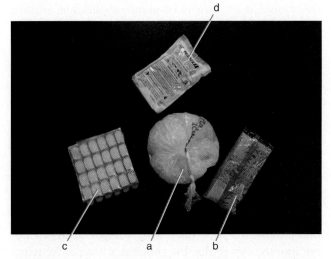

FIGURE 6.13 The four most common types of cold packs are shown here: **(a)** a crushed ice pack, **(b)** a gel pack (cold pack), **(c)** an artificial ice pack (with sheets of ice showing on top), and **(d)** a crushable chemical pack.

Cubed ice is also used. It does not conform to the body as well as crushed ice, however.

Crushed ice packs are also excellent for on-the-field use. They can be prepared before a practice or event, placed in an insulated cooler, and used hours later. Without a phase change, other types of cold packs do not stay cold for not nearly as long.

Crushed ice packs are not effective for home use. They cool to about 1°F (–17°C) in a home freezer, so if applied directly to the skin they will cause tissue damage. They also become solid when frozen in a home freezer, so they do not conform to irregular body surfaces.

You can make an ice pack by placing 1.5–2.5 lb (0.7–1.2 kg) of crushed or cubed ice in a plastic bag. Suck out as much air as possible from the bag, and tie the end in a knot (Fig. 6.14).

Gel Pack

A **gel pack** is a reusable type of cold pack, consisting of water mixed with an antifreeze, such as alcohol, and a gel substance, in a vinyl pouch bag (Fig. 6.13b). The alcohol keeps the water from freezing solid, and the gel gives it body so the water does not slosh around in the pack. They are cooled in a freezer to about 1°F (–17°C).

Gel packs do not cool as effectively as crushed ice, and they are much more dangerous. The water does not freeze, so they do not go through a phase change when applied, and therefore do not withdraw as much heat from the body. But because they are cooled to ~1°F (~17°C), they may cause frostbite if applied directly to the skin (Fig. 6.15). Applying a barrier to protect the skin from the extreme temperature further decreases their cooling effectiveness.

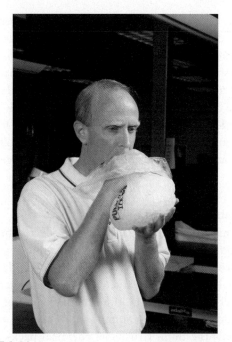

FIGURE 6.14 Remove as much air as possible from a crushed ice pack by sucking it out. Twist it before removing it from your face, and then quickly tie the end of the bag in a knot.

Artificial Ice Pack

An **artificial ice pack** is a vinyl sheet divided into a series of cells 1 × 1.5 in. (3 × 4 cm). The cells are filled with water and a group of cells are enclosed in a nylon covering (Fig. 6.13c). The vinyl sheets were designed to keep fruit and vegetables cool during interstate shipping. (The sheets used for cold packs are subdivided from the much larger sheets used for shipping produce.) Artificial ice packs are frozen in a freezer at 1°F (~17°C), but the nylon

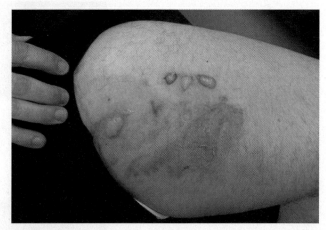

FIGURE 6.15 Frozen gel packs can cause severe skin damage if applied directly to the skin. An individual took a frozen gel pack from our laboratory, without permission, and applied it directly to his skin (thigh) for 90 minutes to treat radiating pain. Blisters began forming that evening and continued to grow until 2 days later when this photo was taken. The skin healed without scaring, but was still mildly sensitive to touch 20 months later.

covering insulates them so the application temperature is close to 32°F (0°C). Artificial ice packs are not as flexible as gel packs, but they are much more flexible than refrozen crushed ice packs. Owing to the nylon covering, they are not as effective in cooling tissue as crushed ice, but they are more effective in cooling than a gel pack because they undergo a phase change. They are preferred for home use because they can be safely applied after cooling in a freezer, are flexible, and go through a phase change as they warm.

Crushable Chemical Pack

A **crushable chemical pack** consists of a thin-walled vinyl pouch of a liquid packaged within a stronger, larger vinyl pouch of dry crystals (Fig. 6.13d). When squeezed with sufficient force, the smaller, inner pouch is broken, leaking its fluid into the larger, outer pouch. The fluid and crystals combine in a chemical reaction that cools the fluid. Crushable chemical packs are not recommended because they neither get the body cold enough nor last long enough to be used in place of crushed ice.[72] There also is a danger of chemical burns if the contents of a chemical pack leak onto the skin. Crushable chemical cold packs should be used only as a last resort.

Frozen Peas

A bag of frozen peas has become a popular form of cryotherapy.[73,74] Advocates claim it is cheap and convenient.[73] But how effective is it? Better than nothing and gel packs,[75,76] not as effective as crushed ice packs or cold water immersion.[75] After a 20-minute application, crushed ice packs reduced ankle temperature 19.6 ± 3.8°C, but the frozen peas decreased it only 14.6 ± 4.2°, a difference of 25%.[75] It is noteworthy that prior to application, the peas were colder (–10°C) than the crushed ice packs (0.1°C). It appears then, that the difference in cooling was due to a greater phase change in the crushed ice packs than did the frozen peas.[75] We recommend that this form of cryotherapy be avoided if possible.

Ice Massage

Ice massage is simply rubbing a frozen ice cube over the tissue (see Fig. 12.2). The most common ice cube is one frozen in 6–8-oz cups, often with a tongue depressor frozen into the cup so that the cube has a handle. We refute the claim that "Ice massage is one of the most effective ways to treat a soft tissue injury."[74] In fact, we recommend that it not be used for immediate care at all. You do not get as great of cooling and cannot apply an elastic wrap for compression during the treatment.

APPLICATION DIRECTLY TO THE SKIN

In general, crushed ice packs are applied directly to the patient's skin (Fig. 6.16).[77,78] A towel or elastic wrap between the ice pack and the body insulates against the full effect of the cold, thereby making the treatment less effective.[42,72,79–81] If used for <60 minutes, most cold packs do not cause frostbite. Frozen gel packs are an exception, however (see Fig. 6.15), and should not be applied directly on the skin. Their temperature might be many degrees below zero and could cause frostbite.

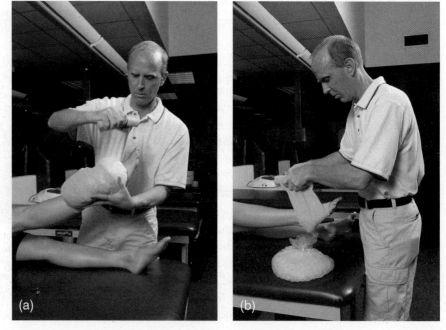

FIGURE 6.16 (a) Apply cold packs directly to the skin. **(b)** A towel or wrap between the cold pack and skin will decrease the effectiveness of cooling.

APPLICATION TIP

FROSTBITE ALERT: WHEN AND WHEN NOT TO APPLY COLD PACKS DIRECTLY TO THE SKIN

Some types of cold packs are too cold to be applied directly to the skin because they will damage the skin. These include frozen gel packs and crushed ice packs using ice frozen in a refrigerator or freezer. Most crushed ice packs are made from ice from an ice machine, which stores the ice just below freezing (30°F or –1°C). But ice from a freezer and gel packs are in the range of –2°F to 5°F (–16°C to –19°C). This is much too cold for the skin and often results in tissue damage.

Placing a towel or elastic wrap between the skin and the cold pack, as many recommend,[7,82] insulates the skin against the cold, decreasing its effectiveness.[72,79–81] (Fig. 6.17) Wet[7,83] or frozen[84] elastic wraps between the skin and cold pack allow the tissue to cool more than dry ones, but not as much as application directly to skin.[79–81]

Most first aid texts recommend against applying ice packs directly to the skin.[7,85] This changed in 2005, however, when the American Academy of Orthopaedic Surgeons and the American Academy of Emergency Physicians text recommended applying crushed ice packs directly to the skin.[86]

Mirkin[78] claimed that ice packs directly on the skin were safe because living tissue will not freeze until its temperature drops below 25°F (–4.3°C), and since an ice pack is 32°F (0°C), it is incapable of causing frostbite. Although he probably was low by 3–5°F (2–3°C) concerning the freezing temperature of skin,[25] he is correct in stating that ice packs can be applied safely to the skin as long as they

are not left on longer than 60 minutes. Long-term application (2–3 days) can lead to nonfreezing tissue damage,[87] which can lead to tissue necrosis that requires partial limb amputation. Where the critical time is between 60 minutes and 3 days is unknown.

We can find no reference to frostbite occurring as a result of a short-term (<60 minutes) crushed ice pack application, nor have we observed frostbite in over 30 years of clinical experience applying crushed ice packs directly to the skin of patients for up to 45 minutes at a time.[25] (See also Chapter 13.) Avoid applying gel packs directly to the skin, however.

LENGTH OF APPLICATION

There is much confusion about how long to apply cold packs. Many incorrectly say to never apply a cold pack for more than 15–20 minutes; that doing so may cause frostbite.[73,74,88,89] Not so; crushed ice packs and ice massage will not cause frostbite, even if applied for an hour. But more importantly, the beneficial effect of immediate care cryotherapy are reduced. This confusion is caused by a lack of understanding of the:

- Desired outcome, or why the cold pack is being used
- Types of cold packs that cause frostbite
- Body's response to various types of cold packs
- Body's response to various lengths of cold application

Immediate Care Versus Transitional and Subacute Care

Cryotherapy for immediate care has entirely different objectives than it does for transitional and subacute care, and therefore how it's applied is different. The goal during immediate care is to decrease metabolism so as to

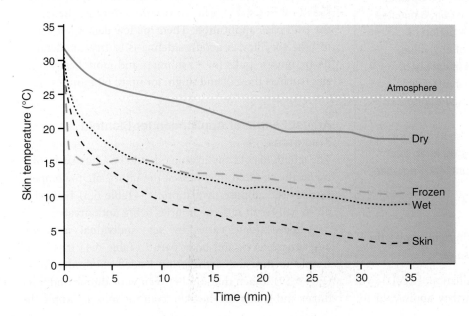

FIGURE 6.17 Applying a crushed ice pack over two layers of a dry, wet, or frozen elastic wrap insulates the body from the cold pack. The most effective cooling occurs when the cold pack is applied directly to the skin. (Source: Adapted from Urban.[80])

minimize secondary metabolic injury (see Figs. 6.3 and 6.4). Decreasing metabolism adequately requires applications of 20–60 minutes, depending on the amount of adipose tissue as determined by skinfold measurements. Limiting application to 15–20 minutes will reduce the effectiveness of the therapy.

Transitional and subacute care use cryotherapy to numb the body part so as to facilitate mobilization. Numbness occurs in 15–20 minutes.[54] Longer applications are unnecessary and a waste of patient and clinician time.

Use Intermitted, Not Continuous Applications

Ice packs should be applied intermittently. Continuous application is both unnecessary and potentially dangerous. Frostbite can occur with continuous application,[87] and the majority of the body rewarms quite slowly following ice pack application.[47,48,90] The beneficial effects of cold application, therefore, remain after the cold packs are removed. Tissue temperature remains depressed after removing the cold modality, so tissue metabolism remains depressed. The body part can be kept cool by applying an ice pack for 30–45 minutes every 2 hours (every hour if the patient is active between applications, such as showering or walking on crutches).

Modality Myth

USING INVALID LENGTHS OF INTERMITTENT COLD APPLICATION

Many clinicians apply ice packs for inappropriate lengths of time, believing their applications are effective. Many applications are less than optimal. Application times for ice packs vary from 6 minutes to continuously for 24–48 hours.[71] A period of 6 minutes is much too short to be of any value, and 24 hours is dangerous. The wide variety of application lengths results from an inadequate theoretical basis for using cryotherapy during immediate care procedures.

For immediate care, application should be for at least 30 minutes, and sometimes up to an hour, depending on the amount of subcutaneous adipose tissue.[41,42]

Most clinicians recommend intermittent applications, even though their reasons for doing so vary:

• Some believe cold-induced vasodilation (CIVD) will increase blood flow to the area if they apply cold for

longer than 10–12 minutes.[91–94] Chu and Lutt[95] felt that initial cold applications should last at least 20 minutes so the body part could pass through a 3–5 minutes period of vasodilation and be in a second period of vasoconstriction. CIVD does not occur during orthopedic injury applications (see Chapter 12), so this logic is incorrect.
• Some fear frostbite[87,91,96] or nerve palsy[97] if they apply cold for too long, which most define as 15–30 minutes. The concept is true, but the time frame is much too short. Applications of up to 60 minutes (for fleshy tissues) are safe.
• Boland[77] felt the application of ice packs for longer than 20–30 minutes was too painful and should not be done. Ice packs for this length are not that painful. Ice immersion can be painful, but immersion is not recommended for immediate care.

There is no direct research on how the length of application affects the amount of tissue damage or subsequent resolution of the injury. The rate of rewarming following application, however, indicates that cold packs should be applied for at least 30 minutes during immediate care.[71] As Figure 6.18 indicates, ankle rewarming following 30, 45, and 60 minutes of ice pack application is significantly slower than following 10 and 20 minutes of ice applications. Thus, metabolism is lowered during the time between intermittent ice pack applications.

The area of the body also affects the length of application. The ankle and forearm temperatures remain depressed for hours after application, while the finger rewarms within minutes (see Fig. 6.12).[46,48] The knee reacts like the ankle and forearm. Thick muscular tissues, such as the thigh, require longer to cool than bony areas, such as the ankle,[45,49] and rewarm more quickly.

Deeper tissues cool more slowly than superficial tissues (see Fig. 6.11). The deeper the injury is, the longer the cold pack application. There are few data upon which to base specifics. A good guideline is to treat moderately fleshy muscle pulls for 45 minutes and more fleshy injuries, such as the calf and thigh, for up to 60 minutes.

Adjust Length of Application for Skinfold Thickness

The length of cold applications should be adjusted according to the skinfold thickness at the injury site to compensate for the adipose insulation.[41,62] (Table 6.3) Failure to do so will result in some injuries being undertreated.

Adipose tissue varies by sex, individual morphology, fitness level, and body part.[43] (Table 6.4) It is fairly simple to measure with spring loaded skinfold calipers (Fig. 6.19). Pinch the skin between your thumb and forefinger and gently lift the skin from the muscle. Apply the

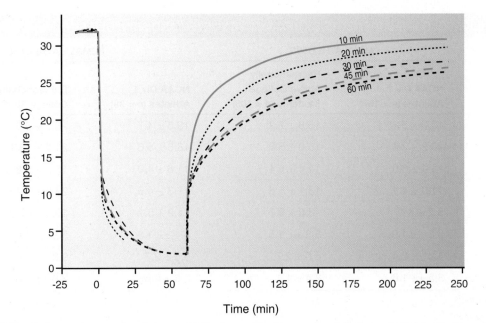

FIGURE 6.18 Ankle cooling and rewarming during and following crushed ice pack applications of 10, 20, 30, 45, and 60 minutes. The quicker rewarming following 10- and 20-minute applications indicates that cold packs should be applied for at least 30 minutes during immediate care. (Source: Adapted from Mlynarczyk.[71])

calipers, read the dial, and then divide the number by 2 (the skinfold between your fingers includes two layers of skin and adipose tissue). We recommend that you apply cold for 30 minutes to injuries.

The data in Tables 6.3 and 6.4 must be considered during immediate care cryotherapy—but cautiously, and only generally. Consider the following:

- The data in Table 6.3 are for muscle 1 cm deep. Ligaments will cool more quickly. Therefore ligament injuries need not be cooled as long as muscle injuries.
- The cooling goal of 44.6°F (7°C) in Table 6.3 was an arbitrary value, chosen to investigate the phenomenon. It is unknown how much of a decrease in metabolism is necessary to minimize secondary metabolic injury. Metabolism is directly related to temperature, however (see Table 6.4),

so it follows that the lower the temperature—without causing tissue damage, the more effective it would be.

- Data in both tables are presented as means ± SD. Statistical theory would predict that 5% of the population would take <9.9 or more than 39.7 minutes to reach the target temperature (mean ± 2SD's). Since there is no way to determine where a specific patient would fit within the range, the data must be interpreted broadly.

We therefore recommend that injuries with up to 20-mm skinfold be treated for ~30 minutes, and those with skinfolds over 20 mm be treated proportionally up to 60 minutes.

RATE OF INTERMITTENT APPLICATION

The question of how long ice packs should be applied involves not just the initial application, but the repeated applications and the time between the applications.

The activity level of the patient determines how quickly subsequent applications should be administered. Generally following the first application, patients will shower and go home. Cold packs should be reapplied immediately after the patient arrives home. If the patient is inactive, however, applications of more than 30 minutes every 2 hours will cause a progressive decrease in the temperature of the ankle.[49]

Because reapplication is usually done by the patient or family or friends, **compliance** is a factor. The more complicated the treatment regimen is, the less likely it will be followed. Recommendations such as "30 minutes on and an hour off" require too much thinking. A simplified

TABLE 6.3 EFFECT OF ADIPOSE TISSUE ON TISSUE COOLING AT 1 CM BELOW THE ADIPOSE TISSUE IN THE THIGH*	
SKINFOLD THICKNESS (MM)	**TIME TO DECREASE TISSUE TEMP 44.6°F (7°C)**
0–10	8.0 ± 3.4 min
11–20	23.3 ± 6.7 min
21–30	37.8 ± 9.6 min
31–40	58.6 ± 11.7 min

*See text about implications of these data to clinical application.

Source: Adapted from Otte et al.[41]

TABLE 6.4	SKINFOLD MEASUREMENTS BY SEX, ACTIVITY LEVEL, AND SKINFOLD SITE, MM (MEAN ± SD)			
	MALE ATHLETES		**FEMALE ATHLETES**	
TREATMENT SITE	**NCAA Div 1 Athletes (n = 157)**	**Recreationally Active College Students (n = 108)**	**NCAA Div 1 Athletes (n = 39)**	**Recreationally Active College Students (n = 85)**
Thigh	13.0 ± 5.4	15.8 ± 7.2	19.5 ± 4.7	25.7 ± 8.5
Deltoid	16.2 ± 2.4	15.0 ± 5.8	18.8 ± 5.6	21.6 ± 13.1
Scapula	13.4 ± 6.0	14.4 ± 5.4	11.6 ± 4.0	15.6 ± 5.8
MCL*	11.0 ± 4.4	13.1 ± 5.6	17.3 ± 4.6	22.0 ± 7.7
Calf	8.2 ± 4.1	13.0 ± 5.7	14.9 ± 5.1	19.0 ±± 7.2
Ulnar groove	5.3 ±± 1.9	5.3 ±± 1.5	5.4 ±± 1.8	5.8 ±± 2.6
Forearm	4.9 ±± 2.4	6.0 ± 2.7	6.5 ± 2.7	9.3 ±± 4.0
ATF†	3.5 ±± 1.6	2.4 ± 1.1	2.6 ± 0.6	2.8 ±± 3.8

*Medial collateral ligament.

†Anterior talofibular ligament.

Source: Adapted from Jutte et al.[43]

DURATION OF THERAPY

Duration, as used here, refers to the calendar or the length of time that intermittent cycles of application-reapplication of cold packs should be continued. In other words, how long should RICES therapy continue? There are no available data to indicate an optimal duration. Most clinicians recommend applications for 12–72 hours, or until the tendency for swelling has passed.[71] One consideration is the severity of the injury. Immediate care procedures can be terminated earlier when treating a mild injury than

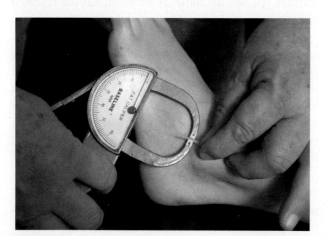

FIGURE 6.19 Skinfold is measured with a spring-loaded caliper.

when treating a severe injury. Another consideration is the therapy chosen for subacute care. It is possible to transition from immediate care to subacute rehabilitation procedures earlier when using a cryotherapeutic technique for rehabilitation than when using a thermotherapeutic technique. But a definitive answer to the question of the optimal duration of cold applications during immediate care awaits further research.

Two examples of cryotherapy techniques for subacute care are cryokinetics and cryostretch. Both combine cryotherapy with exercise. **Cryokinetics** consists of alternating cold immersion and active exercise for rehabilitating acute joint sprains. **Cryostretch** consists of alternating cold application, passive stretch, and resistive muscle contraction for rehabilitating acute muscle strains (see Chapter 13).

For first-degree injuries, transition to one of the above cryotherapy techniques after the initial RICES treatment (30 minutes following the injury) is advisable. For second-degree injuries, continuing RICES treatments until bedtime and after the patient has been evaluated (and possibly x-rayed) the following day is the recommendation. The question is moot for most third-degree injuries because they generally are treated with surgery and/or immobilization until beyond the acute phase.

PREVENTING SWELLING VERSUS REDUCING OR REMOVING IT

Cold is effective in preventing or limiting swelling, but it is of little or no value in removing swelling after it has occurred (see Table 6.2). The cause of edema following traumatic injury is excess free protein in the tissue. As explained

recommendation, that is consistent with the variable application times for various tissues and the data from ankle reapplication,[49,51] is to apply ice packs every 2 hours, rounded to the nearest whole hour (e.g., 2:00, 4:00, 6:00, or 1:00, 3:00, 5:00).

earlier, cold limits secondary injury. With less total injury, there is less tissue debris, less free protein in the tissue, and less edema. Once swelling has occurred, however, it can be removed only by removing the free protein from the extracellular spaces. As long as free protein remains in the tissue spaces, TOP will be abnormally high, thereby retaining excess fluid in the tissue. The only way to permanently remove edema is to remove the excess free protein.

Pieces of free protein, resulting from phagocytosis of protein debris are too large to be absorbed into the circulatory system. They are removed via the lymphatic system, and such removal requires intermittent compression.

The lymphatic system consists of vessels that begin in the tissue and run proximally to the large veins. They have no built-in pumping force, such as the heart, to cause fluid flow. They depend primarily on external compression to force fluid flow (Fig. 6.20). A series of one-way valves allows fluid to flow proximally, but prevents backwash. External compression on the vessel forces valves to open proximately and the fluid to move proximally. When the compression is released, the valves close, preventing fluid from returning distally. This leaves a vacuum at the distal end of the lymph vessel. This vacuum pulls edema (fluid and free protein) into the vessel.[35] Subsequent compression then forces lymph proximately, and the process continues.

Intermittent external force from massage, compression, or lymphedema devices such as the Jobst pump, or the muscle pump, during active exercise stimulates lymph flow.[98,99] Neither heat nor cold applications promote lymph flow. They can be helpful, however, in facilitating one of the other modalities. For instance, with cryokinetics, ice applications decrease pain so that active exercise can begin sooner and be more vigorous. Thus, cold application, which

has no effect by itself, can facilitate active exercise, which in turn compresses lymph vessels and stimulates lymph flow. (Specific techniques for removing swelling by stimulating lymph flow are presented in Chapters 12 and 13.)

Misunderstanding the difference between preventing or limiting swelling and removing it after it has occurred leads many clinicians to use cold applications to "treat" swelling, an effort that is both ineffective and delays proper therapy. An example of this misunderstanding is demonstrated by research on the effects of cold during immediate care that includes patients who were not treated until 12 to 36 hours following their injury.[6,100] Further, this research included reduction in edema as one of the outcome variables. If a patient's treatment is not initiated within an hour or so of the injury, she is not receiving immediate care. And if her treatment is not initiated within 15–20 minutes, she is not receiving optimal immediate care.

Intermittent Versus Continuous Cold and Compression

Cold is always applied intermittently. Applications longer 60 minutes are unnecessary and potentially dangerous.

Compression is applied either intermittently or continuously, depending on the therapeutic goals (see Table 6.2). Preventing swelling during RICES requires continuous application, while removing swelling during transitional or subacute care requires intermittent compression to stimulate lymphatic drainage.

Compression Application Principles

There are three key considerations for applying compression during RICES: what to apply, where to apply it in relation to cold, and how to apply it.

RICES COMPRESSION DEVICES

Elastic wraps are preferred during RICES. When combined with ice packs, they provide more combined cold and compression than other devices (Table 6.5).[101,102] Despite its popularity and ease of application, plastic wrap should not be used during RICES (Fig. 6.21). It does not provide either the compression or the enhanced cooling that an elastic wrap does. Although the ice packs under the plastic wrap and elastic wraps are the same, the greater compression exerted by the elastic wrap assists in providing greater cooling (see earlier discussion).

A Cryo/Cuff is used as a cold/compression device, but it should not be used as an alternative for elastic wraps with ice. Dura*Kold should be used strictly as a cold modality because little compression is given by this device.

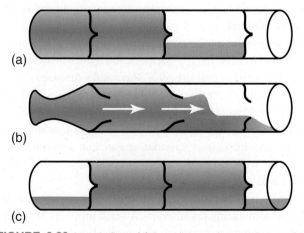

FIGURE 6.20 Lymph flow. **(a)** Lymph vessels contain a series of one-way valves. **(b)** Pressure on the vessel forces fluid to flow proximally. **(c)** Release of the pressure allows some back flow, but the valves close. **(c)** A vacuum in the distal sections draws lymph into the vessel. Ongoing flow occurs from intermittent compression (repeated compression and release).

TABLE 6.5 TEMPERATURE AND COMPRESSION ON THE ANKLE BY VARIOUS TECHNIQUES EXERTED BY VARIOUS COLD AND COMPRESSION TECHNIQUES APPLIED FOR 30 MINUTES[101]

MODALITY	AVERAGE 30 MIN TEMPERATURE	AVERAGE 30 MIN PRESSURE
Cryo/Cuff	13.9 ± 1.8	39.8 ± 6.2
Dura*Kold	14.1 ± 4.1	6.0 ± 2.0
Elastic wrap + ice	7.1 ± 4.8	50.7 ± 21.0
Flexi-Wrap + ice	9.8 ± 5.3	28.6 ± 13.7

Source: Adapted from Danielson et al.[101]

APPLYING ELASTIC WRAPS OVER ICE PACKS

Elastic wraps should be applied over ice packs, as explained earlier, to maximize tissue cooling (see Fig. 6.17). Some clinicians argue that compression is compromised if it is not applied under the ice pack. Compression is not compromised, however; compression over the anterior talofibular ligament is the same whether the elastic wrap is under or over the ice pack, as long as the ice pack is tied so that it maintains a constant volume.[45,103]

STRETCHING ELASTIC WRAPS 75%

We recommend that an elastic wrap be stretched to about 75% of its capacity as it is applied. There is no scientific basis for this recommendation, but it is the naturally selected, or intuitive, stretch that students and professionals apply.[45]

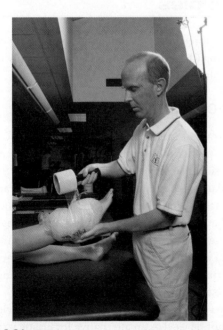

FIGURE 6.21. Plastic wraps are convenient to hold on ice packs, but they do not provide either the compression or the cooling effect of elastic wraps.

Contraindications and Precautions to RICES

Inappropriate use of cryotherapy can cause excessive pain and tissue damage. These fit into five broad categories, cryotherapy that is too cold, cryotherapy that is applied too long,[104] delayed application, cryotherapy applied under excessive compression, and applications to patients who suffer from conditions that cause abnormal responses to the cold.[105] These are discussed in general in this section, and specific contraindication and precautions are listed in the application section later in the chapter.

There is neither a specific temperature nor length of application that causes tissue damage. It is the combination of the two that is dangerous.[106] For example, exposure to −9°F (−4°C) for less than a minute is safe,[107] yet exposure to 45°F (7°C) for 7 days resulted in gangrene. Intermittent ice water immersion (32°F–0°C) for 20–30 minutes is common during rehabilitation of acute ankle sprains. Yet near continuous immersion for 36–72 hours has caused loss of part of the foot.[87,104] Gel packs (which are frozen to about 1°F or −17°C) should never be applied directly to the skin (see Fig. 6.15). Ice water immersion and crushed ice packs should be applied to the skin, but not for longer than an hour.

Elastic wraps applied over a cold pack can be problematic if applied too tightly, especially in thin people and to body parts where the major nerves are superficial, such as the elbow or knee. Do not apply the wrap too tightly. Cases of Temporary **nerve palsy** (local paralysis) from cryotherapy have been reported, but analysis reveals that the combination of a tightly applied elastic wrap and cold pack probably caused the palsy, not the cryotherapy alone.[25] The incidence of such cases is extremely small compared to the numbers of cryotherapy treatments given, so the risk is minimal.

The most common conditions that cause an abnormal response to cryotherapy includes Raynaud's disease, cold hypersensitivity, and urticaria. **Raynaud's disease** is a circulatory disorder caused by cold or emotion, in which the hands, and less commonly the feet, become discolored and painful. Even mild cold exposure, such as reaching into a refrigerator, causes vascular spasm and extreme pain. Patients with these diseases generally know they have them and will refuse cold application.

Cold hypersensitivity is a condition manifested by severe pain during cryotherapy. A small minority of people cannot tolerate any type of cold application for more than a few minutes.

Cold applications can cause urticaria (hives) in some people.[25] A temporary allergic reaction, **urticaria** is characterized by **wheals**, slightly raised, rounded, or flat-topped areas of skin, usually accompanied by burning or intense itching. It can also be caused by exercise, eating certain foods, or from taking certain medicines.

Our experience is that patients with cold urticaria consider it more of a nuisance than a cause for concern. It manifests in patients who have used cold packs previously, often for a number of years. It usually is more intense in the beginning and becomes less severe if the patient continues to receive cold treatments. Our policy is to discuss the situation with patients following the first occurrence and let them decide whether to continue cryotherapy. Most feel the advantages of the cryotherapy outweigh the nuisance of the urticaria, especially as the urticaria decreases in severity over time. Calamine also helps some patients.[108]

Precautions include the following situations where problems could arise if caution is not exercised when using cryotherapy:

- Cardiac disorder
- Compromised local circulation

Electrical Stimulation During Immediate Care

Some clinicians advocate electrical stimulation for the immediate care of orthopedic injuries.[109] We do not recommend this technique at present, for reasons that will become apparent. There have been two schools of thought concerning this issue:

- The mistaken belief that high-volt pulsed current stimulation (see Chapter 16) causes vasoconstriction and therefore limits swelling[110]
- The belief under investigation that sensory-level high-volt pulsed stimulation (see Chapter 16) limits edema development

THE VASOCONSTRICTION THEORY

The belief that high-volt pulsed current stimulation caused vasoconstriction grew out of early marketing efforts by manufacturers who presented pulsed monophasic stimulators as galvanic simulators (see Chapter 16). Because galvanic currents are thought to cause vasoconstriction, presumably these units would do so.[110] But they don't deliver a continuous galvanic current, even though some include the term *galvanic* in their name. So they do not cause vasoconstriction. Also, even if they were vasoconstrictive, the goal of immediate care is to decrease secondary injury, not blood flow.

Another problem is that you sacrifice the full benefits of RICES with this technique. Many apply it by immersing the limb in a tub of ice water and inserting one of the electrodes into the bath. This sacrifices elevation. You also have to sacrifice either compression or some cooling. If you apply an elastic bandage to the limb for compression, the bandage will insulate the limb so there is less cooling. On the other hand, to get full cooling you have to sacrifice compression.

Applying electrical stimulation under the traditional RICES does not solve the problem. The thick rubber electrode will insulate the tissue from the cooling of the ice pack.

THE EDEMA LIMITING THEORY

Limiting edema development by sensory-level high-volt pulsed current stimulation is based on extensive research on small laboratory animals.[109,111–121] The hind limbs of these animals were injured, and the animals were suspended in a sling with the traumatized limbs in a dependent position.[112] The traumatized limbs were immersed in a beaker of water, into which an electrode was placed.

Although research has clearly demonstrated that edema is curbed with high-volt pulsed stimulation, applying this concept is difficult. One problem is that it cannot be used in conjunction with RICES, as scientists suggest doing.[112] Their research suggests that near-continuous treatment is needed throughout the acute inflammatory response.[109,112] A single 30-minute treatment decreases edema for 4 hours but did not significantly decrease long-term edema formation.[67,80,88–90] In addition, the animal model involved no compression or elevation.

Another concern is that the research has not been tested against RICES. Therefore, we do not know whether edema retardation is more, less, or the same as that provided by RICES. Scientists have compared electrical stimulation with cold,[111–113] but the protocols used fail to answer the question. The cold water immersion was at a temperature of 55°F (~13°C), which is not as cold as an ice pack. Also, the electrical stimulation and control were applied with room temperature water (75°F, or 23°C), which is ~15°F cooler than tissue, and so the "control" was a mild form of cryotherapy.

We recommend against using electrical stimulation in place of RICES for immediate care. It might have a place if it is used between ice applications and in conjunction with compression and elevation. Further research will, no doubt, clarify how electrical stimulation can augment RICES.

▮STEPS Application of RICES

▮1▮ STEP 1: FOUNDATION

A. Definition. Procedures used immediately after an acute orthopedic injury to limit the negative sequelae of the injury.

B. Effects
1. Resting the injured structure minimizes aggravating the injury.
2. Ice cools the tissue, thereby minimizing secondary injury. There is less total injured tissue, less tissue debris, less free protein from phagacytosis of the tissue debris, and less edema. It also limits pain and muscle spasm.
3. Compression helps contain edema and increases the cooling effect of ice.
4. Elevation helps lessen the increase in capillary filtration pressure.
5. Stabilization reduces muscle guarding and pain.

C. Advantages. Less total tissue damage and edema

D. Disadvantages. None, if applied correctly

E. Indications. Acute orthopedic or soft tissue injury

F. Contraindications
1. Do not apply cryotherapy directly to the skin for >1 hour continuously; it can cause frostbite.
2. Do not apply cold packs that have been chilled in a freezer directly to the skin (see Fig. 6.15).
3. Do not apply a compression bandage over a chilled gel pack; it can cause frostbite.
4. Do not apply cryotherapy of any type to patients who have any of the following conditions:
   a. Raynaud's or any other vasospastic disease
   b. Cold hypersensitivity, manifested by severe pain
   c. Cardiac disorder
   d. Compromised local circulation

G. Precautions
1. The longer you wait following injury, the less effective it is.
2. Unyielding compression. Despite your best efforts, edema might develop. If the edema is excessive, and the compression is unyielding, the pressure might damage tissue in a manner similar to a *compartment syndrome*, like that which may occur in the lower leg due to excessive exercise.
3. Be extremely cautious when using cryotherapy for treating patients who:
   a. Have certain rheumatoid conditions
   b. Are paralyzed or in a coma
   c. Have coronary artery disease
   d. Have certain hypertensive diseases

4. Be very careful when applying an elastic wrap over a cold pack, especially in thin people and to body parts where the major nerves are superficial, such as the elbow or knee.
5. Be aware that cold applications can cause urticaria (hives) in some people.

▮2▮ STEP 2: PREAPPLICATION TASKS

A. Selecting the proper modality
1. Evaluate the injury or problem to:
   a. Rule out life-threatening situations; if one exists, initiate an emergency action plan.
   b. Collect data about the injury. Once muscle guarding develops, the information you obtain from palpation and stress tests will be decreased.
   c. Perform the evaluation thoroughly but quickly.
2. Check for possible contraindications to cold.

B. Preparing the patient psychologically
1. Explain the procedure.
2. Warn about precautions.
3. Reassure the patient; pain and frustration from the injury are usually very disconcerting.

C. Preparing the patient physically
1. Remove clothing as necessary.
2. Remove bandages, braces, etc. as necessary.
3. Position the patient in a manner that will be comfortable and allow the injury to be elevated.

D. Equipment preparation
1. Make an appropriately sized ice pack.
   a. Place crushed ice in a plastic bag. The bag must be big enough that the finished pack will extend 2–3 in. (5–8 cm) beyond the borders of the injury (Some injuries might require two ice packs.)
   b. Remove as much air as possible from the bag (see Fig. 6.14).
   c. Tie the end of the bag in a knot.
2. Get appropriately sized (width) elastic wrap(s).
   a. For most situations, a 6 in. (15 cm) width is adequate. Never use one smaller than 4 in. (10 cm) for immediate care. Smaller wraps don't adequately cover the area and have a greater tendency to roll up and become a tourniquet.
   b. Double-length or multiple wraps are necessary for applications to the knee, thigh, abdomen, chest, and shoulder.
   c. Get a splint or sling.

3 STEP 3: APPLICATION PARAMETERS

A. Procedures
1. Apply the ice pack so it is centered over the middle of the injury.
    a. Apply directly to the skin.
    b. Shape to the general contour of the body part.
2. Apply the elastic wrap(s) around the ice pack and body part to hold the ice pack in place and to apply compression.
    a. The wrap must extend 2–3 in. (5–8 cm) beyond the borders of the ice pack.
    b. Stretch the wrap to about 75% of its capacity during application.
    c. Secure the end of the wrap with clips or tape, or by tucking it under itself.
3. Check the patient every 5 minutes with a capillary refill (or capillary nail refill) test to see if the wrap is too tight. The test is performed on the finger or toe of the injured limb. It cannot be performed if the nail is covered with nail polish.
    a. Position the patient so the toe or finger is elevated above the level of the heart.
    b. Pinch the nail for a few seconds until the nail bed blanches (turns white), indicating blood flow has been impeded.
    c. Release the pressure and watch for the nail bed to return to its normal pink color. If it takes more than ~2 seconds for the color to return, your wrap is too tight. Loosen it.
4. Also at this time, shake the ice pack to break up the thermal gradient.
5. Apply a splint, sling, or brace to stabilize the injured body part. The goal is to allow muscles surrounding the joint to relax. (see Fig. 6.7)
6. Elevate the limb or situate the patient so that the injury is elevated about 6 in. (15 cm) above the heart.

B. Dosage
1. Use enough ice so that the ice pack(s) and elastic wrap extend 2–3 in. (5–8 cm) beyond the borders of the injury.

C. Length of application
1. Cold, 20–60 min, depending on the injury and the skin-fold of the patient. In general:
    a. 20 minutes for finger
    b. 30 minutes for ankle or arm
    c. 45 minutes for thigh
    d. Add 5 minutes for each millimeter of skin-fold >1 mm.
2. Rest, compression, elevation, and stabilization continuously. Reapply the elastic wrap and stabilization after removing the ice pack.

D. Frequency of application
1. Begin application 5–10 minutes after the injury; immediately after the injury evaluation.
2. Second ice application should be 30–60 minutes later, after the patient has showered and gone home.
3. Apply compression, elevation, rest, and stabilization constantly.
4. Subsequent ice applications every 2 hours until bedtime. Tell the patient not to stay up into the night just to apply RICES.

E. Duration of therapy
1. 30–45 minutes for most first-degree injuries (a single treatment)
2. 12–24 hours for second-degree and third-degree injuries, if followed by a transitional cryotherapy technique, such as cryokinetics or cryostretch

4 STEP 4: POSTAPPLICATION TASKS

A. Equipment replacement; area cleanup
B. Instructions in writing to the patient (Fig. 6.22). These include:
1. Time of appointment for the following day (morning if possible)
2. Resting the injury, that is, not stressing the body part to the point of causing pain. Use a sling or crutches as necessary.
3. Specific times for reapplication of the ice pack
4. *Caution* patient to not reapply more or less frequently than the written instructions specify.
5. Phone number to call if pain or swelling becomes excessive
C. Recording treatment and unique patient responses to treatment

5 STEP 5: MAINTENANCE

A. Routine maintenance. Keep the ice machine in good repair, and replace elastic wraps as they deteriorate.

Extended Immediate Care Procedures
University of Moab Sports Medicine

Your activities during the next 12-72 hours are critical to the resolution of your injury. Failure to follow the following procedures may delay your return to full sport participation by as much as two weeks. Help us to help you by doing the following:

Before leaving the Athletic Training Clinic make sure you have:

_____ Had an initial 30- to 45-minute application of ice, compression, and elevation.

_____ Had a second evaluation of the injury.

_____ Showered.

_____ Had an elastic wrap applied to the injured area.

_____ Been fitted for a sling (if shoulder or arm injury) or crutches (if lower extremity injury).

_____ Received instructions in proper use of the sling or crutches (if fitted with them).

After you return to your dorm/apartment/home:

1. Apply an ice or cold pack to the injury for _40_ minutes at the times circled below. To do this, remove the elastic wrap, put the ice pack directly over the injury, and reapply elastic wrap. The wrap should be snug, but not real tight (remove about 3/4 of the stretch).

    1:00   2:00   3:00 |4:00| 5:00 |6:00| 7:00 |8:00| 9:00 |10:00| 11:00 |12:00|

2. After each _40_ minute ice-pack application, remove the ice pack and **reapply** the elastic wrap (snugly, as above). Following the last ice-pack application, wear the elastic wrap through the night until you return for treatment tomorrow.

3. Keep the injured part above the level of your heart as much as possible (constantly if possible) until you go to bed tonight.

4. Tomorrow, report to:

    The Student Health Center at _____ am/pm

    The Athletic Training Clinic at _10_ am/pm

    _____ at _____ am/pm

    _____ at _____ am/pm

5. AT: _____k.knight_____

6. If you have problems that you feel need immediate attention, call me at _555-1896_

FIGURE 6.22 Giving written instructions to patients after initial RICES treatments increases patient compliance.

The Use of Crutches

Any patient who is unable to walk without a limp should be on crutches. Crutches make it possible for an injured person to walk properly (meaning without pain or a limp) by using the arms to substitute for, or supplement, leg power. Failure to use crutches will result in the following complications:

• Delayed healing. A person limps because the body weight aggravates the injury and causes pain. Neural inhibition results, thereby prolonging the rehabilitation process.

• Compensating muscle problems. The abnormal gait produced by limping causes muscles and other soft tissue surrounding the hip, knee, and/or ankle or the uninjured limb to shorten and tighten. Sometimes the resulting tightness will persist long after the original injury has healed.

Both of these complications can be minimized by the proper use of crutches. Correct crutch use requires:

- The proper fitting of the crutches,
- Selecting the appropriate crutch walking gait,
- Instructing the patient to walk properly with the selected gait
- Observing the patient practicing the gait
- Periodic reevaluation of the patient to ensure that he/she is using the crutches properly

⚠ Modality Myth

CRUTCHES GO IN THE ARMPIT

A common misconception is that crutches should fit into the axillae (armpits) so that the shoulders bear the body weight. This is wrong! The weight of the body must be supported almost entirely by the hands; the remainder is supported by the upper lateral chest wall. Carrying the weight of the body in the axillae can cause contusion or concussion to the nerves of the brachial plexus, resulting in **crutch palsy,** a temporary or permanent loss of either sensation or the ability to move or control movement.

PROPER CRUTCH FITTING

Fitting the crutches to the patient is essential to proper usage. First, adjust the length of the crutches so that there are 2–3 in. between the axillae and the axillary pads (Fig. 6.23a). This adjustment is usually made by removing the two wing nuts and then the two screws near the bottom of the crutches. (Aluminum crutches have a push-button adjustment.) A preliminary adjustment can be made with the patient lying, but the wing nuts should not be tightened until the adjustment has been confirmed with the patient standing.

Second, adjust the handpiece so that the elbow is flexed to ~30° and the wrist is in a comfortable weight-bearing position (Fig. 6.23b). If the position is correct, the patient should lift herself slightly off the floor when pushing down and extending her arms. This adjustment is made by removing the wing nut and screw through the handpiece.

SELECTING THE PROPER GAIT

Selecting the appropriate crutch walking gait depends on how much weight the injured limb can comfortably tolerate. Although there are a number of crutch walking gaits, two are most applicable to lower extremity trauma patients: the non-weight-bearing gait and the partial weight-bearing gait. The **non-weight-bearing gait,** also known as the swing-through gait, is used when the objective is to completely remove weight from one leg or foot (Fig. 6.24a). The

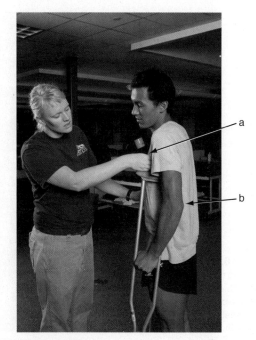

FIGURE 6.23 Crutches are properly fitted when **(a)** there are 2–3 in. between the axilla and axillary pad of the crutch, and **(b)** when the arm is bent about 30°.

injured limb is lifted and the patient walks alternatively on the good leg and the two crutches. This gait should not be used any longer than necessary, though, because it can cause hip and knee tightness as is caused by limping.

The preferred gait for patients with acute orthopedic trauma is the partial weight-bearing gait—also called the *three-point gait* (Fig. 6.24b)—as long as it can be performed pain free. The patient walks as with a normal gait, except for using the crutches to remove just enough weight from the injured limb to eliminate pain and limping. Weight borne by the injured leg will vary from light toe touching to almost full body weight. As the patient's injury heals, more weight is taken by the foot, and less by the hands and crutches.

WALKING INSTRUCTIONS

Instructing the patient in the selected gait is merely telling him when to move the crutches.

- "Think of the crutches as part of your injured limb."
- For the partial weight-bearing gait, "The two crutches are in contact with the ground simultaneously with the injured limb. As you move the injured limb forward, move both the crutches forward also."
- For the non-weight-bearing gait, "Your body weight is totally supported by the uninjured leg while both crutches are placed 12–24 in. in front of the feet. Then transfer your weight to the crutches as you lift your body and swing through to a point 12–24 in. in front of the crutches."

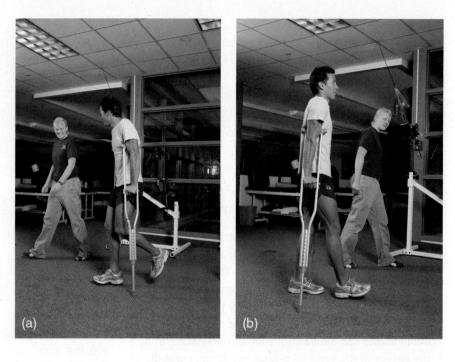

FIGURE 6.24 The purpose of crutch walking is to remove weight from the injured limb or foot. It can be **(a)** total, as with the non-weight-bearing or swing-through gait, or **(b)** partial, as with the partial weight-bearing or three-point gait.

Walking up and down stairs requires special training, because swinging might cause a loss of balance. The following instructions apply no matter which gait the patient uses on level ground:

- For going downstairs: "Begin by lowering the crutches down a step, follow with the injured leg, and then lower the hips down between the crutches. The uninjured leg is brought down last."
- For going upstairs: "The uninjured leg is lifted first, followed by the injured leg, and then the crutches."
- "The phrase 'the good go up to heaven, the bad go down to hell' might help you remember which foot/leg goes first when walking up and down stairs."

The patient should also be instructed not to use a single crutch. With a single crutch, the patient will not stand up straight when walking, and the leaning will cause tightness in the lower back, hip, or knee. Although minimal, the tightness will affect post-injury activities and make the patient susceptible to further injury.

OBSERVING THE PATIENT PRACTICING THE GAIT

Watch the patient walk around long enough until you are satisfied that she has mastered the technique. Going up and down some stairs is part of the practice that should be observed.

PERIODIC REEVALUATION

Periodic reevaluation of the patient should be done so that she will not subconsciously develop a deviant gait pattern that will result in problems after the crutches are no longer needed. This is best done when the patient is unaware that she is being watched. The important thing is for you to make sure that she is walking with as near to a normal gait as possible.

Medicated Ice for Abrasions

Athletes often suffer skin abrasions. An abrasion can become a complicated injury if not handled properly. Proper management includes the standard injury first aid of ice, compression, and elevation to limit pain, swelling, and secondary injury, and also managing potential bacterial contamination.[122]

Neither of the two most popular treatments for abrasions is comprehensive. One treats the injury like a sprain or strain with RICES and ignores the possibility of infection. The other treats the open wound by cleaning it and applying an antiseptic and sterile wound dressing, but ignores the possibility of secondary injury and swelling. MacLeod[122] suggested combining cryotherapy with an antiseptic by applying ice massage to abrasions with medicated ice cups (Fig. 6.25).

A medicated ice cup is sometimes referred to as a medicated popsicle. The povidone-iodine in the ice, like all antiseptics, discourages the formation and propagation of bacteria. The indications, contraindications, and precautions for the povidone-iodine and lidocaine are provided with each medicine.

Ice also acts as an analgesic. Using medicated ice composed of 2% lidocaine produces an even greater analgesic effect, which is necessary when brushing or

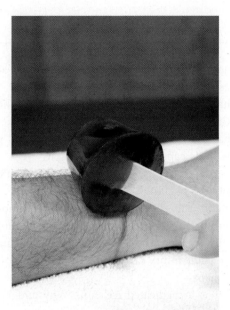

FIGURE 6.25 Ice massage with a medicated ice cup treats abrasions with antiseptic and cryotherapy.

picking dirt and debris out of an open wound. The decrease in pain from the ice and lidocaine also leads to a slowing of the pain-spasm-pain cycle, which helps enhance muscle function around the injury. It is easy to avoid wound infection when the injury is treated early and properly.

PREPARING A MEDICATED POPSICLE

The following materials and medicines are needed to make medicated popsicles:

- Four 2-oz disposable cups
- Plastic stir sticks
- 2% lidocaine
- 10% povidone-iodine
- Distilled or boiled water

Here are the steps:

1. Mix 3 oz of povidone-iodine, 1 oz of lidocaine, and 3 oz of water.
2. Pour the mixture into the four cups.
3. Secure a stir stick vertically in the center of each cup with adhesive tape.
4. Freeze overnight.
5. Clearly label the cups.
6. Isolate the medicated ice cups from other ice cups in the freezer so they are not accidently used for general ice massage (this wouldn't cause problems, but it would be a waste of resources).

HOW TO APPLY MEDICATED ICE

Here are the steps for applying ice massage to an abrasion using medicated ice cups. Do this as soon as possible after the injury:

1. Seek the advice and approval of a physician before applying medicated ice.
2. Hold the stir stick and roll the ice back and forth along the lacerated skin for about 10 minutes. As the ice melts, the medicines will flow into the damaged region and produce analgesic and antiseptic effects.
3. Debride the area (remove foreign materials) with gentle sweeps with a moist gauze pad, picking out foreign material with tweezers.
4. Treat and protect the injured area as you would any open wound, emphasizing sterility.
5. Apply, or instruct the patient to apply, an ice pack for 20–30 minutes each hour until bedtime and apply compression constantly (except when applying or taking off the ice pack) for the first 24–72 hours after the injury.

CLOSING SCENE

If Sammy would have read this chapter, he would realize that there is a lot more to ice application than filling a bag full of ice and putting it on the injury. Among other things, he would have learned the advantages and disadvantages of several types of ice application. He would have learned that applying an ice pack directly to the skin is not only safe but preferred because it provides better cooling than placing a towel or elastic wrap between the skin and the ice bag. He would know how long ice should be applied in various circumstances.

Chapter Reflections

1. Read and ponder each of the following points. Do you feel you have a clear understanding of each concept? If not, reread the appropriate section of the chapter.
   - What is immediate care, and when would you use it?
   - List seven modality myths about the immediate care of orthopedic injuries. For each one, briefly state the myth and the truth.
   - Are immediate care and acute care synonymous? Why or why not?
   - List the stages of acute injury care. Generally when does each occur?
   - What is meant by general time frames for the stages of acute injury care?
   - What does the mnemonic RICES stand for? Briefly describe each element and say why and when each one is most effective.
   - What is swelling, and why and when does it occur?
   - Explain what is meant by this statement: Cold during immediate care is more than swelling control.
   - What are the two most prominent theories about why cryotherapy is used during immediate care. State the major elements of each theory, and their strengths and weakness.
   - What is cold? How is cold transferred from a cold pack to the body?
   - Briefly discuss each of the seven factors that influence the rate of heat conduction from the body to a cold pack.
   - What is meant by the latent heat of fusion? What role does it play in RICES?
   - What is a phase change? How does it apply to cryotherapy?
   - Briefly explain the temperature response to cold pack application. Consider surface, tissue, intra-articular, and rewarming following application.
   - Briefly discuss each of the four major types of cold packs.
   - Should ice be applied directly to the skin? Why and/or why not?

   - What is meant by the depth of target tissue, and how does this apply to RICES?
   - What effect does skinfold thickness have on RICES?
   - What is the basis for stretching an elastic wrap to 75% of its capacity when applying it?
   - What is the difference between preventing and removing swelling?
   - Explain the difference between continuous and intermittent compression, and tell how each is used.
   - Briefly explain the use of crutches during acute orthopedic injury care. Tell why and how you would use them.
   - What is a medicated ice cup? Why and how is it used?
   - Briefly review the five-step process for RICES application.

2. Write three to five questions for discussion with your class instructor, clinical instructor, classmates, and clinical colleagues.

3. Get together with classmates and quiz each other on the concepts of this chapter. Use the points in reflection no. 1 and questions you wrote for reflection no. 2 as a beginning. Explaining concepts out loud to others requires a deeper grasp of the material than feeling you understand it as you read.

4. Once you feel you understand the principles of application of RICES and crutch walking, practice applying RICES using the five-step approach, with a classmate or clinical colleague. Also, fit crutches to a classmate or clinical colleague and instruct them in properly using them. Alternate applying the modalities to each other. When it is being applied to you, listen and observe carefully to determine whether your classmate is using proper application. Consult your notes when the modality is applied to you, and during the first few times you apply the modality to another person. Continue practicing the application until you can do so without using your notes.

Concept Check Responses

CONCEPT CHECK 6.1

The swing gait removes all weight from the injured limb, whereas with the three-point or walking gait, the patient uses the crutches to take enough weight off the injured limb

that he can walk with a normal gait. As the injury heals, the crutches support less and less weight. It is a matter of total rest (undesirable) vs. relative rest (desirable); one case aggravates the injury and the other helps resolve it.

CONCEPT CHECK 6.2

Agree: Cold application is the only element of RICES that limits additional injury. Thus, in a sense it is a preventive measure. It also reduces pain and swelling (edema).

Disagree: Focusing attention on ice application might cause you to think rest, compression, elevation, and stabilization are not that important. This could potentially result in your not using these additional elements, which would be a big mistake. Each of these elements contributes to controlling the injury sequelae.

REFERENCES

1. Matsen FA III, Questad K, Matsen AL. The effect of local cooling on postfracture swelling. A controlled study. *Clin Orthop Relat Res.* 1975;(109):201–206.
2. Sloan JP, Hain R, Pownall R. Clinical benefits of early cold therapy in accident and emergency following ankle sprain. *Arch Emerg Med.* 1989;6:1–6.
3. Bleakley C, McDonough S, MacAuley D. The use of ice in the treatment of acute soft-tissue injury: a systematic review of randomized controlled trials. *Am J Sports Med.* 2004;32(1):251–261.
4. Hubbard TJ, Aronson SL, Denegar CR. Does cryotherapy hasten return to participation? A systematic review. *J Athl Train.* 2004;39(1):88–94.
5. Basur RL, Shephard E, Mouzas GL. A cooling method in the treatment of ankle sprains. *Practitioner.* 1976;216(1296):708–711.
6. Hocutt JE Jr, Jaffe R, Rylander CR, et al. Cryotherapy in ankle sprains. *Am J Sports Med.* 1982;10(5):316–319.
7. Karren KJ, Hafen BQ, Limmer D, et al. *First Aid for Colleges and Universities.* 8th ed. New York: Pearson, Benjamin Cummings, 2004.
8. Altizer L. Strains and sprains. *Orthop Nurs.* 2003;22(6):404–409; quiz 410–401.
9. Bergfeld J, Halpern B. *Sports Medicine: Functional Management of Ankle Injuries.* Kansas City, MO: The American Academy of Family Physicians, 1991.
10. Garrett WE Jr. Muscle strain injuries: clinical and basic aspects. *Med Sci Sports Exerc.* 1990;22(4):436–443.
11. Bennett D. Water at 67 degrees to 69 degrees Fahrenheit to control hemorrhage and swelling encountered in athletic injuries. *J Natl Athl Train Assoc.* 1961;1f:12–14.
12. Järvinen T, Järvinen T, Kääriäinen M, Kalimo H, Järvinen M. Muscle injuries: biology and treatment. *Am J Sports Med.* 2005;33(5):745–764.
13. Gregson W, Black M, Jones H, et al. Influence of cold water immersion on limb and cutaneous blood flow at rest. *Am J Sports Med.* 2011;39(6):1316–1323.
14. Deal DN, Tipton J, Rosencrance E, et al. Ice reduces edema. A study of microvascular permeability in rats. *J Bone Joint Surg Am.* 2002; 84-A(9):1573–1578.
15. Schwartz D, Kaplin K, Schwartz SI. Hemostasis, surgical bleeding, and transfusion. In: Brunicardi F, Anderson D, Billiar T, et al., eds. *Principles of Surgery.* Vol 8. 2nd ed. New York: McGraw-Hill Book Co., 2005.
16. Holloway GA Jr, Daly CH, Kennedy D, et al. Effects of external pressure loading on human skin blood flow measured by 133Xe clearance. *J Appl Physiol.* 1976;40:597–600.
17. Merrick MA, Knight KL, Ingersoll CD, et al. The effects of cold and compression on tissue temperatures at various depths. *J Athl Train.* 1993;28:236–245.
18. Hargens AR. Fluid shifts in vascular and extravascular spaces during and after simulated weightlessness. *Med Sci Sports Exerc.* 1982;15(5):421–427.
19. Kozin F, Cochrane CC. The contact activation system of plasma: biology and pathophysiology. In: Gallin JI, Snyderman R, eds. *Inflammation: Basic Principles and Clinical Correlates.* 3rd ed. Baltimore, MD: Lippincott Williams & Wilkins, 1999.
20. Butterfield T, Best T, Merrick MA. The dual roles of neutrophils and macrophages in inflammation: A critical balance between tissue damage and repair. *J Athl Train.* 2006;41(4):457–465.
21. Merrick MA. Secondary injury after musculoskeletal trauma: a review and update. *J Athl Train.* 2002;37(2):209–217.
22. Knight KL. The effects of hypothermia on inflammation and swelling. *Athl Train.* 1976;11:7–10.
23. Schaser K, Disch A, Stover J, et al. Prolonged superficial local cryotherapy attenuates microcirculatory impairment, regional inflammation, and muscle necrosis after closed soft tissue injury in rats. *Am J Sports Med.* 2007;35(1):93–102.
24. Oliveira NML, Rainero EP, Salvini TF. Three intermittent sessions of cryotherapy reduce the secondary muscle injury in skeletal muscle of rat. *J Sport Sci Med.* 2006;5:228–234.
25. Knight KL. *Cryotherapy in Sport Injury Management.* Champaign, IL: Human Kinetic, 1995.
26. Seiyama A, Shiga T, Maeda N. Temperature effect on oxygenation and metabolism of perfused rat hindlimb muscle. *Adv Exp Med Biol.* 1990;277:541–547.
27. Blair E. *Clinical Hypothermia.* New York: McGraw-Hill Book Co., 1964.
28. Abramson DI, Kahn A, Rejal H, et al. Relationship between a range of tissue temperature and local oxygen uptake in the human forearm. *Lab Clin Med.* 1957;50:789.
29. Hagerdal M, Harp J, Nilsson L, Siesjo BK. The effect of induced hypothermia upon oxygen consumption in the rat brain. *J Neurochem.* 1975;24(2):311–316.
30. Rosenfeldt FL. Myocardial preservation 1987: what is the state of the art? *Aust MZ J Surg.* 1987;57:349–353.
31. Shapiro M, Dunn D. Transplation. In: Brunicardi F, Anderson D, Billiar T, et al., eds. *Principles of Surgery.* Vol 8. 2nd ed. New York: McGraw-Hill Book Co., 2005.
32. Knight K. *Cryotherapy: Theory, Technique, and Physiology.* 1st ed. Chattanooga, TN: Chattanooga Corp., 1985.
33. Wilkerson GB. Management of the acute inflammatory response following joint trauma. *Sports Med Update.* 1992;7(3):12–15, 28.
34. Wilkerson GB. Treatment of ankle sprains with external compression and early mobilization. *Physician Sportsmed.* 1985;13:83.
35. Guyton AC, Hall JE. *Textbook of Medical Physiology.* 10th ed. Philadephia, PA: WB Saunders Company, 2000.
36. Levick JR, Michel CC. The effects of position and skin temperature on the capillary pressures in the fingers and toes. *J Physiol.* 1978;274:97–109.
37. Serway RA, Faughn JS. Energy in Thermal Processes. *College Physics.* 6th ed. Belmont, CA: Brooks/Cole, 2003:332–337.
38. Fisher D, Solomon S. *Therapeutic Heat and Cold.* 2nd ed. Baltimore, MD: Waverly Press, 1965.
39. Barcroft H, Edholm OG. The effect of temperature on blood flow and deep temperature in the human forearm. *J Physiol.* 1943;102:5–20.
40. Knight KL, Bryan KS, Halvorsen JM. Circulatory changes in the forearm during and after cold pack application and immersion in 1 degree C, 5 degrees C, and 15 degrees C water (abstract). *Int J Sports Med.* 1981;2.
41. Otte JW, Merrick MA, Ingersoll CD, Cordova ML. Subcutaneous adipose tissue thickness alters cooling time during cryotherapy. *Arch Phys Med Rehabil.* 2002;83(11):1501–1505.

42. Petrofsky J, Laymon M. Heat transfer to deep tissue: the effect of body fat and heating modality. *J Med Eng Technol.* 2009;33(5): 337–348.

43. Jutte LS, Hawkins J, Miller KC, Long BC, Knight KL. Skinfold Thickness at 8 Common Cryotherapy Sites in Various Athletic Populations. *J Athl Train.* 2012;47(2):170–177.

44. Lide DR. *CRC Handbook of Chemistry and Physics.* 86th ed. Boca Raton, FL: The Chemical Rubber Co., 2005.

45. Varpalotai MA, Knight KL. Pressures exerted by elastic wraps applied by beginning vs advanced student athletic trainers to the ankle vs the thigh with vs without an ice pack. *Athl Train.* 1991;26:246–250.

46. Knight KL, Aquino J, Johannes SM, Urban CD. A re-examination of Lewis' cold-induced vasodilatation-In the finger and ankle. *Athl Train.* 1980;15:248–250.

47. Knight K, Carmody LW. Rewarming of the ankle and forearm following 30 minutes of ice water immersion. Paper presented at the *National Athletic Trainers Association Annual Clinical Symposium,* Nashville, TN, June 1984.

48. Knight KL, Elam JE. Rewarming of the ankle, forearm, and finger after cryotherapy: further re-examination of Lewis' cold-induced vasodilatation. *J Can Athl Ther Assoc.* 1981;8(2):15–17.

49. Palmer J, Knight K. Ankle and thigh skin surface temperature changes with repeated ice pack application. *J Athl Train.* 1996;31:319–323.

50. Mancuso DL, Knight KL. Effects of prior physical activity on skin surface temperature response of the ankle during and after a 30 minute ice pack application. *J Athl Train.* 1992;27:242–249.

51. Post JB. *Ankle Skin Temperature Changes with a Repeated Ice Pack Application.* Terre Haute, IN: Physical Education, Indiana State University, 1991.

52. Waylonis GW. The physiologic effects of ice massage. *Arch Phys Med Rehab.* 1967;48:37–42.

53. Enwemeka CS, Allen C, Avila P, et al. Soft tissue thermodynamics before, during, and after cold pack therapy. *Med Sci Sports Exerc.* 2002;34(1):45–50.

54. Johannes SM, Knight KL. Temperature response during the warming phase of cryokinetics. 1979.

55. Abramson DI, Chu LSW, Tuck S, et al. Effect of tissue temperature and blood flow on motor nerve conduction velocity. *JAMA.* 1966;198:1082–1088.

56. Halar EM, DeLisa JA, Brozovich FV. Nerve conduction velocity: relationship of skin, subcutaneous intramuscular temperatures. *Arch Phys Med Rehabil.* 1980;61:199–203.

57. Hartviksen K. Ice Therapy in Spasticity. *Acta Neurol Scandinav.* 1962;38:79–84.

58. Borken N, Bierman W. Temperature changes produced by spraying with ethyl chloride. *Arch Phys Med Rehab.* 1955;36:288–290.

59. Petajan JH, Watts N. Effects of cooling on the tricps surae reflex. *J Am Phys Med.* 1962;41:240–251.

60. Ochs S, Smith C. Low temperature slowing and cold-block of fast axoplasmic transport in mammalian nerves in vitro. *J Neurobiol.* 1975;6:85–102.

61. Lowden BJ, Moore RJ. Determinates and nature of intramuscular temperature changes during cold therapy. *Am J Phys Med.* 1975;54:223–233.

62. Myrer WJ, Myrer KA, Measom GJ, et al. Muscle Temperature Is Affected by Overlying Adipose When Cryotherapy Is Administered. *J Athl Train.* 2001;36(1):32–36.

63. Lehmann JF, DeLateur BJ. Diathermy and superficial heat, laser, and cold therapy. In: Kottke FJ, Lehman JF, eds. *Krusen's Handbook of Physical Medicine and Rehabilitation.* Philadelphia, PA: WB Saunders Co., 1990:283–367.

64. Johnson DJ, Moore S, Moore J, Oliver RA. Effect of cold submersion on intramuscular temperature of the gastrocnemius muscle. *Phys Ther.* 1979;59:1238–1242.

65. Bocobo C, Fast A, Kingery W, Kaplan M. The effect of ice on intra-articular temperature in the knee of the dog. *Am J Phys Med.* 1991;70:181–185.

66. Wakim KG, Porter AN, Krusen FH. Influence of physical agents and of certain drugs on intra-articular temperature. *Arch Phys Med Rehab.* 1951;32:714–721.

67. McMaster W, Liddle S, Waugh T. Laboratory Cryotherapy influence on posttraumatic limb edema. *Clin Orthop Relat Res.* 1980;150: 283–287.

68. Kern H, Fessl L, Trnavsky G, Hertz H. Kryotherapie: das verlahten der gelenkstemperatur unter eisapplikation: grundlage fur die praktishe anwendung. *Wein Klin Wochenschr.* 1984;22:832–837.

69. Kim YH, Baek SS, Choi KS, Lee SG, Park SB. The effect of cold air application on intra-articular and skin temperatures in the knee. *Yonsei Med J.* 2002;43(5):621–626.

70. MacAuley D. Do textbooks agree on their advice on ice? *Clin J Sport Med.* 2001;11(2):67–72.

71. Mlynarczyk JH. *Skin Temperature Changes in the Ankle During and After Ice Pack Application of 10, 20, 30, 45, and 60 Minutes.* Terre Haute, IN: Physical Education Department, Indiana State University, 1984.

72. Bernards SA, Knight KL, Jutte LS. Surface and intramuscular temperature changes during ice and chemical cold pack application with and without a barrier. *J Athl Train.* 2003;38:S95 (abstract).

73. Plosser L. Cold Call: Icing an injury can speed recovery—if you do it right. From the December 2009 issue of Runner's World. Available at: http://www.runnersworld.com/article/0,7120,s6-241-286--13411-0,00. html. Accessed May, 2012.

74. Quinn E. Ice massage for a sports injury. *About.com.* Available at: http://sportsmedicine.about.com/od/treatinginjuries/qt/icemassage. htm. Accessed May, 2012.

75. Kennet J, Hardaker N, Hobbs S, Selfe J. Cooling efficiency of 4 common cryotherapeutic agents. *J Athl Train.* 2007;43(3):343–348.

76. Chesterton LS, Foster NE, Ross L. Skin temperature response to cryotherapy. *Arch Phys Med Rehabil.* 2002;83(4):543–549.

77. Boland AL. Rehabilitation of the Injured Athlete. In: Strauss RH, ed. *Sports Medicine and Physiology.* Philidelphia, PA: WB Saunders, 1979:226–234.

78. Mirkin G. Hot and cold: when to apply each to a running injury. *Runner.* 1980:22–23.

79. Belitsky RB, Odam SJ, Hubley-Kozey C. Evaluation of the effectiveness of wet ice, dry ice, and cryogen packs in reducing skin temperature. *Phys Ther.* 1987;67:1080–1084.

80. Urban CD. *Application of Ice, Compression, and Elevation to the Lateral Aspect of the Ankle.* Terre Haute, IN: Physical Education, Indiana State University, 1979.

81. LaVelle BE, Snyder M. Differential conduction of cold through barriers. *J Adv Nurs.* 1985;10(1):55–61.

82. Prentice WE. *Arnheim's Principles of Athletic Training.* 12th ed. St Louis, MO: McGraw-Hill, 2006.

83. Klafs C, Arnheim D. *Modern Principles of Athletic Training.* 4th ed. St. Louis, MO: CV Mosby Co., 1977.

84. Wallace L, Knortz K, Esterson P. Immediate care of ankle injuries. *J Orthop Sports Phys Ther.* 1979;1:46–50.

85. National Safety Council. *First Aid and CPR Essentials.* 98–103rd ed. Sudbury, MA: Jones and Bartlett Publishers, 1997.

86. Thygerson A, Gulli B, eds. *First Aid, CPR and AED.* 4th ed. Sudbury, MA: Jones and Bartlett Publishers, 2005.

87. Proulx RP. Southern California frostbite. *J Am Col Emerg Phys.* 1976;5(8):618.

88. Cluett J. How to ice an injury. *About.com.* Available at: http://orthopedics.about.com/cs/sprainsstrains/ht/iceinjury.htm. Accessed May, 2012.

89. Proctor. Reusable frozen "peas" to ice an injury. Available at: http://www.fitlink.com/reusable-frozen-peas-to-ice-an-injury. Accessed May, 2012.

90. Johnson N. *The Effects of Three Different Ice Bath Immersion Times on Numbness (Sensation of Pressure), Surface Temperature, and Perceived Pain.* Provo, UT: Exercise Sciences, Brigham Young University, 2003.

91. Wise D. Application of cold in treating soft tissue injury. *Coaching Sci Update.* 1979:53.

92. Hocutt JE Jr. Cryotherapy. *Am Fam Physician*. 1981;23:141–144.

93. DePodesta M. Cryotherapy in rehabilitation. *Can Athl Train Assoc J*. 1979;6:15–16.

94. Ork H. *Physical Therapy for Sports*. Philadelphia, PA: WB Saunders Co., 1982.

95. Chu DA, Lutt CJ. The rationale of ice therapy. *The Journal of the NATA*. 1969;4:8–9.

96. Hirata I. *The Doctor and the Athlete*. Philadelphia, PA: JB Lippincott Co., 1974.

97. Drez D, Faust DC, Evans JP. Cryotherapy and nerve palsy. *Am J Sports Med*. 1981;9(4):256–257.

98. Man IOW, Lepar GS, Morrissey MC, Cywinski JK. Effect of neuro-muscular electrical stimulation on foot/ankle volume during standing. *Med Sci Sports Exerc*. 2003;35(4):630–634.

99. Mora S, Zalavras CG, Wang L, Thordarson DB. The role of pulsatile cold compression in edema resolution following ankle fractures: a randomized clinical trial. *Foot Ankle Int*. 2002;23(11):999–1002.

100. Rucinski TJ, Hooker DN, Prentice WE, Shields EW, Cote-Murray DJ. The effects of intermittent compression on edema in postacute ankle sprains. *J Orthop Sports Physical Ther*. 1991;14:65–69.

101. Danielson R, Jaeger J, Rippetoe J, et al. Differences in skin surface temperature and pressure during the application of various cold and compression devices. *J Athl Train*. 1997;32:s–76.

102. Tomchuk D, Rubley MD, Holcomb WR, Giadagmoli M, Tarno JM. The magnitude of tissue cooling during cryotherapy with varied Types of compression. *J Athl Train*. 2010;45(3):230–237.

103. Duffley H, Knight K. Ankle compression variability using the elastic wrap, elastic wrap with a horseshoe, Edema II boot, and Air-Stirrup brace. *Athl Train*. 1989;24:320–323.

104. Appenzeller H, Ross CT. Utah: can a student trainer be held to the same standard of care of a physician or surgeon? *Sports Courts*.1984;5:11–13.

105. Harvey CK. An overview of cold injuries. *J Am Podiatr Med Assoc*. 1992;82(8):436–438.

106. Keatinge W, Cannon P. Freezing-point of human skin. *Lancet*. 1960;1:11–14.

107. Granberg P. Freezing cold injury. *Arctic Med Res*. 1991;50(6):76–79.

108. Kendall Demonstration Elementary School Health Services. Severe allergic reaction: hives (Urticaria) protocol. *Gallaudet University*. Available at: http://clerccenter.gallaudet.edu/SupportServices/schoolnurse/hive1b.html. Accessed January, 2006.

109. Dolan MG, Mendel FC. Clinical application of electrotherapy. *Athl Ther Today*. 2004;9(5):11–16.

110. Ralston DJ. High voltage galvanic stimulation: can there be a "state of the art"? *Athl Train*. 1985;(20):291–293.

111. Dolan MG, Thornton RM, Fish DR, Mendel FC. Effects of cold water immersion on edema formation after blunt injury to the hind limbs of rats. *J Athl Train*. 1997;32(3):233–237.

112. Dolan MG, Mychaskiw AM, Mattacola CG, Mendel FC. Effects of cool-water immersion and high-voltage electric stimulation for 3 continuous hours on acute edema in rats. *J Athl Train*. 2003;38(4):325–329.

113. Dolan MG, Mychaskiw AM, Mendel FC. Cool-Water Immersion and High-Voltage Electric Stimulation Curb Edema Formation in Rats. *J Athl Train*. 2003;38:225–230.

114. McKeon PO, Dolan MG, Gandolph J, Grossman K, Koehneke PM. Effects of dependent positioning, cool water immersion and high voltage electrical stimulation on non-traumatized limb volumes. *J Athl Train*. 2003;38(2 Suppl):S-35.

115. Bettany JA, Fish DR, Mendel FC. Influence of high voltage pulsed direct current on edema formation following impact injury. *Phys Ther*. 1990;70(4):219–224.

116. Bettany JA, Fish DR, Mendel FC. High-voltage pulsed direct current: effect on edema formation after hyperflexion injury. *Arch Phys Med Rehabil*. 1990;71(9):677–681.

117. Fish DR, Mendel FC, Schultz AM, Gottstein-Yerke LM. Effect of anodal high voltage pulsed current on edema formation in frog hind limbs. *Phys Ther*. 1991;71(10):724–730; discussion 730–733.

118. Taylor K, Fish DR, Mendel FC, Burton HW. Effect of electrically induced muscle contractions on posttraumatic edema formation in frog hind limbs. *Phys Ther*. 1992;72(2):127–132.

119. Mendel FC, Fish DR. New perspectives in edema control via electrical stimulation. *J Athl Train*. 1993;28(1):63.

120. Taylor K, Mendel FC, Fish DR, Hard R, Burton HW. Effect of high-voltage pulsed current and alternating current on macromolecular leakage in hamster cheek pouch microcirculation. *Phys Ther*. 1997;77(12):1729–1740.

121. Thornton RM, Mendel FC, Fish DR. Effects of electrical stimulation on edema formation in different strains of rats. *Phys Ther*. 1998;78(4):386–393.

122. MacLeod J. Treating abrasions with medicated ice. *Phys Sportsmed*. 1985;13(8).

7

The Healing Process

OPENING SCENE

Sofia suffered a second-degree medial collateral ligament (MCL) sprain to her knee 2 days ago during basketball practice. She is concerned about her condition and asks you, "Why do I have all of this swelling, and when will it go away? How long until my ligament is healed, and what can I do to ensure that it heals as strongly as possible? When can I begin exercising?"

The Repair of Injured Tissue

Whenever tissue has been damaged during injury, it must be repaired. **Repair** consists of processes that replace dead or damaged cells with healthy ones.[1] Repair follows inflammation, after enough of the cellular debris has been removed to allow the repair processes to begin. Therefore, the bigger the hematoma, the longer it takes for repair to begin.

TYPES OF REPAIR: RECONSTITUTION AND REPLACEMENT

There are two types of repair: reconstitution with the same type of cells as were injured, and/or replacement with simpler cells.

Reconstitution occurs in cells that normally have a high rate of turnover (i.e., skin cells, liver cells, etc.). In *perfect reconstitution*, the cells that were damaged are replaced by identical cells, and there remains no evidence that the injury occurred. In *imperfect reconstitution*, most of the damaged cells are replaced by identical cells, but there is some replacement with connective tissue and thus some scar formation.

Replacement with simpler cells results in scar tissue formation. It occurs in connective tissue, muscle tissue, central nervous system tissue, and in any area where the damage is extensive enough to disrupt the basic cellular framework. This type of repair is also known as *repair by connective tissue,* and it can either be primary union or secondary union. *Primary union* occurs in an area with a small laceration or incision, such as a 1/3 in. (1 cm) cut on the chin (Fig. 7.1). It fills and heals very rapidly. *Secondary union* occurs when there is a large gap or hole to be filled, such as a 5-in. (13 cm) gaping laceration. Replacement is much slower and leaves a bigger scar.

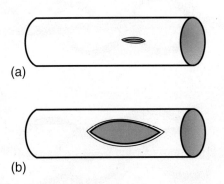

FIGURE 7.1 Replacement, or repair by connective tissue. **(a)** Primary union occurs when the wound is small and the wound edges are close together. **(b)** Secondary union occurs when there is a large gap or hole to be filled, such as a 13 cm gaping laceration. Replacement is much slower and leaves a bigger scar.

 CONCEPT CHECK 7.1. Based on the information presented above, why is it important to close lacerations quickly following an injury? Why is it even more important to quickly close them on the face?

The Phases of Repair

Like the inflammatory response (see Chapter 5), repair is:

- a sequence of hundreds of events that follow one another, but that overlap because they occur at the same time in different parts of the damaged area.[2,3]
- controlled by a complex, precisely coordinated balance of signaling factors (such as growth factors and cytokines) that are expressed and regulated in a temporospatial manner.[3,4]

These events have been organized into phases in various ways. And although the names of the phases differ, the events within the phases are the same. Contemporary authors organize the process into three[3,5] or four[6] phases—the only difference is the inclusion of hemostasis or epithelialization as a separate phase.

1. Hemostasis and inflammation
2. Epithelialization
3. Proliferation
4. Remodeling

HEMOSTASIS AND INFLAMMATION

The hemostasis and inflammation phase of repair is the same as the hemodynamic, leukocyte migration, and phagocytosis phases of the inflammatory response. Some authors consider it a separate phase, so as to emphasize the importance of the vascular responses to healing.[3]

Hemostasis is the arrest or stoppage of bleeding[7]; the opposite of hemorrhaging (see Chapter 5). The platelets within the clot are more than a plug; they release a variety of chemical mediators to signal various healing activities.[3]

This is followed by macrophages scavenging the cellular debris. The circulatory and lymphatic systems (mostly lymphatic) drain away the liquefied cellular remains, which are mostly small particles of free protein. This is very important because the more protein that remains, the bigger the scar will be,[8] a condition known as a **keloid**.[9]

Lymphatic Drainage and Exercise

The lymphatic system is passive; its vessel walls do not contract, nor is there any pressure to cause fluid to move through it, such as provided by the heart to the venous system. The lymphatic system depends on external force to promote fluid movement—for example, distal-to-proximal massage or muscular contraction. As a muscle expands in size during contraction, it squeezes the lymph vessels and forces their contents upstream toward their junction with the vascular system (see Fig. 6.20). Thus manual massage, intermittent compression pumps, or moderate activity during the cellular phase of repair will promote lymphatic drainage and hasten healing.

EPITHELIALIZATION

The process of developing a membranous tissue covering (epithelium) over exposed tissue or organs is called **epithelialization**.[4] In the case of a blister or superficial abrasion, the majority or all of healing is epithelialization. With more severe injuries, it protects the body from assault by outside organisms as the wound proceeds through the remaining wound healing phases.[6]

PROLIFERATION

The **proliferation phase** consists of three major events: angiogenesis (growth of new blood vessels), collagen synthesis (also known as collagenization), and wound contraction (the drawing together of the wound edges).[6]

Angiogenesis

Angiogenesis is a transient phase during which lots of new blood vessels are formed, (which later disappear). These vessels are necessary to deliver the great amounts of oxygen and nutrients to the wound area needed for repair.[6] This phase usually takes 4 to 6 days.

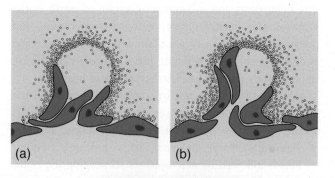
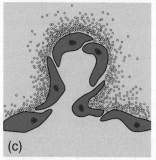

FIGURE 7.2 Capillary budding. New blood vessels are formed as the endothelial cells at a budding site on an existing vessel divide. **(a)** They slide past each other into **(b)** positions distal to their place of origin and **(c)** form a bud.

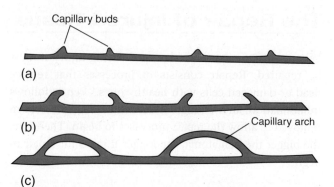

FIGURE 7.3 (a) Capillary arches are formed by numerous capillary buds along a vessel. **(b)** Initially the buds grow randomly into the injured tissue, eventually moving toward each other where **(c)** they join to form a capillary arch. Once the arches form, blood begins flowing through them to supply fibroblasts and oxygen to rebuild the injured tissue.

A process known as **capillary budding** is the primary mechanism of the vascular phase of the repair process (Fig. 7.2). Endothelial cells of existing vessels at the edge of the wound begin to divide. The new cells crawl away from, but keep contact with, the existing vessel. New cells force themselves between existing cells, thus forcing the end cells to advance into the wound area.

Adjacent capillary buds migrate toward one another, meet, form together, and create a **capillary arch** (Fig. 7.3). Blood then begins to flow through the arch, and new budding begins from the arch. Soon a network of these arches, or a **capillary arcade**, is formed (Fig. 7.4). The network eventually develops throughout the entire wound area, providing abundant circulation, which is necessary to support collagenization.

Eventually, after collagen synthesis is completed, and the need for abundant circulation has passed, most of the new vessels will atrophy. A few will form into arterioles, some into venules, and some will remain as capillaries.

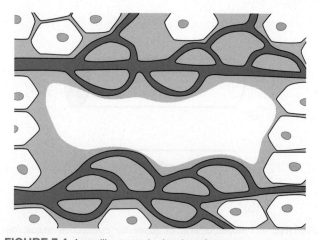

FIGURE 7.4 A capillary arcade develops from numerous capillary arches from the blood vessels on the periphery of the injured tissue. Most of these new vessels will collapse once the tissue is healed and the need for oxygen drastically decreases.

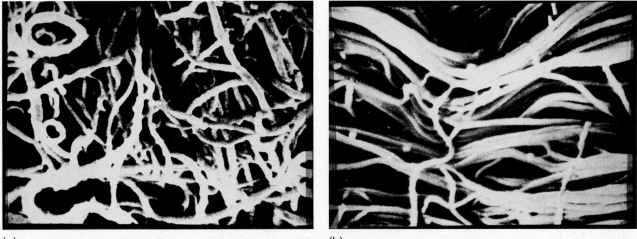

(a)   (b)

FIGURE 7.5 Electron micrographs of human collagen. (**a**) New collagen fibers assemble haphazardly at first. (**b**) The same site weeks later after the collagen has realigned in a parallel fashion. Note how the new collagen appears like a plate of cooked spaghetti, while the more mature collagen looks more like uncooked spaghetti right out of the box. (Courtesy of John Burgfeld, MD.)

Collagen Synthesis

Collagen synthesis or *collagenization* is the process of manufacturing and laying down collagen in the wound space. **Collagen**, a fibrous protein found in all types of connective tissue, is the primary solid substance of ligaments, tendons, and scar tissue. It is made by fibroblasts, cells that migrate along strands of fibrin into the wound area, but do not move far beyond the capillary arcade. They then begin to manufacture fibers of collagen, which extrude haphazardly into the wound space (Fig. 7.5a). Within 4–6 days after the injury, vascularization is maximal, and collagenization is operating at its peak. Most collagen is laid down within 15–20 days after the injury.[10] The wound is not very strong yet; many of the fibers are diagonal or parallel to the wound edges, and, therefore, do little to hold the wound edges together. In time, the collagen will realign so that it is directly from one edge of the wound to the other, making the wound strong (Fig. 7.5b). The collagen strands realign parallel to the *lines of force*, so gentle activity is essential. This realignment sometimes takes up to a year, especially if the patient is inactive.

Collagenization requires great amounts of oxygen.[11,12] Oxygen provides energy (through aerobic metabolism) for the fibroblasts to function and also is an essential building block of collagen. Healing wounds normally do not have all the oxygen that they could use (Fig. 7.6).[12] The amount of collagen accumulated in a wound area, and the tensile strength of skin wounds, are linearly related

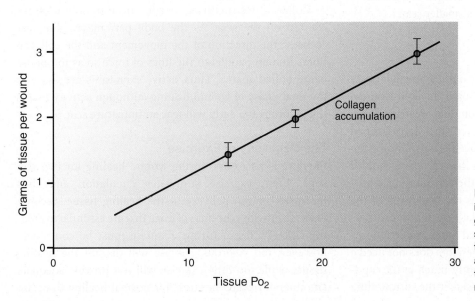

FIGURE 7.6 The need for oxygen in a healing wound is illustrated in this graph of collagen accumulation and tissue (oxygen partial pressure, pO_2). Note the linear relationship between collagen accumulation and pO_2 when pO_2 is less than normal, normal, and higher than normal. (Source: Adapted from Silver.[13])

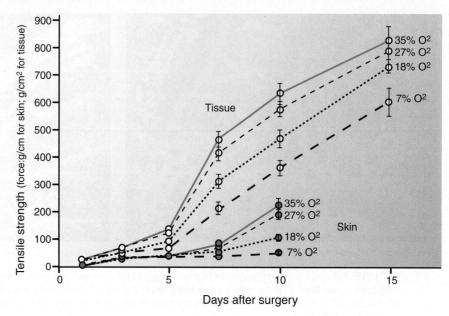

FIGURE 7.7 The effect of changing oxygen supply on wound healing. The more oxygen available, the stronger the wound becomes. (Source: Adapted from Niinikoski.[14])

to the amount of oxygen available to the healing wound[14] (Fig. 7.7). **Tensile strength** is a measure of the amount of longitudinal stress a wound can withstand before tearing apart. Increasing the percentage of oxygen in the air breathed by injured laboratory rats between days 5 and 15 resulted in greater tensile strength of their wounds.[14]

Wound Contraction

Wound contraction pulls the sides of the wound together in an attempt to close it.[6] The primary actor in this process is the **myofibroblast**, a cell that appears as a cross between a fibroblast and a smooth muscle cell. Like a smooth muscle cell, they contain actin and myosin, so they can contract and relax. The more myofibroblasts that are laid down, the smaller the wound is and so the less collagen that is needed to close the wound. This results in a smaller scar.

THE REMODELING PHASE

The remodeling phase consists of two processes that cause the scar to become smaller, more pale (in light-skinned people), and stronger: **contraction** and **restructuring**. A new scar will appear to be quite red (in a light-skinned person) and mounded or raised above the surrounding tissue. With time, the appearance of the scar changes until it is pale and flat or sunken below the surrounding skin.

Contraction, the first process, is the collapsing of the capillary arcade. Collagen is a relatively inactive tissue; once it is laid down, it does not need much oxygen to satisfy its energy requirements, and therefore does not need a great deal of circulation. Consequently, much of the capillary arcade collapses and is compressed by the surrounding

collagen. This accounts for most of the contraction of the scar. Also, with less blood circulating through the wound, the scar appears paler.

In **restructuring**, the second process, the collagen itself is restructured. This occurs concurrently with contraction. The collagen fibers are reorganized from the haphazard way they were laid down to a parallel arrangement (see Fig. 7.5b). This reorganization of fibers causes the scar to become more compact, and thus concave. But compactness is not the major reason reorganization occurs.

Collagen fiber reorganization is necessary to give the scar greater strength. Fibers running parallel to the wound edges will not help keep the edges of the wound together. Only fibers connecting the wound edges strengthen the injured tissue (Fig. 7.8).

Collagen restructuring occurs in response to force exerted on the scar. As the body part moves, the scar "senses" the direction of the movement and the collagen fibers line up parallel to the lines of force so as to oppose being pulled apart.[10] Thus, active exercise is necessary to the final phase of wound healing, although activity that is too vigorous too early will tear an immature scar.

The Necessity of Exercise

Exercise is necessary during wound healing for two reasons. First, exercise stimulates circulation and thus increases oxygen delivery to the healing tissue. Second, exercise provides the lines of force that are essential to guiding collagen restructuring. Exercise must be controlled, however; too vigorous exercise will disrupt the healing tissue, while too little exercise will not provide adequate amounts of oxygen or stress for normal healing to occur.

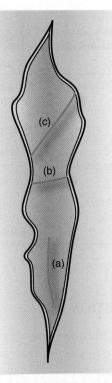

FIGURE 7.8 Model of tissue with a laceration, and newly laid down collagen fibers. The haphazard configuration (see Fig. 7.5a) gives little tensile strength to the wound. In this simplified model, fibers oriented as in (a) are useless in holding the edges of the wound together, whereas those in (b) provide maximal support. Fibers oriented as in (c) give minimal support. The wound gains strength during remodeling as fibers such as (a) and (c) are realigned to be more like fiber (b).

There is a fine line between the amount of exercise that optimizes tissue repair and that which compromises the repair process (see Fig. 1.5).

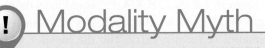

Modality Myth

HEALING TISSUE MUST BE RESTED

Some people believe that healing tissue must be rested in order to prevent tearing the injured tissue. While it is true that too vigorous exercise is counterproductive, complete rest will actually slow or prevent healing (see Fig. 1.5). Moderate, controlled exercise is essential for stimulating collagenization and restructuring of the injured tissue and for maintaining normal nerve function. It also is psychologically beneficial for the patient to be doing something other than waiting for healing to take place.

TRAFFIC AND TRAFFIC CONTROLLERS

Each step in the healing process results from a complex balance of signaling factors and proteins.

Healing Modifiers

The body's natural healing process can be facilitated (speeded up) or hindered (slowed down) in many ways. Obviously, your goal is to help the healing process, so you need to eliminate the hindrances and aid the facilitators. Following are the most common facilitators or modifiers.

IMMEDIATE CARE PROCEDURES

The size of the hematoma affects healing time in two ways: the smaller the hematoma is, the quicker repair can begin and the less there is to repair.[2] Can you affect the size of the hematoma? Yes! Aggressively treating the injury as soon after it occurs as possible (within minutes) can have a major influence (see Chapter 6).

MANAGE PAIN AND THE PATIENT'S REACTION TO PAIN

Pain, patients experience with prior pain, and how they react to the present pain can have wide-ranging effects on the healing process; from hindering and delaying to facilitating and speeding up the healing process.[15,16] Pain is a symptom that does not necessarily correlate directly to injury or illness.[15] A person's response to pain is cultivated, or developed, over time; a concept referred to as "learned pain,"[15,16] and is quite malleable.

It is imperative that you have open conversations about pain throughout the healing process so as to minimize the negative effects of pain on healing and facilitate the positive. These topics are covered in Chapters 8 and 9. (See especially the sections on Dehne's Spinal Adaptation Syndrome, the Placebo Effect, and Learned Pain in Chapter 9).

CLOSING LACERATIONS QUICKLY

Lacerations must be sutured or steri-stripped to close the wound gap, thus allowing healing by primary union. For best results, these procedures should be done within 4 to 6 hours after the wound occurs.

Sutures, Steri-Strips, and Glue

Some surgeons avoid using sutures to close lacerations because implanting sutures into the tissue causes additional tissue injury and invokes additional inflammation as the body tries to destroy the sutures, a foreign substance. Steri-strips (Fig. 7.9) or the newly developed tissue glue are less traumatic to the tissue. But they also are not as effective for athletic injuries, when the athlete continues physical activity, which places additional stresses on the tissue.

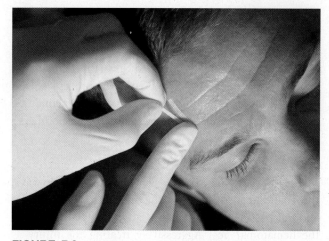

FIGURE 7.9 Steri-strips are effective in holding small wounds together when there is not too much stress on the tissue.

TABLE 7.1	THE ROLE OF THERAPEUTIC MODALITIES IN WOUND HEALING
THERAPEUTIC GOAL	**MODALITIES**
Stimulate healing process	Ultrasound Electrical muscle stimulation Hot packs
Promote lymphatic drainage to hasten the cellular phase of the repair process	Massage Cryokinetics Edema pressure devices
Moderate pain, thereby facilitating therapeutic exercise	Cryokinetics Cryostretch TENS

THERAPEUTIC EXERCISE

Therapeutic exercise can either facilitate or hinder healing (see Fig. 1.5). As discussed earlier, exercise is essential to healing—to both stimulate blood flow during collagenization in order to bring more oxygen to the wound site, and to stimulate and guide the reorienting of collagen fibers during the restructuring phase. Lack of exercise will delay healing. On the other hand, too vigorous exercise will tear the healing tissue and thus delay healing.

✔ APPLICATION TIP

KNOW THE RIGHT EXERCISE AMOUNT

How do you determine how much exercise is enough without going over the line? Remember two principles. First: Pain must be avoided during rehabilitation. Pain during an activity tells you that the patient is exercising too vigorously. Also, pain on the following day tells you that yesterday's exercise was too vigorous. In either case, reduce the amount of exercise. Second: Use progressive resistance exercise. Many patients are reluctant to exercise, thinking exercise will disrupt the healing tissue. Encourage them to begin slow, simple range of motion (ROM) exercises, and progressively increase the complexity.

THERAPEUTIC MODALITIES

The role of therapeutic modalities is to assist the body in its normal healing process (Table 7.1).[17] Some modalities accomplish this task by stimulating healing. Others promote lymphatic drainage, which hastens the cellular phase of the repair process. Still others moderate pain, thereby facilitating therapeutic exercise.

PROPER NUTRITION

Many vitamins and trace elements are essential to healing. Although there is no evidence that supplementing with extra amounts of these substances improves or accelerates healing, a lack of them will hinder the process. People who eat a healthy, normal, well-balanced diet do not need to supplement with multiple vitamins.

HYPERBARIC OXYGEN THERAPY

Hyperbaric oxygen therapy (abbreviated HBOT; Barnett, 2006 #5577; Niezgoda, 2012 #5569)[18–20] OHB,[21] HBO[22–24] involves patients breathing 100% oxygen while sitting or lying in a chamber in which the atmospheric pressure is above 1.4[25] atmospheres absolute (ATA), but typically between 2.0 and 2.5 ATA,[20–22] equal to swimming at a depth of 33 to 39 ft. The result is a 125% increase in the amount of oxygen carried by the blood.[26] In-depth reviews of the physiological mechanisms are available elsewhere.[19–20]

The use of HBO has exploded in the past 20 years, mostly in treating patients with compromised wound healing,[20,22] where loss of function, limb, or life is threatened.[25] Its use in treating sports injuries is controversial, however.[22,27] Although oxygen is an integral component for wound healing,[19] and there are many adherents of HBOT,[26,27] there are equally as many opponents.[24,28,29]

Proponents argue for the therapy on the basis of its theoretical benefits, while opponents argue against it because of its potential risks,[24] high cost, and the lack of clinical or scientific evidence that it speeds healing of wounds that occur in sport.[24]

At present, HBOT is recognized as "adjunctive therapy (to be used) only after there are no measurable signs of healing for at least 30 days of treatment with standard wound therapy and must be used in addition to standard wound care.[25] This obviously is outside the realm of athletic trainer (AT) philosophy, which is to return patients to activity as quickly as possible.

More randomized controlled clinical trials with larger sample sizes must be conducted before hyperbaric oxygen can be established as a safe adjunctive therapy for soft tissue sports injuries.[22–24,30]

CLOSING SCENE

Recall Sofia's questions concerning the healing of her second-degree MCL sprain? You now can answer her. You tell her of your plan of action to get rid of the swelling. By decreasing the size of the hematoma, healing will take place faster. Then after completing a graded exercise program that is rigorous enough to lay down collagen without tearing it, she will be able to return to activity.

Chapter Reflections

1. Read and ponder each of the following points. Do you feel you have a clear understanding of each concept? If not, reread the appropriate section of the chapter.
   - Define repair and its four phases.
   - Explain the relationship between inflammation and repair.
   - Define the two types of repair and how they differ.
   - Explain why exercise is important during tissue repair and the phases of repair during which it is most beneficial.
   - Explain the difference between a capillary arch and a capillary arcade, and describe the role that each one plays in repair.
   - Explain why a scar is red (in light-skinned people) and mounded at one time and pale and sunken at others.
   - Explain what modifiers of inflammation are, and how they can help or hinder repair. Include immediate care procedures; closing lacerations quickly; sutures, steri-strips, and glue; therapeutic exercise; therapeutic modalities; hyperbaric oxygen therapy; proper nutrition.

2. Write three to five questions for discussion with your class instructor, clinical instructor, classmates, and clinical colleagues.

3. Get together with classmates and quiz each other on the concepts of this chapter. Use the points in reflection no. 1 and questions you wrote for reflection no. 2 as a beginning. Explaining concepts out loud to others requires a deeper grasp of the material than feeling you understand it as you read.

Concept Check Responses

CONCEPT CHECK 7.1

The quicker the laceration is closed, the smaller the scar is. The farther apart the wound edges are, the more collagen will be deposited in the space. Minimizing the size of scars is especially important on the face. But there are always some who feel scars are a badge of honor. Don't give patients a choice, just patch them up as quickly as possible.

REFERENCES

1. Chettibi S, Ferguson MWJ. Wound repair: an overview. In: Gallin JI, Snyderman R, eds. *Inflammation: Basic Principles and Clinical Correlates*. 3rd ed. Philadelphia, PA: Lippincott Williams & Wilkins, 1999.
2. Hunt TK, Hopf H, Hussain Z. Physiology of wound healing. *Adv Skin Wound Care*. 2000;13(2 Suppl):6–11.
3. Ozturk F, Ermertcan A. Wound healing: a new approach to the topical wound care. *Cutan Ocul Toxicol*. 2011;30(2):92–99.
4. Raja SK, Garcia MS, Isseroff RR. Wound re-epithelialization: modulating keratinocyte migration in wound healing. *Front Biosci*. 2007;12(May):1249–1268.
5. Park E, Lee SM, Jung I-K, Lim Y, Kim J-H. Effects of genistein on early-stage cutaneous wound healing. *Biochem Biophys Res Commun*. 2011;410:514–519.
6. Sussman C, Bates-Jensen BM. Skin and soft tissue anatomy and wound healing physiology. In: Sussman C, Bates-Jensen BM, eds. *Wound Care: A Collaborative Practice Manual for Health Professionals*. 4th ed. Baltimore, MD: Lippincott Williams & Wilkins, 2012:17–52.
7. Merriam-Webster's Online Dictionary. *Accessed via OneLook Dictionary Search, OneLook.com* [website]. Available at: http://www.merriam-webster.com/dictionary/rehabilitation. Accessed November, 2011.
8. Kushner I, Rzewnicki D. Acute phase response. In: Gallin JI, Snyderman R, eds. *Inflammation: Basic Principles and Clinical Correlates*. 3rd ed. Philadelphia, PA: Lippincott Williams & Wilkins, 1999.
9. Dioufa N, Schally A, Chatzistamou I, et al. Acceleration of wound healing by growth hormone-releasing hormone and its agonists. *Proc Natl Acad Sci U S A*. 2010;107(43):18611–18615.
10. Enwemeka CS. Inflammation, cellularity, and fibrillogenesis in regenerating tendon: implications for tendon rehabilitation. *Phys Ther*. 1989;69(10):816–825.
11. Niinikoski J. Oxygen and wound healing. *Clin Plast Surg*. 1977;4(3):361–374.
12. Ehrlick HP, Grislis C, Hunt TK. Metabolic and circulatory contributions to oxygen gradients in wounds. *Surgery*. 1972:578–583.
13. Silver IA. The measurement of oxygen tension in healing tissue. *Progr Resp Res*. 1968;3:124–135.
14. Niinikoski J. Effect of oxygen supply on wound healing and formation of experimental granulation tissue. *Acta Physiol Scand Suppl*. 1969;334:1–72.
15. Tyrer S. Learned pain behaviour. *Br Med J*. 1986;292(6512):1–2.
16. Sussman C. Preventing and modulating learned wound pain. *Ostomy Wound Manage*. 2008;54(11):38–47.
17. Sussman C, Bates-Jensen B. *Wound Care A Collaborative Practice Manual for Physical Therapists and Nurses*. 2nd ed. Baltimore, MD: Lippincott Williams & Wilkins, 2001.
18. Barnett, A. Using recovery modalities between training sessions in elite athletes: does it help? *Sports Med (Auckland, N.Z.)*. 1996;22(4):219–227.
19. Adkinson C. Hyperbaric oxygen for treatment of problem wounds. *Minn Med*. 2011;94(11):41–46.
20. Niezgoda JA. Hyperbaric oxygen therapy: management of the hypoxic wound. In: Sussman C, Bates-Jensen BM, eds. *Wound Care: A Collaborative Practice Manual for Health Professionals*. 4th ed. Baltimore, MD: Lippincott Williams & Wilkins, 2012:781–791.
21. Drobnic F, Turmo A. Hyperbaric oxygen treatment of musculoskeletal disorders on the sports medicine. State of the art. *Med Clin (Barc)*. 2010;134(7):312–315.
22. Babul S, Rhodes EC. The role of hyperbaric oxygen therapy in sports medicine. *Sports Med (Auckland, N.Z.)*. 2000;30(6):395–403.
23. Ishii Y, Deie M, Adachi N, et al. Hyperbaric oxygen as an adjuvant for athletes. *Sports Med (Auckland, N.Z.)*. 2005;35(9):739–746.
24. Kanhai A, Losito JM. Hyperbaric oxygen therapy for lower-extremity soft-tissue sports injuries. *J Am Podiatr Med Assoc*. 2003;93(4):298–306.
25. CMS. National Coverage Determination (NCD) for Hyperbaric Oxygen Therapy (20.29). *United States Centers for Medicare & Medicaid Services*. Available at: http://www.cms.gov/medicare-coverage-database/details/ncd-details.aspx?NCDId=12&ncdver=3&NCAId=37&NcaName=Hyperbaric+Oxygen+Therapy+for+Hypoxic+Wounds+and+Diabetic+Wounds+of+the+Lower+Extremities&IsPopup=y&bc=AAAAAAAAIAAA&. Accessed June, 2012.
26. Strauss MB. Letter regarding editorial on "Hyperbaric Oxygen Therapy in Sports". *Am J Sports Med*. 1999;27(2):265–266.
27. Staples J, Clement D. Hyperbaric oxygen chambers and the treatment of sports injuries. *Sports Med (Auckland, N.Z.)*. 1996;22(4):219–227.
28. Committee AR. Hyperbaric oxygen therapy in sports (editorial). *Am J Sports Med*. 1998;26(4):489–499.
29. Committee AR. Hyperbaric oxygen therapy in sports (response to letter). *Am J Sports Med*. 1999;27(2):265–266.
30. O'Reilly D, Linden R, Fedorko L, et al. A prospective, double-blind, randomized, controlled clinical trial comparing standard wound care with adjunctive hyperbaric oxygen therapy (HBOT) to standard wound care only for the treatment of chronic, non-healing ulcers of the lower limb in patients with diabetes mellitus: a study protocol. *Trials*. 2011;12(1):69.

Review Questions

Part II

Chapter 5

1. A clot is formed by _____ and platelets.
   a. fibrin
   b. collagen
   c. protocollagen
   d. fibroblasts
   e. both b and c

2. Which of the following cleans up most of the tissue debris during the inflammatory response?
   a. polymorph
   b. macrophage
   c. fibrin
   d. fibroblasts
   e. neutrophils

3. Which of the following is *not* a sign of inflammation?
   a. heat
   b. redness
   c. swelling
   d. loss of function
   e. All of the above are signs of inflammation.

4. Opening of the endothelial walls of blood vessels and capillaries so that blood cells can move out of the blood vessel occurs during which event of inflammation?
   a. leukocyte migration
   b. metabolic changes
   c. neutrophilic changes
   d. vascular changes
   e. permeability changes

5. A local reaction of the body tissues to any irritant is called _____.
   a. primary injury
   b. secondary injury
   c. pathogenic
   d. inflammation
   e. none of the above

6. Contrast the amount of tissue debris in a wound 24 hours after the injury when ice is applied within 5 minutes after the injury occurred with the amount of tissue debris when ice is not used at all. If ice is used, the primary-injury tissue debris will be _____ and the secondary-injury tissue debris will be _____.
   a. less; less
   b. less; more
   c. less; the same
   d. the same; more
   e. the same; less

7. Secondary metabolic injury results from an imbalance between _____.
   a. metabolism and oxygen delivery
   b. metabolism and inflammation
   c. inflammation and oxygen delivery
   d. enzymatic injury and edema
   e. none of the above

Chapter 6

1. Ice, compression, and elevation are indicated for the immediate care of acute injury. What does elevation do that is most beneficial in swelling control?
   a. decreases tissue oncotic pressure
   b. decreases secondary injury
   c. decreases capillary hydrostatic pressure
   d. decreases tissue hydrostatic pressure
   e. decreases external pressure force

2. Which of the following components of capillary filtration pressure is changed the most during the 24 hours after an acute injury as a result of cold pack application immediately after the injury?
   a. capillary hydrostatic
   b. tissue hydrostatic
   c. tissue oncotic
   d. capillary oncotic
   e. external

3. Swelling _____.
   a. and edema mean the same thing
   b. and inflammation and edema mean the same thing
   c. is a sign of inflammation and edema
   d. is a sign of edema but not of inflammation
   e. none of the above

4. The most important physiological effect of cold applications during the immediate care of acute injuries is _____.
   a. decreased circulation
   b. decreased pain
   c. decreased inflammation
   d. decreased metabolism
   e. decreased tissue elasticity

5. Which of the following should be applied directly to the skin during immediate care procedures?
   a. ice packs
   b. cold packs
   c. a wet elastic wrap
   d. a frozen elastic wrap
   e. none of the above

6. During immediate care procedures, compression should be applied to the injury _____.
   a. continuously for 2 hours
   b. continuously until bedtime
   c. for 30 minutes every 2 hours until bedtime
   d. for 30 minutes every hour for the first 24 hours
   e. continuously for at least 24 hours

Chapter 7

1. The forming of new blood vessels is known as _____.
   a. collagenization
   b. cascading
   c. capillary budding
   d. arching
   e. both a and c

2. The phase of repair during which fibroblasts manufacture collagen cells is known as the _____ phase.
   a. cellular
   b. vascular
   c. manufacturing
   d. arching
   e. none of the above

3. Fibroblasts usually lay down collagen _____.
   a. parallel to the wound edges
   b. parallel to the bones
   c. parallel to the lines of force
   d. perpendicular to the lines of force
   e. haphazardly

4. The rate of the contraction or restructuring phase of wound repair can be increased by _____.
   a. increasing the oxygen delivery to the wound
   b. using moderate exercise
   c. using vigorous exercise
   d. both a and b
   e. both a and c

5. Oxygen is important during wound healing because it is used _____.
   a. for energy production
   b. as a raw material for collagen production
   c. to promote capillary arcading
   d. to prevent secondary metabolic injury
   e. both a and b

6. Moderate exercise is _____ during wound healing because it _____.
   a. important; stimulates circulation and, therefore, more oxygen is delivered to the wound
   b. important; stresses the tissue and, therefore, guides restructuring
   c. detrimental; stresses the tissue and, therefore, causes reinjury
   d. detrimental; uses up the oxygen so the wound can't heal
   e. both a and b

Part III

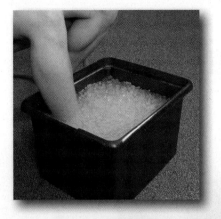

Pain and Orthopedic Injuries

Pain is the primary symptom that causes people to seek treatment. Yet, despite its universality, pain has not been adequately defined and is therefore hard to measure; and at times hard to treat. However, much is known about pain and about the interventions that usually relieve or modify pain. We'll discuss pain as both friend and foe, and try to help you develop a philosophy for using the friendly aspects while avoiding the foe (adverse aspects).

8

Understanding Pain and Its Relationship to Injury

OPENING SCENE

Coach Jiminez comes into the athletic therapy clinic, where you are a student intern, to check on her basketball players prior to practice. She notices Sofia with hot packs on her knees. "What's wrong?" she asks, "Nothin' coach, it just helps the pain and stiffness go away." She then notices Nikki sitting with her foot in a bucket of ice water. "How's that ankle sprain?" she asks. "It's really improving, I can jog without pain after icing it, coach. At this rate I'll be practicing in a couple of days." Madi is on a treatment table with an electrical simulator hooked up to her sore elbow, "to decrease the pain." She then notices one of the AT's stretching Rachel's painful back. Coach Jiminez thinks to herself, "These people sure treat pain in a lot of different ways. It seems very confusing."

What Is Pain?

Pain is the number one reason an athlete or patient seeks treatment.[1] Or is it the suffering that results from pain that causes patients to seek care?[2] Everyone knows what pain is, but few can explain it. In fact, some claim that pain has not been adequately defined or objectively measured.[3,4] Imagine trying to describe the taste of salt to someone who has never tasted it. "Gee, it isn't sweet, and it isn't sour—it's salty." It's very difficult to describe the flavor of salt, but once you've tried it (especially in excess), you know exactly what it tastes like. Pain is somewhat like this, except it has a variety of causes and manifestations. Both pain physiology and pain relief are difficult to analyze and evaluate, and therefore sometimes hard to treat. This chapter will help clear up much of the confusion, however.

There are several definitions of pain. We find this one to be the most useful in understanding the simple pain that occurs with most sports-related injuries such as sprains, strains, and contusions: **Pain** is an unpleasant sensory and emotional experience associated with actual or potential tissue damage or described in terms of such damage.[5,6]

Note, first of all, that pain is an experience associated with, but not necessarily caused by, tissue damage. There is much more to pain than the simple acute pain most people are familiar with; it is a multidimensional response to multidimensional stimuli, and the response intensity and duration are not always correlated to the initial stimulus.[7-9]

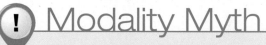

Modality Myth

PAIN IS A STIMULUS-RESPONSE MECHANISM

Many people incorrectly think that pain is a simple stimulus-response mechanism—that injured tissue stimulates a signal that is sent to the brain where it is interpreted as pain. It also is incorrect to think that the level of pain one feels is a direct result of the amount of tissue damage. Pain and the perception of pain are much more complex than the concept of a simple, rigid, stimulus-response system accounts for. To properly manage pain, you must think of it in a much broader context, as a social, emotional, psychological experience that modulates (modifies) the response to the pain-inducing stimulus.

THE FUNCTION OF PAIN: BLESSING-CURSE

Pain is both good and bad, both a blessing and a curse. Its main purpose is good; it protects you by alerting you to danger and stimulating action that prevents or minimizes injury.[10-12] It makes you move differently, think differently, and behave differently.[13] Without pain, people could do many dangerous things without realizing it.[14] Prolonged or chronic pain, however, may result in disability, atrophy, circulatory deficiency, and loss of skill (see Chapter 9) as well as in symptoms like anxiety and depression that result in a marked decrease in the quality of life.[10–12]

- Pain serves as a warning for withdrawal. For example, when one touches a hot object, pain from the heat causes one to immediately pull the hand away.
- Pain alerts a person that something is wrong. For example, the classic arch pain of plantar fasciitis that an athlete experiences when first getting out of bed in the morning is a warning sign. If the pain continues to nag for several mornings, it will prompt him to seek evaluation by a medical professional.
- Pain protects the injured part of the body through muscle guarding (muscle spasm). When a musculoskeletal injury occurs, muscle spasm or guarding usually accompanies the pain. In a sense, the body splints itself to prevent further injury (Fig. 8.1).

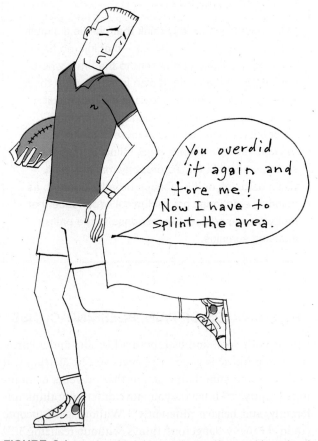

FIGURE 8.1 Imagine this conversation a 40-year-old weekend warrior's body has with itself after a backyard neighborhood flag football game injury: "All right, you old duff—you overdid it again and tore your hamstring. That will teach ya. I guess I'll send a protective muscle spasm down that leg so you don't damage more muscle fibers."

HOW PAIN OCCURS AND ITS EFFECT ON THE BODY

Pain is caused in a variety of ways, although most people think of pain as a response to tissue damage. Certainly, this is the most common type of pain experienced by athletes. It will therefore be the initial focus of this chapter. Understanding this type of pain will provide a foundation for understanding the other types/causes of pain addressed later in the chapter.

Simple pain (acute pain) occurs when your body's alarm system alerts the brain to actual or potential tissue damage. This causes a broad sequence of events, involving many body systems.[13] Each response is aimed at protection and healing. Pain can be so inclusive that you can't think, feel, or focus on anything else. On the other hand, however, if the brain reasons that experiencing pain is not the best for your survival (imagine a wounded soldier hiding from the enemy), you may not experience pain, even though you have suffered a serious injury.

Simple everyday pains, such as from insect bites, sprains, and postural malalignment, are caused by changes in body tissues. The brain concludes that the tissues are under threat and that action is required, including healing behaviors. An added benefit of pain is that it hopefully will protect you from making the same mistakes twice.

If untreated, and sometimes if treated, even simple pain can become chronic, leading to varying levels of nagging discomfort. If you are in pain at this moment, you are not alone. It is estimated that 20% of people have pain that has persisted for more than 3 months.[15]

The manifestation of pain is not always straightforward. After any injury, there may be no symptoms for days, even weeks, and then major pain expresses itself.[16]

Pain is also often manifested as, or accompanied by, a wide variety of sensations, such as burning, throbbing, tingling, prickly, and itchiness.[17] Other rather odd or weird sensations also accompany pain. People report feeling sensations such as it's *strings pulling*, *water running on my skin*, and *ants on me*. These other sensations can make the pain worse.[13]

Clearly, pain is multifaceted and complex; more about this later in the chapter.

Pain Basics: The Language of Pain

This section includes a brief review of terminology necessary for understanding pain and pain relief. This terminology can be confusing because some terms relate to anatomy or structure, others to physiology or function, and some to both. The major elements of the nervous system are outlined in Figure 8.2.

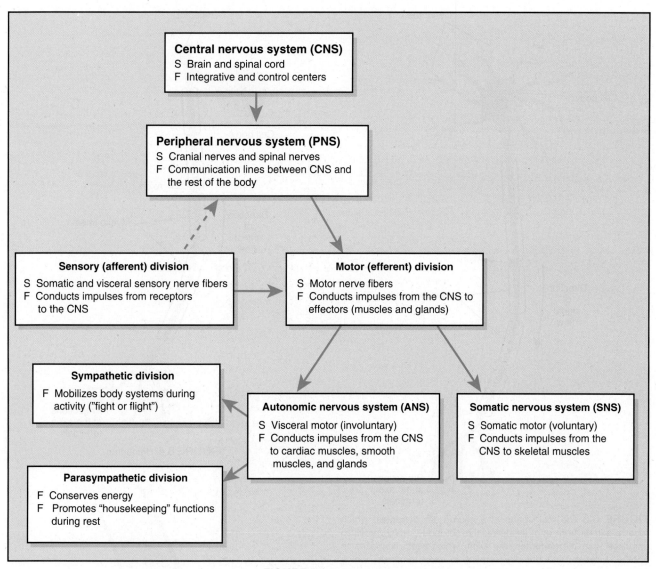

FIGURE 8.2 System chart.

NERVOUS SYSTEM DEFINITIONS: NEUROANATOMY

A. **Nerves**

1. **Neuron** (also known as **nerve cell**): Neurons are the basic functional unit of the nervous system; they are located in the central nervous system (CNS) and the motor division of the peripheral nervous system (PNS). Neurons in the sensory division of the PNS are slightly different (see "Pseudounipolar Neuron" below). All neurons are electrically excitable cells that process and transmit information by electrical and chemical signaling. Their main components are a cell body, dendrites, an axon, and branches that end in axon terminals or twigs (Fig. 8.3).

   There are three classifications of neurons, based on the number of branches that originate from the cell body:

   a. Unipolar (one branch)
   b. Bipolar (two branches)
   c. Multipolar (many branches)

   Neurons send signals or messages to other nerves through an electrochemical process. They are stimulated by terminal axons of other neurons, by the external world (as in a sensory neuron), or by electrotherapy (see Chapters 16 and 17). The signal then travels on the neuron as an electrical signal and stimulates the next nerve through a chemical process (see "Synapse" below). Stimulation of any part of the neuron causes an electrical signal to spread to all parts of the cell distal to the point of stimulation, that is, toward the axon terminals.

2. **Pseudounipolar neuron** (sometimes called a **specialized neuron**, or simply a **neuron**): A sensory neuron in the PNS. Similar to a neuron, but without

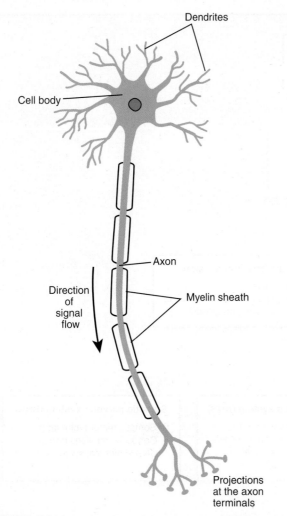

FIGURE 8.3 The main parts of a neuron are dendrites, which receive stimuli from another nerve; the cell body, which receives impulses from the dendrites; the axon, which sends impulses to another location; and branches ending in axon terminals, which release neurotransmitter molecules that either stimulate or inhibit a response in the receiving neuron.

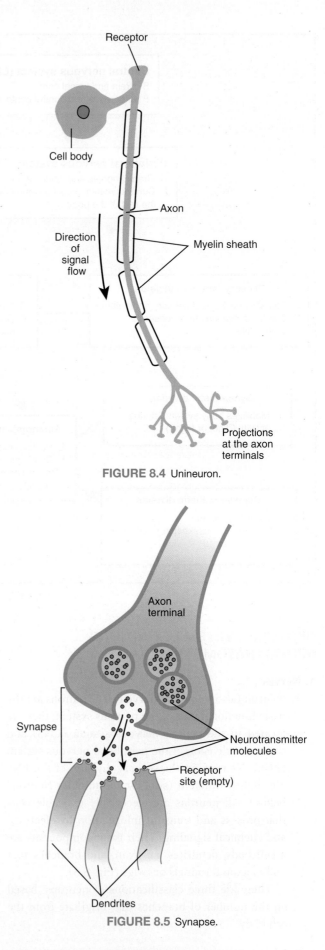

FIGURE 8.4 Unineuron.

FIGURE 8.5 Synapse.

dendrites (Fig. 8.4). These neurons have an axon with two branches that act as a single neuron. One branch, called the *distal process*, runs from the periphery and the other, called the *central or proximal process*, runs to the spinal cord. Impulses may or may not pass through the cell body, which is apart from the axon.

3. **Synapse** (also known as a **synaptic cleft**) (Fig. 8.5): The junction between two neurons; the space between the axon terminal of a *presynaptic neuron* and the cell body or dendrite of a *postsynaptic neuron*. Impulses can cross the synapse in one direction only, because of the locations of the neurotransmitters and receptors. A neuron receiving a postsynaptic signal will be excited, inhibited, or otherwise modulated.

a. **Neurotransmitters**: Chemicals that transmit an impulse across a synapse. They are stored in *vesicles* in axon terminals. Electrical signals traveling down the axon and into the axon terminals cause the vesicles to release the neurotransmitter molecules into the synapse. The chemicals then cross to the cell body or dendrites of the postsynaptic neuron where they fit into specific receptors (see Fig. 8.5).

b. **Lock and key**: A metaphor for the way neurotransmitters interact with dendrites. They have unique shapes that fit specific receptors on dendrites, like a key fits into a lock (Fig. 8.6). Thus, impulses cross a synapse only if the specific neurotransmitter is released that fits the specific receptor.

4. **Nerve fiber**: The dendrites or sensory receptor, axon and axon terminals of a single neuron. It transmits information unidirectionally, via electrical signals, within the brain and spinal cord, or between the brain, spinal cord, and other parts of the body.

5. **Mixed nerve** (also known simply as a **nerve**): A cable-like bundle of nerve fibers of mixed sizes and function in the PNS, similar to a tract or pathway in the CNS. Although the individual nerve fibers within it are unidirectional, the nerve itself is bidirectional because it contains both sensory and motor fibers, which transmit signals in opposite directions.

6. **Dorsal root ganglion** (also known as **spinal ganglion**): A nodule on the dorsal root of the spinal cord that contains the cell bodies of afferent spinal neurons

7. **Sensory receptor**: The first component of the sensory system. Highly specialized sensory nerve endings (sometimes called dendrites) that respond to specific internal or external stimuli. In response to stimuli the sensory receptor initiates *sensory transduction* (conversion) of the stimulus into an electrical signal, which is then sent to the CNS via a sensory nerve.

Humans experience a multitude of senses,[14] and process thousands of incoming messages simultaneously,[18] allowing the CNS to be aware of its surroundings and take appropriate actions.

The number and functioning of senses is so complex that differences of opinion exist in defining what exactly a sense is,[14] and how to classify them. The following system, which classifies sense in three overlapping ways, is sufficient for our needs[18]:

a. By receptor complexity
   i. *Free nerve endings* have little or no physical specialization.
   ii. *Encapsulated nerve endings* are enclosed in a capsule of connective tissue.
   iii. *Sense organs* (such as the eyes and ears) for the special senses (vision, hearing, smell, taste, and equilibrium) or for connective, epithelial, or other tissues

b. By location
   i. *Exteroceptors* are located at or near the surface of the skin and are sensitive to stimuli occurring outside or on the surface of the body. They detect tactile sensations, such as touch, pain, and temperature, as well as vision, hearing, smell, and taste.
   ii. *Interoceptors* (or *visceroceptors*) are located internally and respond to stimuli from visceral organs and blood vessels. These provide sensory input to the autonomic nervous system (ANS).
   iii. Proprioceptors are located in skeletal muscles, tendons, ligaments, and joints. They collect information concerning body position and function, such as joint angle, muscle length, muscle tension, and position of a limb in space.

c. By type of stimulus detected
   i. Mechanoreceptors respond to physical force such as pressure (touch or blood pressure) and stretch.
   ii. Photoreceptors respond to light.
   iii. Thermoreceptors respond to temperature changes.
   iv. Chemoreceptors respond to dissolved chemicals during sensations of taste and smell and to changes in internal body chemistry such as variations of O_2, CO_2, or H^+ in the blood.

B. CNS: The brain and spinal cord
   1. **Hypothalamus**: A structure about the size of a pea. It is the part of the brain that mainly acts as a central monitoring and control station in a variety of the body's activities. It regulates the functions of the

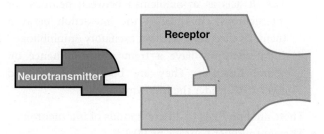

FIGURE 8.6 Lock and key. Neurotransmitters have specific shapes that fit specific receptors, much like a key fitting into a lock. Thus, not all neurotransmitters activate all receptors.

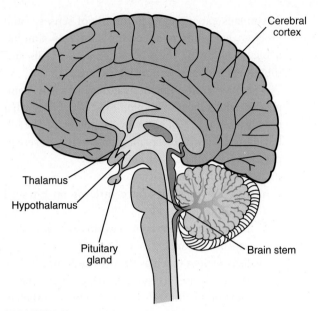

FIGURE 8.7 The brain and brainstem, showing the hypothalamus, thalamus, pituitary, and cerebral cortex.

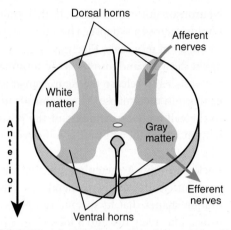

FIGURE 8.8 The spinal cord consists of thousands of individual nerve fibers. Some fibers are covered with myelin, a white insulating substance that makes areas appear white. In the spinal cord, the white matter is myelinated axons. The gray matter is unmyelinated axons, plus neuron cell bodies and dendrites. The pattern of the four areas of unmyelinated fibers makes the gray matter appear to have horns. The dorsal horns are the two horns at the posterior side of the cord. The ventral horns are the two horns at the anterior side. Afferent nerves enter the spinal cord via the dorsal horns, and efferent nerves exit the spinal cord via the ventral horns.

ANS (defined below), and also appears to play a role in mood and motivational states (Fig. 8.7).

2. **Thalamus**: A pair of egg-shaped structures at the top of the brainstem that serve as the main relay center of the brain. Sensations from all the sense organs except the nose are sent to the thalamus, which analyzes the information and relays it on to the higher levels of the brain (cerebral cortex). For example, sensations such as heat, cold, pain, and touch travel along nerves throughout the body to the thalamus, which then relays the signals to the cerebral cortex (see Fig. 8.7).

3. **Cerebral cortex**: The outer part of the brain. It has numerous functions; with respect to pain, it coordinates the signals and determines the intensity and location of the pain. The cerebral cortex also initiates descending pain control mechanisms.

4. **Tract or pathway**: A bundle of nerve fibers in the CNS, having a common origin, termination, and function. (Similar to a mixed nerve in the PNS.) Information can flow in either of two directions on unidirectional fibers:

   a. Descending tracts transmit information from the brain down the spinal cord.

   b. Ascending tracts transmit information up the spinal cord to the brain.

5. **White and gray matter**: Neurons are gray in color. Some, however, are surrounded by a myelin sheath, which is white (see Fig. 8.3). Thus in a cross-sectional slice of the spinal cord the myelinated areas (cord bundles) appear white and the unmyelinated

bundles appear gray; hence, they are called white and gray matter, respectively (Fig. 8.8). The location of the white matter makes the spinal cord cross section look as if it has two sets of back-to-back horns (myelination on neurons increases its speed of conduction):

   a. **Dorsal or posterior horn**: The posterior portion of the gray matter of the spinal cord. Afferent nerves enter the spinal cord through the dorsal horn. It is the first central relay station for somatosensory perception;

   b. **Ventral or anterior horn**: The anterior portion of the gray matter of the spinal cord. Efferent nerves exit the spinal cord through the ventral horn (Box 8.1).

6. **Interneuron** (also called **relay neuron**, **connector neuron**, or **local circuit neuron**): A neuron, entirely within the CNS, that connects afferent and efferent neurons, and other interneurons, in neural pathways and reflex arcs. It acts as a middleman between neurons (or interneurons), modulating the interaction between them. Its effect may be either excitatory or inhibitory.[19]

Interneurons have a tremendous influence on neural function. They are both numerous and diverse. Consider the following:

- There are hundreds of different kinds of interneurons.
- They outnumber neurons by 99:1.[19]
- Neuroscientists estimate that the human brain contains 100 billion (10^{11}) interneurons, each averaging 1000

<table>
<tr><td style="background:#6b6b6b;color:white">BOX 8.1</td><td style="background:#8a8a8a;color:white">MEMORY AID: AFFERENT VERSUS EFFERENT; DORSAL VERSUS VENTRAL</td></tr>
</table>

Here are some memory aids to help you keep the functions of afferent and efferent nerves separate.

- *Afferents Arrive* and *Efferents Exit* the CNS.
- *Efferents* are *Engine* (another name for motor) nerves

To remember where nerves enter and exit the spinal cord, you might think *"ADam and EVe"*:

- *Afferents arrive at the Dorsal horn*
- *Efferents exit from the Ventral horn*

And to remember that dorsal is on the back, think of scenes from movies, such as Jaws, where the dorsal fin of a shark slices through the water as the shark swims near the surface.

synapses with neutrons or other interneurons.[20] So the brain has about 100 trillion (10^{14}) connections.

C. **Peripheral nervous system (PNS):**
1. Nerves that communicate between the CNS and the periphery of the body. There are two types
   a. Cranial nerves interact directly with the brain. They are all sensory nerves, such as the optic and auditory nerves.
   b. Spinal nerves interact with the spinal cord. They can be sensory or motor nerves. Peripheral nerves are classified, and named, according to their size, which is directly correlated with their speed of conduction (Tables 8.1 and 8.2).

2. **Sensory nerves**: Nerves that are activated by physical stimuli acting on them, which then transmit impulses from the periphery, organs, and structures of the body to the CNS. The information it collects and transmits informs the CNS of the state of the body and its external environment. Their neurons are pseudounipolar, their cell bodies are located in the dorsal root ganglion, and they enter the gray matter of the spinal cord via the dorsal horn (see Fig. 8.8).

3. **Motor nerves** (also known as **effector nerves**): Nerves that carry impulses from the CNS (specifically the spine) to effectors such as muscles, organ, or glands. They effect or cause action such as muscle contraction or glandular secretion. Their cell bodies are located in the gray matter of the ventral horn (see Fig. 8.8). There are two types of motor nerves:
   a. **Somatic motor nerves**: Nerves that terminate in skeletal muscle. They are controlled voluntarily.
   b. **Autonomic motor nerves**: Nerves that terminate in smooth muscle, cardiac muscle, glands, and organs. They are controlled involuntarily.

NERVOUS SYSTEM DEFINITIONS: NEUROPHYSIOLOGY

A. ANS: The part of the PNS that controls smooth muscle, cardiac muscle, organs, and glands. It is referred to as *self-controlling* because it functions involuntarily and reflexively. The ANS consists of two physiologically and anatomically distinct, mutually antagonistic branches (meaning they compete with each other for control—only one is active at a time): sympathetic and parasympathetic.

TABLE 8.1 PERIPHERAL NERVE CLASSIFICATION: LETTER SYSTEM

TYPE OF FIBER	DIAMETER (µm)	CONDUCTION VELOCITY (m/s)	GENERAL FUNCTION
A-alpha	39,103	70–120	Alpha motor neurons, muscle spindle primary endings, Golgi tendon organs, touch
A-beta	38,941	40–70	Touch, kinesthesia, muscle spindle secondary endings
A-gamma	38,814	15–40	Touch, pressure, gamma motor neurons
A-delta	38,720	38,851	Pain, crude touch, pressure, temperature
B	38,719	38,789	Preganglionic* autonomic
C	0.1–1	0.2–2	Pain, touch, pressure, temperature, postganglionic* autonomic

*Preganglionic means from the CNS to the ganglia. Postganglionic means from the ganglia to the periphery. A ganglion is a group of nerves outside the CNS.
Source: Adapted from Mann.[111]

TABLE 8.2 PERIPHERAL NERVE CLASSIFICATION: ROMAN NUMERAL SYSTEM

TYPE OF FIBER	DIAMETER (μm)	CONDUCTION VELOCITY (m/s)	GENERAL FUNCTION
Ia	39,070	70–120	Muscle spindle primary endings
Ib	39,039	66–114	Golgi tendon organs
II	38,848	20–50	Touch, kinesthesia, muscle spindle secondary endings
III	38,721	38,826	Pain, crude touch, pressure, temperature
IV	0.1–2	0.2–3	Pain, touch, pressure, temperature

Source: Adapted from Mann.[111]

1. **Sympathetic nervous system**: The branch of the ANS that regulates the body's *fight-or-flight* responses, such as increased heart rate, resulting from stress
2. **Parasympathetic nervous system**: The branch of the ANS that regulates the *rest and digest* responses, such as decreased heart rate and secretion of digestive enzymes

B. Somatic nervous system (SNS): Somatic (efferent) motor nerves and sensory (afferent) nerves
1. **Stimulus** (stimulus is singular, stimuli is plural). The action of one agent on another (e.g., nerve, muscle) that evokes activity in the receiving structure or agent. The activity does not have to be gross activity; it may be nothing more than a change in permeability in a membrane.
   a. **Noxious stimulus**: Stimulus that results in pain; hence it is known as harmful or unhealthy simulation.
   b. **Threshold**: The minimal point at which a stimulus causes an *action potential* (wave of activity) to begin traveling on a nerve. Individual neurons respond in an *all or none* fashion, so the response in a single neuron is the same when the stimulus just barely exceeds a threshold level as it is when the stimulus is many times greater than threshold. Remember, however, that there are many individual neurons with different thresholds within a given area. So a greater stimulus may also evoke a response in adjacent neurons whose threshold is higher. With more nerves responding, the response in the whole tissue would be greater.
   c. **Subthreshold stimulus**: Stimulation below the threshold level. It does not evoke an action potential, but does cause a change in the electrical activity of the tissue.
2. **Response**: A reaction, such as stimulating a neuron, muscle contraction, or secretion of a gland, that results from stimulation

3. **Summation**: A process by which subthreshold stimuli add together to evoke a response
   a. **Temporal summation**: Summed over time. This summation occurs when a number of subthreshold stimuli from the same axon are repeated one after another before the effect of the previous stimulus has dissipated.
   b. **Spatial summation**: Summed over space. This summation occurs when multiple subthreshold stimuli from different axons converge on one cell body simultaneously (Fig. 8.9).
4. **Facilitation**: Enabling a neural response; the opposite of inhibition. For instance, during summation, subthreshold stimuli from one neuron make it easier for another neuron to stimulate a postsynaptic neuron. This is because the neurotransmitter molecules released by the first neuron into the synapse, although not enough to reach threshold, will partially activate the postsynaptic neuron, and therefore it is easier for subsequent neurons to reach threshold.
5. **Inhibition**: Restraining or repressing a neural response; the opposite of facilitation. If, during summation, a presynaptic neuron releases a substance into the synapse that deactivates the neurotransmitter, it will

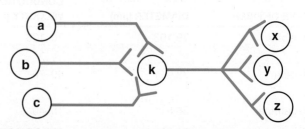

FIGURE 8.9 A simplified model of neural transmission and summation. In reality, there are numerous neurons and thousands of axon terminals and dendrites at each synapse. In this model, neurons a, b, and c synapse with neuron k, which in turn synapses with neurons x, y, and z. Spatial summation occurs if subthreshold stimuli from a, b, and c all arrive at k simultaneously; if the sum of their individual stimuli (the neurotransmitters) is greater than k's threshold, k will respond and send impulses to x, y, and z.

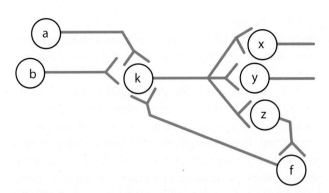

FIGURE 8.10 Positive feedback: Neurons a and b sum to stimulate neuron k, which stimulates neurons x, y, and z. Neuron z stimulates neuron f, which then sums with either a or b to stimulate or inhibit k (depending on whether f releases facilitatory or inhibitory neurotransmitters). If f is facilitatory, either a or b can stimulate k by itself, once the initial stimulus begins the feedback loop. Negative feedback occurs if f inhibits k, in which case the sum of neurons a and neuron b would not reach threshold and k would not be stimulated.

negate the effects of some neurons, thereby preventing impulse transmission or at least making it harder.

6. **Positive feedback**: Activity on a neuron that eventually is returned through a network of interneurons, thereby facilitating further activity on that neuron (Fig. 8.10).

7. **Negative feedback**: Activity on a neuron that eventually is returned through a network of interneurons, thereby inhibiting further activity on that neuron (see Fig. 8.10)

8. **Orders of neurons**: Sensory neurons are labeled for their order in the sensory chain from receptor to the cortex.[21] *First-order neurons* transmit sensory information from the receptor to the dorsal horn of the spinal cord. *Second-order neurons* transmit information from sensory pathways and various reflex networks in the spinal cord to the thalamus. *Third-order neurons* relay information from the thalamus to the cerebral cortex. These three orders correspond to the three levels of neural integration; sensory reception, ascending pathways, and central processing.

9. **Neuromodulation**: The process of modulating neuron activity. Modulate means to temporally modify, alter, or adjust something according to specific parameters or limiting factors, without permanently losing its core characteristics.

NOCICEPTORS AND NOCICEPTION

Nociceptors are specialized nerve endings, or sensory receptors, that respond to potentially damaging stimuli, such as mechanical, thermal, or chemical energy impingement. They respond by activating A-delta and C nerve fibers, which relay the signal to the CNS, where it is interpreted as pain. This process is called **nociception**. Thus nociception is the ability to feel pain.

Pain can also occur without a nociceptive stimulus, however.[22–24] Pain and nociception are closely related, but are not the same. Nociception is an objective event; specific neurophysiological activity in afferent nerve pathways that convey information about tissue damage or other painful stimuli to the brain. Pain, on the other hand, is a subjective, emotional experience that results from the modulation of nociception by a host of factors, including heredity, psychosocial experience, prior pain experience, and general life stress.

There are three types of nociceptors: cutaneous (in the skin), somatic (in joints and bones), and visceral (in body organs).[25] The two most common nociceptors are[6]:

• **Mechanical nociceptors**: Lightly myelinated **A-delta fibers**; activated primarily by strong mechanical displacement of the tissue; also called high-threshold mechanoreceptors

• **Polymodal nociceptors**: Unmyelinated **C fibers**, activated by several different types of stimuli, such as heat, mechanical pressure, or inflammatory chemical mediators produced by tissue injury

In addition, nociceptors have been found in every organ and joint capsule of the body.[25] They are stimulated by **endogenous** (internal) chemicals and by mechanical forces.

COMMON NOXIOUS STIMULI THAT CAUSE PAIN

Various types of stimuli can result in pain. Each of the following stimuli stimulates nociceptors, which are attached to sensory nerves that carry pain signals to the CNS:

• *Mechanical stimulus*: Stimulation caused by pressure on a nerve, often due to swelling or muscle spasm. This is the most frequent type of noxious stimulus seen in sports medicine.

• *Thermal stimulus*: Stimulation caused by radiant heat, such as the ultraviolet rays of the sun or a burn from touching a hot object

• *Electrical stimulus*: Touching a "hot" wire or feeling the "buzz" from poor grounding of a light socket are examples of mild electrical stimuli.

• *Chemical stimulus*: During the inflammatory response, chemical mediators transmit pain through the body to alert you that something is wrong (see Chapter 5). One of these chemicals is bradykinin, probably the most painful substance known. Its molecular composition resembles that of snake venom, and just a tiny amount inserted under the skin with a needle can cause excruciating pain.

THE PATHWAY OF PAIN

Now that you have been briefed on the anatomy and physiology of the nervous system, let's trace the pathway of pain through your body following an injury (Fig. 8.11). Imagine you are putting the shot (throwing it) and accidentally drop the 8-lb piece of iron on your big toe. The pain signal begins with the release of potent chemicals stored near nerve receptors (free nerve endings) in your big toe. These chemicals cause the receptor to generate an electric signal, which is transmitted up the leg on first-order sensory fibers that terminate in the dorsal horn of the spinal cord, a region that runs the length of the spine and receives signals from all over the body.[26]

At the spinal cord, the signal is relayed to a second-order neuron and numerous interneurons.[6] The second-order neuron transmits the signal up the spinal cord to the thalamus where sensations such as heat, cold, touch, and pain first become noticeable. However, you don't know where the pain is located; you only know that there is pain somewhere in your body. Processing of the signals has not yet occurred.

From the thalamus, the pain signal is relayed to the cerebral cortex by the third-order neuron, where it is processed, and the exact *location* and *intensity* of the pain are determined. Bystanders might hear you exclaim, "I have pain in my right big toe and it hurts like heck!" This whole process seems to occur in an instant; the impulse travels from the toe to the brain at an estimated speed of 33 miles per hour![27] (Box 8.2).

Additional manifestations of this injury could include any or all of the following: jerking your leg, rubbing your toe, shaking your foot, swearing (or wanting to swear), dancing a jig, feeling nauseous, and vomiting. Some of these would be caused by interneuron activity and others from signal processing in the brain, and subsequent descending signals. And 6 months later, dropping a heavy

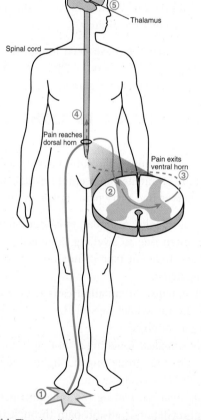

FIGURE 8.11 The simplistic pathway that pain travels through the body. (1) Noxious stimuli initiates a pain signal in the injured toe that travels as an electrochemical impulse along a first-order neuron up the entire length of the leg to the (2) dorsal horn of the spinal cord. (3) The impulse then synapses with the second-order neuron and (4) is then relayed up the spinal cord (4) to the thalamus (5) and then synapses with the third-order neuron and travels to the cerebral cortex (6).

BOX 8.2   PAIN: RELAY RACE OR FOOTBALL SCRIMMAGE?

An extremely simplistic analogy of acute pain is as a relay race with three runners. Think of pain as a baton that is handed to the nociceptor of the first runner (first-order neuron), who runs from the site of injury up to the dorsal horn of the spinal column. The next runner (second-order neuron) carries the baton to the thalamus, and the third runner (third-order neuron) sprints to the finish line in the sensory cortex.

In reality, however, there are many more players than the three runners. A better, yet still somewhat simplistic analogy is a football scrimmage. In this analogy, the football is the pain. The ball is placed in the hands (nociceptors) of the center (first-order neuron), who transfers it to the quarterback (second-order neuron). However, as soon as the center begins moving the ball, many other players (interneurons) jump into action trying to facilitate (offensive players) or inhibit (defensive players) progress of the football. Usually the center is successful in getting the ball to the quarterback (second-order neuron). The quarterback then sweeps the end and moves up field a ways before lateraling the ball to the running back (third-order neuron) who then runs the ball into the end zone for a touchdown, as long as the offensive interneurons outplay the defensive interneurons.

object could cause some, or all of, these same responses, even if it did not hit your toe.

PAIN PERCEPTION AND TOLERANCE THRESHOLDS

Pain perception threshold is the point that a stimulus begins to hurt. The pain tolerance threshold is the point at which a person acts to stop the pain.[28] There are considerable differences in individuals' pain perception and tolerance thresholds. Ethnicity, genetics, and sex influence some of these changes, but there are also wide variations of people within subgroups.[29]

Theories About Pain

Many theories have been proposed to explain responses to noxious (painful) stimuli. Each has adequately explained the knowledge about pain at the time of its inception. But as additional knowledge about pain has been gained, each theory has been proven to be inadequate, and a newer theory is developed that is consistent with all pain knowledge. Because aspects of each major theory carry forward and are part of newer theories, we present the main ideas of the most important theories.

Pain was initially thought to be a spiritual, mystical experience.[30] This began changing after 1644 when Descartes theorized that pain was a disturbance that passed along a single channel of nerve fibers to the brain.[31,32] This was essentially the specificity theory.

THE SPECIFICITY THEORY OF PAIN

The specificity theory stated that when specific nociceptors in the periphery of the body are stimulated, the impulse is carried to the brain via specific nerve pathways, resulting in pain.[33,34] Specific receptors are a physiological fact,[26] but the direct connection between stimulation of the receptors and pain is a weakness of the theory. There is not always a one-to-one relationship between nociceptor firing and nociception. Also, the specificity theory does not account for:

- Many types of fiber stimulation that result in pain
- **Phantom limb pain** (the sensation of pain in a limb that has been amputated)
- Why people react differently to pain
- The fact that pain can be modulated by input from the spinal cord or the brain
- The fact that people and animals have been trained to react favorably to noxious stimuli (i.e., Pavlov's dogs)
- Psychological variables such as past experience and cognition

THE PATTERN THEORY OF PAIN

The pattern theory was a reaction against the specificity theory; it attempted to explain many of the inadequacies of the specificity theory. It denied the existence of specific pain receptors and instead suggested that pain occurred when the rate and pattern of sensory input from generic receptors exceeded a threshold.[33,34] According to this theory, the intensity of nociceptive stimulation evokes a pattern of impulses in nonspecific receptors that is interpreted by the brain as pain. Moreover, a slowly conducting nerve fiber system carries pain, whereas normally this system, and pain, are inhibited by a rapidly conducting nerve fiber system. In pathological conditions, the intensity of stimulation in the slow system becomes much greater, dominates over the fast (inhibitory) system, and results in pain.

There are two main problems with the pattern theory. It is too general, and it does not account for the physiological evidence for the high degree of receptor-nerve specialization. For example, when the eyes (a sensory receptor) are stimulated, they send impulses to the brain via the optic nerve.

THE GATE CONTROL THEORY OF PAIN

Melzack and Wall[33] proposed the **gate control theory of pain** in 1965 to integrate the best of the specificity and pattern theories. Operating at the spinal level, the gate control theory proposed that a gating mechanism, located in the dorsal horn of the spinal cord, allows only one sensation at a time to pass through to the brain (Fig. 8.12).

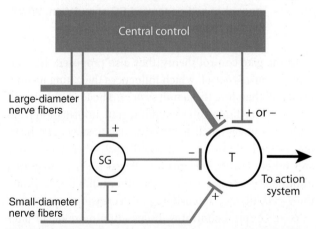

FIGURE 8.12 A model of the three main aspects of the gate control theory of pain. (1) Both large-diameter and small-diameter afferent nerve fibers facilitate the T-cell, which transmits the signal to the action system. (2) A group of cells in the substantia gelatinosa (SG) of the dorsal horn constantly send inhibitory signals to the T-cell. SG cells are facilitated by large sensory nerves and inhibited by small sensory nerves. (3) Central control, located in the brain, can either facilitate (+) or inhibit (–) T-cell transmission. Central control receives signals from both large and small fibers.

The theory recognized that pain and other sensory stimuli travel along both large-diameter and small-diameter nerve fibers, which converge at the **T-cell** (transmission cell), which is the gate. The T-cell determines which impulse will continue up or down the spinal cord and subsequently to other parts of the body (the action system) where various actions will be invoked.

Sharp, stinging pain travels along large fibers, whereas dull, aching pain travels along small fibers. Other sensations also travel along both fiber types. Strong sensory stimulation can control pain by "closing the gate" to pain, as the gate (the T-cell) opens to allow the stronger sensory stimuli to pass through to the action system.

Another aspect of the gate control theory is an inhibitory mechanism located in the **substantia gelatinosa (SG) [tract]** in the dorsal horn of the spinal cord. The SG sends inhibitory interneurons to the T-cell. It is always active, constantly providing self-generated background inhibition to the T-cell. In addition to its self-generated inhibition, the SG is influenced by stimuli from both large and small fibers via interneurons. The two types of fibers have different effects on the SG, and therefore modify the inhibition the SG exerts on the T-cell. Large-fiber stimulation facilitates the SG, thus increasing its inhibition on the T-cell. Small-fiber stimulation, however, inhibits the SG, thereby decreasing the inhibition the SG has on the T-cell.

CONCEPT CHECK 8.1. One of the explanations for the difference in people's pain threshold is that they have differences in the amount of self-generated SG stimulation. Why? Explain the mechanism.

In the gate control theory, they also proposed the concept of *central control*, which influences the gating mechanism and therefore the action system. The idea is that pain centers in the brain collect and integrate information from multiple sources, such as memory, vision, smell, and hearing, as well as the large-fiber and small-fiber nociceptive and other sensory information. Based on the integrated information, central control can either inhibit or facilitate the T-cell, thereby intensifying or decreasing its response to pain. (Central control is discussed in more detail later in the chapter.)

Problems with the Gate Control Theory

The gate control theory led to the development and use of *transcutaneous electrical nerve simulators* (**TENS**) (Fig. 8.13). In turn, responses to TENS revealed several problems with the gate control theory of pain:

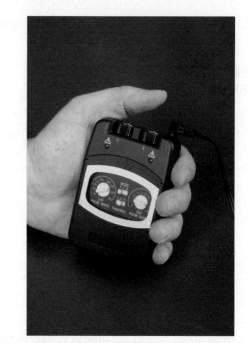

FIGURE 8.13 A typical TENS unit, used to help decrease or change a person's awareness of pain.

- Migraine headache is often relieved by TENS application to the temples. But since the temples are not anatomically related to the spinal column, there is no gating mechanism.
- The gate control theory indicates that you must stimulate the exact dermatome serving the site of pain. Sometimes, however, the placing of electrodes several dermatome levels above or below the pain site is effective in relieving pain. Therefore something other than the gating mechanism must be acting to decrease pain.
- There seems to be a memory associated with chronic pain and its treatment. Sometimes pain is reduced several hours or days following TENS application, rather than during application when the gate should be active.
- Some people are born without the ability to perceive pain, yet they have an overabundance of nociceptors, and neural circuits (Box 8.3).

Other deficiencies of the gate control theory are:

- It cannot account for several chronic pain problems, such as phantom limb pain, why a specific stimulus evokes more or less pain over time, or how the placebo effect works.[31]
- It does not explain the influence of drugs on moderating pain. This is understandable because the bulk of the drug information was discovered after the gate control theory was proposed in 1965. Nevertheless, this deficiency had to be remedied.

BOX 8.3 HOW CAN A THEORY DISPROVE ITSELF? OR THE CIRCULARITY OF SCIENCE

Physicians working with chronic low-back pain patients reasoned that if the gate control theory was correct, strong sensory stimulation to the lower spine would alleviate the pain. They experimented with surgically implanting small electrical stimulators next to the spinal cord. The surgically implanted *dorsal column stimulators* relieved pain for many patients. In an effort to screen those patients who were good candidates for the procedure, they decided to apply stimulators to the surface, reasoning that if it seemed to work, they would surgically implant them. The surface stimulation was as effective as the surgically implanted ones, so they decided that they could eliminate the surgery. Thus transcutaneous nerve stimulators (TNS), later called transcutaneous electrical nerve stimulators (TENS), became standard treatment, and substantiated the gate control theory. In time, however, the success of TENS revealed deficiencies in the gate control theory, thus causing doubts about the theory.

How can this be? The answer lies in an understanding of what theories are. A theory is simply an attempt to explain a group of observed phenomena. Theories are analytical tools for understanding, explaining, and making predictions about a given subject matter.[35] Because theories are abstract and conceptual, they should not be considered right or wrong; rather, they should be discussed as being supported or challenged by observations in the world.

The strength of a theory is determined by the number of observations (or facts) that support it, or that it explains. And often theories have to be modified as new, related observations are made. The best theories are fruitful and lead to new discovery, some of which supports the theory and others which challenge it, or aspects of it.

Does this mean the gate control theory is wrong and should be discarded? No! Even though some of the details were inaccurate, the concept was solid. Like other major theories in science, the gate control theory contains key conceptual ideas that had a powerful impact on pain research, pain theory, and health care. Many of the basic tenets of the gate control theory remain part of today's established pain theories. As one scholar noted concerning the gate control theory, "Ideas need to be fruitful, they do not have to be right."[36] And Melzack's response, "Good theories are instrumental in producing facts that eventually require a new theory to incorporate them. And this is what has happened."[37]

Following are the three major contributions of the gate control theory:

- The dorsal horns are not merely passive transmission stations, but sites where the dynamic activities of inhibition, excitation, and modulation occur.
- Pain cannot be explained by peripheral factors alone.
- The brain is an active system that filters, selects, and modulates multiple inputs.

Alternatives to the Gate Control Pain Theory

Numerous theories were proposed to explain pain following the partial collapse of the gate control theory, the majority of which address the influence of drugs, and/or chronic pain. The most promising and comprehensive are the neuromatrix theory.[9,38] Details of these theories are given later in the chapter, after we discuss the effects of drugs on pain relief and differentiate between pain and the pain experience.

Drugs, Endogenous Chemicals, and Pain Relief

To understand current pain control theories, you need to understand how drugs block pain. **Morphine** blocks pain by filling receptors (the locks) so that the neurotransmitters (the keys) cannot occupy those sites (see Fig. 8.6). Thus, pain signals cannot cross the synapse, and therefore there is no pain.

Scientists discovered **naloxone**, a morphine antidote, which reverses the effect of morphine by bonding with the morphine so that morphine cannot block the neurotransmitter. Naloxone also reverses electrically induced pain relief in rats and acupuncture pain relief in humans.[39] This finding led scientists to hypothesize that pain relief may be related to a morphine-like substance produced in the body. In 1975, three teams of scientists discovered what we now know are two different substances:

- **Enkephalin** (Greek for "in the head"), discovered in Scotland,[40] is similar in molecular structure to morphine and has similar analgesic properties. Found in the brain, spinal cord, and GI tract, enkephalin has a half-life (Box 8.4) of only a few seconds, which means it operates at the spinal cord level rather than circulating through the body. Enkephalin is thought to "block the gate" by interfering with A-delta and C fiber signal transmission to T-cells. It is released through nonpainful

BOX 8.4   HALF-LIFE

Half-life refers to the degradation/decay of a substance, such as an enzyme. It is the time it takes for the substance to decrease by half. Originally, the name described radioactive decay, but it now refers to any quantity that follows a set rate of decay.

A substance, such as endorphins and enkephalin, that decays at a set rate will reduce to 6.25% in 4 half-lives (to 50%, then to 25%, then to 12.5%, and then to 6.25%).

The half-life of a substance helps understand how long it is active. Consider the difference between enkephalin, with a few seconds' half-life and endorphin, with a 4-hour half-life. Enkephalin would be totally inactive within the first minute after it was released, while endorphin would still be 25% active after 12 hours (3 half-lives).

sensory stimuli—that is, low-intensity **sensory TENS**, or gentle massage.

- **Endorphin**, another morphine-like molecule, was discovered simultaneously by two teams of scientists working independently in the United States.[41,42] (The name is from endogenous and morphine.)[43] Produced in the pituitary gland at the base of the brain, endorphin is circulated throughout the body (its half-life is 4 hours). Endorphin exists in several forms, the most active being beta-endorphin. It acts in several different areas of the CNS (including the dorsal horn) to inhibit pain signal transmission and decreases the amount of chemical irritants present in the CNS. Modalities that might release endorphins are acupuncture, Neuroprobe, high-intensity **noxious TENS**, and intense exercise.

These discoveries caused much speculation,[39] including the following: Perhaps people especially sensitive to pain have a deficiency of enkephalin or enkephalin receptors. Perhaps the placebo effect occurs because of increased enkephalin and endorphin in the body.

Two additional substances are also known to be involved in pain relief:

- **Serotonin**: A biochemical messenger and regulator, found primarily in the CNS, GI tract, and blood platelets.[44] It mediates several physiological functions, including neurotransmission. Serotonin influences pain perception via a descending tract system (brain to spinal cord) that inhibits signals from peripheral nociceptors.
- **Dopamine**: A neurotransmitter in the **extrapyramidal system** of the brain, important in regulating movement.

It is also used by the body to synthesize **norepinephrine** and **epinephrine**, major neurotransmitters. It affects brain processes that control movement, emotional response, and the ability to experience pleasure and pain.[45,46] Its effects are much greater than morphine, leading some to call it *dynamite morphine*.[27]

OPIOIDS: ENDOGENOUS OPIATES

An *opioid* is a synthetic **opiate**, a substance that numbs or decreases pain.[47] In reference to pain control, the term is used to denote the body's naturally occurring or endogenous (within the body) pain killers, such as enkephalin, endorphin, serotonin, and dopamine. Opioids operate in different parts of the nervous system, are thousands of times stronger than morphine, and are effective for varying lengths of time.

Pain Perception

Pain is multifaceted and is often confused with other sensations. While it is true that "pain is whatever the experiencing person says it is, existing whenever he says it does,"[48] such a definition is simplistic. In this section, we differentiate pain perception from other related sensations.

PAIN VERSUS PAIN EXPERIENCE

Pain is the brain's response to a neural impulse from a noxious stimulus that aversive events are occurring at a specific anatomical location.[49] For example, a pin prick or a sprained ankle. The pain is perceived as being located at the point of tissue damage, and has other features such as intensity and duration that are attributed to physical objects or quantities.[49] It is referred to as acute pain.

Normally, as healing progresses, noxious stimuli decline and pain sensation diminishes until minimal or no pain is felt.[50] Persistent, intense pain, however, activates secondary mechanisms at the periphery and within the CNS that cause increased sensitivity to pain, exaggerated levels of pain, and pain provoked by normally nonpainful stimuli. Normal functioning is diminished. But of greater concern is the fact that numerous chemical mediators and second-order neurons and interneurons are activated that alter processes in the spinal cord and CNS, which gradually transforms the acute pain to chronic pain.

Chronic pain perception is very different than acute pain perception.[22–24,29] It is driven by genetic factors and many psychosociological factors, such as feelings, beliefs, and memories in addition to noxious input.[51,52] It therefore is referred to as a *pain experience*.

The experience has been described in many ways by a variety of people, including medical clinicians from a host of disciplines, scientists, novelists, entertainers, and politicians. Each tries to describe the experience for their specific group of constitutions, which at times is confusing. In this section, we describe the pain experience in a variety of ways so that you can both understand the complexity of the experience and explain it in simple terms to patients.

PAIN, SUFFERING, AND DISABILITY

Managing chronic pain requires an ability to discriminate between tissue damage, pain, suffering, pain behaviors, impairment, and disability.[53]

Pain and **suffering** are frequently confused.[54] Pain is a physical sensation, an unpleasant signal that something is wrong. Suffering is a state of severe distress, associated with events that threaten to harm the person.[55] It is a cognitive-social behavior that the brain assigns to the pain signal, resulting from its interpretation of the meaning of the signal. Pain is inevitable, but suffering is optional (Buddist proverb). Patients can reduce their level of suffering and the accompanying stress by identifying and changing their irrational thinking, beliefs, and expectations about the pain.

Disability is often a poorly defined, understood, and measured concept.[56,57] It is an umbrella term covering impairments, activity limitations, and participation restrictions.[58] It can be physical, cognitive, mental, sensory, emotional, developmental or combination of these.[58] It is also a legal or social judgment, based in part on medical judgments.[54] Disability can be the source of personal rewards to patients, in sympathy and financial support.

Passive treatment often results in more suffering than should occur, and excessive duration and magnitude of disability.[53,54] Inordinate physical inactivity, feelings of inadequacy, an inability to cope with society, and self-pity contribute to excessive suffering and disability.

THE MULTIDIMENSIONAL NATURE OF PAIN PERCEPTION

In order to understand the full nature of pain, Melzack and Torgeson[7] analyzed the open-ended descriptions of the pain perception of thousands of pain clinic patients. This resulted in 85 unique terms and four dimensions of pain perception: sensory, affective, evaluative, and miscellaneous. See the *McGill Pain Questionnaire* in Chapter 9 for the terms, and the following for descriptions of the dimensions.

- *Sensory* refers to the nature of the noxious stimulus or actual sensation of pain, that is, the conduction of impulses from peripheral sense organs to reflex (spinal) or higher CNS centers. It is what you feel—the source of the pain. It is also known as *sensory/discriminative* because it involves distinguishing it from other sensations and locations. Words patients use to describe the sensory dimension of pain include *throbbing*, *stabbing*, *sharp*, *stinging*, *aching*, and *splitting*.

- *Affective* refers to the emotional or autonomic response to the pain stimulus, such as crying or being very anxious or depressed due to painful experiences. It is influenced by mental state, personality type, goals, desires, and the expectations of the patient. It is also known as *affective/motivational* because it makes you determined to do something. *Tiring*, *sickening*, *frightening*, and *cruel* are words often used to describe the affective dimension of pain.

- *Evaluative* refers to the conscious thought processes concerning the pain stimulus. A patient compares noxious stimulus with past experiences and assigns a meaning to the experience. For example, an athlete who sprains the ankle will compare the present pain to the pain experienced from previous ankle sprains. The athlete will then subjectively judge the overall intensity of the pain. It is also known as *cognitive/evaluative* because it causes you to think carefully about the pain before making a judgment about importance or quality. Words that describe the evaluative dimension of pain include *mild*, *intense*, and *excruciating*.

- *Miscellaneous* is a combination of the other three dimensions. Descriptive words include *cold*, *numb*, *tight*, *nagging*, and *penetrating*.

THE VARIABILITY OF PAIN TOLERANCE

The response to pain varies from person to person, and from episode to episode in the same individual with a similar injury. Sometimes the affective dimension of pain overrides the sensory dimension, giving rise to variations in pain tolerance. For example, a separated shoulder might be very painful to a businessman who fell while playing recreational tennis. He may not be accustomed to this level of pain or the fact that the pain will limit his opportunity to relieve some stress via recreation. Yet professional football players have continued to play with this identical injury, feeling little pain, because the importance of winning the game (the affective dimension) and extensive experience with previous injury (evaluative dimensions). It is, therefore, difficult to analyze and evaluate pain physiology, pain tolerance, or pain relief since each one varies so much from person to person. It is often hard to describe the pain you are experiencing to someone else. Pain is whatever the person experiencing it says it is.

APPLICATION TIP

TREAT THE EFFECTS OF PAIN, AS WELL AS THE CAUSE OF THE PAIN

It is not enough to treat only tissue damage, or the cause of the pain. The social, emotional, and psychological effects of an injury often persist long after the injured tissue has been healed (see "Learned Pain"). These factors, if not addressed, can become the source of additional pain and can prevent the patient from realizing her full physical potential. Treating the social, emotional, and psychological effects of an injury helps maximize the mind-body connection.

CONCEPT CHECK 8.2. The pain experience varies from individual to individual and is influenced by anxiety, distress, and the degree of suffering it causes. One example of this variability occurred during the Battle of Anzio in World War II.[59] The soldiers who fought in this fierce battle suffered broken bones and severe cuts and bruises. The people of the village of Anzio suffered nearly identical wounds, yet the soldiers needed far less morphine than the civilians. Why did the soldiers need fewer painkilling drugs?

LEARNED PAIN

A learned, or conditioned, response that develops from a patient's "pain memories" of physiological and emotional elements of either nociceptive or neuropathic pain experience.[24,60,61] The pain stimuli is indirectly paired with any of an infinite number of environmental or sociological stimuli, even inactivity. Eventually, these secondary stimuli elicit pain.[60]

- Pain anticipation/expectation
- Delayed resolution of the injury
- Inordinate emotional stress associated with the injury (especially if prolonged)
- Inactivity, as in Dehne's spinal adaptation syndrome (above)
- Activity that elicits pain (see "No Pain, No Gain" above)

Pain cannot be reliably measured. Assessment of pain depends on verbal description, nonverbal expressions, specific tests, and our empathy. From this perspective pain is a matter of subjective experience and communication.[4]

BOX 8.5   MODEL VERSUS THEORY

Models are a mental picture of *what is*. Theories *predict or describe what will happen* in specific situations.[62,63]

Scientific models seek to logically and objectively represent objects, phenomena, and physical processes observed from nature or experimentation, but that cannot be directly measured.[63,64] Thus they are simplified reflections of reality; a substitute for direct measurement; an estimate of outcomes. They are not as reliable as direct measurement under controlled conditions, but useful when it is impossible or impractical to perform rigorous experiments.[64]

Scientific theories are well-substantiated explanations of some aspect of the natural world, based on a body of facts, laws, inferences, and tested hypotheses that have been repeatedly confirmed through observation and experiment.[65–67] They are much more than the educated guesses of detective novels, yet less than scientific laws.

Post-Gate Pain Theories

Numerous theories and models have proposed as alternatives to the gate control theory of pain. The first three theories are the most prominent responses to the problems of the gate control theory. The last three are models that attempt to explain the pain experience associated with chronic pain. A brief discussion of the difference between models and laws is in Box 8.5.

THE DESCENDING ENDOGENOUS OPIATE THEORY OF PAIN

This theory suggests that a **descending endogenous opiate system (DEOS)** operates at supraspinal levels (i.e., cortical and subcortical areas) and that the spinal gate originates from above–from supraspinal areas that contain opioid-secreting interneurons (Fig. 8.14). The T-cell, in response to small-fiber pain impulses, sends an impulse to the periaqueductal gray (PAG),[68] which passes it on to the raphe nucleus (RN; Fig. 8.14). The raphe nuclei descend to the dorsal horn of the spinal cord where they regulate the release of enkephalins, which inhibit pain sensation.[69] The PAG also releases enkephalin and seretonin, to help moderate pain.[68]

THE CENTRAL CONTROL TRIGGER THEORY

The **central control trigger theory** is a modification of the gate control theory. It involves the original gating mechanism plus an additional central inhibitory mechanism.

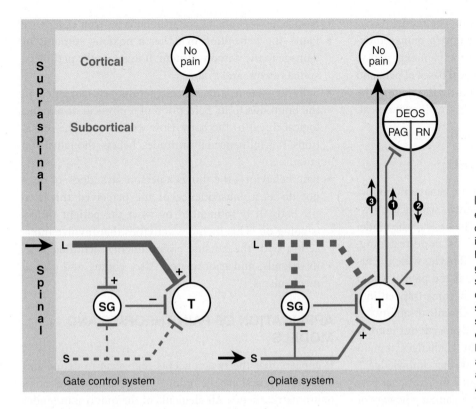

FIGURE 8.14 The descending endogenous opiate system (DEOS) is illustrated on the right. The gate control, on the left, is shown for comparison. L, large fibers; RN, raphe nucleus; PAG, periaqueductal gray matter; S, small fibers; SG, substantia gelatinosa; T, pain-transmitting cells; +, excitatory synapse; −, inhibitory synapse; arrow L, preferential electrical stimulation of large-diameter sensory fibers; arrow S, preferential electrical stimulation of small-diameter sensory fibers; arrows 1 and 2, negative-feedback loop; arrow 3, pathway to the brain. (Source: Adapted from Belanger.[110])

The former modulates the T-cell neurons as originally proposed (i.e., central control) and the latter acts via endorphin and enkephalin. Thus there are at least two different mechanisms of pain control in the spinal column, one local and one via descending tracts.[11,70]

> **?** **CONCEPT CHECK 8.3.** TENS research substantiated the central control trigger theory.[39] A group of 20 patients who achieved TENS pain relief were put into two treatment groups of 10 patients each. One group received TENS over conventional sites and the other group over acupuncture sites. After 3 months of successful pain relief, both groups were given naloxone. The naloxone reversed the pain relief in 6 of the 10 patients in the acupuncture group, but only 1 of the 10 in the conventional stimulation group. Why do you think this happened?

THE NEUROMATRIX THEORY OF PAIN

The **neuromatrix theory of pain** was proposed by Melzack[9,37,38,71,72] as an expansion of the gate control theory[33], incorporating newer information about the endogenous opiate systems and chronic pain. It is now the most comprehensive and dominant theory of pain.

According to the neuromatrix theory, pain is a multidimensional experience produced by characteristic *neurosignature* patterns of nerve impulses generated by a widely distributed neural network in the brain.[9,37,38,71,72] These patterns may be triggered by, or independent of, sensory inputs. Acute pain is evoked by brief noxious inputs that are transmitted to, and processed by, the CNS as described by the gate control theory. Chronic pain, however, occurs with little or no perceptible injury, inflammation, or pathology. Rather, it results from simultaneous modulation by multiple influences, including from a widely distributed neural network in the brain; a neuromatrix. Genetics determines a person's basic neuromatrix, which is then heavily modified throughout life by the convergence of sensory experiences, psychosocial factors, prior pain experience, cognitive and emotional events, and general life stress. Thus, pain is a *biopsychosocial event*,[29,73] resulting from integration and modulation of multidimensional inputs.[74] The response to pain is similarly complex, multidimensional, and unique to each individual.

One example of the power of this theory was a report of a patient with chronic pelvic pain who had obtained no relief from a host of medical and psychiatric therapies.[75] The pain subsided, however, following psychoanalysis that explored multiple factors that impact on the mind-brain-body complex.

THE ORCHESTRA MODEL

The **orchestra model** describes pain as resulting from the integration of input, which it calls *danger messages*, from a combination of tissue processes. The integration is carried out in many parts of the brain. The model recognizes that various cues (e.g., fear, memories, damaged tissues, circumstances) can be a part of the pain experience. It integrates biological and psychological bases of pain and acknowledges that even though the processes occur in the brain, they manifest themselves in very real, anatomical, and biological ways.

THE FEAR-AVOIDANCE MODEL

The fear-avoidance model is a cognitive behavioral model proposed to explain why some individuals with acute low-back pain develop chronic pain.[76,77] The basis of the model is that if acute pain is interpreted as nonthreatening, patients usually continue an active lifestyle, which leads to functional recovery.[78] In contrast, if the pain is (mis) interpreted as threatening, they may become trapped in a vicious cycle of pain-related fear and chronic disability.[79,80]

The fear-avoidance model has advanced our understanding of persistent disability, but challenges remain regarding the clinical application of that knowledge.[80] Also, it needs to more explicitly adopt a motivational perspective, one that is built around the organizing powers of goals and self-regulatory processes.[79]

✔ **APPLICATION TIP**

CHRONIC PAIN IS MORE DIFFICULT TO TREAT THAN ACUTE PAIN

Chronic pain is much more difficult to treat because it often involves more social, emotional, and psychological input than acute pain does. As such, chronic pain can be perpetuated even though the tissue damage that caused the initial acute pain is reduced or even healed. It is important to manage acute pain aggressively and wisely so that it doesn't become chronic pain.

Even physicians appear to be biased toward sensory and against affective qualities when evaluating patients' pain experiences.[24]

THE ONION SKIN MODEL

The **Onion skin model** of pain describes the pain experience as being comprised of four elements, depicted as nested concentric circles, like the layers of an onion, arranged from the inside outward.[2,81] The first three layers are personal, private, internal events; they cannot be observed or objectively measured. The fourth is observable and measurable, and constitutes the patient's and clinician's interpretation of the pain experience.[2,81–83]

- Nociception—initiates and maintains the pain experience
- Pain—the perception of either a noxious stimulus or damage to the nervous system. It involves the periphery, spinal nerves, and brain.
- Suffering—a negative affective response generated in the brain due to its perception of a physical or psychological threat to the body. How we interpret the sensations. It is influenced by attitudes, beliefs, thoughts, and emotions.
- Pain behavior—the things a person says, does, or does not do as a consequence of the perceived threat to the body. It is influenced by what the patient thinks is going on. This includes activities that involve interaction with the outside environment, including family, friends, and team mates. Also, coping and escape mechanisms.

APPLICATION OF PAIN THEORIES AND MODELS

It appears that the two concepts that seem to define and explain pain best are the onion skin model and Melzack's neuromatrix theory. All elements of the onion skin model fit within the neuromatrix theory, but are not explained as clearly. So use both of these concepts to guide your clinical procedures.

More Language of Pain: Types/Classification

There is more to the language of pain than those terms associated with neuroanatomy and neurophysiology. These additional terms are associated with the various types (also called classifications) of pain. Pain has been typed according to a variety of attributes (e.g., its involved anatomy or location, duration, time course, intensity, type of patient, and specific pathology).[84]

To successfully manage pain, practitioners must understand the characteristics of each pain type and how they relate to a patient's individual circumstances. The types are nonexclusive; specific pains generally belong to multiple types/classifications. Following are the most common types of pain:

LOCATION

Pain is often named for the involved anatomical location, such as low-back pain, knee pain, kidney pain, or headache; or by the body system involved, such as neuromuscular pain, vascular pain, or low-back pain.

DURATION

There are three types of pain named for their duration or longevity:

- **Acute pain** lasts up to 1 month. It is brief, short-term (minutes to days), often of rapid onset, and usually well localized and defined. Many describe acute pain as being of high intensity. It usually lasts as long as the noxious stimulation persists.
- **Subacute pain** lasts for 1 to 3–6 months. It usually starts as acute pain.
- **Chronic pain** may start as acute pain, but persists (weeks to years) beyond the usual course of an acute disease or after the injury has healed. The International Association for the Study of Pain defines chronic pain as any pain lasting longer than 3–6 months.[85] It is also associated with a chronic pathological process that causes continuous pain, or in which the pain recurs at intervals for months to years. Often it is pain that is not related to or located at the site of underlying tissue trauma.
  - When pain persists and feels like it is ruining your life, it is difficult to see how it can be serving any useful purpose. But even this pain results because the brain has somehow concluded for some reason or another, often completely subconsciously, that you are threatened and in danger. The trick is finding out why the brain has come to this conclusion.

- Decreased levels of enkephalins and increased numbers and sensitivity of nociceptors have been observed in individuals with chronic pain.[86] In the 1980s, it was estimated that 14% of the US population suffered from chronic pain related to the joints and the musculoskeletal system.[87,88]

The effects of acute and chronic pain on the body are summarized in Table 8.3.

MANIFESTATION

Referred and radiating pain occur at a site other than its origin.

- **Referred pain** is pain at a site other than the actual location of trauma or pathology. Referred pain tends to be projected outward from the source and distally along the extremities or to the shoulders if the pain is from an injury to an abdominal organ such as the spleen or liver. It is perceived in an area that often seems to have little relation to the pathology. For example, a ruptured spleen will often refer pain to the left shoulder. The site of the referred pain is called a **trigger point**.
- **Radiating pain** originates from an irritated nerve root and travels along that particular nerve's **dermatome** (area of skin innervated by a particular nerve). (An understanding of radiating pain is essential for proper electrode placement when administering electrotherapy; see Chapter 10.)

TABLE 8.3   THE EFFECTS OF ACUTE AND CHRONIC PAIN ON THE BODY

DESCRIPTOR	ACUTE PAIN	CHRONIC PAIN
Biological function	Warning	None
Time frame	<1mo	>1 mo
Nerve fiber transmission	A-delta	C fiber
Patient localization	Well localized and defined	Poorly localized
Psychological and environmental influences	Minor role	Prominent role
Verbal descriptors	Sensory (shooting, hot, sharp)	Emotional or motivational
Most frequent affective problem	Anxiety	Abnormal illness or behavior
Symptoms and dysfunction	Present, easily identifiable	Absent or can't identify
Drug intake	None to appropriate use	Misuse and addiction
Physical activity	Diminished with gradual return	Diminished to absent
Social activity	Diminished with gradual return	Diminished to absent
Probability of divorce	Same as average norms	High
Suicide attempt or consideration	No	Yes

INTENSITY

It is common to use a 10-point numeric scale to rate pain intensity where 0 = no pain and 10 is the worst pain imaginable.[84] These numbers are then used to classify the pain into three groups as follows:

- Mild: 4
- Moderate: 5–6
- Severe: 7

ORIGIN

Four general origins of pain have been identified.

- **Nociceptive pain** occurs in response to injury or illness to bodily structures. It involves messages conducted from nociceptors at the site of injury, on efferent nerves up through the spinal cord into the brain, where the messages are interpreted as pain.[61,89]
- **Neuropathic pain** is a complex, chronic pain state that often shows up in illogical ways. It usually is accompanied by tissue damage to the nerve fibers themselves. Thus the nerve fibers become dysfunctional and send incorrect signals to the brain and other pain centers.[61,89]
- **Idiopathic pain** is of unknown origin, meaning there is no identifiable pathology associated with it.[61,89]
- **Learned pain** is a phenomenon that develops from a patient's "pain memories" of physiological and emotional elements of either nociceptive or neuropathic pain experience.[24,60,61] One explanation is that following a specific pain-producing stimuli, such as injury, organic disease, or surgery, the pain stimuli is indirectly paired with any of an infinite number of environmental or sociological stimuli, even inactivity. In time, pain can be elicited by the secondary stimuli, and thus becomes a learned—or conditioned—response, via the classic Pavlovian conditioning of dogs to salivate when they heard the ringing of a bell.[60]

Differentiating between these types of pain is sometimes difficult, but essential to proper management. For example, although opioids are unsurpassed in treating acute and cancer pain, their use in chronic noncancer pain is clearly limited.[89] Also, it appears opioids are ineffective in reducing pain when there is a major affective component (relating to moods, feelings, and attitudes) to the pain or when *learned pain* behavior is the main problem.[89]

Pain Management

The process of managing pain is complex, and it must be tailored to each patient. What works with one patient may not work with another. And what worked with a patient one time may not work later for the same patient with a similar injury. Following are some principles upon which to base your pain management strategies. Specific techniques are discussed in Chapter 9.

PAIN EXPERIENCE MODIFIERS

Many factors modify the pain experience. Following are some of the more common pain modifiers:

- Movement often makes it worse. Nerves are more comfortable in some positions than others. When a nerve is sensitive, you tend to favor postures that avoid putting mechanical load on the affected nerve. For example, you develop a limp, or you might bend over to take stress off your spine, shoulder, and so on. While this may help initially, it is important that we return to normal mechanics as soon as possible before this new posture becomes permanent.
- Stress makes it worse. Nerves, especially damaged ones, can become sensitive to stress-produced chemicals, which can result in a nasty cycle.[90] The brain concludes that you are under threat because of this *unexplained* pain, so it causes an increased production of stress chemicals, which fires danger messages to the brain, which tell the brain that you are under threat, and they cycle repeats.
- Zings. Without warning, movement or even just sustained posture may ignite an injured nerve, causing it to discharge, sometimes repeatedly like the ringing of a car alarm.[17] The sporadic nature of this response can be quite disturbing to patients.[90] It probably is due to dorsal root ganglion involvement,[91] via interneurons.
- Delayed onset. After injury there may be no symptoms for days or even weeks, and then pain appears, apparently unprovoked.[16]
- An itch may occur in skin zones over the painful area.[17,92] Patients describe it as "feeling weird," "like water running on my skin," "prickly," "like ants are crawling on me," or "like strings are pulling."

  Reassure patients that they aren't strange or going crazy, and that the nerves aren't dying or decaying. The nerves are just doing the wrong thing and in many cases are just responding to signals from the brain that tell them that increased sensitivity and better warning are required.

- **Cognitive behavioral strategies** are a set of psychologic behaviors used to modulate a patient's perception or interpretation of a pain sensation or situation.[93] These include meditation, distraction, relaxation, fear, depression, former pain experiences, and family and cultural influences.[4,94,95] They have also been shown to be as effective as ibuprofen in the initial stages of orthodontic treatment.[96]

- Brain imaging studies indicate that these strategies act at numerous sites in the brain.[29,97]

The effectiveness of cognitive behavioral strategies is influenced by a number of factors, including the patient's:

- Attention
- Beliefs
- Conditioning
- Expectations
- Mood
- Emotional response to noxious sensory events[94]

Different cognitive strategies recruit different brain regions to perform the same task: pain modulation.[93]

SEX DIFFERENCES

There are differences in the way men and women experience pain. Although 10 years of laboratory research on healthy individuals have not been successful in producing a clear and consistent pattern of sex differences in human pain sensitivity,[98] clinical research on pain patients indicates:

- Women report more severe levels of pain, more frequent pain, pain of longer duration,[99,100] and occurring in a greater number of body regions.[100]
- Women are more likely than men to experience a variety of recurrent pains,[99,100] such as fibromyalgia, temporomandibular dysfunction, migraine, rheumatoid arthritis, and irritable bowel syndrome.[100]
- Women may be at greater risk for developing several chronic pain disorders[101] and pain-related disability.[99]

And it appears that women are more vulnerable to having health care providers unjustly attribute their pain to the mind (fantasy).[99]

Mechanisms underlying the differences between women and men are currently unknown,[100] but the following factors are proposed as influencing the mechanism:

- Psychosocial factors such as sex role beliefs, pain coping strategies, mood, and pain-related expectancies[101]
- Sex hormones, which are known to affect pain responses[101]
- Interactions between biological, sociocultural, and psychological aspects[100]
- Quantitative and qualitative differences in endogenous pain inhibitory systems[100]
- Influence of gonadal hormones on men[100]
- Exposure to painful visceral events (e.g., menses, labor) during life may contribute to an increased sensitivity to, and greater prevalence of, pain among women[100]

So what are the clinical applications of these data? Pain is a unique personal experience showing variability between sexes.[100] You must treat men and women as individuals. Do not assume their responses to similar injuries will be the same. Although the magnitude of these effects has not been well characterized, there are potentially important practical implications of sex differences in pain responses.[101]

PAIN NEUROMATRIX APPROACH FOR CHRONIC PAIN

This approach is based on the neuromatrix pain theory[9,37,38,102] and the following fundamental principles[103]:

- Pain is produced whenever the brain concludes that body tissue is in danger.
- The purpose of pain is to cause action.
- Pain is a multisystem output that is produced when an individual-specific cortical pain neuromatrix is activated.

When pain becomes chronic, the efficacy of the pain neuromatrix is strengthened via nociceptive and non-nociceptive mechanisms, which means that pain can be produced with less input, both nociceptive and non-nociceptive. The clinical approach, therefore, must focus on decreasing all inputs that the brain might interpret as meaning that body tissue is in danger, and then on progressively activating components of the pain neuromatrix without activating its output. For example, the aim of cryokinetics and cryostretch (Chapter 13) is to numb sensory transmission with cold, and then progressively increase the activity level of the body part.

CENTRAL CONTROL

The concept of central control is key to pain management. Pain is subjective and ultimately at the mercy of the brain. **Central control** is a theory that previous experiences, emotional influences, sensory perception, and other factors influence the response of the brain to nociceptors and thus the perception of pain. Central control collects and stores information related to pain and mediates the body's response to noxious stimuli. Previous experiences and other sensory input influence pain via central control. The following examples illustrate this concept:

1. The sight of blood intensifies the pain experience. The response of an individual (usually a child) to an injury is generally minimal until he notices blood, at which point he responds directly. The noxious stimulus from the injury site was the same before he saw blood, yet

the sight of blood—sensory input to central control via the optic nerve—altered the response to the noxious stimulus.

2. Pain minimized by a rational thought to ignore it. One of our former athletes, a moderately successful wrestler, was plagued with minor nicks and scrapes during his early college career. Two years later, after being a two-time All-American and a world medalist, he paid very little attention to these injuries. When asked what the difference was, he replied that he'd discovered that the difference between a good athlete and a world-class athlete is how they handle pain and adversity. He still got the minor nicks and scrapes, but had learned to ignore them. In other words, minor injuries that were painful early in his career did not cause pain in his later career because of conscious, rational thought (central control). We are not suggesting that an athlete should rationalize away pain, or ignore it. Our point is that central control can greatly influence the perception and management of pain.

3. Psychoanalysis can alleviate long-standing chronic pain. Taylor[75] who reported of a patient with chronic pelvic pain who had obtained no relief from a host of medical and psychiatric therapies. The pain subsided, however, following psychoanalysis, which explored multiple factors that impact on the mind-brain-body complex.

4. Alleviating chronic pain in amputees and spinal chord injured with *mirror therapy* (also known as *motor imagery*), wherein they mentally exercise while their body image is distorted using a mirror to hide their injured or amputated limb and projecting an image of their uninjured limb exercising normally.[104–107] For example, spinal cord–injured patients decreased their neuropathic pain by approximately 65% through imagined walking and "watched themselves" walk with a mirror placed in front of a screen.[105] Patients aligned their own upper body with a film of a lower body walking. Guided imagery and simply watching the film without it appearing to be their injured limb were of minimal value in decasing pain.

Another example of the power of this therapy was an amputee who had the sensation that his nonexistent limb was extremely painful due to being engorged and swollen. With mirror therapy, his normal limb was projected to appear in place of his amputated limb, except the limb was enlarged so it appeared engorged. While exercising the limb, it appeared the two limbs were both moving. The image of the amputated limb was gradually reduced to normal size, and the "pain" the patient was experiencing also decreased. In essence, the brain was reprogrammed.

5. Strength can be developed by merely thinking about performing exercise. Mental training enhances the cortical output signal, which drives the muscles to a higher activation level and increases strength.[108] Two groups of subjects trained for 12 weeks (15 min/day, 5 days/wk) to increase their little finger abduction strength. The group that physically performed the exercises increased strength by 53%. The second group increased strength 35% by performing only "mental contractions" of little finger abduction. Monitoring with surface EMG showed no apparent muscle activity during training. Both groups had significant increases in electroencephalogram-derived cortical potential, shown to be directly related to control of voluntary muscle.

"The primary mechanism underlying the strength increase is a mental training-induced enhancement in the central command to muscle."[108] Thus the brain generated stronger signals to the muscle. And since voluntary muscle force is proportional to the magnitude of brain-to-muscle signal, the greater strength is a consequence of stronger brain activity.

We do not advocate mental training over traditional resistance training for strength development, but this research is further evidence of the impact of central control over the neuromuscular system.

✔ APPLICATION TIP

MANIPULATE THE PLACEBO EFFECT

The concept of central control helps explain how the placebo effect can be so powerful in eliminating pain, and why the attitude and approach of the clinician can have such an important effect on a patient's response to an injury. A cheerful, positive approach by the clinician and the patient can change not only the patient's perception of pain, but the healing process as well.[97,109] A negative, defeatist attitude can have the opposite effect by activating nocebos. Use this powerful tool to enhance the effects of other treatments. (See Chapter 9 for more about the placebo effect.)

THREE LEVELS OF PAIN CONTROL

Three levels for controlling pain have been described, based on the current theories of pain:

1. *Level I, Ascending Influence Pain Control.* Pain relief induced by a gating mechanism occurs during the application of modalities such as traditional TENS, massage, and cryotherapy. This is traditional gate control pain relief.

2. *Level II, Descending Influence Pain Control.* Pain relief modulated by transmissions from higher brain centers, such as in the **raphe nucleus** to the dorsal horn of the spinal cord, which triggers the release of enkephalin and modulates pain. This descending tract is stimulated by noxious stimuli transmitted to the **periaqueductal gray (PAG)** matter in the brain. This model provides a possible explanation for pain relief induced by somewhat painful stimulation of afferent nerves (C fibers), such as acupressure or noxious TENS (delivered at a high intensity and frequency).

3. *Level III, Beta-Endorphin-Mediated Pain Control.* Prolonged stimulation of afferent nerves (A-delta fibers) triggers the release of beta-endorphin by the pituitary gland from connections between the hypothalamus and the raphe nucleus. Since beta-endorphin has a long half-life, this provides long-term stimulation of descending tracts. This model provides a possible explanation for pain relief from modalities such as electroacupuncture and low-frequency motor or noxious TENS.

> **CONCEPT CHECK 8.4.** Ryan, a certified athletic trainer, was covering a youth soccer tournament as part of his clinic's outreach program. A 10-year-old boy came to him complaining of stomach pain. Ryan asked what the boy had for breakfast and how long ago he had eaten, then determined that the pain wasn't related to diet. He then asked the boy if he had been kicked in the stomach. "Yes." The boy said. Ryan then palpated the boy's upper left abdominal quadrant and found that it was rigid. Ryan then asked the boy if he had pain anywhere else. "My left shoulder," the boy replied. Ryan immediately called an ambulance. Why?

CLOSING SCENE

Recall from the chapter opening scene that you are gaining some clinical experience as a student athletic trainer at a high school. Each day prior to basketball practice, one of Coach Jiminez' players applies hot packs to her knees to help relieve the pain and stiffness. Other athletes use electrical stimulation, or ice, to decrease the pain. Why are there so many different treatment therapies for pain reduction? After reading this chapter, you can describe several pain theories, and why external stimuli, such as heat, cold, electricity, and manual pressure, stimulate special nerve fibers that help override the pain message.

Chapter Reflections

1. Read and ponder each of the following points. Do you feel you have a clear understanding of each concept? If not, reread the appropriate section of the chapter.
   - Define pain.
   - Discuss the functions of pain.
   - Discuss and differentiate between neurons, pseudounipolar neurons, and interneurons.
   - Discuss the function and classification of receptors.
   - Differentiate between nerves and nerve fibers.
   - Define nociception and differentiate it from nociceptors.
   - Discuss the common noxious stimuli that cause pain.
   - Discuss the four dimensions of pain.
   - How is pain a friend to the patient and clinician? How is it a foe?
   - Outline the pathway of pain.
   - Discuss the difference between acute and chronic pain.
   - What is the difference between radiating and referred pain?
   - Describe the major points of the specificity and pattern theories of pain.
   - Discuss the gate control theory of pain, four reasons that exposed it as inadequate, and what its major contributions were.
   - Differentiate between pain, pain experience, suffering, and disability.
   - Discuss the types/classification of pain.
   - Discuss the body's internal pain suppressors.

- Discuss central control and how you might apply this concept in managing a patient's pain.
- Discuss the neuromatrix theory of pain and why it is presently the dominant theory of pain.
- Define mirror therapy.
- Define the placebo effect.
- Discuss the onion skin model for pain and how it relates to the neuromatrix theory of pain.
- Define how drugs and endogenous chemicals affect pain relief.

2. Write three to five questions for discussion with your class instructor, clinical instructor, classmates, and clinical colleagues.
3. Get together with classmates and quiz each other on the concepts of this chapter. Use the points in reflection no. 1 and the questions you wrote for reflection no. 2 as a beginning. Explaining concepts out loud to others requires a deeper grasp of the material than feeling you understand it as you read.

CONCEPT CHECK RESPONSES

CONCEPT CHECK 8.1

SG stimulation is self-generated and sent to the T-cell, where it interacts with the facilitatory large- or small-fiber stimulation to determine the reaction. So the more SG, the less the response. Therefore, differences in the amount of background inhibition (SG self-generated) between people will result in a different response to the same noxious stimuli.

CONCEPT CHECK 8.2

Since naloxone is a morphine inhibitor, it must have inhibited endorphin release, indicating that endorphins and/or enkephalins were involved in the pain relief. In the conventional group, naloxone had no effect, indicating that the pain was relieved by something other than endorphin/enkephalin—that is, the gating mechanism. This research indicated that there were two different kinds of TENS analgesia, and at least two different mechanisms of pain control.

CONCEPT CHECK 8.3

The reason the citizens of Anzio needed more morphine than the soldiers was because of the mental stress associated with the battle. Anzio residents also lost homes, jobs, and even loved ones. Although the soldiers didn't lose their homes, they got to go home because of their injuries. The presumed reason why the soldiers needed less morphine than the residents of Anzio for identical injuries (now known as the Anzio effect) was that the wounds to the residents were a source of anxiety, whereas these same wounds to the soldiers meant they were going home.

CONCEPT CHECK 8.4

Let's review the symptoms. The boy got kicked in the stomach, had stomach pain, and had pain in the left shoulder. These symptoms are consistent with a ruptured spleen. He was exhibiting referred pain to the left shoulder (Kehr's sign). This is a true story. When the ambulance arrived at the emergency room, the young man was taken for an x-ray where it was determined that, indeed, he did have a ruptured spleen. The physician took the boy into surgery and removed the spleen. Due to Ryan's knowledge of referred pain patterns, the boy's life was saved.

REFERENCES

1. Turk DC, Melzack R. The measurement of pain and the assessment of people experiencing pain. In: Turk DC, Melzack R, eds. *Handbook of Pain Assessment*. 2nd ed. New York: The Guilford Press, 2001: 3–14.
2. Loeser JD. Pain and suffering. *Clin J Pain*. 2000;16(2 Suppl):S2–S6.
3. Scarcella JB, Cohn BT. The effect of cold therapy on the postoperative course of total hip and knee arthroplasty patients. *Am J Orthop*. 1995;24(11):847–852.
4. Frischenschlager O, Pucher I. Psychological management of pain. *Disabil Rehabil*. 2002;24(8):416–422.
5. Merskey H, Bogduk N. *IASP Task Force on Taxonomy*. 2nd ed. Seattle: IASP Press, 1994.
6. Steeds CE. The anatomy and physiology of pain. *Surgery*. 2009; 27(12):507–511.
7. Melzack R, Torgerson W. On the language of pain. *Anesthesiology*. 1971;34:50.
8. Bond M, Simpson K. *Pain: Its Nature and Treatment*. New York: Churchill Livingstone, 2006.
9. Melzack R. Pain and the neuromatrix in the brain. *J Dent Educ*. 2001;65(11):1378–1382.
10. Usunoff K, Popratiloff A, Schmitt O, Wree A. *Functional Neuroanatomy of Pain*. Berlin, Heidelberg: Springer-Verlag, 2006.
11. Institute of Medicine (US) Committee on Advancing Pain Research, Care, and, Education. *Relieving Pain in America: A Blueprint for Transforming Prevention, Care, Education, and Research*. Washington, DC: National Academies Press (US), 2011.

12. Woolf CJ, Bennett GJ, Doherty M, et al. Towards a mechanism-based classification of pain? *Pain*. 1998;77(3):227–229.

13. Butler D, Moseley L. *Explain Pain*. Adelaide, Australia: Noihtoup Publications, 2003.

14. Wikipedia.com. Sense. Available at: http://en.wikipedia.org/wiki/Sense. Accessed April, 2011.

15. Blyth F, March L, Brnabic A, et al. Chronic pain in Australia: a prevalence study. *Pain*. 2001;89(2-3):127–134.

16. Devor M, Selzer Z. Palophysiology of damaged nerves in realization to chronic pain. In: Wall P, Melzack R, eds. *Text Book of Pain*. Edinburgh: Churchill, Livingstone, 1999.

17. Torebjörk H, Ochoa J. Pain and itch from C fibre stimulation. *Neurosci Abstr*. 1981;7:228.

18. Cliffnotes.com. Sensory Receptors. Available at: http://www.cliffsnotes.com/study_guide/topicArticleId-22032,articleId-21950.html. Accessed April, 2011.

19. Enoka RM. *Neuromechanical Basis of Kinesiology: Chapter 7 Voluntary Movement*. 4th ed. Champaign, IL: Human Kinetics, 2008.

20. Sharma NS. *Molecular Cell Biology*. New Delhi, India: International Scientific Publishing Academy, 2005.

21. Porth CM. *Essentials of Pathophysiology: Concepts of Altered Health States*. 3rd ed. Baltimore, MD: Lippincott Williams & Wilkins, 2010.

22. Charlton JE. *Core Curriculum for Professional Education in Pain*. Seattle: IASP Press, 2005.

23. Tyrer S. Learned pain behaviour. *Br Med J*. 1986;292(6512):1–2.

24. Chen LA, Tudi SR, Deconda D, et al. Is there physician bias against eliciting affective qualities of pain? *J Clin Gastroenterol*. 2010;44(1):9–11.

25. Zimmerman M. Basic physiology of pain perception. In: Lautenbacher S, Fillingim RB, eds. *Pathophysiology of Pain Perception*. New York: Kluwer Academic/Plenum Publishers, 2004:1–24.

26. Willis WDJ. *The Pain System: The Neural Basis of Nociceptive Transmission in the Mammalian Nervous System*. Vol 8. New York: S. Karger, 1985.

27. Silverstein A, Silverstiein V. *World of the Brain*. New York: William Morrow and Co., Inc., 1986:68.

28. Pain, Thresholds. Available at: http://en.wikipedia.org/wiki/Pain#Thresholds. Accessed August, 2012.

29. Gatchel RJ, Peng YB, Peters ML, Fuchs PN, Turk DC. The biopsychosocial approach to chronic pain: Scientific advances and future directions. *Psychol Bull*. 2007;133(4):581–624.

30. Pain, Historical Theories. Available at: http://en.wikipedia.org/wiki/Pain#Historical_theories. Accessed August, 2012.

31. Melzack R. Pain: past, present and future. *Can J Exp Psychol*. 1993;47(4):615–629.

32. DeLeo J. Basic science of pain. *J Bone Joint Surg Am*. 2006;88(Suppl 2):58–62.

33. Melzack R, Wall PD. Pain mechanisms: a new theory. *Science*. 1965;150:971–979.

34. Todd EM, Kucharski A. Pain: historical perspectives. In: Bajwa ZH, Warfield CA, ed. *The Management of Pain*. 2nd ed. New York: McGraw Hill, 2004:1–10.

35. Theory. *Wikipedia*. Available at: http://en.wikipedia.org/wiki/Theory. Accessed May, 2011.

36. Nathan PW. The gate-control theory of pain. A critical review. *Brain*. 1976;99(1):123–158.

37. Melzack R. Evolution of the neuromatrix theory of pain. The Prithvi Raj Lecture: presented at the third World Congress of World Institute of Pain, Barcelona 2004. *Pain Pract*. 2004;5(2):85–94.

38. Melzack R. From the gate to the neuromatrix. *Pain*. 1999;(Suppl 6):S121–S126.

39. Svacina L. *Pain Control #10*. Longmont: Staodynamics Inc, 1977.

40. Hughes J, Smith T, Kosterlitz H, et al. Identification of two related pentapeptides from the brain with potent opiate agonist activity. *Nature*. 1875;258(5536):577–580.

41. Li C, Chung D. Isolation and structure of an untriakontapeptide with opiate activity from camel pituitary glands. *Proc Natl Acad Sci U S A*. 1976;73(4):1145–1148.

42. Simantov R, Snyder S. Morphine-like peptides in mammalian brain: isolation, structure elucidation, and interactions with the opiate receptor. *Proc Natl Acad Sci USA*. 1976;73(7):2515–2519.

43. Loh H, Tseng L, Wei E, Li C. beta-endorphin is a potent analgesic agent. *Proc Natl Acad Sci U S A*. 1876;73(8):2895–2898.

44. Medicine NLo. Medical Subject Headings. National Library of Medicine [web page]. 2004. Available at: http://www.nlm.nih.gov/mesh/2003/MBrowser.html

45. Gear RW, Aley KO, Levine JD. Pain-induced analgesia mediated by mesolimbic reward circuits. *J Neurosci*. 1999;19(16):7175–7181.

46. Wickelgren I. Neuroscience: getting the brain's attention. *Science*. 1997;278(5335):35–37.

47. Stedman's Electronic Medical Dictionary. Philadelphia, PA: Lippincott Williams & Wilkins.

48. McCaffery M, Pasero C, eds. *Pain: Clinical Manual*. 2nd ed. St Louis MO: Mosby, 1999.

49. Aydede M. Pain. In: Zalta EN, ed. *The Stanford Encyclopedia of Philosophy*. 2010. Available at: http://plato.stanford.edu/cgi-bin/encyclopedia/archinfo.cgi?entry=pain. Accessed August, 2012.

50. Voscopoulos C, Lema M. When does acute pain become chronic? *Br J Anaesth*. 2010;105(S1):i69–i85.

51. Wiech K, Ploner M, Tracey I. Neurocognitive aspects of pain perception. *Trends Cogn Sci*. 2008;12(8):306–313.

52. Tracey I, Mantyh PW. The cerebral signature for pain perception and its modulation. *Neuron*. 2007;55(3):377–391.

53. Loeser JD. What is chronic pain? *Theor Med*. 1991;12(3):213–225.

54. Fordyce WE. Pain and suffering. A reappraisal. *Am Psychol*. 1988;43(4):276–283.

55. Bonica JJ. Evolution and current status of pain programs. *J Pain Symp Manage*. 1990;5(6):368–374.

56. Bagraith KS, Strong J, Sussex R. Disentangling disability in the fear avoidance model: more than pain interference alone. *Clin J Pain*. 2012;28(3):273–274.

57. Leonardi M, Bickenbach J, Ustun TB, Kostanjsek N, Chatterji S. The definition of disability: what is in a name? *Lancet*. 2006;368(9543):1219–1221.

58. Wikipedia. Disability. Available at: http://en.wikipedia.org/wiki/Disability. Accessed August, 2012.

59. Beecher H. Pain in men wounded in battle. *Ann Surg*. 1946;123:96–105.

60. Sussman C. Preventing and modulating learned wound pain. *Ostomy Wound Manage*. 2008;54(11):38–47.

61. Arner S, Meyerson BA. Lack of analgesic effect of opioids on neuropathic and idiopathic forms of pain. *Pain*. 1988;33:11–23.

62. Baugh J. Theories vs Models. *blog comments on Physics Forums*. Available at: http://www.physicsforums.com/showthread.php?t=75042. Accessed August, 2012.

63. Box GEP, Draper NR. *Empirical Model-Building and Response Surfaces*. Hoblken, NJ: John Wiley & Sons, 1987:424.

64. Wikipedia. Scientific Modeling. Available at: http://en.wikipedia.org/wiki/Scientific_modelling. Accessed August, 2012.

65. Wikipedia. Scientific Theory. Available at: http://en.wikipedia.org/wiki/Scientific_theory. Accessed August, 2012.

66. Creationism SCoSa, Sciences NAo. *Science and Creationism: A View from the National Academy of Sciences*. 2nd ed. The National Academies Press. Available at: http://www.nap.edu/openbook.php?record_id=6024&page=2. Accessed August, 2012.

67. AAOS Press Room. Q & A on Evolution and Intelligent Design. *Advancing Science Serving Society*. Available at: http://www.aaas.org/news/press_room/evolution/qanda.shtml. Accessed August, 2012.

68. Wikipedia. Periaqueductal gray. *Wikipedia*. Accessed May, 2011.

69. Wikipedia. Raphe nuclei. *Wikipedia*. Accessed May, 2011.

70. Watkins L, Mayer D. Multiple endogenous opiate and non-opiate analgesia systems: evidence of their existence and clinical implications. *Ann NY Acad Sci*. 1986;467:273–299.

71. Melzack R, Coderre TJ, Katz J, Vaccarino AL. Central neuroplasticity and pathological pain. *Ann N Y Acad Sci*. 2001;933:157–174.

72. Melzack R. Pain—an overview. *Acta Anaesthesiol Scand.* 1999; 43(9):880–884.

73. Gatchel RJ. *Clinical Essentials of Pain Management.* Washington, D.C.: American Psychological Association, 2005.

74. Trout K. The neuromatrix theory of pain: implications for selected nonpharmacologic methods of pain relief for labor. *J Midwifery Womens Health.* 2004;49(6):482–488.

75. Taylor G. The challenge of chronic pain: a psychoanalytic approach. *J Am Acad Psychoanal Dyn Psychiatry.* 2008;36(1):49–68.

76. Vlaeyen JWS, Kole Snijders AMJ, Boeren RGB, van Eek H. Fear of movement/(re)injury in chronic low back pain and its relation to behavioral performance. *Pain.* 1995;62(3):363–372.

77. Vlaeyen JW, Linton SJ. Fear-avoidance and its consequences in chronic musculoskeletal pain: a state of the art. *Pain.* 2000;85(3):317–332.

78. Leeuw M, Goossens MlEJB, Linton SJ, et al. The fear-avoidance model of musculoskeletal pain: current state of scientific evidence. *J Behav Med.* 2007;30(1):77–94.

79. Crombez G, Eccleston C, Van Damme S, Vlaeyen JWS, Karoly P. Fear-avoidance model of chronic pain: the next generation. *Clin J Pain.* 2012;28(6):475–483.

80. Vlaeyen JWS, Linton SJ. Fear-avoidance model of chronic musculoskeletal pain: 12 years on. *Pain.* 2012;153(6):1144–1147.

81. Loeser JD. Perspectives on pain. Paper presented at: Proceedings of the First World Congress on Clinical Pharmacology and Therapeutics, London. 1980:316–326.

82. Loeser JD, Cousins MJ. Contemporary pain management. *TMJOA.* 1990;153(4):208.

83. Ducar R. Pain physiology and psychology. Available at: http://www.fchs.ac.ae/fchs/uploads/Files/Semester%201%20-%202011–2012/3971NRS/LECTURE%206%20PDF%20[Compatibility%20Mode].pdf. Accessed August, 2012.

84. Cole BE. Pain management: Classifying, understanding, and treating pain. *Hosp Phys.* 2002;38:23–30.

85. Subcommittee on Taxonomy of the International Association for the Study of Pain. Classification of chronic pain. Descriptions of chronic pain syndromes and definitions of pain terms. *Pain (Suppl).* 1886;3:s1–s226.

86. Leavitt F, Garron D. Psychological disturbance and pain report differences in both organic and non-organic low back pain patients. *Pain.* 1979;7(2):187–195.

87. Osterweis M, Klenman A, Mechanic D. *Pain and Disability: Clinical, Behavior, and Public Policy Prospective - Institute of Medicine, Committee on Pain, Disability, and Chronic Illness Behavior.* Washington, DC: National Academy Press, 1987.

88. Magni G, Caldieron C, Rigatti-Luchini S, Merskey H. Chronic musculoskeletal pain and depressive symptoms in the general population. An analysis of the 1st National Health and Nutrition Examination Survey data. *Pain.* 1990;43(3):299–307.

89. Stein C, Schäfer M, Machelska H. Why is morphine not the ultimate analgesic and what can be done to improve it? *J Pain.* 2000;1(3):51–56.

90. Abbott B, Schoen L, Badia P. Predictable and unpredictable shock: Behavioral measures of aversion and physiological measures of stress. *Psychol Bull.* 1984;96(1)45–71.

91. Neary D, Ochoa J, Gilliatt R. Sub-clinical entrapment neuropathy in man. *J Neurol Sci.* 1975;24(3):283–298.

92. Schmelz M, Schmidt R, Bickel A, Handwerker H, Torebjork H. Specific C-receptors for itch in human skin. *J Neurosci.* 1997;17(20): 8003–8008.

93. Lawrence JM, Hoeft F, Sheau KE, Mackey SC. Strategy-dependent dissociation of the neural correlates involved in pain modulation. *Anesthesiology.* 2011;115(4):844–851.

94. Zeidan F, Grant JA, Brown CA, McHaffie JG, Coghill RC. Mindfulness meditation-related pain relief: evidence for unique brain mechanisms in the regulation of pain. *Neurosci Lett.* 2012;520(2):165–173.

95. Seminowicz DA, Mikulis DJ, Davis KD. Cognitive modulation of pain-related brain responses depends on behavioral strategy. *Pain.* 2004;112(1-2):48–58.

96. Wang J, Jian F, Chen J, et al. Cognitive behavioral therapy for orthodontic pain control: a randomized trial. *J Dent Res.* 2012;91(6): 580–585.

97. Kong J, Kaptchuk TJ, Polich G, Kirsch I, Gollub RL. Placebo analgesia: findings from brain imaging studies and emerging hypotheses. *Rev Neurosci.* 2007;18(3-4):173–190.

98. Racine ML, Tousignant-Laflamme Y, Kloda LA, et al. A systematic literature review of 10 years of research on sex/gender and experimental pain perception - part 1: are there really differences between women and men? *Pain.* 2012;153(3):602–618.

99. Unruh AM. Gender variations in clinical pain experience. *Pain.* 1996;65(2–3):123–167.

100. Lund IN, Lundeberg T. Is it all about sex? Acupuncture for the treatment of pain from a biological and gender perspective. *Acupunct Med.* 2008;26(1):33–45.

101. Fillingim RB. Sex, gender, and pain: women and men really are different. *Curr Rev Pain.* 2000;4(1):24–30.

102. Melzack R. Gate control theory: on the evolution of pain concepts. *Pain Forum.* 1996;5(1):128–138.

103. Moseley GL. A pain neuromatrix approach to patients with chronic pain. *Manual Ther.* 2003;8(3):13–140.

104. Lotze M, Moseley GL. Role of distorted body image in pain. *Curr Rheumatol Rep.* 2007;9(6):488–496.

105. Moseley GL. Using visual illusion to reduce at-level neuropathic pain in paraplegia. *Pain.* 2007;130:294–298.

106. Moseley GL, Wiech K. The effect of tactile discrimination training is enhanced when patients watch the reflected image of their unaffected limb during training. *Pain.* 2009;144:314–319.

107. McCabe CS, Haigh RC, Blake DR. Mirror visual feedback for the treatment of complex regional pain syndrome (Type 1). *Curr Pain Headache Rep.* 2008;12(2):103–107.

108. Ranganathan V, Siemionow V, Liu J, Sahgal V, Yue G. From mental power to muscle power—gaining strength by using the mind. *Neuropsychologia.* 2004;42(7):944–954.

109. Moyers B, Flowers BS, Grubin D. *Healing and the Mind.* New York, NY: Doubleday, 1993.

110. Belanger AY. *Therapeutic Electrophysical Agents: Evidence Behind Practice.* 2nd ed. Baltimore, MD: Lippincott Williams & Wilkins, 2009.

111. Mann MD. The Nervous System in Action [online text &.pdf]. Available at: http://michaeldmann.net/The%20Nervous%20System%20In%20Action.html. Accessed March, 2012.

Relieving Orthopedic Injury Pain

OPENING SCENE

You are an athletic training student intern with the rugby team. A player twists his ankle and limps over to you. "Is it pain or is it injury?" Coach Jones wonders whether the distress that caused his athlete to stop practicing is the result of torn tissue or simply "in the athlete's head." It's a legitimate question, you think to yourself. Torn tissue could be aggravated by practicing. But if the distress is only "in the athlete's head," he could "suck it up" or "gut it out" and continue preparing for the big game. Coach Jones consults with your clinical supervisor to determine whether to let the young man have his pain attended to or if he (the coach) should insist that the athlete return to practice.

The Philosophy and Principles of Pain Relief

Drugs, psychological techniques, surgical procedures, and physical therapy have all been used with varying degrees of success for pain relief, but no single method has been consistently successful.[1] This probably is because pain is multidimensional (see Chapter 7), and clinicians sometimes concentrate on a single aspect of the pain. The clinicians we have known who have been the most successful in alleviating pain are directed by a core philosophy. Principles are more important to them than tools. Their therapy is truly an art. Following are the principles that guide these "pain control artists."

MAKE THE PATIENT THE OWNER OF HIS PAIN

The most important aspect of treating pain is to make sure the patients take ownership for their pain.[2] Following are four things that you can do to help patients take ownership:

- Make sure the injury is thoroughly evaluated and diagnosed.
- Discuss the diagnosis and planned treatment with the patient and often significant others (such as parents or spouse). Make sure they understand the problem and that the planned treatment makes sense, and is something they agree to comply with.
- Make sure that all of the patient's questions are answered.
- Establish goals in consultation with the patient so that you both understand them. These must be physical goals, but could also include social and work goals. There must also be a specific quantifiable way of measuring progress for each goal.

RECOGNIZE THAT PAIN IS MULTIDIMENSIONAL

Pain is a multidimensional response to multidimensional stimuli that can both change over time. Think of it as a social, emotional, psychological experience that modulates the response to a pain-inducing stimulus that can morph over time. The response intensity and duration are not always correlated to the initial stimulus.[3–5]

IGNORE OR LISTEN TO PAIN?

Athletic success requires sacrifice, including ignoring discomfort while meeting a difficult challenge—to push beyond previous best effort (Fig. 9.1). At times an athlete must ignore the pain and persist in spite of it, especially pain associated with exertion nearing personal limits.

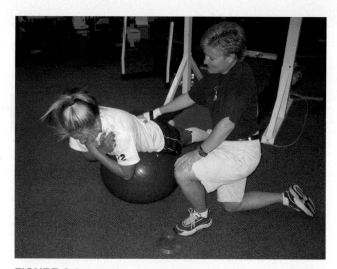

FIGURE 9.1 A patient must work through pain when conditioning but must avoid pain during rehabilitation. Pain during rehabilitation exercises causes neural inhibitions, which decreases flexibility, strength, and other physical activity.

But what about pain associated with injury? Some types of injury pain are just an irritant and must be ignored (Box 9.1). Other types will cause neural inhibitions that decrease neuromuscular functioning (range of motion [ROM], strength, agility, etc.). Persistent painful activity can enhance neural inhibition to such an extent that a permanent physiological block sometimes results. In this case, ignoring pain will prove detrimental to the athlete and result in chronic irritation and temporary loss of skill.

PAIN: DEMANDING DISCIPLINARIAN OR BENEVOLENT BENEFACTOR?

Is pain payback for indiscriminately or accidently pushing your body beyond its limits—a demanding disciplinarian? Or is pain a protective mechanism to keep you from causing further damage—a benevolent benefactor? Either, or both.

The body often mishandles pain. It has a great memory for what it wants to do, but not for why it is doing it.[6,7] Thus, pain often seems to persist long after the cause of

---

BOX 9.1   WORLD CLASS ATHLETE'S PAIN

"The difference between a very good athlete and a world class athlete is how they handle pain from minor nicks and knocks." Bruce Baumgartner made this statement after winning his first international title and prior to winning five Olympic medals, to Ken Knight in response to a question about why he (Bruce) was not spending as much time in the athletic training clinic as he had 2 years previously.

the pain is resolved. It's like that annoying relative who you thought was coming to visit for a few days, but stayed much longer than anticipated. Actually what happens is that the nociceptive pain is replaced by learned pain (see Chapter 8); an extremely annoying relative comes just as another relative is leaving. You must respect pain—use it to guide you—but be tough on it when necessary so that it does not take on a life of its own.

NO PAIN, NO GAIN?

When it comes to conditioning, "no pain, no gain" is absolutely right. But this adage does not apply to rehabilitation. During rehabilitation, the mantra is twofold:

- Ignoring the pain equals no brain, and
- Pandering to pain propagates pain.

Together these statements explain how to apply the statement in the previous paragraph—that you must respect pain and use it during rehabilitation. To ignore pain is not smart because it often leads to more pain and disability. On the other hand, if you eliminate all activity to avoid causing any pain, the pain will take on a life of its own, meaning it takes much less stimulus than normal to evoke a pain response (even minor aches and pains will seem worse than they are).

DEHNE'S SPINAL ADAPTATION SYNDROME

The **spinal adaptation syndrome** is a theory based on a 20-year study of sprains by Ernst Dehne (Box 9.2).[6–9] The logic of the theory is summarized as follows:

- Afferent nociceptive impulses arising from traumatized tissues or tissue in the process of repair alter the integration of CNS excitation at the spinal cord level.
- These alterations result in decreased response to volitional stimuli and increased response to otherwise subliminal peripheral stresses, resulting in involuntary muscle action.
- The altered muscle response through the mediation of vasomotor reaction (dilation or constriction of blood vessels) determines the local chemical environment that produces the process of repair.
- The process of repair is a highly sensitive state. It responds adversely to additional stress and favorably to the reestablishment of central control.
- The spinal adaptation syndrome seems to operate in all conditions connected with inflammation and repair. Covering such a broad spectrum, it is not specific to any one condition. It appears that all tissue in the process of repair has an extremely sensitive nociceptive potential and reacts violently to all additional stress, as well as to stress that would be subliminal in the normal state.

BOX 9.2   ERNST DEHNE, MD: AN ORTHOPEDIC VISIONARY

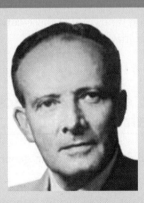

Ernst Dehne[6–9] is often considered the father of modern orthopedic rehabilitation. Although he is relatively unknown, his observations and revolutionary thinking set the stage for the great advances in rehabilitation during the past 30 years. His ideas that were "way out" in the 1950s and 1960s are now standard thinking, although few clinicians are aware of how he has influenced their practices.

Dehne was a German orthopedic surgeon who recognized in the 1930s that the standard practice of long-term cast immobilization (often up to 16 weeks) following orthopedic injury and surgery was detrimental to full recovery.[10,11] Through the years his idea of less immobilization and quicker active use of orthopedically injured limbs grew, in spite of a lack of acceptance by the mainstream medical community. Keith Markey, MD,[12] who served a residency under Dehne, tells of Dehne's frustration with the lack of cooperation by the nursing staff. They were reluctant to follow his orders to get his patients out of bed and walking immediately after surgery. It was so bad that Dehne would sometimes pound on their desk or on an empty hospital bed or table with a baseball bat as he urged them to follow his orders.

Although Grant[13] and Hayden[14] do not mention Dehne in their classic papers on cryokinetics (see Chapter 13), they worked one floor below him at Brook Army Hospital in San Antonio and treated many of his patients. Their "experiment" with ice and early active exercise grew, no doubt, from Dehne's philosophy of immediate mobilization.

The competitive influence of volitional impulses tends to inhibit and eventually to terminate the nociceptive interference at the spinal cord level.

In short, the theory holds that nociceptive impulses from traumatized tissue inhibit motor functions and tissue repair, but that voluntary activity can reestablish central control and prevent this inhibition. In other words, prolonged inactivity following an injury will lead to neural inhibition that could become permanent.

RESETTING CENTRAL CONTROL DURING REHABILITATION

Removing the pain sensation following injury is not enough; you must also get rid of the effects of the pain—that is, reset the system (reset central control). Consider the following analogy.

A plane at Chicago's O'Hare International Airport has a tire blowout during takeoff. Parts of the plane break off as it skids along, leaving the runway littered with debris and luggage. The runway is shut down while crews remove the damaged plane and debris. Within 6 hours the runway is cleaned and can be put back into service (*the pain is removed*).

All is not back to normal, however; thousands of passengers are stranded in the terminal because their flights were cancelled. Tens of thousands of additional passengers are stranded in airports around the world because their flights to Chicago were cancelled or delayed. Business meetings have to be rescheduled, sports and cultural activities rescheduled because teams, performers, and support personnel didn't arrive in time, hotel reservations changed, family activities changed, and so on. It may take weeks or months to get things back to normal, to fix the effects of the blown-out tire in Chicago (*reset central control*).

The concept of resetting central control must be part of the therapy for dealing with pain and injury. Immobilization and injury can cause a physiological block that can become permanent if not handled properly. You must get the whole orchestra playing in unison. If the flutes and violas are just half a beat off, they create discord and noise rather than great soothing music. The following example from one of our athletes illustrates this principle.

Case 9.1 illustrates this principle.

CASE STUDY 1: RESET CENTRAL CONTROL

A gymnast suffered an eversion ankle sprain. Weeks after the injury he was pain-free while walking, had good muscular strength, but could not stick a dismount because of excruciating pain. He had been an All-American the year before and was extremely frus-trated. Everything else was normal. He was referred to one of us (KK) for consultation. After reviewing the case and evaluating the injury, we concluded that the initial injury had healed, and the need was to reset central control via a series of graded skill activities. Although he was an all-arounder, we concentrated on vaulting, his best event, as follows:

- Approach the pommel horse at 50% speed and jump upon the horse into a sitting position.
- Run at 75% speed, straddle the horse, and land on the other side without a flip.
- Repeat the previous step, at 90% speed.
- Approach at 90% speed, do a simple flip over the horse, and land on the mat.
- Approach at 90% speed and perform the easiest vault that would score points.

He performed each of these events pain-free, and as you might expect, with a bigger grin following each one. We told him to do nothing else but to return that evening (the team had a meet), go through normal warm-ups, and then perform the same series of activities just prior to the vault competition. Again there was no pain during any of the jumps/vaults. He competed without pain and scored just under his all-time best. The following Monday, and thereafter, he practiced all events without pain or disability.

This case illustrates both the effects of the spinal adaptation syndrome and the need to reset central control following injury. Make these concepts part of your pain and injury management.

Sources of Orthopedic Injury Pain

Pain sources fall into one of four general classes (see Chapter 7):

1. Nociceptive Pain. Most acute orthopedic or sports injuries occur in response to injury or illness to bodily structures. Nociceptors at the site of injury initiate messages that are then conducted on efferent nerves up through the spinal cord into the brain, where the messages are interpreted as pain.[15,16] Acute orthopedic injury pain results from the stimulation of nociceptors by the following:
   a. Injured tissue (mediator release)
   b. Edema pressure
   c. Stretching injured tissue
   d. Muscle spasm pressure

2. Neuropathic Pain. A complex, chronic pain state that usually is accompanied by tissue damage to the nerve fibers themselves. Thus the nerve fibers become dysfunctional and send incorrect signals to the brain and other pain centers.[15,16] It often shows up in illogical ways. Chronic orthopedic injury pain occurs due to:
   a. Acute nerve damage, such as with a stinger or pinched nerve, in which the nerve is crushed, compressed, stretched, or severed
   b. Otherwise normal activity in a tissue that becomes sensitized from disuse following injury
   c. Surgery that involves neural tissue. One example is amputation, that often results in phantom limb pain.
   d. Numerous conditions (such as alcoholism, chemotherapy, nutritional deficiencies, or diabetes) that cause nerves to become dysfunctional
3. Learned Pain. A learned, or conditioned, response that develops from a patient's "pain memories" of physiological and emotional elements of either nociceptive or neuropathic pain experience.[16,17] The pain stimuli is indirectly paired with any of an infinite number of environmental or sociological stimuli, even inactivity. Eventually these secondary stimuli elicit pain.[17] Thus pain can be evoked without noxious input.[18]
   a. Pain anticipation/expectation
   b. Delayed resolution of the injury
   c. Inordinate emotional stress associated with the injury (especially if prolonged)
   d. Inactivity, as in Dehne's Spinal Adaptation Syndrome (above)
   e. Activity that elicits pain (see "No Pain, No Gain" above)
4. Idiopathic Pain. Unknown origin, meaning there is no identifiable pathology associated with it.[15,16] This pain will drive you batty in trying to locate a cause.

The Placebo Effect and Pain Relief

Derived from the Latin for "I shall please," **placebo** is a medicinally inactive substance given as a medicine for its suggestive effect or to satisfy the patient's demand for medicine. It is most often thought of as a mock intervention (such as a sugar pill instead of aspirin) that brings about a desired response (pain relief), but has no physiological effects. Patients think they are receiving an actual dose of medicine when they are not, and the psychological effects of their expectations of benefit are responsible for the result.[19] For example, 35% of postoperative pain, diabetes, and chronic headache patients obtain relief as a result of placebos.[20,21] In a multicenter study of patients with ulcers, 76% of sufferers obtained relief with Tagamet therapy, but 63% obtained relief from taking a placebo.[22]

The benefits or effects of placebo occur in response to many types of interventions in addition to taking medically inactive substances.[20] This concept is known as the **placebo effect**—a measurable, observable, or felt improvement in health not attributable to treatment. Psychological factors, particularly the clinician's and the patient's expectations of pain relief, contain powerful therapeutic value in their own right, in addition to the effects of the procedure itself.[23,24] Additional mechanisms, such as learning or conditioned reflex,[25] cognitive modulation,[26] and neurotransmitter reaction,[27] result in a placebo effect. All of these mechanisms fit into the concept of central control (see Chapter 7).

On the negative side, one reason quackery abounds is because of the placebo effect. The so-called snake oil salesmen convince their clients that they have a powerful medicine, when in reality the medicine is inert. Another disadvantage relates to research. Sometimes patients will get better due to chance or belief in the intervention. That's why good research often requires a large number of subjects to help separate those who get better because of the placebo effect from those who get better from the intervention being studied.

The placebo effect is a powerful, dynamic, robust, and widespread phenomenon.[28] It is not a "nontreatment." Brain mapping with advanced MRI scanners indicate that activity in pain-sensitive brain regions is altered by placebos.[29] A placebo does not interfere with the body's ability to sense pain but instead affects how the brain modulates its interpretation of the body's signals.[29–31] Thus a person's state of mind and previous experiences have a strong effect on descending tract pain control.[32] Clinicians should take advantage of the placebo effect in treating patients (Box 9.3).

PSYCHOLOGICAL ASPECTS AND A POSITIVE ATTITUDE

Psychological and emotional influences surrounding an injury can have a great impact on pain treatments and patient response. For example, if a starting senior guard on the basketball team suffers an anterior cruciate ligament (ACL) sprain, the emotional aspect of this injury—causing him to miss the rest of his college career—will make the immediate pain almost unbearable. If, however, the same injury happened to a third-string sophomore, the emotional impact might be less if he feels he has two additional years to play, and thus the pain will probably be less than that of his senior team mate.

Another important aspect to consider is if a patient is negative toward treatment and rehabilitation, the body's healing processes will not work as well. Having a positive the same manner. If a technique isn't working after three or four treatments, try something else. Change methods when necessary; sometimes the body adapts to the treatment method and the method becomes ineffective. Here are two examples:

- Some athletes are sensitive to cold and so cryokinetics is not possible (see Chapter 13). TENS can be used rather than the cold to facilitate exercise.[33]
- A football wide receiver suffered from a moderate-plus quadriceps contusion. Although he initially responded well to cryostretch treatments (see Chapter 13), after 2 or 3 days, the cold no longer facilitated therapeutic exercise. The athletic trainer then switched his treatment to TENS and exercise. He continued to progress for another couple of days and then plateaued. He was then treated with analgesic balm and therapeutic exercise for 2 days, and then went back to the cryostretch. He continued the rotation through the three techniques for pain relief as the athletic trainer continued the therapeutic exercise until he was able to perform pain-free.

DIRECT VERSUS INDIRECT PAIN RELIEF

There are two main approaches to treating orthopedic injury pain: direct and indirect. The direct method of pain relief addresses the pain itself. The application of TENS to a sprained ankle to gate the pain or release endogenous opiates is an example of direct pain relief.

The indirect method focuses on removing the cause of pain. For example, if a basketball player with an ankle sprain is experiencing pain from the pressure of edema on nociceptors, using an intermittent compression pump and elevation will reduce the swelling in this area and thus

attitude toward injury care helps the body respond to the treatment more favorably (Box 9.4), and lessens the development of learned pain.

Use a Variety of Techniques

It is important to have a variety of pain relief methods at your disposal. Just as all patients do not respond to pain in the same way, not all patients respond to treatments in relieve the pain. Preventing learned pain is also an indirect method of pain relief.

Tools for Relieving Pain

A variety of techniques are available to relieve pain (Fig. 9.2). Differences in injury and in patient response will dictate differences in therapeutic approaches, so clinicians need to be skilled in using a number of techniques. It's essential to remember that the tool is not as important as the philosophy of the approach. And the keystone of that philosophy is to reset central control.

Many of the following tools are used simultaneously. For example, cryotherapy and exercise are used interchangeably in cryokinetics and cryostretch (see Chapter 13) to incrementally restore full pain-free activity.

IMMOBILIZATION

Immobilization is used to decrease pain in many situations, especially in the early stages of rehabilitation. It allows torn tissue to begin healing, and structurally intact but irritated tissues to "quiet down." Prolonged inactivity is dangerous, however, and can result in prolonged disability (see Fig. 1.5). Patients should transition to controlled activity as quickly as possible. Managing this process is an art.

THERAPEUTIC EXERCISE

Low-level, controlled therapeutic exercise decreases edema-induced pain by stimulating lymph flow, thereby reducing mechanical pressure on nociceptors. Isometric contractions interspersed with static stretching relieve pain by reducing muscle spasm (see Chapter 13).

Therapeutic exercise should be relatively pain-free. It is acceptable if the activity is mildly uncomfortable, but

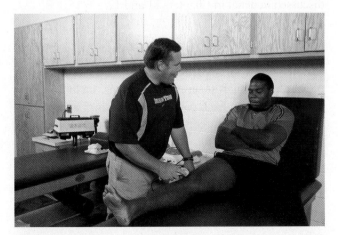

FIGURE 9.2 Therapeutic modalities modulate pain so that patients can begin therapeutic exercise.

serious discomfort is a warning from the body that something is wrong. Therapeutic exercise or activity during rehabilitation should not evoke the same type of pain that was experienced when the injury occurred.

COUNTER-IRRITANTS

Counter-irritants are substances that irritate the skin when applied, causing mild skin inflammation. The irritation closes the gate on mild pain in muscles, joints, or internal organs. In essence, the counter-irritant causes the brain to switch its attention from the mild pain to the counter-irritant. Counter-irritation is perhaps one of the oldest[34] and simplest methods of pain relief. Examples are:

- Ethyl chloride spray
- Hot water bottle
- Ice packs
- Vibration
- Tactile stimulation (pressure)
- Neuromuscular electrical stimulation (NMES)
- Static electricity
- Analgesic balms

The use of most of the above counter-irritants is straight forward. Analgesic balms are an exception. Claims of their effects are often misstated and they are at times misused. Therefore we will discuss them in more detail.

Analgesic Balms

Analgesic balms make up most of the counter-irritants used by the public (e.g., Sports Cream, Ben Gay, Icy Hot, Flex-all). An **analgesic balm** is an externally applied drug that has a topical analgesic, anesthetic, or anti-itching effect by depressing cutaneous sensory receptors, or a topical counter-irritant effect by stimulating cutaneous sensory receptors.

There are several over-the-counter analgesic lotions, creams, and patches that patients can use to reduce aches and pains. The active ingredients in most of these topical analgesics are menthol, methyl salicylate, and capsaicin, used singly or in combination with one or both of the others.

Menthol is an alcohol obtained from oil of peppermint and derived from the mint plant. Menthol is classified as an irritant that produces a cooling sensation when used at 1.25–16%. Menthol is included in analgesic balms to provide a sensation of cold, although some patients describe a cool burning sensation. The amount of menthol in many OTC topical analgesics ranges from 1–16%.

Methyl salicylate is wintergreen oil, produced synthetically or from the distilled leaves of sweet birch. Methyl salicylate is classified as an irritant that produces redness when used at 10–60%. It is included in analgesic balms to provide a sensation of heat. For methyl salicylate to be classified as an active ingredient, it needs to constitute 10–60% of the product.

Capsaicin is a derivative of the hot-pepper plant and is an irritant included in analgesic balms to provide a sensation of heat.

Scientists have studied the effects of topical analgesics in reducing pain associated with delayed-onset muscle soreness.[35] Pain perception was measured with a visual analog scale (VAS) 48 hours after eccentric exercise. Subjects were then divided into three groups: placebo, menthol/methyl salicylate, and capsaicin (an irritant included in analgesic balms to provide a sensation of heat). The treatments were applied over the most painful area for 5 minutes and then removed. Subjects in the menthol/methyl salicylate group experienced a significant reduction in pain compared to the other two groups.

Using an animal model, scientists reported that administration of menthol (1.9%) to the skin surface of contracting muscles decreased autonomic responses to static muscle contractions.[36] This effect was independent of higher brain processing and strongly suggests that menthol application to the skin has analgesic effects on pain signals located in the muscle.

Scientists who have performed research on products that contain either menthol or methyl salicylate as an active ingredient have reported that these products produce no significant increase in muscle or skin temperature.[37] How do these products provide the sensations of heat or cold, and how do they relieve pain?

The mechanism by which menthol works has not been well understood until recently.[35,38] It seems that some of the same receptors in the skin that respond to cold stimuli (temperatures between 46 and 86°F (8 and 30°C) also respond to menthol.[35] Because the same receptor is stimulated by both cold and menthol, patients might notice a sensation of cooling, or burning cold, after the menthol application.[35] These sensations, in turn, may reduce the amount of pain they experience.[39]

The fact that these products don't increase or decrease the temperature does not mean that they are ineffective. They may help reduce pain in two ways. First, as these chemicals (menthol or methyl salicylate) stimulate the cutaneous sensory receptors, pain signals may be altered at the dorsal horn of the spinal cord. Second, the action of massaging the analgesic cream into the area, and the stimulating effects of the counter-irritant, may increase large-diameter afferent nerve input. Indeed, topically applied external analgesics appear to provide some benefit for pain relief. In fact, the American College of Rheumatology supports these agents as primary therapy for disorders such as osteoarthritis of the knee and promote their use before relying on therapy using NSAIDs (nonsteroidal anti-inflammatory drugs).[40]

THERMOTHERAPY

Pain reduction is probably the most frequent indication for the use of heat in a therapeutic setting.[41] Topical heat is effective for reducing pain associated with rheumatoid arthritis,[42,43] adhesive capsulitis,[44] and neck and back **trigger point pain**[45] (a hypersensitive area or site in muscle or connective tissue, usually associated with myofascial pain syndromes). Experimental research on patients with low-back pain has demonstrated that topical heat provided greater pain relief and resulted in lower disability for 24 hours after thermotherapy application, compared to no treatment.[46] Similar effects were also shown in the treatment of trapezius myalgia with low-level topical heat.[47] Heat's pain-relieving qualities are related to its ability to increase local blood flow,[48–50] promote the relaxation of soft tissue,[49–51] and reduce muscle spasm.[52–54]

Erasala et al.[50] used Doppler ultrasound to demonstrate increased blood flow in the trapezius muscle following topical thermotherapy. This increased blood flow is thought to "wash away" chemical irritants such as bradykinin. In addition to increased blood flow, heating is also believed to cause a counter-irritant effect through the stimulation of cutaneous nerves, specifically **thermoreceptors**, sensory receptors that respond to heat or cold.[49] As a result of thermoreceptor activity, both sedation and relaxation are facilitated, which often leads to pain modulation.[41,49] Although the mechanisms underlying these phenomena are not completely understood, both the gate control theory and a decrease in the response rates of specific nerves (axons of gamma motor neurons) that supply muscles have been proposed as possible mechanisms for the decreased pain and muscle relaxation that occurs with the application of thermotherapy.[41,49,55]

Finally, as a muscle spasm is relaxed, pressure on nociceptors is lessened, thereby leading to a reduction in pain, called reduction of the pain-spasm-pain cycle. Thermotherapy is discussed in detail in Chapters 11 and 12.

ELECTROTHERAPY

Various forms of electrical nerve stimulation devices provide pain relief in several conditions, including osteoarthritis,[56,57] low-back pain,[58,59] neck pain,[60] and postoperative orthopedic surgery pain.[61–63] Electrical stimulating currents are thought to reduce pain in three ways:

- By reducing muscle spasm (relaxing the muscle) and thereby removing mechanical pressure on nerves that initiate pain
- By releasing endogenous opiates at pain receptor sites
- By stimulating nonpainful nerves, thus gating, or modulating, the pain

  Electrotherapy is discussed in Chapter 10.

CRYOTHERAPY

Cold is perhaps the most effective modality available, certainly more effective than heat applications in relieving pain during acute care.[64] Heat, however, appears to be superior in decreasing dull pain that is common the day following extreme exertion or toward the end of subacute care. Here are two guidelines[65]:

- Treat specific acute injuries with cryotherapy, but general aches and pain with a warm whirlpool or hot tub.
- In a subacute injury, if pain prevents normal ROM or gait, use ice to facilitate exercise; if ROM and gait are normal, use heat applications to relieve the dull aches.

Cryotherapy: Powerful Pain Medicine

In the 1940s, Allen and associates[66,67] used cold applications (ice packs and immersion for 1–5 hours) as the only analgesic for limb amputation. Cold applied to the leg can prevent tooth pain resulting from the electrical stimulation of teeth fillings and laser-evoked pain.[20,28] Postoperative medication and complications are minimized following orthopedic surgery when cold is applied.[68]

Cryotherapy is also effective in minimizing chronic pain induced by repetitive strain. Baseball pitchers who immersed their arms in ice water following a simulated game were more accurate and could throw with greater velocity in a subsequent game 3 or 4 days later.[69,70]

The most common use of cold with acute orthopedic injury is to modulate the pain of sprains, strains, and contusions in order to facilitate therapeutic exercise (Fig. 9.3).[13,14,71–74] The discovery of this technique, known as cryokinetics, in the mid-1960s dramatically changed the approach to the rehabilitation of sprains, strains, and contusions. These concepts are discussed in greater detail in Chapters 13 and 14.

Pain Resulting from Cold Immersion

Immersion in a slush bucket, with the water temperature near 34°F (1°C) is very painful during the first few sessions. For this reason, some clinicians avoid using certain cryotherapy techniques. But this rationalization is detrimental to patients. They quickly adapt to cold induced pain and find that faster recovery more than compensates for the initial cold-induced pain.

PSYCHOLOGICAL TOOLS

A variety of psychological behaviors modulate a patient's perception or interpretation of a sensation or situation. These behaviors are involved in both the manifestation and treatment of pain. The sight of blood may exacerbate pain from a simple wound. Learned pain is psychological behavior gone astray. And as the placebo effect attests, belief in a therapeutic regimen can have a powerfully

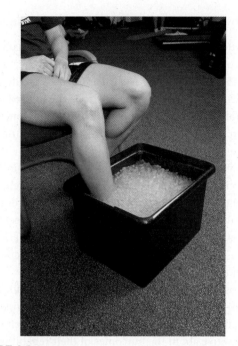

FIGURE 9.3 Cryokinetics, the alternating of cold application and therapeutic exercise, is a powerful technique that combines the pain-modulating effects of both cold and controlled, progressive therapeutic exercise.

positive effect on the outcome of the therapy. Doubt can have the opposite effect.[20]

Following are selected psychological tools for your pain relief tool box.

- Goals/expectations. Clinician and patient expectations of pain relief is powerful medicine.[23,24] Discuss each element of the rehabilitation process with the patient and agree on specific long-term, mid-range, and short-term goals.
- Biofeedback. Measure performance of the short-term goal activities, and discuss the results with the patient. For example, mark specific end points for flexion and extension, tell the patient to touch the endpoints during each repetition, and measure the time—to the nearest second—that it takes to perform 10 pain-free repetitions. Emphasize that they must be pain-free. If the activity is not performed properly, don't count it—and tell the patient that it does not count.
- Cognitive strategies. A variety of psychological behaviors are effective in modulating a patients perception, or interpretation, of a sensation or situation.[75,76] These are not gimmicks used to fool the gullible; their physiological basis is being revealed by measuring and correlating patterns of brain activation during application of the various strategies.[29–32,75,79] The effectiveness of various cognitive strategies differs among individuals, however. Individuals recruit different brain regions to perform the same task.

Following are some representative cognitive strategies:

a. Attentional modulation. Distract the patient by requiring her to concentrate on another sensory modality, such as visual, auditory, or tactile stimulus.[26] Talk to your patient, stroke the injured or contralateral limb. You might also have her concentrate on breathing by breathing in through the nose and out through the mouth.

b. Meditation.[77] The mind and body can be trained so as to increase mental calmness and physical relaxation, improve psychological balance, cope with illness, or enhance overall health and well-being. Techniques may involve a specific posture, focused attention, or an open attitude toward distractions. Specific techniques are available on the Internet.[78,79]

c. Positive attitude. Clinicians should maintain a positive and upbeat attitude and behavior during interactions with patients, and encourage patients to be positive about the outcomes of their rehabilitation.[28] Don't allow patients to dwell on previous negative injury rehabilitation experiences that they or acquaintances have experienced.

d. Social interaction. Maintain normal social interaction as much as possible.

Monitoring and Assessing Pain Relief During Rehabilitation

Pain must be monitored throughout the rehabilitation process. As discussed in Chapter 1, pain during an activity indicates the activity is too strenuous or complex; residual pain, or pain the next day, indicates that the previous day's activity was too strenuous. Activities that result in pain during rehabilitation will hinder the rehabilitation process by inducing neural inhibition.

Because pain tolerance varies from person to person and the perception of pain is subjective, pain itself is difficult to measure, and pain relief is hard to quantify. The best assessment tools are questionnaires and scales that quantify a person's subjective evaluation of the pain. Most instruments measure a single quality of pain, such as intensity. One scale, the McGill Pain Questionnaire, measures multiple qualities of pain. These are the most common pain assessment instruments:

- Number scale
- Verbal rating scale
- VAS
- Graphic rating scale
- McGill Pain Questionnaire

THE NUMBER SCALE

Number scales are used to measure pain intensity. They consist of a range of numbers (such as 0–10) and descriptors associated with some or all of the numbers (Fig. 9.4). Patients are instructed to select the number that best describes their pain. For example, 0 means no pain, and 10 means pain so severe that the patient feels a need to go to the hospital.

THE VERBAL RATING SCALE

Verbal rating scales consist of a group of descriptors but no numbers. For example, patients may be asked to rate their pain as absent, mild, moderate, or severe, or their pain relief as none, slight, moderate, or good. Verbal rating scales are thought to be insensitive to slight changes.[80,81]

Circle the word and/or number that best describes the intensity of your pain:

0	Nothing at all
0.5	Very, very weak (just noticeable)
1	Very weak
2	Weak (light)
3	Moderate
4	Somewhat strong
5	Strong (heavy)
6	
7	Very strong
8	
9	
10	Very, very strong (almost maximal)
	Maximal

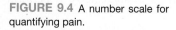
FIGURE 9.4 A number scale for quantifying pain.

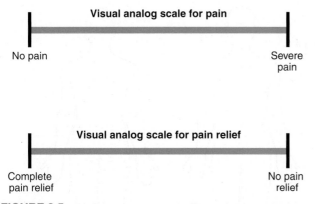

FIGURE 9.5 A VAS for assessing pain. The patient makes a vertical slash on a 100-mm line where she feels her pain is.

THE VISUAL ANALOG SCALE

The **visual analog scale (VAS)** consists of a line of specific length, usually 100 mm (4 in.), with contrasting descriptors at either end of the line. Descriptors may indicate any quality of pain, such as "no pain" and "severe pain," "annoying" and "unbearable," "dull" and "sharp" (Fig. 9.5). There are no numbers displayed on the line. The patient simply makes a vertical slash on the line where she feels her pain is. The clinician then measures from the left side of the scale to the slash to assess the pain. The measurement in mm is then converted to a percentage. The VAS is thought to represent a robust, sensitive, and reproducible measure of pain.[81–83]

One area of contention concerning the VAS is whether to allow patients to see previous results when assessing subsequent pain. For example, if you wanted to assess the effectiveness of a single treatment or a course of treatments, you would measure pain before and after treatment. Knowledge of the first measurement will influence the subsequent measurement. A purist would say that the two measurements must be independent. Yet the subjective nature of assessing pain almost demands that assessing change be done from the perspective of the initial assessment. We favor the latter.

 CONCEPT CHECK 9.1. You use a TENS unit to treat a patient with elbow pain and want to see how effective your treatment is at relieving pain. What could you use to measure pain relief? How would you know if you are making progress?

THE GRAPHIC RATING SCALE

The **graphic rating scale** is a horizontal line similar to the VAS with anchor points at each end and descriptors spread along the line (Fig. 9.6). It is administered and scored the same as the VAS. Some feel is it a better scale than the VAS because it is more sensitive to intensity,[84] is easier to use,[85] and has greater within- and between-subject reliability.[85]

THE McGILL PAIN QUESTIONNAIRE

The **McGill Pain Questionnaire** is the most complex of the pain measurement tools. It uses pictures, scales, and words to help patients describe sensory and affective aspects, as well as magnitude and changes in their pain. Instructions on how to use this questionnaire are found in Figure 9.7.

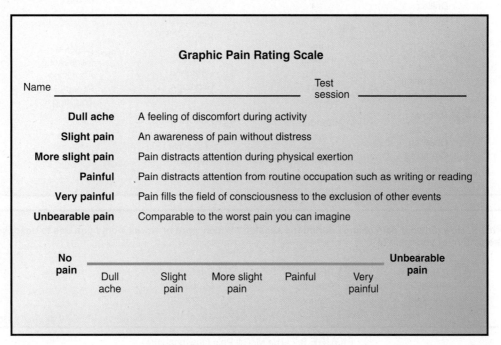

FIGURE 9.6 The graphic rating scale.

Part 1. **Where is your pain? Circle the area of greatest pain.**

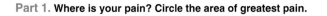

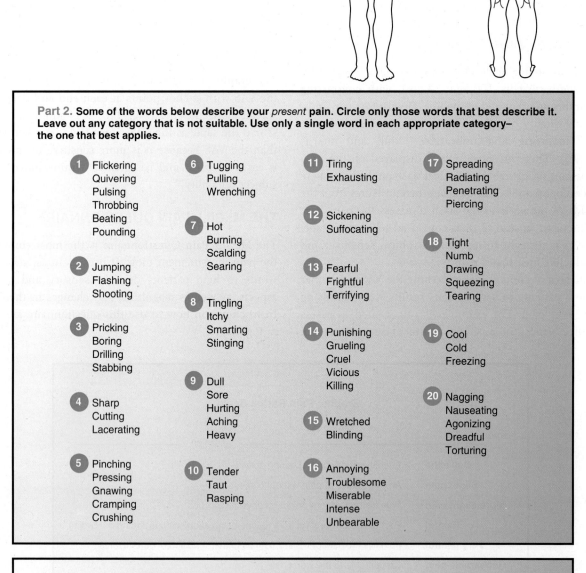

Part 2. **Some of the words below describe your *present* pain. Circle only those words that best describe it. Leave out any category that is not suitable. Use only a single word in each appropriate category– the one that best applies.**

1. Flickering
Quivering
Pulsing
Throbbing
Beating
Pounding

2. Jumping
Flashing
Shooting

3. Pricking
Boring
Drilling
Stabbing

4. Sharp
Cutting
Lacerating

5. Pinching
Pressing
Gnawing
Cramping
Crushing

6. Tugging
Pulling
Wrenching

7. Hot
Burning
Scalding
Searing

8. Tingling
Itchy
Smarting
Stinging

9. Dull
Sore
Hurting
Aching
Heavy

10. Tender
Taut
Rasping

11. Tiring
Exhausting

12. Sickening
Suffocating

13. Fearful
Frightful
Terrifying

14. Punishing
Grueling
Cruel
Vicious
Killing

15. Wretched
Blinding

16. Annoying
Troublesome
Miserable
Intense
Unbearable

17. Spreading
Radiating
Penetrating
Piercing

18. Tight
Numb
Drawing
Squeezing
Tearing

19. Cool
Cold
Freezing

20. Nagging
Nauseating
Agonizing
Dreadful
Torturing

Part 3. **How did your pain change during the session? Which word or words would you use to describe the pattern of your pain?a**

31. Continuous
Steady
Constant

32. Rhythmic
Periodic
Intermittent

33. Brief
Momentary
Transient

FIGURE 9.7 The McGill Pain Questionnaire.

CLOSING SCENE

Recall from the chapter opening scene, that you are the student athletic trainer assigned to the rugby team. A player twists his ankle and limps over to the staff AT, obviously in pain. His coach asks if the player actually has an injury that would sideline him, or if he can play through the pain. The staff AT informs Coach Jones that she will evaluate the ankle to determine the extent of the injury. You will also use a pain assessment scale to determine the extent of the pain and to recommend when the athlete will be able to return to practice.

Chapter Reflections

1. Read and ponder each of the following points. Do you feel you have a clear understanding of each concept? If not, reread the appropriate section of the chapter.
   - Discuss the relative effectiveness of drugs, psychological techniques, surgical procedures, and physical therapy for pain control.
   - Why is it important to develop a philosophy about pain and pain relief?
   - Discuss each of the following principles of pain relief, including how each contributes to your philosophy of pain control:
     - Make the patient the owner of his pain
     - Recognize that pain is multidimensional
     - Ignore or listen to pain
     - Pain: Demanding disciplinarian or benevolent benefactor?
     - No pain, no gain
     - Dehne's spinal adaptation syndrome
     - Resetting central control during rehabilitation
   - Give an example of the application of each of the previous pain relief principles when treating patients.
   - What is the placebo effect?
   - What effect does a positive attitude have on pain control?
   - Name four sources of orthopedic injury pain, and briefly discuss the mechanism of each one.
   - Differentiate between direct and indirect pain relief.
   - Discuss the use of each of the following tools for relieving pain:
     - Therapeutic exercise
     - Counter-irritants
     - Thermotherapy
     - Electrotherapy
     - Cryotherapy
     - Psychological tools
   - Discuss the concept of assessing pain and quantifying pain relief.
   - Discuss the advantages and disadvantages of the following pain scales: Number scale, Verbal rating scale, VAS, Graphic rating scale, McGill pain Questionnaire.

2. Write three to five questions for discussion with your class instructor, clinical instructor, classmates, and clinical colleagues.

3. Get together with classmates and quiz each other on the concepts of this chapter. Use the points in reflection no. 1 and the questions you wrote for reflection no. 2 as a beginning. Explaining concepts out loud to others requires a deeper grasp of the material than feeling you understand it as you read.

Critical Thinking Response

The VAS would help measure pain relief. You know if you are making progress by subtracting the current treatment's score from the previous treatment's score. For example, prior to your treatment the patient made a mark on the line at 66 mm from the left anchor point. After the treatment, she makes a mark 22 mm from the left anchor point.

(66 – 22 = 44, or a 67% reduction in pain).

REFERENCES

1. Svacina L. *Pain Control #10*. Longmont: Staodynamics Inc, 1977.
2. Butler D, Moseley L. *Explain Pain*. Adelaide, Australia: Noihtoup Publicatios, 2003.
3. Melzack R, Torgerson W. On the language of pain. *Anesthesiology*. 1971;34:50.
4. Bond M, Simpson K. *Pain: Its Nature and Treatment*. New York: Churchill Livingstone, 2006.
5. Melzack R. Pain and the neuromatrix in the brain. *J Dent Educ*. 2001;65(11):1378–1382.
6. Dehne E. The spinal adaption syndrome (a theory based on the study of sprains). *Clin Orthop*. 1955;5:211–220.
7. Dehne E, Torp RP. Treatment of joint injuries by immediate mobilization. Based upon the spinal adaptation concept. *Clin Orthop*. 1971;77:218–232.
8. Dehne E. Injuries to Ligaments of Elbow (Allgemeine Folgen von Banderrissen und Spatfolgen des medialen Banderrisses am Ellbogen sowle Vorschlage zu Dessen Behandlung). *Dtsch. Z. Chir*. 1934;243:716–723.
9. Dehne E. The rationale of early functional loading in the healing of fractures: a comprehensive gate control concept of repair. *Clin Orthop Rel Res*. 1980:146:18–27.
10. Dehne E. Physiological consideration in treatment of tears of ligaments of the knee (Beurteilung und Behandlung der Verletzungen desBandapparates am Knie unter Zugrundelegung einer mechanistischen oder einer physiologischen Betrachtungsweise). *Arch Orthop Unfallchir*. 1938;39:319.
11. Dehne E. Subluxation of the ankle (Ein Fall von unvollstandiger Luxation des Talus als Folge wiederholter Verletzungen im oberen Sprunggelenk). *Zentralbl Chir*. 1933;60:688.
12. Markey KL. personal communication with Ken Knight; 1985.
13. Grant AE. Massage with ice (cryokinetics) in the treatment of painful conditions of the musculoskeletal system. *Arch Phys Med Rehabil*. 1964;44:233–238.
14. Hayden CA. Cryokinetics in an early treatment program. *J Am Phys Ther Assoc*. 1964;44:990–993.
15. Stein C, Schäfer M, Machelska H. Why is morphine not the ultimate analgesic and what can be done to improve it? *J Pain*. 2000;1(3):51–56.
16. Arner S, Meyerson BA. Lack of analgesic effect of opioids on neuropathic and idiopathic forms of pain. *Pain*. 1988;33:11–23.
17. Sussman C. Preventing and modulating learned wound pain. *Ostomy Wound Manage*. 2008;54(11):38–47.
18. Wiech K, Ploner M, Tracey I. Neurocognitive aspects of pain perception. *Trends Cogn Sci*. 2008;12(8):306–313.
19. Charlton JEE. *Core Curriculum for Professional Education in Pain*. Seattle, WA: IASP Press, 2005.
20. Wall PD. The Placebo and the Placebo Response. In: Wall PD, Melzack R, eds. *Textbook of Pain*. Edinburgh: Churchill Livingstone, 2003:1297–1308.
21. Wall PD. The placebo and the placebo response. In: Wall PD, Melzack R, eds. *Textbook of Pain*, 1984:1297–1308.
22. Kirsch I, Sapirstein G. Listening to prozac but hearing placebo: a meta-analysis of antidepressant medication. *Preven Treat*. 1998:1.
23. Kirsch I. Specifying nonspecifics: psychological mechanisms of placebo effects. In: Harrington A, ed. *The Placebo Effect: An Interdisciplinary Exploration*. Cambridge, MA: Harvard University Press, 1999:166–186.
24. Voudouris N, Peck C, Coleman G. The role of conditioning and expectancy in the placebo response. *Pain*. 1990;43:121–128.
25. Montgomery C, Kirsch I. Classical conditioning and the placebo effect. *Pain*. 1997;72:107–113.
26. Villemure C, Bushnell M. Cognitive modulation of pain: how do attention and emotion influence pain processing. *Pain*. 2002;95:195–199.
27. Amanzio M, Benedetti F. Neuropharmacological dissection of placebo analgesia: expectation-activated opiod systems versus conditioning-activated subsystems. *J Neurosci*. 1999;19:484–494.
28. Gustafson D. Categorizing pain. In: Aydede M, ed. *Pain: New Essays on its Nature and the Methodology of its Study*. Cambridge, MA: The MIT Press, 2005:219–241.
29. Wager T, Rilling J, Smith E, et al. Placebo-induced changes in FMRI in the anticipation and experience of pain. *Science*. 2004;303:1162–1167.
30. Wager TD, Nitschke JB. Placebo effects in the brain: Linking mental and physiological processes. *Brain Behav Immun*. 2005;19:281–282.
31. Kong J, Kaptchuk TJ, Polich G, Kirsch I, Gollub RL. Placebo analgesia: findings from brain imaging studies and emerging hypotheses. *Rev Neurosci*. 2007;18(3–4):173–190.
32. Tracey I, Mantyh PW. The cerebral signature for pain perception and its modulation. *Neuron*. 2007;55(3):377–391.
33. Peppard A, Riegler H. Ankle reconditioning with TNS. *Phys Sportsmed*. 1980;8:105–106.
34. Gammon GD, Starr I. Studies on the relief of pain by counterirritation. *J Clin Invest*. 1941;20:13–20.
35. McKemy D, Neuhausser W, Julius D. Identification of a cold receptor reveals a general role for TRP channels in thermosensation. *Nature*. 2002;416:52–57.
36. Ragan BG. Menthol based analgesic balm attenuates the pressor response evoked by muscle afferents. *J Athl Train*. 2003;38(S34).
37. Draper D, Trowbridge C, Wells A, Egget D. The ThermaCare HeatWrap increases paraspinal muscle temperature greater than the IcyHot Patch and the mentholatum patch. *J Athl Train*. 2003;38:S45.
38. Zucker C. A cool ion channel. *Nature*. 2002;416:17–18.
39. Hill J, Sumida K. Acute effect of two topical counterirritant creams on pain induced by delayed-onset muscle soreness. *J Sport Rehabil*. 2002;11:202–208.
40. Kuritzky L. Topical analgesics: are they underused? *Hosp Pract*. 1997:131–132.
41. Bell GW, Prentice WE. Infared modalities (therapeutic heat and cold). In: Prentice WE, ed. *Therapeutic Modalities in Sports Medicine*. St. Louis, MO: Times Mirror/Mosby College Publishing, 1998:174–177, 190–191.
42. Hawkes J, Care G, Dixon JS, Bird HA, Wright V. Comparison of three physiotherapy regimens for hands with rheumatoid arthritis. *Br Med J (Clin Res Ed)*. 1985;291(6501):1016.
43. Ayling J, Marks R. Efficacy of paraffin wax baths for rheumatoid arthritic hands. *Physiotherapy*. 2000;86:190–201.
44. Miller MD, Wirth MA, Rockwood CA Jr. Thawing the frozen shoulder: the "patient" patient. *Orthopedics*. 1996;19(10):849–853.
45. McCray RE, Patton NJ. Pain relief at trigger points: comparison of moist heat and shortwave diathermy. *J Orthop Sports Phys Ther*. 1984;5:175–178.
46. Steiner D, Erasala GN, Hengehold DA, Goodale MB, Weingand KW. Continuous low-level heat therapy for acute muscular low back pain. Paper presented at: American Pain Society 19th Annual Scientific Meeting, Atlanta, GA. 2000.
47. Steiner D, Erasala GN, Hengehold DA, Goodale MB. Continuous low-level heat therapy for trapezius myalgia. Paper presented at: American Pain Society 19th Annual Scientific Meeting, Atlanta, GA. 2000.
48. Abramson DI, Mitchell RE, Tuck S, Bell Y, Zayas AM. Changes in blood flow, oxygen uptake and tissue temperatures produced by the topical application of wet heat. *Arch Phys Med Rehabil*. 1961;42:305–318.
49. Belanger AY. *Evidence-Based Guide to Therapeutic Physical Agents*. Baltimore, MD: Lippincott Williams & Wilkins, 2002.
50. Erasala GN, Rubin JM, Tuthill TA, et al. The effect of topical heat treatment on trapezius muscle blood flow using power Doppler ultrasound. Paper presented at: APTA Physical Therapy 2001, 2001.
51. Lehmann JF, Masock AJ, Warren CG, Koblanski JN. Effect of therapeutic temperatures on tendon extensibility. *Arch Phys Med Rehab*. 1970;51:481–487.

52. Cordray YM, Krusen EM. Use of hydrocollator packs in the treatment of neck and shoulder pains. *Arch Phys Med Rehab.* 1959;40:105–108.

53. Fountain FP, Gersten JW, Sengir O. Decrease in muscle spasm produced by ultrasound, hot packs, and infrared radiation. *Arch Phys Med Rehab.* 1960;41:293–298.

54. Lehmann J, DeLateur BJ. Therapeutic heat. In: Lehman J, ed. *Therapeutic Heat and Cold.* 4th ed. Baltimore, MD: Williams and Wilkins, 1990:437–442.

55. Lehmann JF, Brunner GD, Stow RW. Pain threshold measurements after therapeutic application of ultrasound, microwaves and infrared. *Arch Phys Med Rehabil.* 1958;39(9):560–565.

56. Taylor AG, West BA, Simon B, Skelton J, Rowlingson JC. How effective is TENS for acute pain? *Am J Nurs.* 1983;83(8):1171–1174.

57. Zizic TM, Hoffman KC, Holt PA, et al. The treatment of osteoarthritis of the knee with pulsed electrical stimulation. *J Rheumatol.* 1995;22(9):1757–1761.

58. Melzack R, Vetere P, Finch L. Transcutaneous electrical nerve stimulation for low back pain. A comparison of TENS and massage for pain and range of motion. *Phys Ther.* 1983;63(4):489–493.

59. Cheing GL, Hui-Chan CW. Transcutaneous electrical nerve stimulation: nonparallel antinociceptive effects on chronic clinical pain and acute experimental pain. *Arch Phys Med Rehabil.* 1999;80(3):305–312.

60. Nordemar R, Thorner C. Treatment of acute cervical pain—a comparative group study. *Pain.* Feb 1981;10(1):93–101.

61. Arvidsson J, Eriksson E. Postoperative TENS pain relief after knee surgery: objective evaluation. *Orthopedics.* 1986;9:1346–1351.

62. Jensen JE, Conn RR, Hazelrigg G, Hewett JE. The use of transcutaneous neural stimulation and isokinetic testing in arthroscopic knee surgery. *Am J Sports Med.* 1985;13(1):27–33.

63. Cornell PE, Lopez AL, Malofsky H. Pain reduction with transcutaneous electrical nerve stimulation after foot surgery. *J Foot Surg.* 1984;23(4):326–333.

64. Chapman CE. Can the use of physical modalities for pain control be rationalized by the research evidence? *Can J Physiol Pharmacol.* 1991;69:704–712.

65. Knight KL. *Cryotherapy in Sport Injury Management.* Champaign, IL: Human Kinetics, 1995.

66. Allen FM. Reduced temperature in surgery, I: surgery of limbs. *Am J Surg.* 1941;52:225–237.

67. Crossman LW, Ruggiero WF, Hurley V, Allen FM. Reduced temperature in surgery, II: amputation for peripheral vascular disease. *Arch Surg.* 1942;44:139–156.

68. Schaubel HJ. The local use of ice after orthopedic procedures. *Amer J Surg.* 1946;122(5).

69. Carbajal FJ, Nelson DO. The effect of cold pack application on the recovery from pitching a baseball. *Athl J.* 1967;47:8–11,85–86.

70. Kato D. Effect of static stretch and ice immersion on pitching performance after induced muscle performance. Thesis, Indiana State University, Terre Haute, 1985.

71. Juvenal JP. Cryokinetics, a new concept in the treatment of injuries. *Scholast Coach.* 1966;35:40–42.

72. Hocutt JE Jr, Jaffe R, Rylander CR, Beebe JK. Cryotherapy in ankle sprains. *Am J Sports Med.* 1982;10(5):316–319.

73. Behnke RS, Blackwell HJ, Nicolette RL, Moore RJ. Ice therapy. Paper presented at: NATA Convention; June 1967, 1967.

74. Moore RJ, Nicolette RL, Behnke RS. The therapeutic use of cold (cryotherapy) in the care of atheltic injuries. *J Natl Athl Train Assoc.* 1967;2(1):6.

75. Lawrence JM, Hoeft F, Sheau KE, Mackey SC. Strategy-dependent dissociation of the neural correlates involved in pain modulation. *Anesthesiology.* 2011;115(4):844–851.

76. Wang J, Jian F, Chen J, et al. Cognitive behavioral therapy for orthodontic pain control: a randomized trial. *J Dent Res* 2012;91(6):580–585.

77. Zeidan F, Grant JA, Brown CA, McHaffie JG, Coghill RC. Mindfulness meditation-related pain relief: Evidence for unique brain mechanisms in the regulation of pain. *Neurosci Lett.* 2012;520(2):165–173.

78. Medicine NCfCaA. Meditation: An Introduction. *US Batuibak Ubstutytes if Health.* Accessed Aug 2012.

79. Staff MC. Meditation: A simple, fast way to reduce stress. Available at: http://www.mayoclinic.com/health/meditation/HQ01070/. Accessed Aug 2012.

80. Ohnhaus E, Adler R. Methodological problems in the measurement of pain: a comparison between the verbal rating scale and the visual analogue scale. *Pain.* 1975;1:379.

81. Huskisson E. *Pain Measurement and Assessment.* New York, NY: Raven Press, 1983.

82. Scott J, Huskisson E. Vertical and horizontal analogue scales. *Ann Rheum Dis.* 1979;38:560.

83. Carlsson AM. Assessment of chronic pain. I. Aspects of the reliability and validity of the visual analogue scale. *Pain.* 1983;16:87–101.

84. Denegar CR, Perrin DH. Effect of transcutaneous electrical nerve stimulation, cold, and a combination treatment on pain, decreased range of motion, and strength loss associated with delayed onset muscle soreness. *J Athl Train.* 1992;27:200–206.

85. Jensen MP, Karoly P, Braver S. The measurement of clinical pain intensity: a comparison of six methods. *Pain.* 1986;27(1):117–126.

Review Questions   Part III

Chapter 8

1. Which theory about pain by Melzack and Wall proposes a mechanism, located in the dorsal horn of the spinal cord, that allows only one sensation at a time to pass through to the brain?
   a. central control
   b. gate control
   c. endogenous opiate
   d. pattern
   e. specificity

2. Pain that is brief, short term, and often of rapid onset and high intensity is called _____.
   a. chronic pain
   b. acute pain
   c. radiating pain
   d. referred pain
   e. phantom pain

3. Pain that persists a month beyond the usual course of an acute disease or a reasonable time for an injury to heal (also described as continuous pain) or that recurs at intervals for months to years is known as _____.
   a. chronic pain
   b. acute pain
   c. radiating pain
   d. referred pain
   e. phantom pain

4. Pain that is felt at a site other than the actual location of a trauma, that tends to be projected outward from the torso and distally along the extremities, and that is perceived in an area that often seems to have little relation to the pathology is known as _____.
   a. chronic pain
   b. acute pain
   c. radiating pain
   d. referred pain
   e. secondary pain

5. A pain theory that considers previous experiences, emotional influences, sensory perception, and other factors as influencing the transmission of the pain messages and thus the perception of pain is called _____.
   a. central control
   b. gate control
   c. endogenous opiate
   d. pattern
   e. specificity

6. In what part of the body is the pain gate located?
   a. cerebral cortex
   b. brainstem
   c. ventral horn
   d. substantia gelatinosa
   e. none of the above

7. What are the voluntarily controlled nerves that transmit impulses from the central nervous system (CNS) to the periphery of the body and terminate in skeletal muscle?
   a. somatic motor nerves
   b. autonomic motor nerves
   c. somatic sensory nerves
   d. autonomic sensory nerves
   e. all of the above

8. The body's naturally occurring painkillers are referred to as _____.
   a. endogenous opiates
   b. T cells
   c. nociceptors
   d. dopamines
   e. morphine

9. Which of the following is not an endogenous opiate?
   a. enkephalin
   b. endorphin
   c. serotonin
   d. bradykinin
   e. none of the above

Chapter 9

1. Which pain assessment tool is a scale that consists of no numbers but is a 100-mm line with contrasting descriptors, such as "no pain" and "severe pain," on the anchor points at the ends of the line.
   a. number scale
   b. verbal rating scale
   c. visual analog scale
   d. graphic rating scale
   e. McGill Pain Questionnaire

2. Which pain measurement tool uses pictures, scales, and words to help patients describe sensory and affective aspects as well as magnitude and changes in their pain?
   a. number scale
   b. verbal rating scale
   c. visual analog scale
   d. graphic rating scale
   e. McGill Pain Questionnaire

3. A medicinally inactive substance or mock intervention given to a patient to bring about a desired response and satisfy the patient's demand for medicine is known as _____.
   a. a counterirritant
   b. a placebo
   c. an irritant
   d. central control
   e. a sugar pill

4. Which of the following is false with respect to exercise and pain?
   a. Therapeutic exercise should be relatively pain free.
   b. It is acceptable if the exercise is moderately uncomfortable as long as swelling does not increase.
   c. Therapeutic exercise or activity during rehabilitation should not evoke the same type of pain that was experienced when the injury occurred.
   d. Pain during an activity indicates the activity is too strenuous or complex.
   e. Sharp pain after an activity indicates the activity is too strenuous or complex.

5. Activities that result in pain during rehabilitation will hinder the rehabilitation process by inducing _____.
   a. neural inhibition
   b. the spinal adaptation syndrome
   c. central control
   d. proprioceptors
   e. swelling

6. Electrical stimulating currents are thought to reduce pain by all of the following except by _____.
   a. reducing muscle spasm, hence relaxing the muscle
   b. releasing endogenous opiates at pain receptor sites
   c. releasing morphine-like drugs from the thalamus
   d. stimulating the nonpainful nerves
   e. modulating neural inhibition

7. The most common use of cold with acute orthopedic injury is to modulate the pain of sprains, strains, and contusions to facilitate _____.
   a. reduction of swelling
   b. healing
   c. therapeutic exercise
   d. reduction of spasm
   e. endorphin release

Part IV

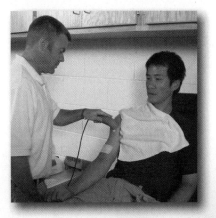

Therapeutic Heat and Cold

Therapeutic heat and cold form the bulk of the traditional therapeutic modalities. Heat modalities have historically been the workhorse of rehabilitation. For decades, clinicians thought that heat applications increase blood flow, thereby carrying away injury wastes and bringing nutrients to rebuild damaged tissue. This does occur. A more powerful reason for therapeutic heat has emerged, however. It now appears that the primary purpose of heat application is to facilitate therapeutic exercise (specifically stretching) and reduce general soreness.

Cryotherapy has emerged as a powerful rehabilitative tool as well, although many people still think of cold only for immediate care to prevent swelling. Cold facilitates active exercise, especially during the early stages of acute orthopedic injury rehabilitation. Thus, therapeutic exercise can begin sooner and progress more quickly.

The chapters in Part IV contain a rich smattering of history, because the past forms the foundation of the present and future. You will also find many references to our research. After more than a combined 30 years of clinical experience, 65 years of research, and the pursuit of thousands of clinical questions, we are quite passionate about understanding and explaining the proper application of therapeutic heat and cold. We hope to impart some of this passion to you as you expand your theoretical understanding and practical skills to improve the health of your patients.

Part IV begins with Chapter 10 on the principles of heat as it applies to thermotherapy, including what it is and why it is used therapeutically. This foundation is essential for understanding how to properly use therapeutic heat and cold. In addition, advances in the use of these modalities require this foundational knowledge. Much of this chapter is a review of concepts taught in a basic physics class.

In Chapter 11, we cover the application of numerous superficial heat modalities. The theoretical basis and application of the two most effective deep-heating modalities (ultrasound and diathermy) are in Chapters 14 and 15.

In Chapter 12, we discuss the theoretical basis for the use of cryotherapy beyond immediate care and dispel many of the myths concerning its use. We also present a concise list of principles of when to use heat and cold therapeutically. Application techniques for the most common uses of cryotherapy for acute orthopedic injury rehabilitation beyond immediate care are in Chapter 15.

Principles of Heat for Thermotherapy

OPENING SCENE

You are in the athletic training clinic, taping an athlete's ankle. You overhear Andrew, a staff AT talking to a baseball player. Andrew suggests a regimen of heat therapy for the player's chronic case of supraspinatus tendinitis (shoulder). The athlete asks, "What kind of heat treatment? Is there a difference between using a whirlpool, hot pack, or ultrasound? What causes the difference?" How would you answer these questions?

Defining Thermotherapy

Thermotherapy is the therapeutic use of heat; the application of a device or substance with a temperature greater than body temperature, thus causing heat to pass from the thermotherapy device to the body. **Cryotherapy** is the therapeutic use of cold; the application of a device or substance with a temperature less than body temperature, thus causing heat to pass from the body to the cryotherapy device.

Heat is a form of energy produced by the movement of atoms and molecules. All substances with a temperature above *absolute zero* (–450°F, –273°C) possess heat. Technically, there is no such thing as cold; **cold** is the absence of heat, or something that has less heat than one would desire.

Temperature is the measure of an object's ability to spontaneously give up energy. It is used to indicate the level of molecular motion associated with heat.

 CONCEPT CHECK 10.1. Is it hot or cold? In the fall, if the temperature drops down to 40°F (4.5°C), you think it's cold out and put on a jacket. In the spring, if the temperature gets up to 40°F (4.5°C), you think it's warm out and shed your coat. Why is your perception of the temperature different between the fall and spring when the temperature is the same?

SUPERFICIAL AND DEEP HEAT

There are two classifications of thermotherapy, superficial and deep. **Superficial thermotherapy** is the application of modalities to the surface of the body that heat primarily the surface tissues (<1 cm; Table 10.1). We should note, however, that *superficial thermal modalities* will heat tissues deeper than 1 cm, but the amount of heating is not enough to evoke the desired therapeutic effects. Hot packs, whirlpool, and paraffin are examples of superficial thermal modalities. These modalities heat primarily by conduction and infrared radiation.

Deep thermotherapy is the application of modalities that cause a *tissue temperature rise (TTR)* in deeper tissues (3–4 cm). Ultrasound and diathermy are the primary deep thermal modalities. They heat by conversion and radiation. Diathermy radiation has different characteristics than infrared radiation and therefore evokes different physiological effects.

Transferring Heat to and from the Body

Therapeutic heat and therapeutic cold applications use one of three types of heat transfer between the therapeutic modality and the body: conduction, convection, or radiation. Conversion is sometimes considered as a type of heat transfer, although this is a misnomer, as discussed below. Heat is always transferred from the object of higher temperature to the object of lower temperature.

CONDUCTION

Conduction is heat transfer between two objects of uneven temperatures after coming into contact with each other. In the human body, conduction occurs on the cellular level, as hotter, rapidly moving, or vibrating atoms and molecules interact with cooler, neighboring atoms and molecules, transferring some of their energy (heat) to the cooler atoms. Given enough time, the process occurs until the objects reach thermal equilibrium, meaning they are at the same temperature. Examples of modalities that transfer heat by conduction are hot packs, whirlpool, ice packs, and slush buckets. Conduction is the most frequently used method of heat transfer in physical medicine.

A **thermal gradient** always develops when heat is transferred by conduction. This means there is a gradual change in temperature from the interior of one object to the interior of the other object (Fig. 10.1). The slope of the gradient becomes less with time as heat is withdrawn from deeper within the warmer object and heat increases deeper in the cooler object. Results from one of our hot pack studies illustrate the thermal gradient in tissue. After a hot pack was applied to the quadriceps for 20 minutes, temperature had risen 6.5°F (3.6°C) at a depth of 1 cm but thereon 1.4°F (0.8°C) at 3 cm.[1] See Table 10.1 for additional examples of thermal gradients in tissue as it is heated with superficial thermal agents.

Many factors affect the rate of heat conduction between various therapeutic modalities and the patient. These were discussed in Chapter 6 in relation to cold and are listed below:

- The temperature differential between the body and the modality
- The dissipation of tissue heat and/or modality heating
- The heat storage capacity of the modality
- The size of the modality
- The amount of tissue in contact with the modality
- The length of application
- Individual patient variability

CONVECTION

Convection is the transfer of heat to or from an object by the passage of a fluid or air past its surface (from a physics standpoint, air is a fluid). Central heating and cooling of a vhome or building are examples of heat transfer by convection. Examples of modalities that transfer heat by convection are whirlpool and fluidotherapy. A whirlpool transfers heat by both conduction and convection.

TABLE 10.1   TEMPERATURE CHANGES DUE TO APPLICATION OF VARIOUS THERMAL MODALITIES

MODALITY	PARAMETERS	DEPTH (CM)	TISSUE	DURATION	TEMP CHANGE (°C)	REFERENCE
Hot pack		1	Triceps surae	15 min	3.6	Draper et al.[1]
		2	Quadriceps	10 min	0.8	Morris[2]
		2	Quadriceps	20 min	2.0	Morris[2]
		2	Quadriceps	30 min	3.0	Morris[2]
		3	Triceps surae	15 min	0.8	Draper et al.[1]
Whirlpool	40.6°C	1.5	Triceps surae	20 min	2.8	Myrer et al.[3]
Contrast ther	40.6°C/15.6°C	1.5	Triceps surae	20 min	0.4	Myrer et al.[3]
	41°C/10°C	1.5	Triceps surae	20 min	0.44	Wertz et al.[4]
Topical heatwrap	Kneewrap	5	Knee jt capsule	120 min	2.6	Mitra et al.[5]
	Backwrap	1.5	Paraspinals	120 min	2.7	Draper & Trowbridge[6]
	Backwrap	1.5	Paraspinals	150 min	1.8	Draper & Trowbridge[7]
	Backwrap	2	Paraspinals	120 min	1.1	Trowbridge et al.[8]
	Kneewrap	1.5	Vastus med	120 min	3.2	Mitra et al.[5]
Shortwave diathermy	Pulsed at 48 W	2	Suprailiac fat	20 min	7.2	Draper & Castel et al.[9]
	Pulsed at 48 W	3	Triceps surae	20 min	4	Draper et al.[10]
	Pulsed at 48 W	3	Triceps surae	20 min	4.6	Garrett et al.[11]
	Pulsed at 48 W	5	Knee capsule	20 min	3.2	Draper et al.[12]
Ultrasound, 1 MHz	1 W/cm²	2.5	Triceps surae	10 min	2	Draper et al.[13]
	1 W/cm²	5	Triceps surae	10 min	2	Draper et al.[13]
	1.5 W/cm²	2.5	Triceps surae	10 min	3	Draper et al.[13]
	1.5 W/cm²	5	Triceps surae	10 min	3	Draper et al.[13]
	1.2 W/cm²	4	Triceps surae	10 min	2.5	Anderson et al.[14]
	1.5 W/cm²	2.5	Triceps surae	12.5 min	4	Rose et al.[15]
	1.5 W/cm²	3, 5	Triceps surae	10 min	3.2	Ashton et al.[16]
	1.5 W/cm²	5	Triceps surae	12.5 min	3.5	Rose et al.[15]
	1.5 W/cm²	5	Triceps surae	10 min	4	Draper et al.[17]
	1.5 W/cm² gel	3	Triceps surae	10 min	4.8	Draper & Sunderland[18]
	1.5 W/cm², water bath	3	Triceps surae	10 min	2.1	Draper & Sunderland[18]
	1.5 W/cm²; 2 ERA	4	Triceps surae	10 min	3.5	Chudleigh et al.[19]
	1.5 W/cm²; 6 ERA	4	Triceps surae	10 min	1.3	Chudleigh et al.[19]
	1.6 W/cm²; BNR 2.3:1	3	Triceps surae	10 min	3	Draper[20]
	1.6 W/cm²; BNR 2.4:1	3	Triceps surae	9 min	4.5	Draper[20]
	1.6 W/cm²; BNR 7.7:1	3	Triceps surae	8.8 min	4.2	Draper[20]
	1.5 W/cm², ice	3	Triceps surae	15 min ice; 10 min US	0.6	Rimington et al.[21]
	1.5 W/cm², ice	5	Triceps surae	5 min ice; 10 min US	1.8	Draper et al.[17]

TABLE 10.1 TEMPERATURE CHANGES DUE TO APPLICATION OF VARIOUS THERMAL MODALITIES (*Continued*)

MODALITY	PARAMETERS	DEPTH (CM)	TISSUE	DURATION	TEMP CHANGE (°C)	REFERENCE
Ultrasound, 3 MHz	1.4 W/cm	2	Triceps surae	5 min	3.3	Anderson et al.[14]
	1.5 W/cm²	1.2	Triceps surae	6 min	5.3	Draper & Ricard[22]
	1 W/cm²	1	Fat (tricep)	10 min	8.4	Draper et al.[23]
	1 W/cm²	1	Patellar tendon	4 min	8.3	Chan et al.[24]
	1 W/cm², gel	1	Lateral ankle	10 min	7.7	Bishop et al.[25]
	1 W/cm², gel pad	1	Lateral ankle	10 min	6.7	Bishop et al.[25]
	Delta 4, 1.2 W/cm²	1, 2.5	Triceps surae	5.5 min	4.4	Wells et al.[26]
	0.5 W/cm²	0.8	Triceps surae	10 min	3	Draper et al.[13]
	0.5 W/cm²	1.6	Triceps surae	10 min	3	Draper et al.[13]
	1 W/cm²	0.8	Triceps surae	10 min	6	Draper et al.[13]
	1 W/cm²	1.6	Triceps surae	10 min	6	Draper et al.[13]

BNR, beam nonuniformity ratio; ERA, effective radiating area; US, ultrasound.

RADIATION

Radiation, also called *radiant energy*, is the transfer of energy in the form of rays, waves, or particles, often from a central source. All substances with a temperature above absolute zero radiate heat to a substance of lower temperature through infrared rays. The sun heats the Earth, in part by radiation of infrared rays. The heat you feel coming off asphalt pavement on a hot summer day is also caused by infrared radiation. Microwave diathermy, laser, infrared (heat) lamps, and ultraviolet lamps are the most common examples of therapeutic modalities that use radiation to transfer heat. Radiation and electromagnetic waves are discussed in greater depth later in the chapter.

CONVERSION

Conversion is the process by which a form of energy other than heat (electricity, chemical, mechanical, etc.) is converted to heat within the body. It is not a form of heat transfer, however, even though deep tissues are heated by this process, and it is an essential part of thermotherapy. Another form of energy—not heat—is transferred from outside into the body, so it is not heat transfer. Examples of modalities that heat by conversion are ultrasound and shortwave diathermy.

Conversion is the only way of increasing the temperature of deep tissues to therapeutic levels. Both conduction and convection deliver heat to the surface of the body, which is then conducted into the body. But most of the heat is dissipated by subcutaneous circulation before it can substantially increase deeper temperatures. The depth of penetration of deep heat depends on the modality and on the physiological and anatomical characteristics of the individual body part.

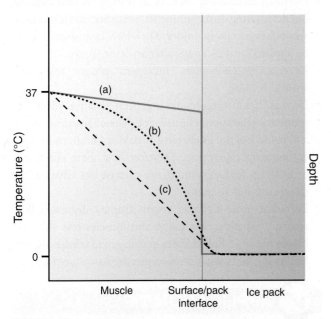

FIGURE 10.1 A thermal gradient develops over time due to heat transfer between two objects of different temperatures in contact with each other. The three lines in this illustration represent the development of a muscle thermal gradient over time as a result of the application of a cold pack. The three lines represent the interface between the two objects, *(a)* immediately upon contact, *(b)* after the passage of time, and *(c)* after the passage of additional time.

Modality Myth

HEAT IS NECESSARY FOR REHABILITATION BECAUSE IT INCREASES BLOOD FLOW AND PROMOTES HEALING

Increasing blood flow is beneficial during healing, and local heat applications do increase blood flow. However, therapeutic exercise increases blood flow many times more than heat applicatoins do. Therefore, therapeutic exercise is more important than heat applications in increasing blood flow during rehabilitation. Exercise has other, sometimes more important, effects on rehabilitation: (1) it provides intermittent compression (called the muscle pump) that promotes lymphatic drainage to remove tissue debris and swelling from the injury site, and (2) it helps decrease neural inhibition, and thus reestablishes normal neuromuscular motor patterns.

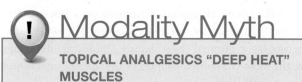

Modality Myth

TOPICAL ANALGESICS "DEEP HEAT" MUSCLES

Several over-the-counter topical analgesics (e.g., Cramergesic, Bengay, Icy Hot, Atomic Balm, Red Hot) claim to provide heat to muscles. Also known as *analgesic balms* and *counter-irritants*, these products are formulated as creams, balms, or ointments. They contain substances such as menthol, methyl salicylate, or hot pepper plant extracts (capsaicin) that cause a sensation of warmth on the skin and a slightly increased blood flow to the skin. They do not, however, substantially increase skin or muscle temperature (see Fig. 11.16). Skin and 2-cm deep intramuscular temperature were <2.7°F (1.5°C) and 1°F (0.5°C), respectively.[1]

The active ingredients (menthol, capsaicin, etc.) irritate the skin so as to give the sensation of heat. The irritation is often intense enough that it gates pain. Thus, the name counter-irritation; the irritation of the balm counters (overrides) the irritation (pain) of the injury or disease. The effect is local, that is, affecting signals from tissue receptors rather than involving higher cortical processing.[2,27,28,29]

The Therapeutic Use of Heat

Traditionally, the primary reason heat was used as a therapeutic agent was to increase blood flow to the injured body part. In the process of carrying away the heat, blood also delivers nutrients to the area and carries metabolites and other waste products away. It is assumed that these latter two functions increase the rate of healing of the injury, although the theory has never been tested. Another argument against the traditional reason for applying thermotherapy is that active exercise increases blood flow much more than therapeutic heat and therefore delivers more oxygen and nutrients to the tissue and carries away more waste.

Therapeutic heat modalities are indispensable for other reasons, however. They promote relaxation, relieve general soreness, and facilitate connective tissue stretching. Also, you can use therapeutic heat modalities to target increased blood flow to a specific area, such as the knee of a patient that is too sore to warm up on a treadmill.

PHYSIOLOGICAL EFFECTS OF HEAT

A major reason for using therapeutic modalities is to stimulate an increased rate of normal functions. The TTR caused by thermotherapy results in the following:

- *Increased circulation*: 1½ to 2 times normal resting blood flow
- *Increased metabolism*: beneficial during wound healing, but devastating during immediate care because it increases secondary metabolic injury. Therefore, heat should never be applied until 2–3 days after an acute injury.
- *Increased inflammation*: increased phagocytosis and wound healing
- *Decreased pain (analgesia)*: a general sedative effect that promotes relaxation; effective for general soreness, aches, and pains, but not as effective as cold applications in moderating acute injury pain. Therefore, it is not as effective as cryotherapy for facilitating active exercise (see Chapter 12).
- *Decreased muscle spasm*
- *Decreased tissue stiffness*: Thermotherapy decreases fluid viscosity, which makes joints and muscles less stiff, and causes the cross-linked fibers in collagen to release, thereby facilitating the elongation of connective tissue (see Fig. 7.5).

✔ APPLICATION TIP

WHEN TO USE HEAT AND COLD

Therapeutic heat is most effective in decreasing general soreness and in preparing soft tissues for stretching and joint mobilization. Therapeutic cold is most effective in relieving pain and inhibition in acutely injured soft tissue, thereby facilitating therapeutic exercise.

HEAT SINKS

Regardless of the cause of local TTR, circulation to the area removes heat and thereby prevents local thermal damage (cooking the tissue). Heat is carried by the blood to **heat sinks**, areas of the body that can accept and dissipate great amounts of heat. The two primary heat sinks in the human body are the lungs and skin. The lungs dissipate heat through respiration, and the skin dissipates heat through perspiration and radiation.

As long as the heat sinks dissipate the heat at least as quickly as heat is added to the body by the modality, the application is safe. If, however, heat is added to the body faster than it is dissipated, the body part will gradually increase in temperature, and local heat injury can result. This is why it is a contraindication to apply heat to areas of compromised circulation, such as the feet of a patient with diabetes. If the heat application gets too warm, inadequate blood flow to cool the tissue can result in overheating and associated tissue destruction.

✔ APPLICATION TIP

WHIRLPOOL TEMPERATURE DEPENDS ON HEAT SINKS

The maximal safe water temperature of a whirlpool is determined by the amount of the body that is immersed in the bath (see Chapter 11). The concept of heat sinks explains why. If only a foot or arm is in the bath, about 5% of the body surface is absorbing heat and about 95% acts as a heat sink to dissipate heat. At the other extreme, if the patient is immersed up to the neck, 95% of the body surface is absorbing heat and 5% dissipates heat. In the latter case, a very small area must dissipate a very large amount of heat being added to the body. Thus, the following principle: The more of the body that is in a whirlpool bath, the lower the temperature should be.

GENERAL HEAT CONTRAINDICATIONS

In most situations, the application of topical heat is safe. There are, however, three general heat contraindications, or contraindications to all forms of heat application. In addition, there are specific contraindications to specific thermal modalities, which will be discussed in later chapters. The general contraindications are:

1. Do not apply any form of heat to an acute injury within the first 48–72 hours of injury. Increased metabolism, stimulated by the heating, will cause an increase in secondary metabolic injury if heat is applied too soon to an acute injury.
2. Do not apply any form of heat to an area with compromised circulation. Inadequate blood flow results in inadequate cooling, and the tissue could suffer heat injury.

3. Do not apply any form of heat to an area with compromised sensation. The same problem potentially exists as with compromised circulation. If the body cannot detect the increasing temperature of the heat application, it may not respond with increased circulation to the area.

Radiation and Electromagnetic Waves

Much of this section is a review of principles taught in a basic physics class. This material will help you understand the principles upon which ultrasound, diathermy, lasers, infrared lamps, and ultraviolet lamps are based and why they are used therapeutically. This information will help you avoid being a knobologist (see Chapter 1).

CONFUSING TERMINOLOGY

Don't be confused by the following terms: radiation, radiant energy, electromagnetic waves, and electromagnetic radiation. They are used interchangeably and although they represent slightly different concepts, they are similar. It would be less confusing if there were a single term, but such is not the case. There apparently is no reason for using one term over another. Unfortunately, this is just one of many examples of inconsistency in the English language.

Understanding scientific notation and the metric system will help you understand radiation. If you need a review, the basics are in Boxes 10.1 and 10.2, and Concept Check 10.2 will test your knowledge.

 CONCEPT CHECK 10.2. Which is bigger, 23×10^2 or 3×10^3?

BOX 10.1 SCIENTIFIC NOTATION

Scientific notation is a way of expressing very large numbers—for example, 6.98×10^4. In this example, it consists of a coefficient (6.98) multiplied by 10 raised to an exponent (4). To convert this to a real number, multiply the 10 by the number of the exponent: $6.98 \times 10 \times 10 \times 10 \times 10 = 69,800$. A simple way to multiply by tens is to just move the decimal point to the right, adding extra zeroes as needed. If the exponent is negative (10^{-4}), move the decimal point to the left. Here are three more examples:

- $3 \times 10^8 = 300,000,000$
- $1 \times 10^2 = 100$
- $10^3 = 1 \times 10^3 = 1000$

ABBREVIATIONS	MEANING	VALUE
K	kilo	10^3 or 1000
M	mega	10^6 or 1,000,000
c	centa	10^{-2} or 1/100
m	milli	10^{-3} or 1/1000
u	micro	10^{-6} or 1/1,000,000
um	millimicro	10^{-9} or 1/1,000,000,000
n	nano	10^{-9} or 1/1,000,000,000
A	angstrom	10^{-10} or 1/10,000,000,000

SIMILARITIES AND DIFFERENCES AMONG FORMS OF RADIATION

As mentioned earlier, radiation propagates energy through empty space as **electromagnetic waves**, which take many forms, including heat, light, electricity, x-rays, and cosmic rays (Fig. 10.2). Forms of radiation have the following in common:

- All are called electromagnetic waves.
- All are caused by minute (pronounced **mi**' nute) particles moving through space.
- All travel as sinusoidal waves.
- All travel at the same linear speed in space, which is 186,000 mi./s or 3×10^8 m/s. Linear speed means average speed from beginning to end; computed as the linear or straight line between the two points, divided by the time to move from beginning to end. Of course, no electromagnetic waves travel linearly; but the concept is important in understanding them.

The various forms of radiation have these main differences:

- Some forms are visible (such as light).
- Some forms are audible (such as radio waves).
- Some forms you can feel (such as electricity and infrared).
- Some forms can pass through you (such as x-rays).
- Each form has different energy.
- Each form has a unique wavelength and a unique frequency.

The differences between various forms of radiation result from their different energy levels, which result from their specific wavelengths and frequencies (see Fig. 10.2).

ELECTROMAGNETIC WAVES

Electromagnetic waves consist of oscillating electric and magnetic fields at right angles to one another and at right angles to the propagation direction (Fig. 10.3). Individual electromagnetic waves, although dual in nature, behave as a single wave and are often represented as such. Each has a unique wavelength and frequency.

Wavelength is the distance, expressed in meters or centimeters, of one repetition of the wave (Fig. 10.4). **Frequency** is the rate of passage of crests on the wave form expressed in cycles per second or hertz (Hz). Even though all electromagnetic waves are sinusoidal waves with the same linear speed, they travel differently. As either wavelength or frequency changes, the other one changes proportionally in the opposite direction; as one increases, the other one decreases. This is so because the linear speed is constant. Therefore, wavelength multiplied by frequency will always equal 186,000 mi./s, or 3×10^8 m/s. The giant and dwarf analogy presented in Box 10.3 helps explain this principle.

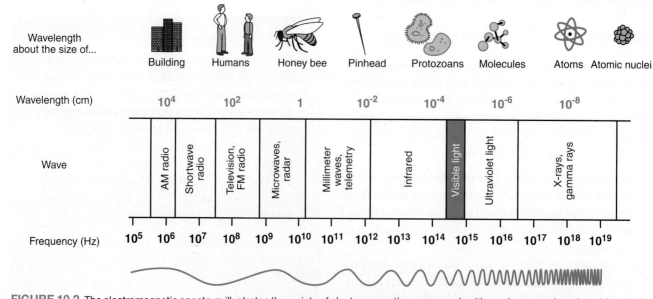

FIGURE 10.2 The electromagnetic spectrum illustrates the variety of electromagnetic waves, each with a unique wavelength and frequency.

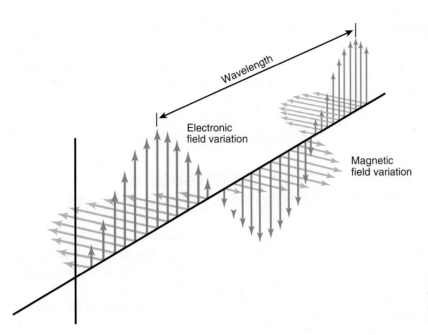

FIGURE 10.3 Electromagnetic waves consist of oscillating electric and magnetic fields at right angles to one another and at right angles to the propagation direction.

If you know either the wavelength or the frequency, you can compute the other. For example, if a particular electromagnetic wave had a wavelength of 186,000 mi., its frequency would be 1 cycle per second or 1 Hz. If its wavelength was 1 mi., its frequency would be 186,000 Hz.

 CONCEPT CHECK 10.3. (a) If an electromagnetic wave was 6200 mi. long, what would its frequency be? (b) If another wave had a frequency of 2000 Hz, what would its wavelength be?

CLASSIFICATION OF ELECTROMAGNETIC WAVES

Because every electromagnetic wave form has a unique wavelength and unique frequency, waves can be classified according to either wavelength or frequency. There is no convention as to which is used. Some are classified by wavelength, others by frequency, and some by both. Electricity and radio waves are examples of electromagnetic waves that are classified according to frequency. Lasers are classified by wavelength. Diathermy is named for its wavelength (e.g., shortwave), but it is classified by its frequency, which sometimes causes confusion (see Chapter 15).

✔ **APPLICATION TIP**

THE THERAPEUTIC EFFICACY OF LASERS IS WAVELENGTH SPECIFIC

The body responds differently to electromagnetic waves of different wavelengths, so one laser does not fit all purposes (see Chapter 20). You cannot use your TV remote control to heal orthopedic injuries.

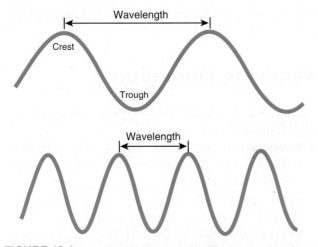

FIGURE 10.4 Two sinusoidal waves with different wavelengths.

BOX 10.3 THE GIANT AND DWARF ANALOGY

The relationship between wavelength and frequency is illustrated with an analogy of a foot race between a giant and a dwarf. Imagine that the NBA's tallest center (perhaps 7 ft 6 in.) and shortest guard (say 5 ft 4 in.) raced from baseline to baseline on a basketball court. Assume they tie. If the center's stride length is 6 ft, he traveled the distance in 16 strides. The guard's stride length is only 4 ft, so it took him 24 strides. So it is with electromagnetic waves; the shorter the wavelength, the greater the frequency.

PROPERTIES OF ELECTROMAGNETIC WAVES

The two most important properties of electromagnetic waves in relation to therapeutic modalities are their energy and their inertia. Both are a function of the photon, a particle produced by molecular motion.

Photons

A **photon** is the basic unit of radiant energy. The amount of energy in photons is a function of the frequency of the electromagnetic wave that produced it, so photons of a given frequency will always have the same amount of energy. There is no such thing as half a photon of energy; photons of a given frequency always occur in precisely the same-sized energy chunks.

Photons do posses differing amounts of energy, however. Since a photon's energy is a function of the frequency of the electromagnetic wave, the greater the frequency (or shorter the wavelength), the more energy it has. Thus, x-rays have much greater energy than radio waves. The energy at lower frequencies is so small that it has no therapeutic value.

Reflection, Refraction, Transmission, and Absorption

Photons possess inertia, so they exert pressure on any object or substance they strike. All electromagnetic waves move in a straight line until they come into contact with some other substance. One, or a combination, of four things will then occur (Fig. 10.5):

1. **Reflection**. As waves hit the substance, they bounce back; there is no penetration of the substance. The angle of reflection is determined by the angle of the strike.
2. **Refraction**. The waves bend as they pass through the substance; an example is light through a prism. The amount of bending depends on the frequency of the waves.

3. **Transmission**. The wave is transmitted through the substance. Transmission can be complete, such as with γ-rays through a door, or partial, such as x-rays through an arm. The depth of penetration is a function of the energy of the waves.
4. **Absorption**. Partially transmitted waves are absorbed by the tissues and turned into heat.

Thermal Effects of Electromagnetic Waves

All electrical currents cause a rise in temperature in the substance through which they flow because of the conversion of electricity to heat. The amount of heat produced is defined by the principles of Joule's law:

- Heat produced is directly proportional to the square of the current strength.
- Heat produced is directly proportional to the resistance of the conductor.
- Heat produced is directly proportional to the duration of the passage of a current.

Two examples are the incandescent light bulb and electrical fuse (Fig. 10.6). (1) In a light bulb, carbon or tungsten filaments are high resistance; as electricity passes though it, the resistance causes the filament to heat, which appears as light. (2) As current flows through the metal filament of the fuse (whose melting point is lower than that of the wires and other components of the circuit), it generates heat in the fuse. If the heat becomes excessive, it will melt the metal, thus breaking connection between the two ends of the fuse and breaking the circuit. Thus, the the wires of the circuit are preserved from excessive heat.

THE INFLUENCE OF TISSUE RESISTANCE

The tissues of the body possess varying resistances. This should mean that tissues with higher resistance would heat up more, but it's not so. Electricity flows along the path of least resistance.

Applying Radiation

The following laws and principles relate to the application of all forms of radiation:

- **Inverse square law**. $I = 1/d^2$. The intensity (I) of radiation is inversely proportional to the distance squared (d^2). Thus, decreasing the distance between the source and the patient will cause an exponential increase in its intensity. For example, decreasing the distance by half increases the intensity fourfold (Fig. 10.7). Because moving the source closer to the body greatly intensifies

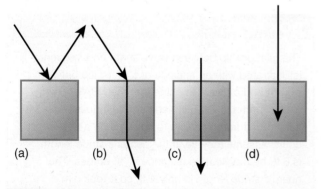

FIGURE 10.5 The possible responses of electromagnetic energy when it comes in contact with matter. The *arrows* represent the movement of photons. **(a)** Reflection, **(b)** refraction, **(c)** transmission, and **(d)** absorption. See text for details.

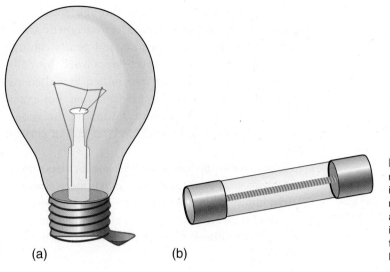

(a)   (b)

FIGURE 10.6 The thermal effects of an electrical current are illustrated here. **(a)** As current flows through an incandescent light bulb, the resistance of the metal filament causes heat that is manifested as light. **(b)** In a fuse, as current passes through the fuse, the metal filament in the middle heats. If the current is too strong, it heats to the point that the metal rod melts and the circuit is broken.

the radiation delivered to the body, small errors in placement of therapeutic modalities such as infrared lamps (see Chapter 11) and microwave diathermy (see Chapter 15) can easily burn patients. This is one of the reasons these modalities are dangerous and should be avoided.

- **Cosine or right-angle law.** The optimum radiation occurs when the source of the radiation is perpendicular to the center of the surface of the area to be radiated. When the source is at an angle, some of it is reflected to the side rather than moving into the tissue (Fig. 10.8). The amount of transmission is a function of the angle of application: full effects are achieved at 90°; 86% at 60°, and only 50% when radiation is applied at 30°.
- **Law of Grotthus-Draper.** Waves must be absorbed in order to be beneficial. Also known as the *principle of photochemical activation* and the *Draper law*, this law was proposed in the nineteenth century to define the effect of photons in stimulating photochemical reactions in a substance.[27]

It had nothing to do with heat. However, since not all of the absorbed light brings about chemical action, most of the "excess" absorbed energy is converted into thermal energy. So indirectly the law applies to heat as well.

Another interpretation of this law that can reasonably be applied to therapeutic modalities is that there is an inverse relationship between the amount of energy absorption and the depth of penetration of the energy. Energy that is absorbed by superficial layers is no longer available to deeper-lying tissues. This law explains why the effects of laser and infrared radiation are only superficial.

- **Arndt-Schultz principle.** There is an optimal amount of energy absorption per unit of time that is beneficial. Less than this amount will not cause a reaction, and more than this amount will be detrimental. The old adage that "more is better" applies only up to a point, as far as therapeutic modalities are concerned.

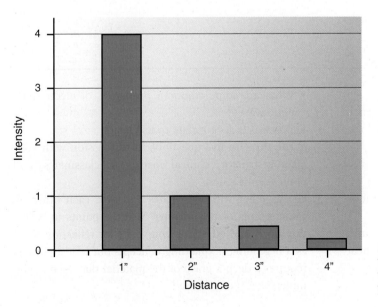

FIGURE 10.7 The inverse square law is demonstrated in this bar graph. Since the intensity of electromagnetic radiation is equal to $1/d^2$, the intensity increases exponentially as the distance between the source and the patient decreases.

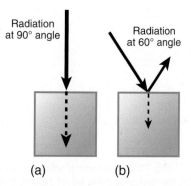

FIGURE 10.8 The effects of the cosine or right-angle law. **(a)** When radiation is at a 90° angle, meaning perpendicular to the surface, all of it transmits; **(b)** when applied at a different angle, some of the radiation is reflected.

Acoustic Waves

Acoustic waves (sound, ultrasound) are not electromagnetic waves. They differ from electromagnetic waves in two dramatic ways:

- Acoustic waves transmit best through solids, and not at all through a vacuum. Electromagnetic waves transmit best through a vacuum and poorly through solids. Electromagnetic waves are slowed by collisions. Acoustic waves are transmitted by collisions; as density increases, so does transmission. For example, ultrasound will transmit: 0.3 mm in the atmosphere, 1.5 mm in soft tissue, and 3.5 mm in cortical bone.

- Acoustic waves do not travel as fast as electromagnetic waves; in fact, they travel much more slowly—a few hundred thousand m/sec (10^5) as opposed to 10^8 m/s for electromagnetic waves. As in electromagnetic waves, linear speed equals wavelength times frequency.

? **CONCEPT CHECK 10.4.** Why must the head of an ultrasound unit be in good contact with the body?

CLOSING SCENE

Recall from the chapter opening scene that Andrew, a staff AT, suggested a regimen of heat therapy for a baseball player's chronic supraspinatus tendinitis. The athlete wondered if there was a difference in the heating effects produced by a whirlpool, hot pack, and ultrasound. You now know that whirlpools and hot packs produce moderate heat in the superficial tissues, while ultrasound can generate even greater amounts of heat into the deep tissues. Since the supraspinatus is a fairly deep muscle underneath the deltoids, you conclude that ultrasound or diathermy would be the modality of choice for heating this deep structure.

Chapter Reflections

1. Read and ponder each of the following points. Do you feel you have a clear understanding of each concept? If not, reread the appropriate section of the chapter.
   - What is heat?
   - Explain why heat is used therapeutically.
   - What are the general indications and contraindications to the therapeutic use of heat?
   - Define conduction, convection, radiation, and conversion and describe how they relate to heat transfer.
   - Provide an example of radiant energy.

   - What are some common properties of electromagnetic waves?
   - When is it appropriate to use heat?
2. Write three to five questions for discussion with your class instructor, clinical instructor, classmates, and clinical colleagues.
3. Get together with classmates and quiz each other on the concepts of this chapter. Use the points in reflection no. 1 and questions you wrote for reflection no. 2 as a beginning. Explaining concepts out loud to others requires a deeper grasp of the material than feeling you understand it as you read.

Concept Check Responses

CONCEPT CHECK 10.1

The sensation of being hot or cold is relative. In the summer, you get used to the temperature being hot, so 40°F (4.5°C) is colder than what you are used to and you interpret it as being cold. During the winter the opposite is true. You get used to it being cold, and since 40°F (4.5°C) is hotter that what you have been used to, you interpret it as being warm.

CONCEPT CHECK 10.2

$23 \times 10^2 = 2300$. $3 \times 10^3 = 3000$, So 3×10^3 is bigger than 23×10^2.

CONCEPT CHECK 10.3

Remember that wavelength times frequency equals 186,000 mi./s. So:
(a) frequency = 30 Hz (186, 000 mi./s ÷ 6200 mi. = 30 Hz).
(b) wavelength = 93 mi. (186, 000 mi./s ÷ 2000 Hz = 93 mi.)

CONCEPT CHECK 10.4

Ultrasound is a mechanical wave that cannot be transmitted through air. Therefore, if the transducer is not in complete contact with the skin and coupling agent, the energy will not be transmitted.

REFERENCES

1. Draper DO, Harris ST, Schulthies SS, et al. Hotpack and 1 MHz ultrasound treatments have an additive effect on muscle temperature increase. *J Athl Train.* 1998;33:21–24.
2. Morris AK. *Moist Heat Pack Re-Warming Following 10, 20, 30 min Application.* Provo, UT: Exercise Science, Brigham Young University, 2003.
3. Myrer JW, Draper DO, Durrant E. Contrast therapy and intramuscular temperature in the human leg. *J Athl Train.* 1994;29:318–322.
4. Wertz AS, Myrer JW. Intramuscular and subcutaneous temperature changes in the human leg due to contrast hydrotherapy. *J Athl Train.* 1997;32(2 Suppl):S33.
5. Mitra A, Draper DO, Hopkins T, Anderson MA. Application of the ThermaCare Knee Wrap results in significant increases in muscle and intracapsular temperature. *J Athl Train.* 2005;40:S88–S89.
6. Draper DO, Trowbridge CA. Continuous low-level heat therapy: what works, what doesn't. *Athl Ther Today.* 2003;8:46–48.
7. Draper D, Trowbridge CA. The thermacare heatwrap increases skin and paraspinal muscle temperature greater than the curaheat patch. *J Athl Train.* 2004;39:S93.
8. Trowbridge C, Draper DO, Feland JB, Eggett D. The thermacare air-activated heat wrap heats paraspinal muscles greater than two menthol-based pain patches. *J Orthop Sports Phys Ther.* 2004;34: 549–558.
9. Draper, Castel, et al. *J Appl Toxicol.* 1998;s-70.
10. Draper DO, Knight KL, Fujiwara T, Castel JC. Temperature change in human muscle during and after pulsed short-wave diathermy. *J Orthop Sports Phys Ther.* 1999;29(1):13–18; discussion 19–22.
11. Garrett CL, Draper DO, Knight KL. Heat distribution in the lower leg from pulsed short-wave diathermy and ultrasound treatments. *J Athl Train.* 2000;35(1):13–22.
12. Draper, et al. *J Appl Toxicol.* 2005;s.
13. Draper DO, Castel JC, Castel D. Rate of temperature increase in human muscle during 1 MHz and 3 MHz continuous ultrasound. *J Orthop Sports Phys Ther.* 1995;22(4):142–150.
14. Anderson M, Eggett D, Draper D. Combining topical analgesics and ultrasound, Part 2. *Athl Ther Today.* 2005;10(2):45–47.
15. Rose S, Draper DO, Schulthies SS, Durrant E. The stretching window part two: rate of thermal decay in deep muscle following 1-MHz ultrasound. *J Athl Train.* 1996;31:139–143.
16. Ashton DF, Draper DO, Myrer JW. Temperature rise in human muscle during ultrasound treatments using flex-all as a coupling agent. *J Athl Train.* 1998;33:136–140.
17. Draper DO, Schulthies S, Sorvisto P, Hautala A-M. Temperature changes in deep muscles of humans during ice and ultrasound therapies: an in vivo study. *J Orthop Sports Phys Ther.* 1995;21(3): 153–157.
18. Draper D, Sunderland S. Examination of the law of Grotthus-Draper: does ultrasound penetrate subcutaneous fat in humans? *J Athl Train.* 1993;28:246–250.
19. Chudleigh D, Schulthies S, Draper D, Myrer J. Muscle temperature rise during 1 MHz ultrasound treatments of two and six times the effective radiating areas of the transducer. *J Athl Train.* 1998; 33(2):s-11.
20. Draper DO. A breakthrough on comfortable ultrasound treatments: Beam non-uniformity ratio is only half of the equation. Paper presented at National Athletic Trainer's Association Annual Symposium; S-25,Kansas City, MO, 1999.
21. Rimington SJ, Draper DO, Durrant E, Fellingham G. Temperature changes during therapeutic ultrasound in the precooled human gastrocnemius muscle. *J Athl Train.* 1994;29:325–327.
22. Draper DO, Ricard MD. Rate of temperature decay in human muscle following 3 mhz ultrasound: the stretching window revealed. *J Athl Train.* 1995;30:304–307.
23. Draper D, Abergel P, Castel J. Rate of temperature change in human fat during external ultrasound: Implications for liposuction. *Am J Cosmetic Surg.* 1998;15(4):361–367.
24. Chan AK, Myrer JW, Measom GJ, et al. Temperature changes in human patellar tendon in response to therapeutic ultrasound. *J Athl Train.* 1998;33(2):130–135.
25. Bishop S, Draper DO, Knight KL, Feland JB, Eggett D. Human-tissue temperature rise during ultrasound treatments with the aquaflex gel pad. *J Athl Train.* 2004;39(2):25–30.
26. Wells A, Draper D, Vincent W. The regression equation of the omnisound 3000p is valid: ultrasound treatments should be temperature dependent not time dependent. *J Athl Train.* 2004;39(2):s-24.
27. Fang H-Y. Environmental Geotechnology Dictionary [website]. Available at: http://www.iseg.giees.uncc.edu/dictionary.cfm, 2006.
28. Ichiyama RM, Ragan BG, Bell GW, Iwamoto G. Effects of topical analgesics on the pressor response evoked by muscle afferents. *Med Sci Sport Exerc.* 2002;34(9):1440–1445.
29. Brewer A, McCarberg B, Argoff C. Update on the use of topical NSAIDs for the treatment of soft tissue and musculoskeletal pain: a review of recent data and current treatment options. *Phys Sports Med.* 2010;38(2):62–70.

11

Superficial Thermotherapy Application

Chapter Outline

OPENING SCENE

Michael and Eric are athletic trainer wantabees. During their first day of observation in the Athletic Training Clinic, they noticed numerous patients in the whirlpool bath and many with hot packs on their shoulders and legs. As they talked about it, Michael remembered the bags of corn that his grandmother heated in the microwave and applied to her neck. Michael remarked that his grandfather's house often had a menthol smell from the "heating" ointment his grandfather applies to his arthritic knees each morning. Many questions arose during their conversation. Why are there so many forms of heat treatments? Do they heat the same? Are there different advantages and disadvantages for using various heating agents? What heat modality would be the best to use under certain circumstances? How much heat does the "heating" ointment actually produce?

Superficial Thermotherapy

Superficial thermotherapy includes modalities that effectively heat only the surface tissues up to about 1 cm (see Table 10.1). The most commonly used modalities are the whirlpool, hot pack, paraffin bath, and electrical heating pads. Infrared lamps are sometimes used as heat modalities, although we do not recommend infrared lamps because they burn too easily. And those heating ointments? They do not substantially increase tissue temperature, but do provide counter-irritation, which can gate pain. This is reflected in the official classification of these ointments; they are known as topical analgesics, despite advertisements that they provide deep heat.

PHYSIOLOGICAL EFFECTS

In general, these modalities heat the surface about 6–8°F (3–5°C) and muscles 3–5°F (2–3°C) at depths <2 cm (see Table 10.1). Blood flow doubles, and metabolism increases. Superficial thermotherapy decreases pain, but not enough to facilitate active exercise. Soreness, however, is decreased during resting and activity. Table 11.1 summarizes these effects and their efficacy in rehabilitating acute and chronic injuries.

Although most of the research on these modalities was conducted prior to 1970, some work has been done since then, and it is included as appropriate throughout this chapter.

ACUTE INJURY REHABILITATION

Historically, acute injuries were treated with ice for 24–72 hours and then with heat applications. If applied too early, thermotherapy will exacerbate swelling. The theory for heat application was that it stimulated increased blood flow, which increased the removal of tissue debris from the injury site and promoted healing by increasing the delivery of nutrients to the injury site. Much of the therapeutic modality research in the 1940s through 1970s concentrated on the modality's effects in increasing blood flow. This theory is now much less importance to physical rehabilitation clinicians, however.

Heat has taken a back seat to exercise as the dominant acute injury rehabilitation modality. First, tissue debris are removed from the injury site via the lymphatic system, which is stimulated by intermittent compression, such as is applied by rhythmic muscle contraction and relaxation (see Chapters 5 and 6). Second, exercise is much more effective in enhancing blood flow than heat is, 15–20 times more. And when combined with cryotherapy, it can begin much earlier, usually within 24 hours of the injury occurrence (see Chapters 12 and 13).

What then is the role of heat applications? It is usually beneficial (more so than cryotherapy) in reducing or reversing:

- General soreness/aching, which often occurs the day following intense activity such as an athletic contest
- General soreness/aching that transitions from acute pain 6–10 days following sprains, strains, and contusions
- Reversing joint motion that is restricted following surgery, long-term immobilization, or inactivity. To be effective, it must be combined with joint mobilization or stretching (see Chapters 14 and 15).

CHRONIC INJURY REHABILITATION

There are two types of chronic injuries: overuse and recurring. Recurring injuries are simply repeated acute injuries and are treated the same as acute injuries.

Overuse injuries, such as bursitis and tendinitis, are more difficult to resolve. Both heat and cold have been suggested for treatment.

TABLE 11.1 THE EFFICACY OF HEAT APPLICATIONS DURING ORTHOPEDIC INJURY CARE

PHYSIOLOGICAL RESPONSE	EFFICACY DURING IMMEDIATE CARE OF ACUTE INJURIES*	EFFICACY DURING REHABILITATION	
		Acute Injuries	Chronic Injuries
Increased circulation	Nil	Positive	Positive
Increased metabolism	very negative†	Nil	Nil
Increased inflammation	Positive	Positive	Negative
Decreased pain (anesthesia)	Positive	Nil‡	Positive
Decreased muscle spasm	Positive	Positive	Nil
Decreased tissue stiffness	Nil	Nil	Positive
Overall	Negative	Nil	?

?indicates that the overall effects of chronic injuries are unknown.

*There is no immediate care of chronic injuries.

†Promotes secondary metabolic injury.

‡Often does not facilitate active exercise.

Whirlpool Application

STEP 1: FOUNDATION

A. Definition. A **whirlpool** is a large body of either hot or cold water that is forcibly circulated or "whirled" about in its container (Fig. 11.1).

B. Effects
1. Hydrotherapy: The buoyancy of water supports the body or body part, providing a sort of suspended animation, thereby allowing easy exercise.
2. Physical massage, provided by the whirling water and air
3. Convective heating or cooling provided by whirling water
4. Temperature effects
   a. Hot water will cause:
      i. Conductive heating, a superficial increase in temperature
      ii. A superficial increase in blood flow
      iii. Decreased muscle spasm through analgesia
      iv. Whole-body relaxation through analgesia (if the whole body is treated)
      v. Increased metabolism
   b. Cold water will cause:
      i. Conductive cooling, a decreased temperature that will penetrate further than heat
      ii. Decreased blood flow
      iii. Contraction or tightness of connective tissue around muscles and joints
      iv. A decrease in pain
      v. Decreased metabolism

C. Advantages
1. Can treat the whole body
2. Provides irregular surfaces with total contact
3. Temperature stability of water; it loses (or gains) heat very slowly.

4. Can provide multiple treatments simultaneously, if treatments involve the limbs (e.g., two to four patients can dangle their legs in the whirlpool at the same time)
5. The force of the water massage can be regulated from quite vigorous to very gentle.
6. Allows range of motion exercises during treatment

D. Disadvantages
1. Causes a person to feel weak or lethargic (if the majority of the body is treated with heat)
2. Increased edema (if hot water is used) when a limb is in a dependent position (lower than the rest of the body)
3. Possibility of infection
4. Messy and noisy
5. Not portable

E. Indications
1. General whole-limb or whole-body stiffness or soreness (i.e., occurring early in a sports season, when practice sessions occur two or three times daily, or when you perform an unaccustomed activity for 3 or 4 days)
2. Whenever superficial heat is desired
3. As a supplement to other treatments

F. Contraindications
1. General heat contraindications. Avoid using:
   a. 24–48 hours after an acute injury
   b. If circulation is compromised
   c. If sensation to the area is compromised
2. Avoid treating a person with a high fever (>101°F, or 38.3°C).

G. Precautions
1. Do not leave a patient in the whirlpool unattended; she might become lethargic enough to faint and drown.
2. Do not allow a patient to turn the whirlpool on or off while in the whirlpool.
3. Clean the tank before and after treating someone with an infectious wound.
4. Keep clothing and bandages out of the whirlpool.
5. Do not let a whirlpool treatment substitute for a more beneficial treatment (e.g., therapeutic exercise).

STEP 2: PREAPPLICATION TASKS

A. Make sure whirlpool is the proper modality for this situation.
1. Reevaluate the injury/problem. Make sure you understand the patient's condition.

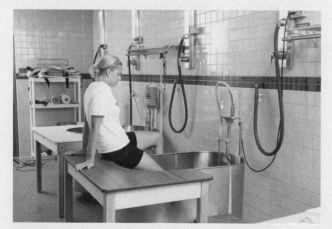

FIGURE 11.1 A typical whirlpool.

2. If whirlpool was previously used, review the patient's response to the previous treatment.
3. Confirm that the objectives of therapy are compatible with whirlpool.
4. Make sure whirlpool is not contraindicated in this situation.

B. Equipment preparation. Prepare the equipment before preparing the patient.
   1. Close the drain.
   2. Select the temperature.
      a. For cryotherapy: 50–60°F (10–15.5°C)
      b. For thermotherapy: 100–108°F (37.7–42.2°C) for the whole body; 105–112°F (40.5–44.4°C) for an extremity
   3. Fill the whirlpool approximately two-thirds full of water; the level depends on the body part being treated.
      a. Cover the agitator intakes by at least 2 in. (5 cm) of water.
      b. Plan ahead; if someone is going to sit down in the whirlpool, this will raise the level of the water. Don't fill so high that it will overflow.
      c. Agitator pressure will raise the level of the water.
      d. Check the temperature while filling, and adjust the hot or cold water as necessary.
   4. If the whirlpool is already filled, check the temperature and adjust as necessary.
   5. Check the whirlpool electrical system (Box 11.1).
      a. It must be grounded via a GFI (Box 11.2).
      b. The electrical cord must be intact: no cracked or frayed sections.
      c. The electrical cord must be off the floor.
      d. Make sure the on–off switch is insulated and out of reach of a patient in the whirlpool.
   6. Add disinfectant if necessary.
      a. Especially if treating a person with open wounds
      b. It can be a psychological aid to patients who are anxious about "catching something" from patients who previously used the whirlpool.

Note: Disinfectants react with extremely hard water to form clusters of scummy bubbles. The scum is not unsanitary, but it gives the appearance of being so. It can be eliminated by adding an antacid to the water.

   7. Check the equipment operation before allowing the patient to get into the tank (unless you have just used the equipment to treat another patient).
      a. Turn on the turbine.
         i. Make sure the water intakes are well covered.
         ii. Adjust the water pressure and air bubbles to soft flow.
         iii. Make sure the air intakes on the motor are not covered.
      b. Turn off the turbine.

BOX 11.1   THE WHIRLPOOL ELECTRICAL SYSTEM

A whirlpool must be hard-wired into an electrical supply. Observe the following guidelines:

1. The on–off switch should be on a wall remote from the whirlpool, far enough away that a patient cannot reach the switch from within the whirlpool.
2. The electrical cord connecting a whirlpool to an electrical source should be hard-wired into the source rather than plugged into an outlet.
3. The cord between the whirlpool and electrical source should be enclosed in electrical conduit.

The above measures will minimize damage to the electrical system, which could result in an electrical fault and possibly causing a patient's death. Although these measures and a GFI may be redundant, with electricity and water, it is best to be safe.

C. Preparing the patient psychologically
   1. Explain the procedure to the patient, including the following:
      a. The combining effects of water and massage action
      b. The physiological effects of heat or cold
      c. The water will be warm (or cold).
      d. The water should be comfortable (unless very cold).
      e. The massage should be comfortable.
      f. The action of the turbine is to add air to the water and to force water to move (whirl) in the tank.
   2. Check for, and warn the patient about, precautions.
D. Preparing the patient physically
   1. Have the patient remove clothing as necessary.
      a. A rolled-up shirt sleeve or pants leg will often get wet.
      b. Gym shorts and T-shirt or swimming suit are best.

BOX 11.2   GFI'S FOR PREVENTING ELECTROCUTION

All therapeutic modalities involving electricity and water must be plugged into a GFI-protected outlet (see Figures. 16.2 and 16.3). As explained in Chapter 16, GFIs detect ground faults and interrupt the flow of current. Patients have been electrocuted during whirlpool treatments (usually when the whirlpool was turned on while the patient was in the water). Never give a whirlpool treatment unless the whirlpool is plugged into a GFI. (See Chapter 9 to review how GFIs work.)

2. Remove all bandages, tape, braces, etc.
3. Position the patient in the whirlpool tank.
   a. Make sure the seat is secure, if a seat is being used.
   b. If the patient is sitting outside the tank, make sure the edge of the tank is padded to prevent cutting off the circulation to an arm or a leg.
   c. The patient should be comfortable.

3 STEP 3: APPLICATION PARAMETERS

A. Procedures
   1. Turn on the turbine before the patient gets into the water.
   2. Help the patient into the whirlpool tank, if necessary.
   3. Adjust the turbine height and readjust the patient (Fig. 11.2).
   4. Adjust the direction of flow of the water.
      a. For maximum force, position the body part directly in line with and about 1 foot (30 cm) from the turbine.
      b. For minimum force, direct the turbine to the side of the tank opposite the body part to be treated.

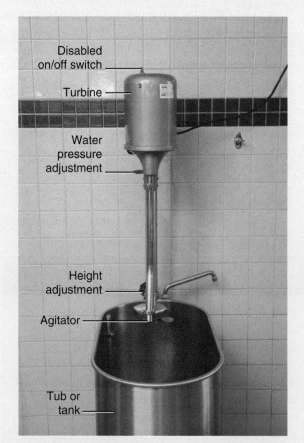

FIGURE 11.2 Components of a whirlpool agitator unit.

c. Adjust the water pressure.
d. Adjust the air flow.

5. Do not leave the patient unattended. If two or more patients are using the whirlpool simultaneously, they can watch each other for signs of lethargy.
6. Turn off the turbine before the patient gets out of the water. The water level may fall below the intake hole when the patient gets out.

B. Dosage
   1. See temperature selection in step 2.
C. Length of application
   1. Treatments usually last 10–20 minutes.
   2. If the patient becomes dizzy, tired, nauseated, or overheated, terminate the treatment.
D. Frequency of application
   1. One or two times daily
E. Duration of therapy
   1. Varies, depending upon phase of injury, and desired effects

4 STEP 4: POSTAPPLICATION TASKS

A. Instructions to the patient
   1. Schedule the next treatment.
   2. Instruct the patient about the level of activity and/or self-treatment prior to the next formal treatment.
   3. If the patient has just finished a warm full-body whirlpool, he/she should rehydrate.
B. Record of treatment, including unique patient responses
C. Whirlpool and area cleanup
   1. Wipe water off benches and clean up the floor.
   2. Drain the tank at the end of the day, after cleaning the inside of the turbine shaft.
      a. Clean the inside of the turbine shaft by adding disinfectant to the water, lowering the shaft to its lowest position, and turning on the motor for 5 minutes, causing the disinfected water to flow through the inside of the shaft.
   3. Clean and disinfect the whirlpool daily, or after five to eight treatments, if used infrequently.

5 STEP 5: MAINTENANCE

A. Keep the equipment clean and polished. Do not use an abrasive cleaner on the whirlpool tank; it will scratch the stainless steel, causing tiny grooves in which staphylococci (bacteria) can grow.
B. Check the electrical cord for fraying.

Hot Pack Application

STEP 1: FOUNDATION

A. Definition. A **hot pack** is a form of moist superficial heat applied with one of the following (Fig. 11.3):
  1. *Hot water bottle:* used for centuries, but it does not stay warm very long (<5 minutes).
  2. *Kenny packs:* a wool pack that is steam-heated and spun dry. It has intense initial heat but cools quickly (5 minutes).
  3. *Hot towel:* a towel dipped in hot water and wrung out. Stays warm 5–10 minutes. Effectiveness time has been increased by adding a heat source such as an electric pad (plastic coated) or heat lamp. Caution: This is not recommended; it burns too easily.
  4. *Hydrocollator pack:* a silica encased in a canvas pack
     a. The gel absorbs great amounts of water and thus retains heat for long periods of time (Fig. 11.4).
     b. Can hold heat up to 30 minutes if heated to 140–160°F (60–70°C)
     c. Towel wrapping provides a temperature of about 115°F (45°C) to the skin.
     d. As the pack cools, layers of towel are removed. Thus, the temperature presented to the skin remains at about 115°F (45°C).

B. Effects (those of conductive heating):
  1. Superficial increase (100%) in circulation
  2. Increased metabolism
  3. Muscle relaxation through analgesia

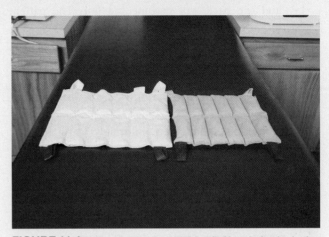

FIGURE 11.4 Hot packs before hydration (**left**) and after hydration (**right**). Notice the difference in volume, indicating the amount of water absorbed by the silica.

C. Advantages
  1. Ease of application
  2. Local heat without heating the whole body
  3. Can provide multiple treatments
  4. Relatively inexpensive
  5. Can treat over an open wound without fear of spreading germs to others
  6. Durability
  7. Portable; the patient can move around.
  8. Heats surface and intramuscular tissues more than paraffin[1]

D. Disadvantages
  1. Weight of the pack may be uncomfortable in some situations.
  2. Time consuming; packs must be reheated between uses.
  3. Packs are difficult to contour to some body parts.
  4. Effects are only superficial: a temperature increase of 6.5°F (3.6°C) at 1 cm depth and a tissue temperature increase of 1.4°F (8°C) at 3 cm depth[2]
  5. Difficult to perform range-of-motion exercises with the pack on the body
  6. The effects of heat are short-lived; the tissue cools quickly.[1,3–5]

E. Indications
  1. Any place local heat is desired
  2. As a supplement to other treatment

F. Contraindications
  1. General heat contraindications

G. Precautions
  1. Never place a bare (unwrapped) pack on a patient.
  2. Do not prepare a hot pack on a patient; the initial single layer of towel is not enough insulation, and you may burn the patient.

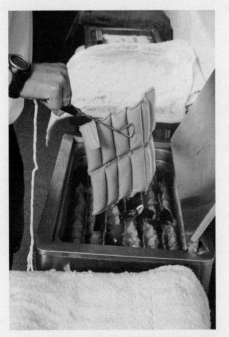

FIGURE 11.3 A hot pack being removed from its heating unit.

3. Do not let a patient sit or lie on a hot pack; the heat will not be able to dissipate into the atmosphere, and the pack will become too hot. The patient might get burned.

4. Keep checking on the patient to make sure the pack does not get too hot (packs are initially cool until the heat penetrates through).

5. Keep removing layers of toweling as the hot pack cools.

6. Hot packs should be comfortably warm but not hot; may burn if blood does not carry heat away

7. It usually takes several minutes for a person to feel the warmth.

8. Report immediately if the hot packs become too hot.

2️⃣ STEP 2: PREAPPLICATION TASKS

A. Make sure hot packs are the proper modality for this situation.
   1. Reevaluate the injury/problem. Make sure you understand the patient's condition.
   2. If a hot pack was applied previously, review the patient's response to the previous treatment.
   3. Confirm that the objectives of therapy are compatible with hot packs.
   4. Make sure hot packs are not contraindicated in this situation.

B. Preparing the patient psychologically
   1. Explain the procedure to the patient, including the following:
      a. Heat will increase blood flow and relax the muscles.
      b. It should be comfortable.
      c. Relax and enjoy it.
   2. Check for, and warn the patient about, precautions.

C. Preparing the patient physically
   1. Clothing need not be removed, but it will get damp if the hot pack is placed over it. Let the patient decide.
   2. Position the patient in a comfortable position, one that he/she can remain in for 15–20 minutes. Lying down is usually best.

D. Equipment preparation
   1. Make sure the heating unit is set at the proper temperature, 140–160°F (60–70°C). The warmer it is, the more it can heat the skin but also the more toweling you must have initially so the *interface temperature* (temperature presented to the skin) is about 115°F (45°C).
   2. Have adequate toweling available (terry cloth towels and/or terry cloth hydrocollator pack covers; Fig. 11.5).

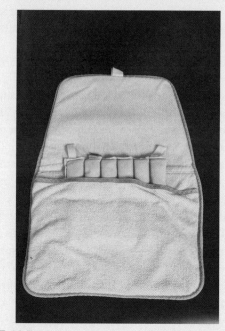

FIGURE 11.5 Hot pack covers contain four layers of terry cloth. They are folded over a hot pack and secured with Velcro straps.

   a. Hot pack covers are more convenient than towels because you do not have to spend time preparing them. But layers cannot be removed as the hot pack cools, so the treatment cannot last as long.
   b. Individual towels give greater control because you can remove layers of the towel as the hot pack cools and thus maintain the interface temperature at 115°F (45°C) longer.
   3. Several hours before treatment:
      a. Presoak new packs for 12–24 hours to absorb a sufficient amount of water.
      b. Water should cover the packs at all times. (Add water only when there is time for it to heat up; end of day or first thing in the morning is a convenient time.)
      c. Preheat the packs for 2–3 hours if the water is cold, 30 minutes if the water is hot.[4]
   4. Immediately before treatment:
      a. Decide whether to use a towel or hot pack cover.
      b. Place a towel or hot pack cover on the table, not on the patient.
      c. Remove the pack from the heating unit.
         i. Do not reach into the water; use tongs or a hook to lift the pack out of the water.
         ii. Allow the excess water to drip into the tank.
         iii. Close the lid of the heating unit so that other packs will stay hot.
      d. Prepare the pack on the table, not on the patient.
         i. Place the hot pack in the middle of the cover, fold the other side over, and attach the Velcro fasteners. Or:

ii. Place the hot pack in the middle and at the end of the towel (Fig. 11.6a).

iii. Fold the sides of towel lengthwise over the pack (Fig. 11.6b).

iv. Fold the towel end-over-end over the hot pack until it is used (Fig. 11.6c).

3️⃣ STEP 3: **APPLICATION PARAMETERS**

A. Procedures
1. Place the folded pack on the patient. *Caution*: Never let a patient lie or sit on a hot pack; the heat cannot dissipate and can cause burning.
2. Place another towel over the pack to keep the heat from dissipating into the air.
3. Check the patient every 4–5 minutes.
   a. Add an extra towel between the pack and the patient if the pack is too hot.
   b. Remove a layer of toweling if the pack is too cool, or change the hot pack if using a hot pack cover.
B. Dosage
1. Within the comfort limits of the patient
C. Length of application
1. 20–25 minutes

D. Frequency of application
1. Application can be repeated two or three times per day if separated by 3–4 hours.
E. Duration of therapy
1. Varies, depending upon phase of injury and desired effects

4️⃣ STEP 4: **POSTAPPLICATION TASKS**

A. Instructions to the patient
1. Schedule the next treatment.
2. Instruct the patient about the level of activity and/or self-treatment prior to the next formal treatment.
B. Record of treatment, including unique patient responses
C. Equipment replacement and cleanup
1. Return the hot pack to the heating unit immediately after the treatment. Delaying its return will prolong reheating.
   a. Return packs to the heating unit according to a specific rotation system (Box 11.3).

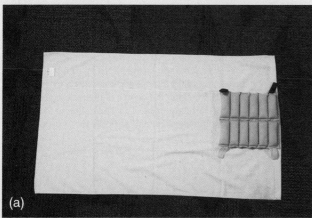

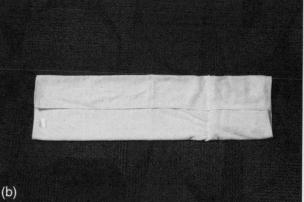

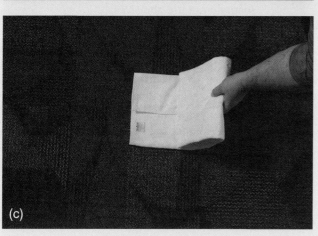

FIGURE 11.6 Preparing a hot pack for application. **(a)** Place the pack at the end of the towel, **(b)** fold the sides of the towel lengthwise over the pack, or **(c)** fold the towel end-over-end over the hot pack until it is used.

BOX 11.3 A HOT PACK ROTATION SYSTEM

A system for rotating the use of hot packs is essential for ensuring that each treatment involves the pack that has warmed/rewarmed the longest. This is especially important in very busy clinics. Without such a system, a single hot pack might be used over and over again without adequately rewarming between treatments, while packs that are at maximum temperature remain unused.

An effective system is the use of colored tabs on one side of the hot packs (use a laundry pen to color the tabs). The following instructions apply to a four-pack heating unit, but the same system can be used in eight-pack units:

1. Remember two principles:
   a. Orientation is front to back of the heating unit.
   b. Look for the first color change.
2. Start the day with all four hot packs placed in the heating unit so the same color tabs are sticking up.
3. For a treatment, select the first hot pack after a color change. For example, for the first treatment of the day, all tabs will be the same color and so you take the first one. But later in the day, if the first two packs are black and the third and fourth are white, you would select the third one. If you had two black-tabbed packs, a blank slot (one was in use), and a white-tabbed pack in slot 4, you would choose the white-tabbed pack (Fig. 11.7).
4. After a treatment, return the pack to the first open slot so that the tabs on top are the same color as the packs before it (toward the front) and opposite of the packs after it (toward the back) (Fig. 11.8).

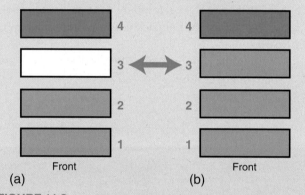

FIGURE 11.7 Hot packs in a heating unit. Note the difference in colors of the first two (*black*) and last two tabs (*white*).

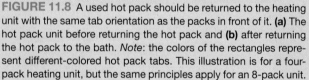

FIGURE 11.8 A used hot pack should be returned to the heating unit with the same tab orientation as the packs in front of it. **(a)** The hot pack unit before returning the hot pack and **(b)** after returning the hot pack to the bath. *Note:* the colors of the rectangles represent different-colored hot pack tabs. This illustration is for a four-pack heating unit, but the same principles apply for an 8-pack unit.

2. Return the towels (or covers) to the drying rack. Exceptions:
   a. If treating a patient with an infectious disease, launder the towel before using it on another person.
   b. If it is the end of the day, towels must be laundered.

5 STEP 5: MAINTENANCE

A. Regular equipment cleaning
   1. Clean the heating unit at least once a month.
      a. Remove the packs and rack.
      b. Drain the water.
      c. Clean the tank with a mild disinfectant and soap; do not use abrasives.
      d. Replace the rack, packs, and water.
B. Routine maintenance
   1. Keep the water level in the heating unit above the top of the packs. Always add water at the end of the day so it has time to heat. Adding water during the day may reduce the temperature of the bath and hot packs.
   2. Do not allow the packs to dry out. Always return them to the heating unit.
   3. Check the thermostat, yearly, for proper operation by inserting an external thermometer in the heated water.

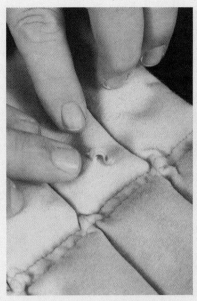

FIGURE 11.9 Example of a breach of the canvas due to excessive wear and tear of a hot pack in a hot pack cell that allows the gel to ooze out.

C. Simple repairs
  1. Watch the packs for loss of gel, usually as a result of wear to, or ripping of, the canvas pack cover (Fig. 11.9).
      a. When this occurs, slit the individual damaged cell, remove the gel by squeezing, wash the inside of the cell with water, and rewarm the pack for continued use.
      b. Hot packs can be used with up to three or four missing cells.

Paraffin Bath Application
5 STEPS

1 STEP 1: FOUNDATION

A. Definition. A **paraffin bath** is a form of moist superficial heat applied by forming a paraffin "glove" around the affected body part (Fig. 11.10). There are two similar techniques, immersion and dip and wrap, explained below in step 3, Application Parameters.
B. Effects (those of conductive heating; similar to hot packs):
  1. Superficial increase in circulation
  2. Increased metabolism
  3. Muscle relaxation through analgesia

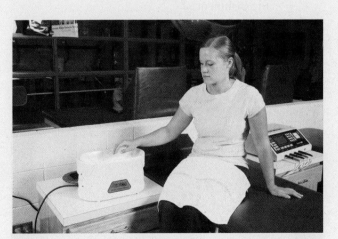

FIGURE 11.10 A patient dipping her hand into a paraffin bath.

C. Advantages
  1. Ease of application
  2. Local heat without heating the whole body
  3. Softens the skin; water tends to dry it.
  4. Uniform heating; all surfaces of the treated part are heated at one time.
  5. Relatively inexpensive
D. Disadvantages
  1. Hand heating is less than with a hot pack, even in the web spaces between fingers.[1]
  2. Can only treat hands and feet
  3. Messy and sometimes smells somewhat badly
  4. Tends to accumulate dirt and debris from the skin
  5. Cannot observe the treated area during treatment
  6. Effects are not long lasting.
  7. Cannot perform range-of-motion exercises during treatment
E. Indications
  1. Local heat to the feet and hands
  2. As a supplement to other treatment
F. Contraindications
  1. General heat contraindications
  2. Cannot apply over infections, rashes, or open lesions
  3. Burns or new scars
G. Precautions
  1. Check the temperature of the paraffin before applying.
  2. The skin must be dry; water droplets may result in burns.

3. Small scratches must be covered.
4. Avoid the seepage of hot paraffin beneath the initial application. This can occur in the following situations:
   a. If you go above the first immersion line on subsequent immersions
   b. If cracks develop in the glove, usually caused by moving the body part

2 STEP 2: PREAPPLICATION TASKS

A. Make sure a paraffin bath is the proper modality for this situation.
   1. Reevaluate the injury/problem. Make sure you understand the patient's condition.
   2. If a paraffin bath was used previously, review the patient response to the previous treatment.
   3. Confirm that the objectives of therapy are compatible with paraffin.
   4. Make sure a paraffin bath is not contraindicated in this situation.
B. Preparing the patient psychologically
   1. Explain the procedure to the patient, including the following:
      a. The paraffin will feel hot, but it will not burn.
      b. It should be comfortable.
   2. Check for, and warn the patient about, precautions.
C. Preparing the patient physically
   1. Remove all clothing, jewelry, bandages, etc., from the area to be treated. (If a ring cannot be removed, cover it with several layers of gauze and then tape it.)
   2. Make sure the skin is clean and dry.
   3. Cover any small scratches.
   4. Place a towel over any clothing that may get soiled from treatment.
D. Equipment preparation
   1. Several hours before treatment:
      a. Prepare the paraffin by either of these two methods:
         i. Mix seven parts wax with one part mineral oil. The mineral oil lowers the melting point of the wax to about 126°F (52°C). Paraffin above 130°F (55.4°C) will burn.
         ii. Purchase premixed paraffin. It comes in blocks (about the size of a gallon of milk) or chips (about the size of potato chips). Place in the heated container and the solid wax will slowly melt.
      b. Use a candy thermometer to check the temperature after all the wax is melted.
      c. Adjust the temperature if it is too hot (add mineral oil) or too cool (add wax). A light scum will form if the temperature is right (Fig. 11.11).
   2. Immediately before treatment:
      a. Check the temperature.

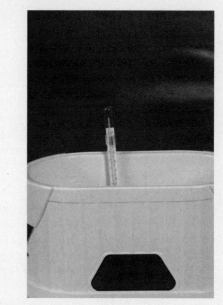

FIGURE 11.11 Using a candy thermometer to check the temperature in a paraffin bath. Note the light scum on top of the paraffin.

3 STEP 3: APPLICATION PARAMETERS

A. Procedures
   1. Dip the body part into the paraffin bath and quickly pull it out.
   2. Allow the paraffin to cool until it solidifies (it will turn milky white in color within 10 seconds) (Fig. 11.12).
   3. Repeat steps 1 and 2 until there is a *glove* of 7–12 layers of paraffin.
   4. The treatment finishes in one of two ways:
      a. Dip and wrap technique. Cover the area with cellophane wrap or a plastic bag and then with a towel. Sit or lie with the hand held in a motionless position.
      b. Immersion technique. Returned the gloved hand to the bath and hold it there for the duration of the treatment.

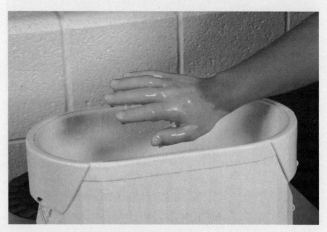

FIGURE 11.12 Paraffin cooling on the hand of a patient.

B. Dosage
   1. 7–12 layers of paraffin
C. Length of application
   1. 20–25 minutes
D. Frequency of application
   1. Application can be repeated two or three times per day if separated by 3–4 hours.
E. Duration of therapy
   1. Varies, depending upon phase of injury and desired effects

 STEP 4: POSTAPPLICATION TASKS

A. Instructions to the patient
   1. Schedule the next treatment.

   2. Instruct the patient about the level of activity and/or self-treatment prior to the next formal treatment.
B. Record of treatment, including unique patient responses
C. Equipment removal; patient cleanup
   1. Peel the paraffin from the body part, and discard it or put it into the bath. Some consider the used paraffin soiled and unsuitable for further use.

5 **STEP 5: MAINTENANCE**

A. Check the paraffin bath periodically for scum or foreign material. Remove any foreign material.
B. Replace the paraffin as it is used.

5 STEPS Do Not Apply Infrared Lamps

1 **STEP 1: FOUNDATION**

A. Definition. Heat from an **infrared (IR) lamp** is a form of superficial heat that radiates from a heat lamp or an IR lamp. Two types, called *near IR* and *far IR*, have been used therapeutically.
B. Effects (those of conductive heating):
   1. Superficial increase in circulation
   2. Increased metabolism
   3. Muscle relaxation through analgesia
C. Advantages
   1. Ease of application
   2. Local heat without heating the whole body
   3. Very inexpensive. An IR bulb can be purchased in any department store.

D. Disadvantages
   1. Burning. It is very easy to burn someone with an IR lamp.
   2. Not as effective as hot packs and paraffin baths
   3. Not portable
E. Indications
   1. None. It is too easy to burn.
F. Contraindications
   1. The danger of easily burning patients and the availability of better forms of superficial heat contraindicate the use of this modality.
G. Precautions
   1. We recommend against using an infrared lamp.
   2. If you choose to use an IR lamp, make sure you have a full understanding of the inverse square law and the cosine law (see Chapter 11).

 CONCEPT CHECK 11.1. A gymnast is experiencing some general soreness in her shoulder and desires some heat application prior to practice. Which would be the most appropriate modality and why?

 CONCEPT CHECK 11.2. A concert pianist is experiencing some general soreness in her right hand and desires a heat application prior to tonight's concert. Which would be the most appropriate modality and why?

Other Superficial Heating Devices

There are many other types of devices for applying superficial heat. The most prominent of these for orthopedic and sports medicine use are fluidotherapy, electric heating pads, portable heat pads, and topical analgesics. Fluidotherapy and electric heating pads perform very much like the traditional thermotherapy devices discussed earlier in this chapter. The other two are quite different.

The active ingredients (menthol, capsaicin, etc.) irritate the skin so as to give the sensation of heat. The irritation

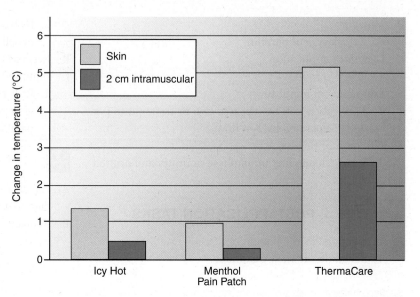

FIGURE 11.13 The results of a 2-hour treatment with a topical analgesic patch that claims to heat muscle and a portable heat wrap. (Source: Trowbridge et al.[6])

is often intense enough that it gates pain. Thus, the name counter-irritation, the irritation of the balm counters (overrides) the irritation (pain) of the injury or disease. The effect is local, that is, affecting signals from tissue receptors rather than involving higher cortical processing.[7,8]

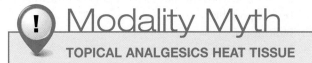

! Modality Myth

TOPICAL ANALGESICS HEAT TISSUE

Several over-the-counter topical analgesics (e.g., Cramergesic, Bengay, Icy Hot, Atomic Balm, Red Hot) claim to provide heat to muscles, some even advertize *deep heat*. Also known as *analgesic balms* and *counter-irritants*, these products are formulated as creams, balms, or ointments. They contain substances such as menthol, methyl salicylate, or hot pepper plant extracts (capsaicin) that cause a sensation of warmth on the skin and a slightly increased blood flow to the skin. They do not, however, substantially increase skin or muscle temperature (Fig. 11.13). Skin and 2-cm-deep intramuscular temperature were <2.7°F (1.5°C) and 1°F (0.5°C), respectively.[6]

FLUIDOTHERAPY

Fluidotherapy is a convection-type heating modality—a dry whirlpool of sorts—that is used to treat the extremities.[9–12] It consists of a rectangular cabinet through which warm air is circulated via a heater and air pump located beneath the cabinet (Fig. 11.14). A bed of very fine solid particles (finely ground corn cobs, called cellulose of Cellex, or glass beads) are placed in the bottom of the cabinet (Fig. 11.15). When the warmed air is forced through the particles, they become suspended in the airstream and take on the characteristics

of a fluid. Patients "submerse" an arm or leg into the airstream through a sleeve, similar to submersing a limb into a hot water whirlpool. And like a whirlpool, patients are treated with heat and a massaging effect, both of which can be controlled for patient comfort. Temperature typically ranges between 39 and 48°C (102–118°F).[13]

Fluidotherapy was developed in the early 1970s by Henley, an American chemical engineer, as an alternative to moist thermal therapeutic modalities such as hot packs, whirlpools, and paraffin bath.[10,11,14] Henley claimed his new dry thermal agent transfers a greater quantity of heat to superficial areas. A somewhat controversial study from his group supports this claim (see Table 11.2). We agree with those who criticized the study[15–17] because the whirlpool temperatures of 102°F (38.9°C) were considerably lower than typical used for treating limbs. In addition, not all therapeutic applications of fluidotherapy are at its highest temperature. Nevertheless, it is at least comparable to other superficial heating modalities.[9]

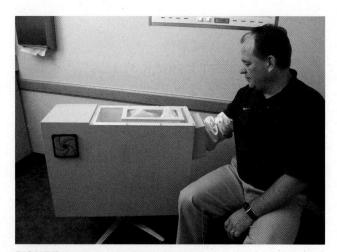

FIGURE 11.14 Fluidotherapy treatment.

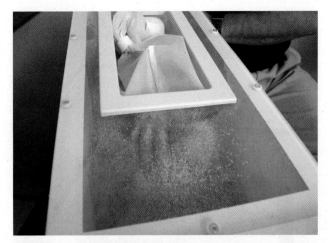

FIGURE 11.15 Inside of a fluidotherapy unit. Note the circulating fine solid particles and arm in the sleeve.

An advantage of fluidotherapy over hot packs and the dip method of paraffin treatments is that it maintains its temperature throughout the treatment. It also can be over bandages and splints, although its heading effects may be diminished by the devices.[18] Fluidotherapy appears to be popular in hand therapy.[19,20]

Surgical and nonsurgical management of upper extremity disorders benefits from the collaboration of a therapist, the treating physician, and the patient. Hand therapy plays a role in many aspects of treatment, and patients with upper extremity injuries may spend considerably more time with a therapist than with a surgeon. Hand therapists coordinate edema control; pain management; minimization of joint contractures; maximization of tendon gliding, strengthening, and work hardening; counseling; and ongoing diagnostic evaluation. Modalities used to manage hand injuries include ultrasound, splinting, fluidotherapy (Chattanooga Group, Chattanooga, TN), cryotherapy, various electrical modalities, phonophoresis, and iontophoresis.[20]

Currently there are three models of the device, allowing for treating varying sizes and numbers of limbs.

• The smallest is a single extremity device that can treat one hand, wrist, elbow, ankle, or foot. It holds 30 lb of Cellex (ground corn cobs; sometimes referred to as cellulose particles).

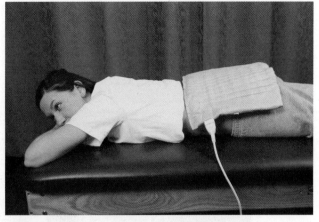

FIGURE 11.16 An electrical heating pad.

• The largest device is also a single extremity device but can treat a knee in addition to the hand, wrist, elbow, ankle, or foot. It holds 60 lb of Cellex.
• The medium-sized device is a dual extremity device that can treat two hands or feet simultaneously. It holds 40 lb Cellex.

Don't confuse this device with the very common practice in South America of treating patients with magnetized water by spiritual healers, which is also known as fluidotherapy.[21]

ELECTRICAL HEATING PADS

Electrical heating pads are an economical (about $30) alternative to a moist hot pack (Fig. 11.16). Once heated, it heats tissue about the same as a moist hot pack,[22] but does not need a hot water bath to prepare it for application, and you don't have to worry about rewarming between applications. It also is an excellent device to send home with a patient who needs additional treatments.

It is commonly believed that moist heating devices heat better than dry heating devices. This was not the case in our single research study.[22] Further investigation will clarify this point, but if the electric hot pad is preheated, or applied for over 30 minutes, it will heat as much as or more than a 20-minute moist hot pack. There is no need to apply a moist towel and plastic barrier under the electric heating pad as some recommend.

TABLE 11.2	TEMPERATURE RISE RESULTING FROM APPLICATION OF 3 SUPERFICIAL THERMAL MODALITIES		
MODALITY	**MODALITY TEMPERATURE**	**MAXIMUM TEMPERATURE RISE**	
		Jt Capsule	**Muscle @ 0.5 cm**
Fluidotherapy	47.8°C (118°F)	9.0°C (16.2°F)	5.3°C (9.5°F)
Paraffin wax	Not given	7.5°C (13.5°F)	4.5°C (8.1°F)
Water bath	38.9°C (102°F)	6.0°C (10.8°F)	4.3°C (7.7°F)

Source: Borrell et al.[11]

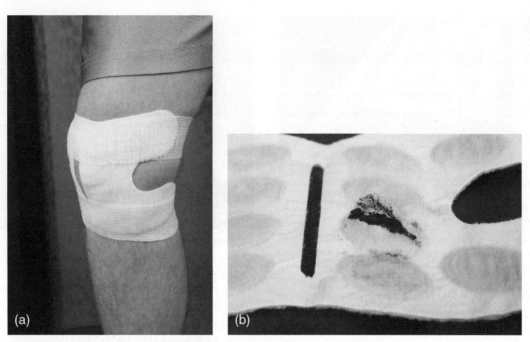

FIGURE 11.17 (a) A ThermaCare portable heat wrap applied to the knee. **(b)** It is composed of disks of iron, charcoal, and salt woven into a paper wrap.

Caution is advised when using electrical heating pads. Many cases of death and burning have been reported to the U.S. Product Safety Commission and the U.S. Food and Drug Administration.[23] Most problems appear to occur due to one of the following:

- Cracked or frayed electrical cords
- Cracked or worn pads
- In infants or the elderly
- When left on while the patient is sleeping

PORTABLE HEATING PRODUCTS

Portable heating devices (e.g., ThermaCare) use chemical reactions to produce long-lasting, low-level heating.[24] ThermaCare heat wraps are disks composed of iron, charcoal, and salt in a paper wrap (Fig. 11.17). When the wrap is exposed to oxygen in the air, an *exothermic reaction* occurs, which produces a low level of heat (104°F, or 40°C) on the skin that lasts for 8 hours (Fig. 11.13).[6]

CLOSING SCENE

In response to your grandfather's questions in this chapter opening scene, you explain that the ingredients in the topical ointment he uses do not actually heat or cool muscles, they just provide a hot or cool sensation. This irritation, in a sense, stimulates nerves that help override the pain signals. You tell him about thermal agents that actually produce heat, such as whirlpool, hot packs, and portable heat wraps. By analyzing the advantages and disadvantages of each modality, you can provide some sources of heat that are appropriate for his arthritic knees.

Chapter Reflections

1. Read and ponder each of the following points. Do you feel you have a clear understanding of each concept? If not, reread the appropriate section of the chapter.
   • Discuss whirlpool application, including foundational information, preapplication tasks, application procedures, postapplication tasks, and maintenance.
   • Discuss hot pack application, including foundational information, preapplication tasks, application procedures, postapplication tasks, and maintenance.
   • Discuss paraffin bath application, including foundational information, preapplication tasks, application procedures, postapplication tasks, and maintenance.
   • Tell why infrared lamps are contraindicated as a heating modality.
   • Discuss portable heating devices and how they compare with other superficial heating devices.
   • Discuss why it is incorrect to classify topical analgesics as heating devices.

2. Write three to five questions for discussion with your class instructor, clinical instructor, classmates, and clinical colleagues.

3. Get together with classmates and quiz each other on the concepts of this chapter. Use the points in reflection no. 1 and questions you wrote for reflection no. 2 as a beginning. Explaining concepts out loud to others requires a deeper grasp of the material than feeling you understand it as you read.

4. Once you feel you understand the principles of application of whirlpool, hot packs, and paraffin baths, practice applying each, using the five-step approach, with a classmate or clinical colleague. Alternate applying the modalities to each other. When it is being applied to you, listen and observe carefully to determine whether your classmate is using proper application. Consult your notes when the modality is applied to you, and during the first few times, you apply the modality to another person. Continue practicing the application until you can do so without using your notes.

Concept Check Responses

CONCEPT CHECK 11.1

Probably the best form of heat for the shoulder is a hot pack. Paraffin would be very messy to apply to this area, and the patient would need to immerse her whole body in a whirlpool in order to target the shoulder.

CONCEPT CHECK 11.2

Probably the best form of heat for this condition is paraffin glove since it can treat the peaks (knuckles) and valleys (palm and between knuckles) of the hand. After the 15-minute treatment, the patient removes the wax and puts it back in the container. The athletic trainer can then massage the hand. Another option is a small whirlpool since it can treat the peaks (knuckles) and valleys (palm and between knuckles) of the hand. The last choice would be the hot pack, since it cannot conform to the peaks and valleys of the hand.

REFERENCES

1. Wilson J, Knight K, Hawkins J, Long B. Dip-wrap paraffin wax and moist heat pack application and the subsequent rise in tissue temperatureS (abs). *J Athl Train.* 2007;42(Suppl):S45.
2. Draper DO, Harris ST, Schulthies SS, et al. Hotpack and 1 MHz ultrasound treatments have an additive effect on muscle temperature increase. *J Athl Train.* 1998;33:01–02.
3. Smith K. *The Effects of Silica Gel Hot Packs on Human Muscle Temperature.* [Masters]. Provo, UT: Exercise Sciences, Brigham Young University, 1994.
4. Kaiser DA, Knight KL, Huff JM, Jutte LS, Carlson P. Hot-Pack Warming in 4- and 8-Pack Hydrocollator Units. *J Sports Rehabil.* 2004;13(2):103–113.
5. Morris A. *Moist Heat Pack Rewarming Following 10, 20, 30 min Application.* Provo, UT: Exercise Sciences, Brigham Young University, 2003.
6. Trowbridge C, Draper D, Feland JB, Eggett D. The ThermaCare air-activated heat wrap heats paraspinal muscles greater than two menthol-based pain patches. *J Orthop Sports Phys Ther.* 2004;34: 549–558.
7. Ichiyama RM, Ragan BG, Bell GW, Iwamoto G. Effects of topical analgesics on the pressor response evoked by muscle afferents. *Med Sci Sport Exerc.* 2002;34(9):1440–1445.
8. Brewer A, McCarberg B, Argoff C. Update on the use of topical NSAIDs for the treatment of soft tissue and musculoskeletal pain: a review of recent data and current treatment options. *Phys Sports Med.* 2010;38(2):62–70.
9. Aetna Inc. Clinical Policy Bulletin: Fluidized Therapy (Fluidotherapy). Available at: http://www.aetna.com/cpb/medical/data/400_499/0450. html. Accessed January, 2012.
10. Borrell RM, Henley EJ, Ho P, Hubbell MK. Fluidotherapy: evaluation of a new heat mod. *Phys Med Rehabil.* 1977;58(2):69–71.

11. Borrell R, Parker R, Henley E, Masley D, Repinecz M. Comparison of in vivo temperatures produced by hydrotherapy, paraffin wax treatment, and fluidotherapy. *Phys Ther.* 1980;60(10):1273–1276.

12. Belanger AY. *Therapeutic Electrophysical Agents: Evidence Behind Practice.* 2nd ed. Baltimore, MD: Lippincott Williams & Wilkins, 2009.

13. Mich&others, Michlovitz SL, others? Therapeutic heat. In: Michlovitz SL, Nolan TP, Bellew JW, eds. *Modalities for Therapeutic Intervention.* 5th ed. Philadelphia, PA: F.A. Davis Co., 2011.

14. Valenza J, Rossi C, Parker R, Henley E. A clinical study of a new heat modality: fluidotherapy. *J Am Podiatry Assoc.* 1979;69(7):440–442.

15. Clinkingbeard KA. And the heat goes on (letter). *Phys Ther.* 1981;61(7):1063.

16. Clinkingbeard KA. Heat from fluidotherapy. *Phys Ther.* 1981;61(3):391.

17. White GT. Heat still on (letter). *Phys Ther.* 1981;61(6):927.

18. Michlovitz SL, von Nieda K. Heat and cold modalities. In: Behrens B, Michlovitz SL, eds. *Physical Agents Theory and Practice.* 2nd ed. Philadelphia, PA: FA Davis; 2006:36–54.

19. Herrick RT, Herrick S. Fluidotherapy. Clinical applications and techniques. *Ala Med.* 1992;61(12):20–25.

20. Dorf E, Blue C, Smith B, Koman L. Therapy after injury to the hand. *J Am Acad Orthop Surg.* 2010;18(8):464–473.

21. Lucchetti G, Lucchetti A, Bassi R, Nobre M. Complementary spiritist therapy: systematic review of scientific evidence. *Evid Based Complement Alternat Med.* 2011;2011:835–945.

22. Wood C, Knight K. Dry and moist heat application and the subsequent rise in tissue temperatures. *J Athl Training.* 2004;39:S91.

23. Dijkman B, Abouali J, Kooistra B, et al. Twenty years of meta-analyses in orthopaedic surgery: has quality kept up with quantity? *J Bone Joint Surg Am.* 2010;92(1):48–57.

24. Draper D, Trowbridge C. Continuous low-level therapy; What works and what doesn't. *Athl Ther Today.* 2003;8(5):46–48.

Cryotherapy Beyond Immediate Care

OPENING SCENE

A group of first year athletic training students were visiting in the athletic training clinic about their therapeutic modality class.

During a basketball game, your shooting guard sprains his ankle. After a through evaluation, your clinical instructor diagnoses it as a moderate ankle sprain, and asks you to apply RICES. You apply an ice pack and elastic wrap to the area. The CI tells you to stay with the athlete while she goes back to check on the game. After 15 minutes, a student athletic trainer from the host team comes into the room and asks if you need any help. He then asks how long you are going to ice the ankle. You say 30–45 minutes. The student's eyes get wide and he says, "You're kidding. Don't you know about the hunting response?" When you shake your head no, he continues, "After about 15 minutes of ice application, the blood vessels will dilate, so you don't want to ice the area for any longer than 15 minutes to avoid vasodilation." You wonder to yourself as you scratch your head, "Is he right?"

Cryotherapy: Not Just Immediate Care

There is a common misconception that you treat injuries with cold for the first 24–72 hours and then treat them with heat. For many injuries, cryotherapy extends beyond immediate care. Rehabilitation progresses more quickly because therapeutic exercises can be used earlier and are more effective when they are alternated with cold applications. Additional therapeutic uses of cryotherapy beyond immediate care include reducing spasticity, minimizing surgical complications, and preserving organs for transplantation.

How and why cold is used during rehabilitative cryotherapy is different from how and why it is used during immediate care. A lack of understanding of these differences has led to confusion about use of cold and led to improper applications. Thus we chose to separate our discussion of cryotherapy into separate sections of this book.

⦿ Modality Myth

There are numerous myths about the use of cryotherapy. Some of these were presented in Chapter 6. Additional ones are exposed in this chapter, including the following:

- The major reason for cryotherapy is to decrease blood flow.
- Acute injuries are treated with cold for the first 24–72 hours and then with heat.

- Cold should always be applied for ____ (fill in the blank).
- The application of cryotherapy is essentially the same regardless of why it is being applied.
- Cold increases circulation if applied for longer than 15–20 minutes, through the process of cold-induced vasodilation, or the hunting reaction.
- Research proves that cold-induced vasodilation occurs during athletic injury rehabilitation.
- Contrast bath therapy reduces swelling through a milking action caused by alternating vasodilation (from the heat) and vasoconstriction (from the cold).
- Heat applications decrease pain and allow active exercise during the early acute stages of orthopedic injury.

CRYOTHERAPY CONFUSION

The versatility of cryotherapy has caused great confusion among those who use it without an adequate understanding of its scientific and theoretical basis. Confusion has resulted in various definitions and in numerous opinions about why certain cryotherapeutic techniques should be used, their proper application, and the response of body tissues when they are used. See Box 12.1 for one example.

The debate over how long ice should be applied illustrates how confusion has led to the improper use of cryotherapy. Some clinicians claim cryotherapy should be applied for only 20 minutes, while others claim treatments of <30 minutes are ineffective. Both are correct–depending on when and why the cold is applied. Cold is used during

BOX 12.1 HEAT OR COLD? PATIENT EXPECTATIONS

"Quack, quack, quack," is a phrase I (KK) have heard at two stages in my career. In both cases it was uttered by patients under my care as a commentary on my competence in treating their athletic injuries. The comment was first expressed in the early 1970s when I began using cryokinetics to rehabilitate joint sprains. Many Weber State athletes were convinced I was incompetent. "Everyone knows you use heat after the first 24–72 hours to treat injuries," they would say. I hasten to add, however, that none of my cryokinetics patients were among the detractors.

Later in my career, in the early 1980s, after the cryotherapy revolution, I was again accused of being incompetent when I applied a hot pack to an Indiana State patient with an extremely sore ankle. "Don't you know you treat injuries with cold?" I was asked. It had come full circle.

My philosophy had not changed in the intervening years, but my philosophy was more comprehensive than that of the athletes I was treating, so my actions did not meet their expectations. The use of therapeutic heat and cold depends on the situation.

immediate care to limit secondary injury (see Chapter 6); therefore, applications of 30 minutes or longer are needed to lower metabolism in the underlying tissues. However, the goal in intermediate care is to decrease pain to facilitate active exercise, and localized numbing can be achieved in 12–20 minutes.

 CONCEPT CHECK 12.1 How is using cold to manage swelling an example of cryotherapy confusion?

As with all modalities, it is essential that any cryotherapy begin with a clear understanding of the goal of the therapy and of the differing physiological responses of the body to cold applications. To obtain the maximum benefit from any therapeutic modality, you must understand the specific needs of the patient and the physiological response to specific modalities. You must also understand that cryotherapy involves more than cold applications, and that both the cold and the noncold portions of the therapy differ depending on the therapeutic goals. There are numerous local physiological responses to cold applications, including decreased temperature, metabolism, inflammation, circulation, pain, and spasm,

and increased tissue stiffness. Some of these responses are beneficial, others detrimental, during various phases of injury management.

Cryotherapeutic modalities are used for a wide range of objectives. So referring to an individual specific technique as cryotherapy leads to confusion and ambiguity. To avoid the confusion, refer to individual techniques by their names. Think of the term "cryotherapy" only in a broad sense, as an umbrella covering the specific techniques.

EXAMPLES OF CRYOTHERAPY

Cryotherapy literally means "cold therapy." Therefore any use of ice or cold application for therapeutic purposes can be considered cryotherapy. Stated another way, cryotherapy is the therapeutic application of any device or substance to the body that results in the withdrawal of heat, thereby lowering tissue temperature. Thus, each of the following techniques is a type of cryotherapy:

- Ice or cold pack application for the immediate care of acute injuries
- Running cold water over a burn
- Cryokinetics (alternating cold applications with active exercise)
- Cryostretch (alternating cold applications with muscle stretching)
- Cold water baths (cold whirlpool or immersion in a slush bucket)
- Ice massage
- Treating trigger points with ice massage
- Postsurgical ice or cold pack applications
- Lowering whole-body temperature to induce hypothermia prior to organ transplant surgery
- Cryosurgery (applying –76°F [–60°C] probes or spraying liquid nitrogen on tissue to freeze and destroy it)

CRYOTHERAPEUTIC TECHNIQUES

Cryotherapeutic techniques can be grouped into five major categories, based on the objectives for using them:

- *Immediate care*: cooling acutely injured musculoskeletal tissue immediately after the injury as part of first aid (see Chapters 5 and 6)
- *Post–immediate care*: cooling tissue during rehabilitation of various musculoskeletal pathologies as an adjunct to other therapy, usually exercise
- *Surgical adjunct*: cooling tissue prior to, during, or after surgical procedures
- *Cryosurgery*: freezing tissue for surgical purposes
- *Miscellaneous*: techniques that do not fit into one of the above four categories

Immediate Care Cryotherapy

The objective during immediate care procedures is two-fold: removing the cause of the injury and minimizing the adverse sequelae. A **sequela** is an effect that follows, or results from, an injury. Except in the case of a burn, cold applications have no effect on removing the cause of the injury, but they have a great effect on minimizing secondary injury and thereby decreasing total injury (see Chapter 6).[1]

Post–Immediate Care Cryotherapy

The main benefit of cold application during post–immediate care is that it decreases pain and/or muscle spasm and thereby allows earlier mobilization. The sooner therapeutic exercise begins, the better the patient is for three reasons:

- The proper use of exercise speeds the healing process.[2–4]
- The lack of exercise during the early stages of rehabilitation may result in permanent disability.[5,6]
- Function is restored sooner, which is beneficial physically and psychologically.

Caution must be observed though; too vigorous exercise can also result in permanent disability. The optimum conditions for healing depend on a very fine balance between returning to full normal function at the earliest possible time and protecting the injury from overstress and reinjury[6] (see Fig. 1.5).

The major cryotherapeutic techniques used during post–immediate care are:

- Cryokinetics
- Cryostretch
- Connective tissue stretch
- Cold compression devices
- Contrast baths

These are explained in greater detail later in this chapter. Detailed application procedures are in Chapter 13.

Surgical Adjunct Cryotherapy

Cryotherapy is often used prior to, during, and after surgical procedures. The objective is the same as during immediate care of acute injuries: lowering metabolism in order to minimize secondary injury.

Cryosurgery

Cryosurgery is a surgical technique that uses ultra-low temperature probes (–4 to –94°F, or –20 to –70°C) to freeze tissue and thereby destroy it.[7,8] Its use is beyond the scope of this book.

Miscellaneous Techniques

Techniques for decreasing menstrual cramps and pain, reducing cold sores, and easing painful injections are examples of cryotherapeutic techniques. Descriptions are outside the scope of this book; they can be found elsewhere.[1]

The Physiological Effects of Cold Application

The physiological responses to cold can be summarized or grouped into nine categories[1]:

- Decreased temperature
- Tissue destruction
- Increased or decreased inflammation
- Decreased metabolism
- Decreased or increased pain
- Decreased muscle spasm
- Increased tissue stiffness
- Decreased arthrogenic muscle inhibition (AMI)
- Decreased circulation

DECREASED TEMPERATURE

Immediately upon the application of cold, heat begins moving from the tissue into the cold modality, resulting in decreased tissue temperature. In severe cooling (–4 to –94°F, or –20 to –70°C), tissue is destroyed, as in cryosurgery. For treating orthopedic injuries, the tissue is usually cooled to a surface temperature of 33–50°F (1–10°C). This degree of cooling causes the tissue responses listed above, except for tissue destruction.

Temperature changes are neither immediate nor uniform throughout the tissue. Heat moves by conduction between adjacent layers of cells (see Chapter 10). Heat first moves from surface tissue into the cold modality. As the surface temperature decreases, heat is conducted from subcutaneous tissues to the surface, which results in heat conduction from intermediate tissues to the subcutaneous tissues, and so on until heat is being conducted in stages from the very deep tissues (if the cold modality remains on long enough and doesn't warm up too quickly).

After a few minutes, a thermal gradient develops in the tissue (see Fig. 10.1). This gradient remains after the cold modality is removed. In fact, because of the gradient and heat conduction, deeper tissue temperature continues to decrease after the modality is removed, or the body is removed from the modality, as is the case with ice water immersion.

Thermal gradients can also develop in the modality. The clinician should shake a cold pack and swirl the water in an ice immersion bucket every 5 minutes or so to break up the gradient. Patients will notice the difference.

CONCEPT CHECK 12.2 A patient immerses his foot in an ice water bath and holds it still for 5–10 minutes. He then moves the foot and is surprised that it feels colder and a bit more painful. Why the change in sensations?

TISSUE DESTRUCTION

Tissue destruction occurs at extreme temperatures (–4 to –94°F, or –20 to –70°C), such as with liquid nitrogen or the application of a gel pack applied directly on the skin. The liquid nitrogen application is generally intentional so as to remove unwanted tissue, such as warts. The gel pack is usually accidental, as in Figure 6.15.

INCREASED OR DECREASED INFLAMMATION

It is commonly thought that one of the benefits of cryotherapy in treating acute injury is to decrease inflammation. This is probably not true for two reasons: (1) inflammation is necessary for resolution of the injury (see Chapter 6), and (2) there has been very little research on the acute inflammatory response.

Cryotherapy research involving inflammation has concentrated on arthritis, the healing of surgical wounds, and inflammation induced by injecting various substances under the skin. In these situations, inflammation has been decreased[9–11] or delayed—that is, it is reduced during cryotherapy but then runs its full course after rewarming.[12–15] But these situations are quite different from the inflammatory response during acute trauma.

DECREASED METABOLISM

There is a direct relationship between tissue temperature and metabolism (see Fig. 6.4). The more the cooling, the greater the decrease in metabolism.[1]

DECREASED OR INCREASED PAIN

Cold is a very effective and underused modality for pain.[16] Although there is clear experimental evidence that cold decreases pain,[17] many clinicians do not appreciate its value, especially during acute injury care. By numbing a muscle or joint, active exercise can be used earlier in the rehabilitation process.[18–21]

Understanding the relationship between cryotherapy and pain begins with the recognition that pain from three origins is involved:

- *Cold pain*: Caused by the application of intense cold, usually ice water immersion. Patients quickly habituate to it, so it is only a problem during the first few treatment sessions. Cold pain is a nuisance; it serves no useful purpose. But it is not a reason for avoiding treatments such as cryokinetics.
- *Residual pain*: Caused by the injury (damaged tissue and pressure on nerve endings by swelling and by inflammatory chemicals, such as bradykinins and prostaglandins). Residual pain precludes exercising, but can be neutralized by cold-induced numbness. This is the key to cryokinetics, which allows early exercise following joint sprains.
- *Reinjury pain*: Caused by stressing tissues to the point of reinjuring them. Reinjury pain is not affected by numbness, and therefore is a safety valve when using cryokinetics. Respect it and respond to it. Reduce the intensity of the patient's activity when she feels reinjury pain.

Cold pain rarely occurs during immersion in water lower than 59°F (15°C), and rarely during other cold applications, such as ice massage and ice packs. Immersion in water near 32°F (0°C) is very painful during its first use.[1] Patients quickly habituate to cold pain, however, so it is a manageable problem. Efforts to minimize cold pain during ice immersion have led to the following application adjustments:

- The development of a neoprene toe cap.[22] The toe cap eliminates pain in the toes and forefoot, which accounts for over 50% of the pain during ice immersion.[23] We recommend them.
- Refraining from using cryokinetics. This is unfortunate because cryokinetics is a powerful tool, and cold pain is temporary. Its intensity decreases dramatically after the first immersion and continues to decrease after subsequent immersions. Most patients feel no pain during ice water immersion after 2–3 days of cryokinetic treatments.
- The use of warmer water. Although warmer water is less painful, it is not as effective in numbing the injured limb,[24] and so the effectiveness of the treatment is decreased. We recommend against this practice.

✔ APPLICATION TIP

ICE WATER IMMERSION SHOULD BE IN 32–33°F (0–1°C) WATER

Pain is most effectively reduced with immersion in 32–35°F (0–2°C) ice water. Always have your patient wear a toe cap to moderate the cold-induced pain.

DECREASED MUSCLE SPASM

Muscle spasm is a tightness in the muscle. It is of gradual onset and usually not particularly painful. It results from an increase in the baseline tone (neurological activity) of the muscle. Muscle spasm is not muscle cramping. A **muscle cramp**, commonly called a *charley horse*, is a sudden, intense, painful, tetanic muscle contraction. It is short-lived, usually lasting <20 seconds.

Muscle spasm is decreased by cold applications, although the specific mechanism is unknown.[1] Three mechanisms have been suggested, each of which probably plays a role:

• Decreased nerve conduction[1,25–27]
• Breaking the pain-spasm-pain cycle.[28–31] This mechanism is undoubtedly effective and part of the explanation: Remove the cause of the spasm, and the spasm disappears.
• A neural mechanism. This hypothesis is based on the following:
    Cooling a skin flap (cut in a U and lifted from the body) without cooling the underlying muscle causes a decrease in tonic stretch reflexes in the muscle.[32]
    Reflex responses decrease quickly following cold application.[33,34]
    Sympathetic nervous system stimulation causes a significant decrease in *muscle spindle* afferent discharge during stretching.[35]

Whatever the mechanism, cold is effective in diminishing the muscle spasm that accompanies most acute strains and sprains. Its effectiveness is increased when combined with stretching, as is the case with the cryostretch technique.

INCREASED TISSUE STIFFNESS

Cooling tissues causes them to become more stiff (less elastic) and more resistant to movement, due to a combination[36] of increased viscosity of joint synovial fluid,[37–40] decreased muscle power,[40,41] and decreased connective tissue elasticity.[41–43] Some feel this contraindicates exercise following cryotherapy, fearing tissues will tear. We disagree. Fine motor skills are hindered, but gross motor movement is not.[1,44]

DECREASED ARTHROGENIC MUSCLE INHIBITION

Arthrogenic muscle inhibition (AMI) is an ongoing reflex inhibition of muscles surrounding a joint, caused by distension or damage to that joint.[45] AMI can occur in the absence of pain,[45] such as from injecting saline in the knee, and is reversed or disinhibited by TENS and cryotherapy.[46] In this model, cryotherapy also facilitates the motor neuron pool, but TENS does not.[46] Perhaps one of the most exciting results of this research is that cryotherapy facilitated the resting motor neuron pool (motor neurons available to be stimulated) above baseline measures during cooling and during the 30 minutes[47,48] and 60 minutes after cryotherapy.[48]

It appears that cryotherapy may not only reverse inhibition following injury, but also facilitate muscular activity

above normal levels. This research is still in its infancy, and much remains to be discovered concerning the effects of cryotherapy on muscle inhibition. The possibilities are exciting to contemplate.[49]

DECREASED CIRCULATION

There is great confusion concerning the circulatory effects of cold applications. There are reports that indicate cold applications result in both increased and decreased blood flow, although those who have proposed increased blood flow have had either nonexistent or arbitrary explanations for when blood flow increases and decreases.

Most of the confusion about the circulatory response of cold has resulted from an inappropriate application of the concept of **cold-induced vasodilation (CIVD)**. Even though there is ample evidence that cryotherapy used in treating orthopedic injuries deceases rather than increases blood flow, the concept of CIVD persists. Because of the resilience of the CIVD concept, a detailed discussion follows.

Cold-Induced Vasodilation: Facts and Fallacies

Cold-induced vasodilation (CIVD) is the dilation of blood vessels (increase in circumference) as a result of cold applications. Popular thought, however, is that CIVD causes an increase in blood flow as a result of cold applications.[1] While some have claimed that CIVD increases blood flow more than heat applications do, this is not the case.[50]

The term CIVD was coined by Lewis[51] in 1930 to explain temperature fluctuations in the finger during and after ice water immersion. The success of cryokinetics, the alternating of cold applications and active exercise, in the mid 1960s led to claims that CIVD caused increased blood flow at one of two possible times (see Fig. 12.1):

• During application, sometimes called the **hunting response**
• Following application, sometimes called the *rebound effect*

Many accepted the CIVD concept without question, and despite the confusion about when CIVD occurs.

There is also confusion about when during injury management CIVD occurs. There is no question that cold applications during immediate care cause vasoconstriction and decreased blood flow. Yet some believe that post-acute cold applications cause vasodilation and increased blood flow. For these two factors to occur, the body would have to somehow know what the therapeutic goal was. A more rational explanation is that CIVD does not occur during sports injury therapy, as the evidence indicates.

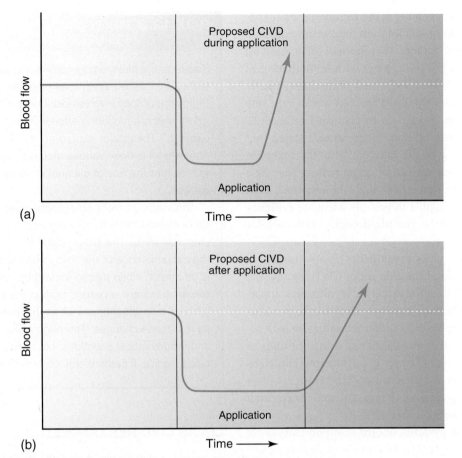

FIGURE 12.1 Proponents of CIVD as an explanation for enhanced rehabilitation have suggested that cold applications cause blood flow to increase, either (**a**) during application or (**b**) following application. We disagree with both hypotheses, as explained in the text.

THE HISTORY AND DEVELOPMENT OF THE CIVD CONCEPT

A brief timeline of the CIVD concept is shown in Box 12.2. Grant, a physiatrist[18] and Hayden, a physical therapist,[19] introduced cryokinetics in 1965 for rehabilitating acute musculoskeletal injuries occurring during army basic training. Their articles included dramatic statistics of the "striking" success of CIVD. Grant proposed that early movement and restoring normal function are the keys to reducing symptoms, and that using ice is simply for relieving pain and allowing such early movement.[18]

BOX 12.2	A TIMELINE OF THE CIVD CONCEPT TO EXPLAIN THE SUCCESS OF CRYOTHERAPY
1930	Lewis[51] coined term to explain finger temperature fluctuations during and after CWIs.
1965	Grant[18] and Hayden[19] developed cryokinetics but did not explain why it worked.
1967	Moore et al.[52] suggested CIVD as a possibility but offered no evidence to support the suggestion.
Late 1960s	Considered an extreme idea.
Mid-1970s	Probable; too much success with cryokinetics to ignore the possibility.
Early-1980s	Absolute; cryotherapy had swept the athletic training world and was popular in physical therapy.
Mid-1980s	Doubtful; research did not support the concept, but did support the theory that exercise was the key.
Early-1990s	Improbable. Evidence against CIVD continued to build.
Today	Many still believe. Apparently they have not read, or they ignore, the evidence.

Athletic trainers began using the technique, and experienced much quicker rehabilitation than with traditional heat applications.[52-54] One AT reported on a football player who returned to full contact with no limitation of motion in <72 hours after a sprained ankle that normally would have kept him sidelined for 2–3 weeks.[53] In one of the first attempts to explain mechanisms to account for this quicker rehabilitation, Moore et al.[52] stated that cold prepares the area for exercise, and that exercise was important to the success of cryokinetics. They also introduced the idea that CIVD might be involved, even though they were not able to provide adequate evidence to substantiate CIVD as the physiological rationale for cryokinetics.[52]

During the next 7 years, cryokinetics became a standard in sports medicine, and the concept of CIVD became the standard explanation for the success of cryokinetics, apparently because CIVD more closely resembled the previous theory that heat applications promote healing by increasing blood flow to carry away debris and bring nutrients to the healing wound (see Chapter 11). Numerous clinicians wrote as if CIVD were a proven fact.[29,55-59] However, they did not present original data; they just quoted the research and opinions of others.

The major points of evidence quoted to support CIVD are the following:

- Research of Lewis[51]
- Research of Clark et al.[60]
- A feeling of warmth occurs during ice water immersion.
- Cold applications cause the tissue to turn red.
- Rehabilitation is quicker with cryokinetics than with thermotherapy. Since thermotherapy promotes healing by increasing blood flow, cryokinetics must also, many thought.

One of the first attempts to substantiate the occurrence of CIVD during cryokinetics involved measuring ankle blood flow during six combinations of heat, cold, and exercise[50]; using strain-gauge plethysmography (Box 12.3). There was no CIVD, in fact just the opposite—blood flow decreased during a 25-minute cold pack application and remained depressed for the 20 minutes following application that blood flow was measured (Fig. 12.2). Blood flow during combined cold and exercise (cryokinetics) had greater increases than with cold alone, with control (meaning no treatment), and with heat pack application. This supported Grant's hypothesis that exercise is the key to cryokinetics success and that cold acts only to facilitate exercise. This study[50] stimulated a reexamination of the studies of Lewis[51] and Clarke et al.[60] to determine why the results appeared to differ from theirs.

BOX 12.3 STRAIN-GAUGE PLETHYSMOGRAPHY FOR MEASURING BLOOD FLOW

Strain-gauge plethysmography is a standard technique for measuring total blood flow to a limb. Plethysmography involves occluding a limb's venous return (without hindering arterial inflow), causing it to expand.[73] The rate of expansion is a function of the rate of arterial flow. Various methods have been used to measure the rate of expansion, including strain gauges.

Strain-gauge plethysmography uses a very thin rubber tube filled with mercury and attached to electrical wires. The strain gauge is 5–10% less than the circumference of the limb to be measured, so it is on stretch when placed around the limb. A small electrical current is passed though the strain gauge. When it is lengthened (as when the limb expands), its resistance changes. Thorough calibration and mathematical equations, blood flow can be calculated as a percent change in limb volume.

LEWIS CIVD REEXAMINED

As noted, Lewis[51] introduced the concept of CIVD in a 1930 paper. He reported a series of experiments in which he measured finger temperature—not blood flow—in a single individual. A typical experiment involved one finger, with adjacent fingers as controls (Fig. 12.3). The fingers rested on a cork platform above a beaker of ice water. After baseline measurements, the experimental finger was immersed into the beaker through a hole in the cork. Resulting data were neither combined nor statistically analyzed. Here are the key points about this paper:

- At 6 minutes following 15 minutes of immersion in 44.6°F (7°C) water, the right second finger (R2) temperature was 50°F (10°C) warmer than the control (R3) finger. The temperature remained at this level for 10 minutes and then gradually returned toward control, but it was still 35.6°F (2°C) above control 1 hour after immersion.
- These data appear to provide unquestionable support for CIVD. A closer evaluation of the data, however, following research by Knight et al.,[61] revealed that the control finger was maintained at 66.2°F (19°C), probably because the room temperature was quite cold (see RT at bottom right of Fig. 12.3). The experimental finger rose to 84.2°F (29°C) following immersion. Normal finger temperature is 86–93.2°F (30–34°C). Therefore, the

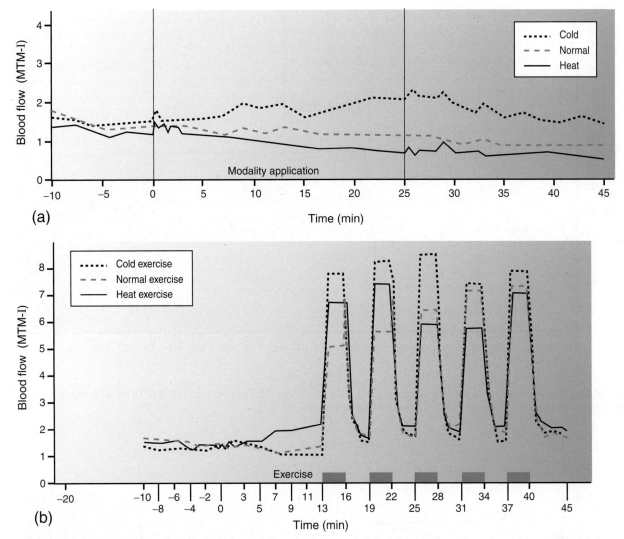

FIGURE 12.2 The first challenge to the idea that CIVD occurred during cryokinetics. (**a**) Note that blood flow decreased during the 25-minute cold pack application and remained depressed for 20 minutes following application. (**b**) Blood flow during the exercise conditions was much greater than during hot pack application limb. MTM-I = mm of blood flow per 100 mm of tissue, or percent blood flow, at the specific time of measurement. (Source: Knight and Londeree.[50])

experimental finger warmed toward normal but began cooling again without ever reaching what would be considered normal temperature.

Lewis recognized that the after-effect occurred only when the fingers and room were at what he called a "suitable" initial temperature, which was much colder than what would be considered normal.

Following three studies using Lewis's methods, except at room temperature and involving the finger and other body parts, we concluded that:

- The finger returns to normal within 10–20 minutes, but ankle temperature remains depressed (average of 50°F, or 10°C) for an extended period of time.[61]
- Following 30 minutes[62] and 40 minutes[63] of immersion, the forearm and ankle require in excess of 2.5 hours to

return to within 1.8°F (1°C) of the contralateral control limb (Fig. 12.4).

- Lewis results occurred during extreme conditions (in very cold rooms) that resulted in the experimental and control fingers being much colder than those of patients undergoing rehabilitation in modern-day clinics. Also the finger responds more dramatically than the ankle and forearm, so results from research on the finger cannot be generalized to the majority of sports injuries.

Lewis also reported that during prolonged cold water immersion (CWI) (for 2 hours), finger temperature oscillated, a phenomenon he called the hunting reaction, also known as the hunting response. At one time, he reported, there was a sixfold increase. This caused some[57]

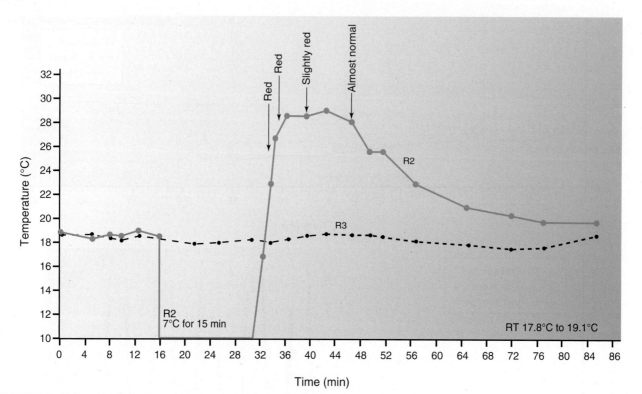

FIGURE 12.3 Finger temperatures during and following immersion of a finger (R2) in a beaker of 44.6°F (7°C) ice water for 15 minutes. The control finger (R3) remained on a cork platform above the beaker. (Source: Lewis.[51])

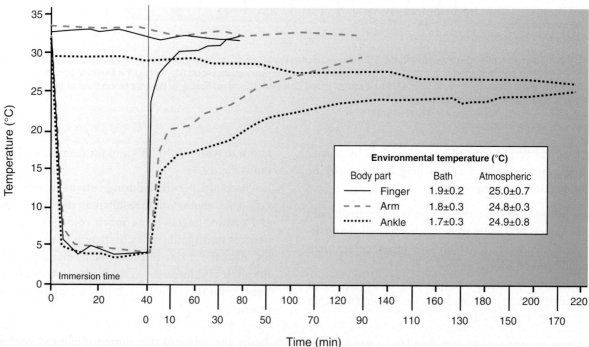

FIGURE 12.4 Rewarming of the finger, forearm, and ankle following 40 minutes of immersion in ~35.6°F (2°C) water. At no time did the temperature exceed either the control (contralateral limb) or preimmersion temperatures. Note that the finger rewarmed much more quickly (~20 minutes) than either the forearm or ankle, which required more than 2.5 hours to return to within 33.8°F (1°C) of the contralateral control. (Source: Knight et al.[63])

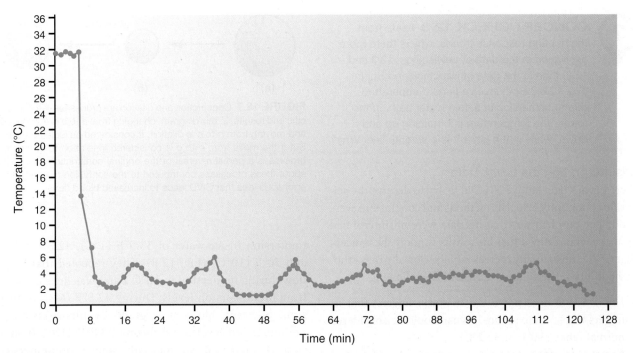

FIGURE 12.5 The hunting reaction, or hunting response: oscillations in finger temperature during immersion in crushed ice. Note that the oscillations occur only after a profound decrease in temperature, and their magnitude is small compared to preimmersion temperature. (Source: Lewis.[51])

to conclude that cold caused greater blood flow than heat applications. A close examination of the data indicates this interpretation was in error (Fig. 12.5). The sixfold oscillation was from 35.6°–53.6°F (2°C–12°C) and occurred only after an initial decrease from approximately 87.8°F (31°C). Moreover, most oscillations were between 35.6°F and 42.8°F (2°C and 6°C).

The hunting response may only be a measurement artifact. In the course of one experiment, Knight et al.[61] noticed

that finger temperature rose as Lewis had described, but quickly fell when the finger was moved. We incorporated this into another experiment in which we asked subjects to hold their ankles very still for 20 minutes of immersion.[23] Then when they moved their ankles (while still in the water), the temperature decreased (Fig. 12.6, toe cap group). The hunting response is the result of a water temperature gradient, not a physiological response, and it does not result in increased blood flow to the immersed body part.

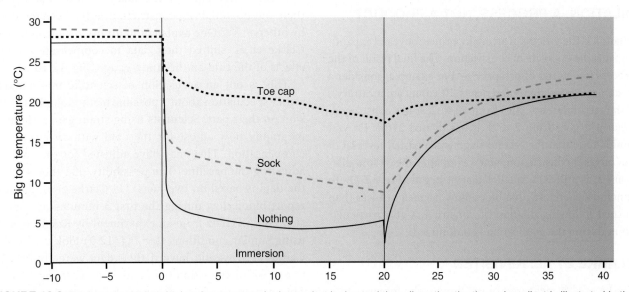

FIGURE 12.6 The hypothesis that the hunting response is due to developing and then disrupting the thermal gradient is illustrated in the toe cap group (see text for details). (Source: Nimchick and Knight.[23])

CONCEPT CHECK 12.3 Aside from the hunting response trends, why is there more oscillation in the data of Lewis (Figs. 12.3 and 12.5) than in the data of Nimchick and Knight (Fig. 12.6)? Both involve finger temperature during immersion in a cold water bath. In the former the temperature is bouncing up and down, while in the latter it is a smooth line. Why?

Misinterpreting the Lewis Data

Were Lewis's data faulty? No. Did he try to deceive the scientific community? No. His methods and conclusions were solid. The problem was that his data were misinterpreted by those who claimed that his results support the concept that CIVD substantially increases blood flow during orthopedic injury rehabilitation. Consider the following.

- Lewis' CIVD does not occur in warm fingers, that is, fingers whose temperature is what would be considered normal (above 90°F, or 32.2°C).
- There is not a direct correlation between blood flow and finger temperature.[64]
- Apparently the enthusiasm to explain the rapid rehabilitation, coupled with the pervading theory that rehabilitation was the result of blood flow, overshadowed careful examination of his work.
- The hunting response is a measurement artifact, occurring when a thermal gradient builds and then is interrupted.

CONCEPT CHECK 12.4 How can you prevent making errors in judgment when interpreting the research related to clinical techniques?

DILATION: A PROCESS, NOT A PRODUCT

Dilation is the process of an organ, orifice, or vessel expanding; it is the opposite of constriction. The final result of the process is a matter of perspective. For example, consider a structure whose circumference is 10 (units are arbitrary). If the circumference goes from 10 to 2, it has constricted. Then if it goes from 2 to 5, it has dilated 250%. Or you could argue that the second stage was a partial reversal of the original constriction, since even after the "250% dilation," it is still 50% smaller than it began (Fig. 12.7). To conclude, therefore, that blood flow is greater or less than normal following dilation or constriction at a particular point during the application is unfounded.

CLARKE ET AL. REVISITED

Clarke et al.[60] measured blood flow to the forearm with strain-gauge plethysmography during 45 minutes of

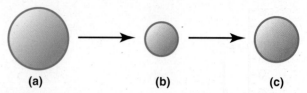

FIGURE 12.7 Constriction and dilation are processes without specific end results. In this diagram, changing from *a* to *b* is constriction and moving from *b* to *c* is dilation, if considered as isolated events. But if the move from *b* to *c* is considered in relation to *a*, the later process is a partial reversal of the original constriction. Confusion about these processes contributed to the confusion that led to the erroneous idea that CIVD leads to increased blood flow.

immersion in ice water of 33.8°F (1°C), 42.8°F (6°C), and 50°F (10°C) (Fig. 12.8). They reported that blood flow during immersion in 10°C water was little changed from preimmersion levels. During 42.8°F (6°C) immersion, however, blood flow gradually increased above preimmersion levels, and during 33.8°F (1°C) immersion it increased substantially above preimmersion levels.

The results of Clarke et al. are in sharp contrast to those of others who have reported blood flow to be less than normal during the following:

- Forearm immersion in 39.2°F (4°C) water for 192 minutes[65]
- Cold packs applied to the ankle for 25 minutes[50] (see Fig. 12.2)
- Forearm immersion in 33.8°F (1°C), 42.8°F (6°C), 50°F (10°C), and 59°F (15°C) water baths for 45 minutes[66] (Fig. 12.9)
- Gel pack application to the ankle for 20 minutes[67]

A major problem with the data of Clarke et al. is that there was no initial vasoconstriction, as has been reported by others.[65,68–73] One explanation for discrepancies is that Clarke et al. shifted their data to compensate for the effects of the cold on the strain-gauge (Fig. 12.10).

This is not an accusation of scientific misconduct, rather speculation about a possible methodological decision on their part. Scientists using strain gauge plethysmography now adjust for the cold with an electronic compensation. They may have adjusted for the cold by adjusting the baseline. The possibility that they shifted the data is based on two facts: (1) Clarke et al. did not report blood flow during the first 3 minutes of immersion, and (2) data from an experiment by Knight et al.[66] using similar conditions (see Fig. 12.9) look much like Clarke et al. would have if their data were "returned" to a preshifted position (compare Figs. 12.9 and 12.10). This explanation also accounts for the lack of initial vasoconstriction.

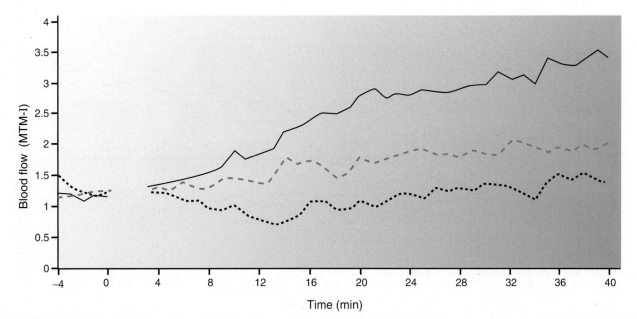

FIGURE 12.8 Forearm blood flow during 40 minutes of immersion in ice water baths. Note the lack of a control condition and the 3-minute gap at the beginning of immersion. This is a composite graph drawn from data obtained by averaging the four individual graphs (each representing a single subject).MTM-I = mm of blood flow per 100 mm of tissue, or percent blood flow, at the specific time of measurement. (Source: Adapted from Clarke et al.[60])

FEELING OF WARMTH

Most people experience four sensations during cold application: pain, warming or burning, aching or tingling, and numbness.[1] The warming sensation has been attributed to CIVD.[57] But neither a surface nor a subcutaneous temperature increase accompanies changes in sensation during ankle immersion in ice water (Fig. 12.11).[74] Both temperatures decreased throughout the time that subjects reported feeling a warming sensation. Apparently the feeling of warmth is a psychological sensation rather than a physiological sensation.

SKIN REDNESS

The skin turns bright red during cold application, which some attribute to CIVD.[57] This phenomenon has not been investigated, so any explanation is speculative. One

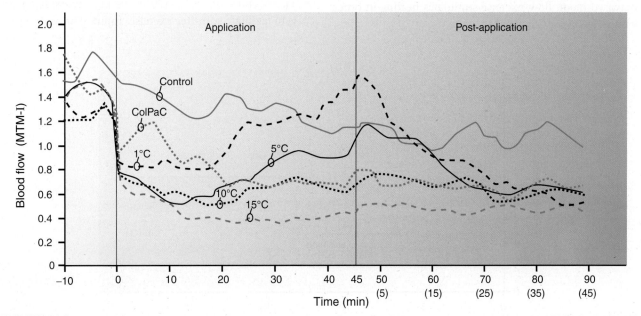

FIGURE 12.9 Forearm blood flow during and after 45 minutes of cryotherapy. Black lines represent immersion in 33.8°F (1°C), 41°F (5°C), and 50°F (10°C) water baths. *Blue lines* represent immersion in 59°F (15°C) water, gel pack, and control. MTM-I = mm of blood flow per 100 mm of tissue, or percent blood flow, at the specific time of measurement. (Source: Knight et al.[66])

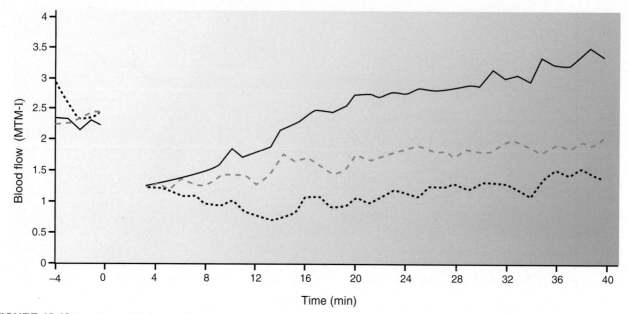

FIGURE 12.10 The data of Clarke et al.[60] as they may have appeared prior to being adjusted (see text for details). MTM-I = mm of blood flow per 100 mm of tissue, or percent blood flow, at the specific time of measurement. Note the similarity between these data and the black lines in Figure 12.9.

proposed explanation is that due to lowered tissue metabolism during cold applications, oxygen exchange between the tissues and capillaries is decreased. The result is more highly oxygenated blood (which appears redder) in the skin's venous system.[38]

INCREASED RATE OF HEALING

The success of cryokinetics is due to exercise. Exercise increases blood flow to a greater degree than either heat or cold applications (Fig. 12.12).[50] But in addition to increased blood flow, exercise stimulates healing in other ways as well (see Chapter 7).

CONCLUSIONS ABOUT CIVD AND CRYOKINETICS

Based on a critical reexamination of the literature concerning CIVD following a series of studies by Knight and associates, we conclude the following:

• CIVD does not lead to increased blood flow during or following therapeutic applications of cold. Those who claimed it did were too hasty in developing a theory to explain the success of cryokinetics.

• The purpose of cold applications post–immediate care is to facilitate pain-free exercise. Injury pain and muscle

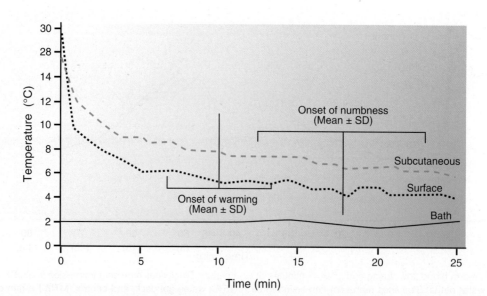

FIGURE 12.11 Although patients may report a warming sensation during ice immersion, these data clearly indicate no increase in tissue temperature during the warming sensation. SD = Standard deviation. (Source: Johannes and Knight.[74])

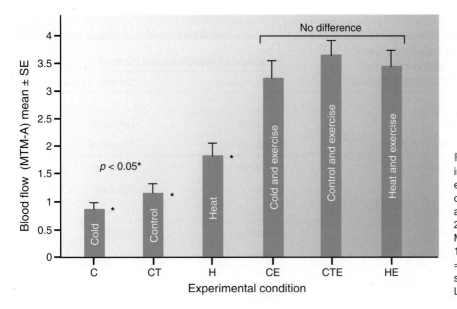

FIGURE 12.12 Average blood flow during six treatments clearly demonstrates that exercise is more effective than either heat or cold in increasing blood flow. Data are averages of 45-minute treatments that included 25 minutes of modality application each. MTM-A = Average mm of blood flow per 100 mm of tissue, or percent blood flow. SE = Standard Error of the Mean. Data are the same as in Figure 12.2. (Source: Knight and Londeree.[50]).

spasm are decreased, thereby allowing exercise to begin earlier and progress faster.

- Exercise is the key to rehabilitation. Without properly executed therapeutic exercise, cold applications will hinder rather than promote rehabilitation.
- Moore et al.[52] stated that one of the purposes of their paper was to encourage other researchers to continue studying the physiological mechanisms involved in cryokinetics. It has.
- Nathan,[75] commenting on the gate control theory of pain, stated that ideas need to be fruitful, but they don't necessarily have to be right. The same can be said about CIVD during therapeutic applications of cold. Although the idea that CIVD results in increased blood flow has proven to be false, it has been very fruitful. It has led to a greater understanding of the physiological basis of cold and rehabilitation, and has therefore served us well.

Heat Versus Cold: When and Why

Each of the physiological responses discussed above occurs when cold is applied to the body. As mentioned earlier, not all of them are beneficial, however, and a response that helps reach one therapeutic goal may not be desirable or useful for reaching another goal. The specific modality you use and how you apply it will make a difference in the physiological response and thus the therapeutic effect. Therefore, it is important to understand both the response and its efficacy (desirability) during various phases of orthopedic injury care. Table 12.1 presents the physiological responses of local tissue to therapeutic applications

of heat and cold, along with their efficacy during various phases of orthopedic injury management.

IMMEDIATE CARE OF ACUTE INJURIES

Decreased metabolism is the most important physiological response to cold during immediate care procedures because it limits secondary injury.[1,76,77] Decreasing circulation is actually detrimental at this time, because it reduces oxygen delivery and therefore contributes to secondary metabolic injury. The benefits from decreased metabolism, however, are so much greater than the detrimental effects of decreased circulation that the net result of cold applications is positive. In addition, cold is beneficial during these procedures because it decreases muscle spasm and pain.

Heat applications are contraindicated during immediate care because increased metabolism will promote secondary metabolic injury, thereby increasing the total injury.

SUBACUTE CARE OF ACUTE INJURIES

Decreased circulation, metabolism, and inflammation, along with increasing tissue stiffness are all detrimental to acute injury rehabilitation.[15,78] During this period, the tissue needs increased circulation and metabolism. Decreased pain and spasm are, of course, desirable. From a mathematical standpoint (summing the positive and negative effects) there is no benefit to using cryotherapy during rehabilitation. This is true for some cryotherapeutic techniques; however, the exercise component of cryokinetics provides benefits that more than compensate for the decrease in circulation and metabolism caused by the cold.[6,28,50,79]

TABLE 12.1   THE EFFICACY OF HEAT AND COLD APPLICATIONS DURING ORTHOPEDIC INJURY CARE

PHYSIOLOGICAL RESPONSE	EFFICACY DURING IMMEDIATE CARE OF ACUTE INJURIES*	EFFICACY DURING REHABILITATION	
		Acute Injuries	Chronic Injuries
OF COLD			
Decreased circulation	Nil	Negative	Negative
Decreased metabolism	Very positive†	Negative	Negative
Decreased inflammation	Negative	Negative	Positive
Decreased pain (anesthesia)	Positive	Positive‡	Positive
Decreased muscle spasm	Positive	Positive	Nil
Increased tissue stiffness	Nil	Negative	Negative
Overall	Positive†	Positive‡	?
OF HEAT			
Increased circulation	Nil	Positive	Positive
Increased metabolism	Very negative§	Nil¶	Nil
Increased inflammation	Positive	Positive	Negative
Decreased pain (anesthesia)	Positive	Nil¶	Positive
Decreased muscle spasm	Positive	Positive	Nil
Decreased tissue stiffness	Nil	Nil	Positive
Overall	Negative	Nil	?

*There is no immediate care of chronic injuries.

†Inhibits secondary metabolic injury.

‡Allows/requires active exercise.

§Promotes secondary metabolic injury.

¶Often does not facilitate active exercise.

Exercise does the following:

- Increases blood flow to a much greater extent than that which results from heat applications.[50]
- Retards the development of adhesions.
- Reverses neural inhibitions[80] and thus facilitates increased activity.
- Activates the lymphatic system,[81–83] the primary system for removing tissue debris from injured tissue.[84] Since lymphatic flow requires muscular action to pump the fluid, active exercise is essential for proper functioning.

INCREASED TISSUE STIFFNESS

Pain usually prevents active exercise for many days after even minor joint sprains.[28,80,85] Therefore, cold-induced pain relief enables the performance of active exercise much earlier than would otherwise be possible.[28,86,87] Because increased tissue stiffness hinders active exercise, it is considered a negative effect during rehabilitation.

Heat applications are not as effective as cold applications in facilitating exercise following an acute orthopedic injury.[88] Because exercise following heat applications usually causes a return of the pain and muscle spasm that were present beforehand. This does not seem to be true with chronic injuries. In addition, heat is effective in relieving general muscle soreness.

Cryokinetics can begin much earlier than thermal therapy.[86,89,90] Thermotherapy requires waiting until the circulation is restored, to avoid causing additional secondary metabolic injury. This usually takes 48–72 hours following an injury; whereas cryokinetics can begin 1–24 hours post-injury.[89]

LATE SUBACUTE CARE

Within 10–15 days after an acute injury, pain becomes more of a dull soreness than a sharp stabbing pain. Soreness responds better to heat than cold. Decreased range of motion can result from either muscle spasm or contracted connective tissue. Therefore treat muscle spasm with cold; and treat connective tissue with a combination of heat, stretching, and cold.

CHRONIC OR OVERUSE INJURIES

There is no immediate care for overuse injuries. Since the onset of these injuries is gradual, there is little vascular collapse and therefore little fear of secondary metabolic injury.

Issues surrounding the rehabilitation of chronic injuries are a source of confusion.[91-93] Generally there is minimal or no muscle spasm, and pain occurs only during extended activity. An overactive inflammatory response would indicate cold applications to decrease the inflammation. However, there is no evidence that cold is beneficial.

A popular therapy for tendinitis is the application of hot packs before, and cold packs after, practice or exercise. But evidence neither supports nor refutes this regimen.

Although ultrasound applications applied twice daily for 10 days might be effective, there is no documented evidence to support the claim; it is strictly our clinical impression based on experience with baseball players and gymnasts.

Cryotherapeutic Techniques for Transition and Subacute Care

The five most popular cryotherapy techniques used for transition and subacute care of acute orthopedic injury are discussed below. Each has specific indications; the techniques are not interchangeable. Specific application procedures for four of the techniques are in Chapter 14.

CRYOKINETICS FOR ACUTE JOINT SPRAIN REHABILITATION

Cryokinetics is a systematic combination of cold applications to numb the injured body part and graded, progressive, active exercise.[20,52] Cryokinetics is the most effective form of cryotherapy for rehabilitation of ligament sprains. Especially effective for ankle sprains, the technique can be used for any acute musculoskeletal joint injury. Cryokinetics allows rehabilitation to begin much sooner than traditional thermotherapy, and it can shorten rehabilitation time by days or even weeks.[18,19,94,95]

Pain-Free Exercise
Pain-free exercise is the key to cryokinetics.[1,20,52] The purpose of cold applications is pain reduction, to make active exercise possible.

Safety Valve
Unlike local anesthetic injections of pain-numbing drugs, such as procaine, cold does not totally inhibit the body's pain-sensing mechanism. Cold relieves residual pain (pain

from damaged tissue, pressure from swelling on nerves, etc.) thereby facilitating active exercise. But if the exercise becomes so vigorous that further damage might result, the body responds with a pain sensation. Thus, cryokinetics has a built-in safety valve: Pain from numbness indicates the exercise is too vigorous and activity level must be decreased (as long as the limb is properly numbed with ice application).

Psychological Preparation
The initial numbing during the first treatment session is usually difficult for the patient, and he/she will experience intense pain before the body part numbs. But the body quickly adapts to the pain, so subsequent ice applications are much less intense.[96,97] You must prepare the patient for the initial intense pain. Make sure he/she understands these important points:

- The pain is only temporary; it will not occur during subsequent cold applications.
- The benefits of the treatment, primarily decreased disability time, greatly outweigh the temporary discomfort.
- Shorter disability time is the main benefit of the cold.
- Patients who are not prepared for the intense cold and pain at the first immersion sometimes refuse to continue the treatment. See Chapter 14 for cryokinetics application procedures.

CRYOSTRETCH FOR ACUTE MUSCLE INJURIES

While cryokinetics is especially effective for treating acute joint sprains, it is not the best treatment for acute muscle strains. Muscle strains should be passively stretched. The cryostretch technique combines cold and passive stretching. It should be used during the early phases of muscle strain rehabilitation and followed by cryokinetics, as explained later in this chapter.

The cryostretch technique is dynamite for reducing low-grade muscle spasm, and most muscle injuries (strains and contusions) result in some degree of muscle spasm or tightness. In fact, many mild muscle "pulls" are actually muscles in spasm rather than torn muscle fibers.[98] In either case, the first step in rehabilitation is reducing the spasm and reestablishing pain-free range of motion.

Cryostretch combines three techniques for reducing muscle spasm: cold application, static stretching, and isometric contraction (the hold-relax technique of *proprioceptive neuromuscular facilitation [PNF]*).[99,100] While cryostretch is similar to cryokinetics in that exercise is performed while the body part is numbed, it differs in the number of exercise sets (three in cryostretch vs. five in cryokinetics) and in the exercise itself. During cryostretch exercises, the injured muscle is alternately statically stretched and isometrically contracted.

Cryostretch begins with cold application, typically ice massage, ice packs, or large cold packs. Following numbness, and interspersed with renumbing, are three exercise bouts of about 2.5 minutes. Each *exercise bout* consists of two 65-second sets of exercise with a 20-second relaxation period between sets. An *exercise set* consists of alternating static stretch with three repetitions of isometric contractions (hold-relax). See Chapter 14 for application procedures.

CONNECTIVE TISSUE STRETCH

The **connective tissue stretch** is a combination of heat application, long-term passive stretch, and cold applications. It is used to increase joint flexibility following prolonged immobilization during which connective tissue contractures have developed. Heat causes collagen fibers to relax, stretch lengthens the collagen fibers, and cold enables the collagen fibers to reattach in a lengthened position. See Chapter 14 for application procedures.

LYMPHEDEMA PUMPS

Lymphedema pumps, known formerly as *intermittent compression pumps*, *cold compression devices*, *pneumatic compression pumps* and *intermittent compression devices* are devices for providing intermittent compression to a body segment. The device consists of a boot or sleeve that fits over an extremity, a pump, hoses connecting the pump to the sleeve, and often a small ice water bath. The pump forces air or chilled water into the sleeve, applying pressure to the joint. The pump is controlled by a timing mechanism that turns it on and off, causing the sleeve or boot to intermittently inflate and deflate. The changes in sleeve pressure force lymphatic and venous drainage and thus reduce edema.

Cryokinetics is preferred for edema reduction because the rate of inflation/deflation of lymphedema pumps is much slower than the muscle pump provided by cryokinetics. Also, with cryokinetics you get the additional benefits of active exercise. See Chapter 14 for application procedures.

CONTRAST BATH THERAPY

Contrast bath therapy involves alternating immersion of the injured body part in hot and cold water baths. The traditional theory is that the alternating hot and cold baths cause alternating vasodilation and vasoconstriction, which pumps edema from the tissue. The time of application of the two baths varies greatly. Numerous ratios of hot to cold have been suggested, including 4:1, 3:1, 3:2, 5:2, and 5:5 minutes.[1,101]

The theory that contrast therapy helps to pump out edema has so many holes in it that we do not recommend the technique. For example:

- Edema is reduced by removing free protein from the tissue. This is done via the lymphatic system, not the vascular system (see Chapter 5).
- Even if edema was reduced via the vascular system, the tissue temperature changes are not great enough to cause significant vascular reactions.[101–103]
- Even if the temperature changes were great enough to effect vascular changes, the venules, capillaries, and lymph vessels do not contain muscles to be affected by the temperature changes. They therefore could not constrict and dilate with contrasting temperatures.
- Even if the technique caused vascular or lymphatic pumping, cryokinetics would cause many more pumps. Consider: a ratio of 3:1 would induce a pump each 4 minutes or 15 pumps in an hour. During 1 hour of cryokinetics, a patient would actively exercise for 15 minutes. During each exercise repetition, muscle contraction will pump the venous and lymphatic systems. They would perform 20–30 pumps per minute, or 20–30 times more than each minute in a contrast bath.

Another theory is that alternating sensations during the alternating applications of heat and cold cause a decrease in pain that allows more activity following the contrast bath therapy. This theory is flawed, however.[1] There is no change in numbness in uninjured subjects when contrast therapy is used.[99]

Recovery Cryotherapy

Cryotherapy is increasingly being used to help athletes recover from the rigors of their workout or competition more quickly.[104–107] Baseball pitchers have been icing their arms for decades. Runners were next to adopt the practice,[104,108] and now increasing numbers of football, elite soccer, rugby, and professional cycling athletes are using "cold plunging" as well; crediting it with helping them recover more quickly.[108,109] Scientists struggle to find a rationale theory to explain why the technique is beneficial,[110] but the technique is gaining momentum. Is this an example of technique proceeding theory (see Chapter 2), or of "herd mentality?".

The two primary modes of recovery cryotherapy are whole body cryotherapy (WBC) and cold water immersion (CWI). Both techniques were first used to treat injury and disease.

BASEBALL PITCHERS

Ice immersion after pitching baseballs appears to enhance recovery. Pitchers who applied cold packs or immersed their elbows in ice water and applied ice packs to their shoulders for 20 minutes threw with greater velocity and were more accurate 3–4 days later than when they had no treatment.[111-113] Cryotherapy also enhanced shoulder range of motion 24 hours later.[114]

WHOLE BODY CRYOTHERAPY

Whole-body cryotherapy (WBC) is the most expensive and dangerous recovery method. It involves a brief exposure (2–3 minutes) to very cold air (–110° to –140°C; –166° to –220°F) in temperature-controlled chambers, which range from—two to three progressively colder rooms[115] that can accommodate up to six people[116] to a one-person chamber the size of a phone booth.[116] The concept was developed in Japan in 1978 and then developed for therapy in Poland.[116] Originally it was intended for treating rheumatic and spastic diseases; to allow patients to move pain free, and therefore to benefit from the therapeutic exercise. It is used in sports medicine to improve recovery from exhaustive practice and competition.[108,110,117,118]

The chambers are cooled with a refrigeration unit,[115] dry ice,[116] or liquid nitrogen.[119] Clients/patients wear several pairs of gloves, a face mask, a woolly headband to protect the ears, and dry socks.[108,115,116,119]

At least one world-class athlete suffered frostbite to the bottom of both feet during WBC. He neglected to put on totally dry socks before entering the chamber, and the sweat in the socks he was wearing froze and then froze his feet—unfortunately just before a world meet.[108]

Scientific reports are conflicted on the use of WBC; it appears that it:

- Is of no benefit[120]
- Can be beneficial in males for increasing anaerobic capacity in speed and strength sports[121]
- Seems to have a positive effect on aerobic, but often not for anaerobic, performances[104]
- May be beneficial after a series of 20 treatments[118]
- Is effective in reducing the inflammatory process[122]

In summary:

- Evidence is weak and may be negative.[123]
- Further evidence is needed,[124] especially from large-scale trials.[105]
- It is not harmful unless used improperly.[110]

COLD WATER IMMERSION

CWI is simple to apply to single or small groups of athletes and a little more difficult for large groups because of the time required to treat all of the athletes.[106] All that is needed is a barrel deep enough for a person to stand in it up to the waist or thighs. Whirlpools are often used. Larger athletic training clinics have large immersion pools that can be chilled. Cattle drinking troughs have been used for large-scale, on-the-field treatments.[116]

There is a discrepancy between duration of treatments in performance research (15–20 minutes) and actual athlete use, which may be as little as 30 seconds.[106] Like WBC, the evidence for CWI is mixed; positive reports indicate that CWI:

- Immediately after prolonged intermittent shuttle running reduced some indices of exercise-induced muscle damage[125]
- Decreased stiffness and creatine kinase on days 2 and 3 following application
- Promoted faster acute recovery of maximal anaerobic performances after an intermittent exhaustive exercise[126]
- Reduced decrements to isometric leg extension and flexion strength 48-hour post-exercise[126]
- Reduced muscle soreness ratings[126,127]
- Intermittent (5 × 1 minute at 10°C) CWI reduced the perception of fatigue and enhanced restoration of some match-related performance measures during a 4-day tournament.[128]
- Six-minute treatment assisted acute recovery from high-intensity running.[129]
- Repeated exercise performance in heat may be improved when a short period (5 minutes) of CWI is applied during the recovery period.[130]

Negative research results indicated that CWI had a:

- Negative effect on neuromuscular function[107]
- Possible negative effects on performance following 15-minute gel pack application immediately following sprint-interval training[131]
- No effect on perception of tenderness and strength loss[132]
- No benefit from a single 10-minute bout (10°C) after a damaging bout of exercise on exercise-induced muscle damage[133]
- Not effect on physical test performance or indices of muscle damage and inflammation when applied immediately postmatch, but does reduce the perception of general fatigue and leg soreness between matches in tournaments[134]
- Three 1-minute apps in ice water were ineffective.[135]
- Not as effective as LED light therapy short-term postexercise recovery[136]

Like WBC, further performance-orientated research is required to determine whether water immersion is beneficial to athletes.[106]

TO USE OR NOT TO USE

It appears that the use of cryotherapy to enhance recovery from fatiguing physical performance is based on anecdotal information, with limited research on actual performance.[106] There is a definite psychological benefit to athletes who are convinced that it is beneficial.[106,108,109] In the words of an elite rugby player, "I'd be lying if I didn't say it was a pretty savage experience, but the other side of the coin is that it is definitely working and allowing us to train in a way that would be impossible under normal conditions."[116]

Highly trained athletes and their coaches seek every advantage they can find to improve their performance. There are hints in the scientific literature that recovery cryotherapy is effective. But regardless of what science indicates, until there is evidence that it is beneficial, or some winning athlete or team proposes something better, the technique will continue to be used. And the general public will follow, as evidenced by the opening of a cryotherapy chamber that caters to recreational athletes opened in Northern California in 2011.[108]

Comparing Heat and Cold for Rehabilitation

Some clinicians feel that cryotherapy is better than thermotherapy during rehabilitation because the temperature change during application is many times greater with cold than with heat. This is not true. This false idea developed because the core temperature was used to compute the changes. But therapeutic modalities are applied most often to the extremities, so the differential should be computed from extremity temperature, which is lower than core temperature (Table 12.2). For instance, the absolute change in temperature between a cold whirlpool and the core is 6.3 times as great as the change from a warm whirlpool and the

core 66.2°F versus 37.4°F (19°C vs. 3°C). When computing the difference between extremity temperature and hot and cold whirlpool temperatures, the change with cold is only twice as great 42.8°F versus 53.6°F (6°C vs. 12°C).

✔ APPLICATION TIP

CRYOTHERAPY: POWERFUL THERAPY BEYOND IMMEDIATE CARE

Cryotherapy is extremely powerful during immediate care and beyond. But we don't want to give the impression that it is the answer to rehabilitation of all orthopedic injuries. For acute sprains and strains, cryotherapy, in the form of cryokinetics or cryostretch, should follow RICES treatments and continue well into the post-acute phase of rehabilitation. Heat helps reduce general soreness and must be used to prepare collagen tissue for stretching and joint mobilization. Both thermotherapy and extended cryotherapy have their place.

WHEN TO USE COLD AND WHEN TO USE HEAT

Based on our personal research, reading, and clinical experience, we offer the following opinions:

- Cold applications must always be used for the immediate care of acute injuries.
- Cold applications are more effective in facilitating exercise during the rehabilitation of acute orthopedic injuries.
- Muscle spasm is relieved more quickly with cold and stretching than with heat and stretching.
- Chronic inflammatory conditions should respond well to ultrasound (twice a day) and with either superficial heat or cold. Some individuals respond better to superficial cold, while others respond better to superficial heat. Treat

TABLE 12.2 TEMPERATURE DIFFERENTIALS DURING CRYOTHERAPY AND THERMOTHERAPY			
		CHANGE IN TEMPERATURE FROM	
	NORMAL TEMPERATURE	**Core**	**Extremities**
Core	98.6°F (37°C)		
Human extremities	86–93°F (30–34°F)		
SUPERFICIAL HEAT			
Hot packs	115°F (45°C)	16.4°F (+8°C)	+22 to 29°F (+11 to 15°C)
Whirlpool	105°F (40°C)	6.4°F (+3°C)	+12 to 19°F (+6 to 10°C)
SUPERFICIAL COLD			
Immersion	34°F (1°C)	64.6°F (−36°C)	−52 to 59°F (−29 to 33°C)
Cold pack	41°F (5°C)	57.6°F (−32°C)	−45 to 52°F (−25 to 29°C)
Whirlpool	65°F (18°C)	33.6°F (−19°C)	−21 to 28°F (−12 to 16°C)

the symptoms with whatever modality is most comfortable for the patient.

- Connective tissue contractures resulting from immobilization (2 weeks or longer) must be treated with heat followed by stretching or mobilization.
- General soreness is best treated with a warm whirlpool.
- Subacute joint sprains (4–14 days post-injury) that remain sore, but that allow the patient to exercise, should be treated with heat prior to exercise or practice and cold afterwards.

> **✔ APPLICATION TIP**
>
> **THERAPEUTIC GOALS DETERMINE SELECTION OF THERAPEUTIC MODALITIES**
>
> The recommendations for when to use cold and when to use heat illustrates the principle that the choice of what therapeutic modality to use should be a matter of matching therapeutic goals with the body's response to the modality. Remember the SAID principle from the first chapter?

CLOSING SCENE

The AT student in the opening scene tells you to apply ice to an injured player's ankle for no longer than 15 minutes. His rationale was that after 15 minutes, CIVD will occur and this might add to the swelling. You correct him and explain why CIVD is a flawed theory, but that this does not negate the use of cryotherapy beyond immediate care. Further, you explain why facilitating therapeutic exercise is much more powerful that inducing increased blood flow.

Chapter Reflections

1. Read and ponder each of the following points. Do you feel you have a clear understanding of each concept? If not, reread the appropriate section of the chapter.
   - Define cryotherapy.
   - Why is there confusion concerning cryotherapy?
   - Explain the profile of temperature changes during cold applications, including differences between surface and deep temperatures, and thermal gradients in the tissue and modality.
   - Describe the relationship between immediate care and post–immediate care cryotherapy during orthopedic injury management. Include the theory, goals, and application of cryotherapy during each phase.
   - Why is there confusion about cryotherapy during immediate care and post–immediate care of orthopedic injuries?
   - In the relationship between pain and cryotherapy, how can cryotherapy both cause and relieve pain?
   - Name the nine major physiological responses to cryotherapy, and briefly explain the mechanism of each.
   - Discuss strategies to minimize pain during cryotherapy.
   - What is the difference between coping with, and habituation to, cold-induced pain? Discuss strategies for both during cryotherapy.
   - Describe CIVD—what it is, when it occurs, and why clinicians are confused about its role in orthopedic injury management.
   - Discuss the efficacy of heat and cold (including the influence of each physiological response) when used during immediate care and acute care of orthopedic injuries.
   - What are the criteria for selecting which therapeutic modality to use?
   - Define and briefly discuss when and how you would use cryokinetics, cryostretch, connective tissue stretch, contrast bath therapy, and lymphedema pumps.
2. Write three to five questions for discussion with your class instructor, clinical instructor, classmates, and clinical colleagues.
3. Get together with classmates and quiz each other on the concepts of this chapter. Use the points in reflection no. 1 and questions you wrote for reflection no. 2 as a beginning. Explaining concepts out loud to others requires a deeper grasp of the material than feeling you understand it as you read.

Concept Check Responses

CONCEPT CHECK 12.1

Cold (RICES) is essential immediately after an injury, and extending for 10–24 hours to decrease secondary injury. Many continue to use it for days following the injury in an effort to reduce the swelling. The later efforts are futile, however. First of all, swelling is a process, not an entity. Swelling is the result of a shift in capillary filtration pressure due to extracellular free protein. To reduce the swelling, you must remove the excess extracellular free protein. This requires stimulating the lymphatic system via some type of intermittent compression, such as active exercise, massage, a lymphedema pump, or electrical muscle stimulation.

CONCEPT CHECK 12.2

If the foot is held still in an ice water bath, a temperature gradient develops in the water, making the water near the body warmer than the rest of ice water bath. If the patient then moves his foot (or if you swirl the water), the gradient is broken up and the water near the foot becomes colder. The decrease in temperature of the local environment elicits a pain response.

CONCEPT CHECK 12.3

Figures 12.3 and 12.4 represent data from a single subject; Figure 12.6 presents averaged data from 12 subjects. Temperatures of individual subjects in the later study oscillated just as much as in the former, but since the fluctuation occurred at slightly different times, averaging them together smoothed the line. For example, consider three consecutive measurements in each of three subjects: (subject a) 2, 4, 2; (subject b) 3, 3, 4; and (subject c) 4, 2, 3. Each of the three subjects is oscillating; in fact, the second reading of subject a is twice as much as the first

and third readings. When the data are averaged, however, they are 3, 3, 3, which would graph as a straight line. Remember when reading experimental results that the data presented represent an average of many individuals. A second important consideration is that patients are not average, meaning that individual patients are not going to respond exactly like the average.

CONCEPT CHECK 12.4

You can prevent interpretation errors by actively thinking. Don't be naive or cynical. As the 16th century philosopher Francis Bacon taught, read not to contradict and refute, nor to believe and take for granted, but to weigh and consider.

We all want to be able to justify or explain why we do something, not only for our own curiosity, but to explain what we are doing to our patients. Unfortunately, many clinicians accept dubious claims of theory and pass them on. This is especially true of claims by salespeople. Most are honorable, but there are "snake oil peddlers" among them. And even the honorable inadvertently share misinformation.

Be sure to check references when you read journal articles. References are sometimes misinterpreted and then passed on. For example, McMaster[137] is often quoted as a source for applying cold for 20 minutes during immediate care, but his source is an article by Knight and Londeree[50] about cryokinetics. So research concerning cryotherapy for pain control was improperly used to reference cryotherapy for immediate care where the goal is decreased metabolism, and then passed on by many others who did not check the original reference.

Another point about references is their content. A reference to specific research on a topic is stronger than to an opinion, even if the opinion is by a prominent scientist or clinician.

REFERENCES

1. Knight KL. *Cryotherapy in Sport Injury Management.* Champaign, IL: Human Kinetics, 1995.
2. Jarvinen M. Immobilization effect on the tensile properties of striated muscle: an experimental study in the rat. *Arch Phys Med Rehabil.* 1977;58(3):123–127.
3. Jarvinen M. Healing of a crush injury in rat striated muscle. 2. a histological study of the effect of early mobilization and immobilization on the repair processes. *Acta Pathol Microbiol Scand A.* 1975;83(3):269–282.
4. Hurme T, Kalimo H, Lehto M, Jarvinen M. Healing of skeletal muscle injury: an ultrastructural and immunohistochemical study. *Med Sci Sports Exerc.* 1991;23:801–810.
5. Kvist H, Jarvinen M, Sorvari T. Effect of mobilization and immobilization on the healing of contusion injury in muscle. A preliminary report of a histological study in rats. *Scand J Rehabil Med.* 1974;6(3):134–140.
6. Dehne E. The rationale of early functional loading in the healing of fractures: a comprehensive gate control concept of repair. *Clin Orthop Relat Res.* 1980;(146):18–27.
7. Buch B, Papert AI, Shear M. Microscopic changes in rat tongue following experimental cryosurgery. *J Oral Pathol.* 1979;8(2):94–102.
8. Marcove RC, Weis LD, Vaghaiwalla MR, Pearson R. Cryosurgery in the treatment of giant cell tumors of bone: a report of 52 consecutive cases. *Clin Orthop Relat Res.* 1978(134):275–289.
9. Boykin JV, Jr, Crute SL. Mechanisms of burn shock protection after severe scald injury by cold-water treatment. *J Trauma.* 1982;22(10):859–866.

10. Rippe B, Grega GJ. Effects of isoprenaline and cooling on histamine induced changes of capillary permeability in the rat hindquarter vascular bed. *Acta Physiol Scand.* 1978;103(3):252–262.

11. Harris ED Jr, McCroskery PA. The influence of temperature and fibril stability on degradation of cartilage collagen by rheumatoid synovial collagenase. *N Engl J Med.* 1974;290(1):1–6.

12. Svanes K. Studies in hypothermia I. The influence of deep hypothermia on the formation of cellular exudate in acute inflammation in mice. *Acta Anaesthesiol Scand.* 1964;8:143–156.

13. Svanes K. Studies in hypothermia II. The influence of deep hypothermia on the formation of fluid exudate in acute inflammation in mice. *Acta Anaesthesiol Scand.* 1964;8:157–166.

14. Dorwart BB, Hansell JR, Schumacher HR. Effects of heat, cold and mechanical agitation on crystal-induced arthritis in the dog. *Arthr Rheum.* 1973;16(4):563–571.

15. Abakumova E. Effect of hypothermia on wound healing. *Stomatologiia.* 1978;57:19–21.

16. McCaffery M. *Nursing Management of the Patient with Pain.* Philadelphia, PA: JB Lippincott Co., 1979.

17. Chapman CE. Can the use of physical modalities for pain control be rationalized by the research evidence? *Can J Physiol Pharmacol.* 1991;69:704–712.

18. Grant AE. Massage with ice (cryokinetics) in the treatment of painful conditions of the musculoskeletal system. *Arch Phys Med Rehabil.* 1964;44:233–238.

19. Hayden CA. Cryokinetics in an early treatment program. *J Am Phys Ther Assoc.* 1964;44:990–993.

20. Knight KL. Ankle rehabilitation with cryokinetics. *Phys Sportsmed.* 1979;7(11):113.

21. Knight KL. Cryokinetics in rehabilitation of joint sprains. *J Can Athl Ther Assoc.* 1981;8(3):17–18.

22. Tovell J. Ice immersion toe cap. *Athl Train.* 1980;15:33.

23. Nimchick PSR, Knight KL. Effects of wearing a toe cap or a sock on temperature and perceived pain during ice water immersion. *Athl Train.* 1983;18:144–147.

24. Jutte LS, Konz S, Knight KL. A 15 min immersion in 1°C water produces greater numbness than immersion in 4°C Or 10°C water. *J Athl Train.* 2012; In review.

25. Everall M. Cold therapy. *Nurs Times.* 1976;70:144–145.

26. Haines J. A study into a report on cold therapy. *Physiotherapy.* 1970;56:501–502.

27. Raptou AD. Cryotherapy: a brief review. *South Med J.* 1968;61:625–627.

28. Kraus H. Prevention and treatment of skiing injuries. *J Trauma.* 1961;1:457–463.

29. Chu DA, Lutt CJ. The rationale of ice therapy. *J Natl Athl Train Assoc.* 1969;4:8–9.

30. Travell J, Rinzler SH. The myofascial genesis of pain. *Postgrad Med.* 1952;11:425–434.

31. Ashby EC. Abdominal pain of spinal origin. *Ann R Coll Surg Engl.* 1977;59:242–246.

32. Wolf SL, Knutsson E. Effects of skin cooling on stretch reflex activity in triceps surae of the decerebate cat. *Exp Neurol.* 1975;49:22–35.

33. Lane L. Localized hypothermia for relief of pain in musculoskeletal injuries. *Phys Ther.* 1971;51:182–183.

34. Wolf SL, Letbetter WD. Effect of skin cooling on spontaneous EMG activity in triceps surae of the decerebrate cat. *Brain Res.* 1975;91:151–155.

35. Hunt C. The effect of sympathetic stimulation on mammalian muscle spindles. *J Physiol.* 1960;151:332–341.

36. Johns RJ, Wright V. Relative importance of various tissues in joint stiffness. *J Appl Physiol.* 1962;17:824–828.

37. Fox W. Human performance in the cold. *Hum Factors.* 1967;9:203–220.

38. Licht S. History of therapeutic heat and cold. In: Lehman JF, ed. *Therapeutic Heat and Cold.* 3rd ed. Baltimore, MD: Williams & Wilkins, 1982:1–34.

39. Giesbrecht G, Bristow G. Decrement in manual arm performance during whole body cooling. *Aviation Space Environ Med.* 1992;63:1077–1081.

40. LeBlanc JS. Impairment of manual dexterity in the cold. *J Appl Physiol.* 1956;9:62–64.

41. Vincent M, Tipton M. The effects of cold immersion and hand protection on grip strength. *Aviat Space Environ Med.* 1988;59:738–741.

42. Lehmann JF, Masock AJ, Warren CG, Koblanski JN. Effect of therapeutic temperatures on tendon extensibility. *Arch Phys Med Rehabil.* 1970;51:481–487.

43. Warren CG, Lehman JF, Koblanski JN. Elongation of rat tail tendon: effect of load and temperature. *Arch Phys Med Rehabil.* 1971;52:465–474.

44. Evans TA, Ingersoll CD, Knight KL, Worrell TW. The effects of cold application on functional agility. *J Athl Train.* 1995;30:231–234.

45. Hopkins JT, Ingersoll CD. Arthrogenic muscle inhibition: a limiting factor in joint rehabilitation. *J Sport Rehabil.* 2000;9:135–139.

46. Hopkins J, Ingersoll CD, Edwards J, Klootwyk TE. Cryotherapy and transcutaneous electric neuromuscular stimulation decrease arthrogenic muscle inhibition of the vastus medialis after knee joint effusion. *J Athl Train.* 2002;37(1):25–31.

47. Hopkins JT, Ingersoll CD, Krause BA, Edwards JE, Cordova ML. Effect of knee joint effusion on quadriceps and soleus motoneuron pool excitability. *Med Sci Sports Exerc.* 2001;33(1):123–126.

48. Hopkins JT, Stencil R. Ankle cryotherapy facilitates soleus function. *J Orthop Sports Phys Ther.* 2002;32(12):622–627.

49. Ingersoll CD, Palmeiri RM, Hopkins JT. A joint dilemma. *Rehabil Manag.* 2003;16(1):38–42.

50. Knight KL, Londeree BR. Comparison of blood flow in the ankle of uninjured subjects during therapeutic applications of heat, cold, and exercise. *Med Sci Sports Exerc.* 1980;12:76–80.

51. Lewis T. Observations upon the reactions of the vessels of the human skin to cold. *Heart.* 1930;15:177–208.

52. Moore RJ, Nicolette RL, Behnke RS. The therapeutic use of cold (cryotherapy) in the care of athletic injuries. *J Natl Athl Train Assoc.* 1967;2(1):6.

53. Juvenal JP. Cryokinetics, a new concept in the treatment of injuries. *Schol Coach.* 1966;35:40–42.

54. Behnke RS, Blackwell HJ, Nicolette RL, Moore RJ. Ice therapy. Paper presented at: NATA Convention; June 1967.

55. Behnke R. Cryotherapy and vasodilation. *Athl Train.* 1973;8:106.

56. Behnke R. Cold vasodilatation. *Athl J.* 1973;106.

57. Edwards AG. Increasing circulation with cold. *J Natl Athl Train Assoc.* 1971;6:15–16.

58. Wise DD. Ice and the athlete. *Physiother Can.* 1973;25:213–217.

59. Abraham WM. Heat vs. cold therapy for the treatment of muscle injuries. *Athl Train.* 1974;9:177.

60. Clarke RSJ, Hellon RF, Lind AR. Vascular reactions of the human forearm to cold. *Clin Sci.* 1958;17:165–179.

61. Knight KL, Aquino J, Johannes SM, Urban CD. A re-examination of Lewis' cold-induced vasodilatation-In the finger and ankle. *Athl Train.* 1980;15:248–250.

62. Knight K, Carmody LW. Rewarming of the ankle and forearm following 30 minutes of ice water immersion. Paper presented at the *National Athletic Trainers Association Annual Clinical Symposium,* Nashville, TN, June 1984.

63. Knight KL, Elam JE. Rewarming of the ankle, forearm, and finger after cryotherapy: further re-examination of Lewis' cold-induced vasodilatation. *J Can Athl Ther Assoc.* 1981;8(2):15–17.

64. Edwards M, Burton AC. Correlation of heat output and blood flow in the finger, especially in cold-induced vasodilation. *J Appl Physiol.* 1960;15:201–208.

65. Abramson DI, Chu LSW, Tuck S, et al. Effect of tissue temperature and blood flow on motor nerve conduction velocity. *JAMA.* 1966;198:1082–1088.

66. Knight KL, Bryan KS, Halvorsen JM. Circulatory changes in the forearm during and after cold pack application and immersion in 1 degree C, 5 degrees C, and 15 degrees C water (abstract). *Int J Sports Med.* 1981;4:1–2.

67. Taber C, Countryman K, Fahrenbruck J, LaCount K, Cornwall MW. Measurement of reactive vasodilation during cold gel pack application to nontraumatized ankles. *Phys Ther.* 1992;72:294–299.

68. Aizawa Y, Shibata A, Tajiri M, Hirasawa Y. Reflex vasoconstriction to a cold stimulus for non-invasive evaluation of neurovascular function in man. *Jpn Heart J.* 1979;20:301–305.

69. Barcroft H, Edholm OG. The effect of temperature on blood flow and deep temperature in the human forearm. *J Physiol.* 1943;102:5–20.

70. Bonney GLW, Hughes RA, Janus O. Blood flow through the normal human knee segment. *Clin Sci.* 1952;11:167–181.

71. Folkow B, Fox RH, Krog J, Odelram H, Thoren O. Studies on the reactions of the cutaneous vessels to cold exposure. *Acta Physiol Scand.* 1963;58:342–354.

72. Greenfield ADM, Shephard JT. A quantitative study of the response to cold of the circulation throughout the fingers of normal subjects. *Clin Sci.* 1950;9:323–334.

73. Knight K. Comparison of blood flow in normal subjects during therapeutic applications of heat, cold, and exercise of therapeutic levels. Doctoral Dissertation, University of Missouri-Columbia, 1977.

74. Johannes SM, Knight KL. Temperature response during the warming phase of cryokinetics. *Indiana Interagency Research Symposium,* Terre Haute, IN, May 1979.

75. Nathan PW. The gate-control theory of pain. A critical review. *Brain.* 1976;99(1):123–158.

76. Langohr JL, Rosenfield L, Owen CR, Cope O. Effect of therapeutic cold on the circulation of blood and lymph in thermal burns. *Arch Surg.* 1949;59(80).

77. Leadbetter WB. An introduction to sports-induced soft-tissue inflammation. In: Leadbetter WB, Buckwalter JA, Gordon SL, eds. *Sports-Induced Inflammation.* Chicago, IL: American Academy of Orthopaedic Surgeons, 1990:3–23.

78. Lundgren C, Muren A, Zederfeldt B. Effect of cold-vasoconstriction on wound healing in the rabbit. *Acta Chir Scand.* 1959;118:1–4.

79. Hill P. Effects of heat and cold on the perineum after episiotomy/laceration. *J Obstet Gynecol Neonatal Nurs.* 1989;18:124–129.

80. Dehne E, Torp RP. Treatment of joint injuries by immediate mobilization. Based upon the spinal adaptation concept. *Clin Orthop.* 1971;77:218–232.

81. Bohlen HG. The microcirculation and the lymphatic system. In: Rhoades RA, Tanner GA, eds. *Medical Physiology.* 2nd ed. Baltimore, MD: Lippincott Williams & Wilkins, 2003:262–275.

82. Havas E, Parviainen T, Vuorela J, et al. Lymph flow dynamics in exercising human skeletal muscle as detected by scintography. *J Physiol.* 1997;504(Pt 1):233–239.

83. Porth CM. *Pathophysiology.* 7th ed. Baltimore, MD: Lippincott Williams & Wilkins, 2004.

84. Johnson MG. Potential role of the lymphatic vessel in regulating inflammatory events. *Surv Synth Path Res* 1983;1:111–119.

85. Dehne E. The rationale of early functional loading in the healing of fractures. *Clin Orthop Relat Res.* 1979;146:18–27.

86. Handling KA. Rehabilitating athletic injuries with cryotherapy. *Joperd.* 1982;53:338–340.

87. Starkey JA. Treatment of ankle sprains by simultaneous use of intermittent compression and ice packs. *Am J Sports Med.* 1976;4(4):142–144.

88. Lehmann JF, deLateur BJ. Cryotherapy. In: Lehman JF, ed. *Therapeutic Heat and Cold.* 3rd ed. Baltimore, MD: Williams & Wilkins, 1982:563–602.

89. Behnke RS. Cold therapy. *Athl Train.* 1974;9:178–179.

90. Lehmann JF. *Therapeutic Heat and Cold.* 4th ed. Baltimore, MD: Williams & Wilkins, 1990.

91. Stanish WD, Gunnlaugson B. Electrical energy and soft-tissue injury healing. *Sportcare Fitness.* 1988;9:12.

92. O'Connor FG, Sobel JR, Nirschl RP. Five-step treatment for overuse injuries. *Phys Sportsmed.* 1992;20:128–130, 135–142.

93. Puffer J, Zachazewski J. Management of overuse injuries. *Am Fam Physician.* 1988;38:225–231.

94. Barnes L. Cryotherapy — putting injury on ice. *Phys Sportsmed.* 1979;7(6):130–136.

95. Hocutt JE, Jr, Jaffe R, Rylander CR, Beebe JK. Cryotherapy in ankle sprains. *Am J Sports Med.* 1982;10(5):316–319.

96. LeBlanc J, Potvin P. Studies on habituation to cold pain. *Can J Physiol Pharmacol.* 1966;44:287–293.

97. Carman KW, Knight KL. Habituation to cold-pain during repeated cryokinetic sessions. *J Athl Train.* 1992;27:223–230.

98. Peppard A. Myotonic muscle distress: a rationale for therapy. *Athl Train.* 1974;8:166–169.

99. Knott M. *Proprioceptive Neuromuscular Facilitation, Patterns and Techniques.* 2nd ed. New York, NY: Harper & Row, 1968.

100. Knight KL. Cryostretch for muscle injuries. *Phys Sportsmed.* 1980;8(4):126.

101. Cotts BE, Knight KL, Myrer JW, Schulthies S. Contrast-bath therapy and sensation over the anterior talofibular ligament. *J Sports Rehabil.* 2004;13(2):114–121.

102. Myrer JW, Draper DO, Durrant E. Contrast therapy and intramuscular temperature in the human leg. *J Athl Train.* 1994;29:318–322.

103. Myrer JW, Measom G, Durrant E, Fellingham GW. Cold- and hot-pack contrast therapy: subcutaneous and intramuscular temperature change. *J Athl Train.* 1997;32(3):238–241.

104. Ranalli GF, Demartini JK, Casa DJ, et al. Effect of body cooling on subsequent aerobic and anaerobic exercise performance: a systematic review. *J Strength Cond Res.* 2010;24(12):3488–3496.

105. Lateef F. Post exercise ice water immersion: is it a form of active recovery? *J Emerg Trauma Shock.* 2010;3(3):302.

106. Wilcock IM, Cronin JB, Hing WA. Physiological response to water immersion: a method for sport recovery? *Sports Med (Auckland, N.Z.).* 2006;36(9):747–765.

107. Peiffer JJ, Abbiss CR, Nosaka K, Peake JM, Laursen PB. Effect of cold water immersion after exercise in the heat on muscle function, body temperatures, and vessel diameter. *J Sci Med Sport.* 2009;12(1):91–96.

108. Reynolds G. Freezing Athletes to Speed Recovery, New York Times, Wednesday, September 7, 2011. Available at: http://well.blogs.nytimes.com/2011/09/07/freezing-athletes-to-speed-recovery/?ref=health. Accessed January, 2012.

109. Call J. BYU football: Bronco Mendenhall pleased with progress, lack of injuries, as camp winds down. Available at: http://www.deseretnews.com/article/765597728/BYU-football-Bronco-Mendenhall-pleased-with-progress-lack-of-injuries-as-camp-winds-down.html?pg=2. Accessed August, 2012.

110. Banfi G, Melegati G, Barassi A, d'Eril GM. Effects of the whole-body cryotherapy on NTproBNP, hsCRP and troponin I in athletes. *J Sci Med Sport.* 2009;12(6):609–610.

111. Carbajal FJ, Nelson DO. The effect of cold pack application on the recovery from pitching a baseball. *Athl J.* 1967;47:8–11,85–86.

112. Kato D. *Effect of static stretch and ice immersion on pitching performance after induced muscle performance* [Thesis], Indiana State University, Terre Haute, 1985.

113. Gircheck L, Knight KL. Static stretch and ice immersion improved varsity collegiate pitching performance after induced muscle soreness. Unpublished paper: a Thesis. 2630.

114. Yanagisawa O, Miyanaga Y, Shiraki H, et al. The effects of various therapeutic measures on shoulder range of motion and cross-sectional areas of rotator cuff muscles after baseball pitching. *J Sports Med Phys Fitness.* 2003;43(3):356–366.

115. Zimmer MedizinSystems. Cryo Therapy Chamber. Available at: http://www.zimmerusa.com/cryo_chamber.html. Accessed August, 2012.

116. ESPNscrum Staff. Warburton pushes through pain barrier. *ESPNScrum.* Available at: http://www.espnscrum.com/wales/rugby/story/143011.html. Accessed August, 2012.

117. Banfi G, Lombardi G, Colombini A, Melegati G. Whole-body cryotherapy in athletes. *Sports Med (Auckland, N.Z.).* 2010;40(6):509–517.

118. Lubkowska A, Szygula Z, Chlubek D, Banfi G. The effect of prolonged whole-body cryostimulation treatment with different amounts of sessions on chosen pro- and anti-inflammatory cytokines levels in healthy men. *Scand J Clin Lab Invest.* 2011;71(5):419–425.

119. Wikipedia. Cryotherapy; Cryogenic chamber therapy. Available at: http://en.wikipedia.org/wiki/Cryotherapy. Accessed August, 2012.

120. Costello J, Algar L, Donnelly A. Effects of whole-body cryotherapy (−110°C) on proprioception and indices of muscle damage. *Scand J Med Sci Sports.* 2012;22(2):190–198.

121. Klimek AT, Lubkowska A, Szyguła Z, Chudecka M, Fraczek B. Influence of the ten sessions of the whole body cryostimulation on aerobic and anaerobic capacity. *Int J Occup Med Environ Health.* 2010;23(2):181–189.

122. Pournot H, Bieuzen FO, Louis J, et al. Time-course of changes in inflammatory response after whole-body cryotherapy multi exposures following severe exercise. *Plos One.* 2011;6(7):e22748.

123. Yamane M, Teruya H, Nakano M, et al. Post-exercise leg and forearm flexor muscle cooling in humans attenuates endurance and resistance training effects on muscle performance and on circulatory adaptation. *Eur J Appl Physiol.* 2006;96(5):572–580.

124. Barnett AJ. Using recovery modalities between training sessions in elite athletes: does it help? *Sports Med.* 2006;36(9):781–796.

125. Bailey DM, Erith SJ, Griffin PJ, et al. Influence of cold-water immersion on indices of muscle damage following prolonged intermittent shuttle running. *J Sports Sci.* 2007;25(11):1163–1170.

126. Pournot H, Bieuzen F, Duffield R, et al. Short term effects of various water immersions on recovery from exhaustive intermittent exercise. *Eur J Appl Physiol.* 2011;111(7):1287–1295.

127. Ingram J, Dawson B, Goodman C, Wallman K, Beilby J. Effect of water immersion methods on post-exercise recovery from simulated team sport exercise. *J Sci Med Sport.* 2009;12(3):417–421.

128. Rowsell GJ, Coutts AJ, Reaburn P, Hill-Haas S. Effect of post-match cold-water immersion on subsequent match running performance in junior soccer players during tournament play. *J Sports Sci.* 2011;29(1):1–6.

129. Versey NG, Halson SL, Dawson BT. Effect of contrast water therapy duration on recovery of running performance. *Int J Sports Physiol Perform.* 2012;7(2):130–140.

130. Peiffer JJ, Abbiss CR, Watson G, Nosaka K, Laursen PB. Effect of a 5-min cold-water immersion recovery on exercise performance in the heat. *Br J Sports Med.* 2010;44(6):461–465.

131. Nemet D, Meckel Y, Bar-Sela S, et al. Effect of local cold-pack application on systemic anabolic and inflammatory response to sprint-interval training: a prospective comparative trial. *Eur J Appl Physiol.* 2009;107(4):411–417.

132. Eston R, Peters D. Effects of cold water immersion on the symptoms of exercise-induced muscle damage. *J Sports Sci.* 1999;17(3):231–238.

133. Jakeman JR, Macrae R, Eston R. A single 10-min bout of cold-water immersion therapy after strenuous plyometric exercise has no beneficial effect on recovery from the symptoms of exercise-induced muscle damage. *Ergonomics.* 2009;52(4):456–460.

134. Rowsell GJ, Coutts AJ, Reaburn P, Hill-Haas S. Effects of cold-water immersion on physical performance between successive matches in high-performance junior male soccer players. *J Sports Sci.* 2009;27(6):565–573.

135. Sellwood KL, Brukner P, Williams D, Nicol A, Hinman R. Ice-water immersion and delayed-onset muscle soreness: a randomised controlled trial. *Br J Sports Med.* 2007;41(6):392–397.

136. Leal Junior EC, de Godoi V, Mancalossi JL, et al. Comparison between cold water immersion therapy (CWIT) and light emitting diode therapy (LEDT) in short-term skeletal muscle recovery after high-intensity exercise in athletes–preliminary results. *Lasers Med Sci.* 2011;26(4):493–501.

137. McMaster WC. Cryotherapy. *Phys Sportsmed.* 1982;10(11):112–119.

13

Cryotherapy Application for Post–Immediate Care

OPENING SCENE

After reading about cryokinetics in the previous chapter, you decide to give it a try on Andrew, one of your patients, who suffered a second-degree ankle sprain yesterday. You prepare the container of ice water and slowly have him immerse his foot in the slush. You are not prepared for what happens next! He lifts his leg out of the water and yells, "This is too cold!" You have read about how effective cryokinetics is, and you want to continue the treatment. What can you do to help Andrew effectively get through the session?

Transition and Subacute Care Cryotherapy Techniques

In Chapters 6 and 12, we discussed the differences between cryotherapy for immediate care and for transition and post–immediate care. In Chapter 6, we discussed RICES application techniques for immediate care. In this chapter, we present application techniques for transition and post–immediate care.

Acute transition care begins once secondary injury stops. The goal is to facilitate therapeutic exercise by numbing the body so that active exercise can proceed pain-free. The two most common methods for local numbing are ice water immersion and ice massage. Occasionally an ice bag is used. Its construction and application are covered in Chapter 6.

ICE WATER IMMERSION

Ice water immersion, also called *ice bath immersion* and sometimes inappropriately called *ice water submersion*, is not simply immersing an extremity in a pail of ice water. While proper use of the technique is not complicated, there are a few tricks that improve its usefulness:

1. Use a container that is large enough for the extremity to fit, but that is not big and bulky. Also, a plastic or rubber container works better than a metal container. Since the metal container gets very cold, it is painful if the foot comes in contact with the edge of the metal container.

2. Fill the container with ice first and then add water. This will result in a bath temperature between 32 and 34°F (0–1°C). Warmer water may be less painful during the initial treatment, but does not numb the tissue as well.[1]

3. Help the patient adapt to the initial cold pain. He may become discouraged with the treatment if you leave him alone to think about the pain. Following are strategies that will diminish the pain sensation.

4. Give the patient a choice before beginning the treatment. For example, "We can use cryokinetics, which will be quite painful during the initial immersion but will get you back in 2–4 days. Or we can use the traditional heat treatments, which will not be painful and get you back in 2–3 weeks. Which would you prefer?"

5. Assure the patient that subsequent bouts of this session and subsequent sessions will be much less painful.[2] Point out that after a few days, he will feel little or no pain from the cold.

6. Use a toe cap when treating foot, ankle, or lower leg sprains (Fig. 13.1). It will minimize the pain if worn during immersion.[3,4] Most of the pain during ankle immersion is in the toes. The toe cap keeps the toes warm and, therefore, relatively pain-free, but has no effect on the uncovered portions of the foot and ankle.[4] Thus, it does not interfere with the benefits of the treatment. Patients are much more comfortable with a toe cap than without it.

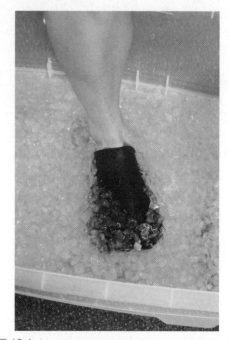

FIGURE 13.1 A neoprene toe cap helps decrease pain during ice water immersion.

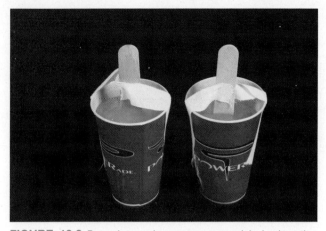

FIGURE 13.2 Preparing an ice massage popsicle by inserting a tongue depressor into the water prior to freezing. Note the tape used to hold the handle in the center during freezing.

7. Talk to the patient continuously during the initial immersion.[5] Any topic that will take his mind off the cold is appropriate. It doesn't matter if you exaggerate or downplay the potential pain; just talk about something.[5]

8. Make sure the patient goes through multiple immersion bouts during the first session. Subsequent bouts are much less painful than the first immersion.[2] Realizing this, patients are more likely to continue the treatments.

ICE MASSAGE

Ice massage is massage with ice, consisting of stroking a body part (usually a muscle) with a large ice cube or "popsicle" (6–8 oz). Here are tips for using ice massage:

1. Prepare ice cubes or popsicles by freezing water in paper drinking cups. The only difference between the two is that one has a tongue depressor inserted prior to freezing (Fig. 13.2).

2. To keep the patient from eating the ice, put a few drops of liquid soap into the cup before freezing.

3. Massage the muscle by grasping the ice cube with a towel or the handle of the tongue depressor and slowly stroking the muscle (Fig. 13.3a). Discontinue when the muscle is numb (10–20 minutes).

4. Numbness can be increased by adding resistance to the massage.[6] Do this by placing a 5–10-lb Olympic plate weight over the ice cube. Use the weight as a handle to maneuver the ice over the muscle (Fig. 13.3b).

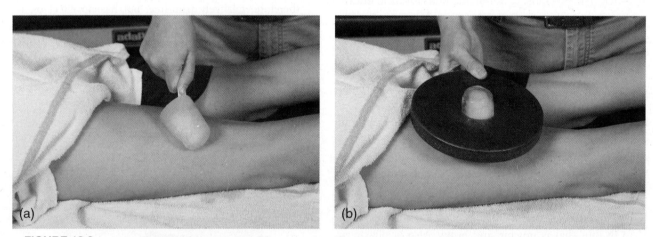

FIGURE 13.3 Ice massage with **(a)** a popsicle or **(b)** an ice cube with a plate weight to add pressure to the area for faster numbing.

5 STEPS | Application of Cryokinetics for Joint Sprains

1 STEP 1: FOUNDATION

A. Definition. **Cryokinetics** is a combination of cold applications and active exercise (Fig. 13.4).[7]

B. Effects
   1. Cold decreases pain and arthrogenic muscle inhibition, thus allowing exercise.
   2. Ice moderates arthrogenic muscle inhibition.
   3. Exercise stimulates increased blood flow.
   4. Exercise reestablishes neuromuscular functioning.
   5. Stresses induced by exercise influence collagen deposition and fiber orientation during repair.

C. Advantages
   1. It allows exercise much sooner than normally would be the case.
   2. Exercise
      a. Retards muscular atrophy
      b. Retards neural inhibitions
      c. Reduces swelling dramatically through muscular milking action
   3. Ice is inexpensive; exercise is free.

D. Disadvantages
   1. The extreme cold is very painful during the initial ice immersion of the first session. (The patient usually adapts, and subsequent immersions of the specific body part are not as painful.)
   2. Melting ice can be messy.

E. Indications
   1. Ankle sprains
      a. Cryokinetics is more effective on ankle sprains than any other injury.
      b. Cryokinetics is more effective on ankle sprains than any other technique for treating the ankle.
   2. Finger sprains
   3. Shoulder sprains
   4. Other joint sprains

F. Contraindications
   1. Any exercise or activity that causes pain
   2. Use of ice on a person who is hypersensitive to cold

G. Precautions
   1. Pain must be used as a guideline. The patient should not consciously or willfully overcome or "gut out" pain.
   2. When treating lower extremity injuries, the patient might limp if she is not regularly reminded to refrain from limping. Limping could lead to overuse injuries to surrounding and contralateral structures.
   3. There may be an increase in pain 4–8 hours after treatment.

2 STEP 2: PREAPPLICATION TASKS

A. Make sure cryokinetics is the proper modality for this situation.
   1. Reevaluate the injury/problem. Make sure you understand the patient's condition.
   2. If cryokinetics was applied previously, review the patient's response to the previous treatment.
   3. Confirm that the objectives of therapy are compatible with cryokinetics.
   4. Make sure cryokinetics is not contraindicated in this situation.

B. Preparing the patient psychologically
   1. Explain the four sensations that the person will go through during ice immersion:
      a. Pain will be very intense during the first application, but will lessen considerably during subsequent treatments.
      b. Warming
      c. Ache or numbing
      d. Numbness—relative anesthesia
   2. Explain that the extreme cold will be very painful during the first application. But also explain that the advantages of the treatment compensate for the discomfort (exercise will be possible, so rehabilitation will proceed much more quickly.)

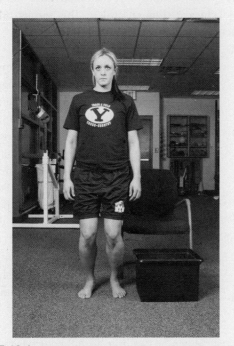

FIGURE 13.4 In a cryokinetics treatment, a patient actively exercises following cold-induced numbing.

C. Preparing the patient physically
   1. Remove necessary clothing (if ice massage is used, the ice will melt and create a puddle of water).
   2. Position the patient so she is comfortable.
D. Equipment preparation
   1. Have a container and ice or popsicle available.
   2. A toe cap is helpful, but not necessary.
   3. Have a towel if ice massage is used, to sop up the melting ice

3 ⬛ STEP 3: APPLICATION PARAMETERS

A. Procedures
   1. Numb the body part by applying ice to the injured area:
      a. Immersion in ice water is preferred, but if that method is not possible, use:
         i. Massage with ice cubes (made in 6–8 oz paper cups)
         ii. Ice bag (ice in a plastic bag)
         iii. Ice packs (ice folded in a towel)
      b. The ice application lasts through four sensations (listed above) and takes 10–20 minutes. However, the patient's sensation is more important than the length of application. When the patient reports numbness, begin exercising; continued cold application wastes time.
         i. Some people (about 10–20%) cannot judge when they are numb. If the patient does not report numbness after 20 minutes (5 minutes when renumbing), assume that pain is sufficiently decreased, and proceed with the exercise phase of the treatment.
      c. Help the patient endure the initial cold pain. She might become discouraged if left alone to think about the pain. Avoid this by talking continuously during the initial immersion to distract attention from the discomfort.[5]
         i. Use a toe cap when treating lower limb injuries. It will substantially reduce pain.
      d. Alternative: If cold applications fail to provide enough pain relief for exercise, try TENS or NEMS.
   2. Exercise the area, as explained below, for as long as it remains numb (about 3 minutes).
   3. Reapply the ice until numbness is again reached (about 3–5 minutes).
   4. Exercise the injured area, alternating with ice immersion and numbness at least five times during each treatment.
   5. Exercising, not the ice, causes rehabilitation.
      a. Remember, numbing serves no purpose other than to allow the body part to actively exercise.

6. Principles of cryokinetic exercises:
   a. All exercise should be:
      i. Active—performed by the patient
      ii. Progressive (increasing in both intensity and complexity)
      iii. Pain-free. Never use an exercise or motion that causes pain. If a particular exercise does cause pain, return to the former activity level.
   b. Exercise as long as the body part is numb, usually 2–3 minutes. As the numbness begins to wear off, reapply the cold. (Renumbing will only take 3–5 minutes.)
   c. Begin with simple range of motion (ROM) activities and progress through full activity, or sport-specific drills.
   d. Exercise must be performed without pain and in a normal, rhythmic, coordinated fashion.
   e. Constantly encourage the patient to progress to the next level of activity (as long as all exercise is performed properly). With some injuries, progression through full activity will take place in a single treatment session, while with others it may take weeks.
   f. The time spent performing an activity or the number of repetitions is not important. The key to cryokinetics is the ability to perform exercise of increasing difficulty properly and without pain.
7. This example of an exercise progression for an ankle sprain can be used as a model for similar progressions for other joints. The exercise progression begins with a basic ROM movement and successively becomes more difficult until full activity is achieved. For an athlete, this means full sport activity, without restrictions.
   a. Non-weight-bearing ROM (Fig. 13.5a)
      i. Perform plantar flexion, dorsiflexion, inversion, eversion, and circumduction (pointing toes to ground, toward nose, to right, to left, and moving in a circle) with the ankle to the limits of motion and/or pain. Exercises such as writing the alphabet with the big toe or picking up a marble with the toes are other ways of requiring the patient to go through an active ROM.[8]
      ii. Move on to the next step when full pain-free ROM is achieved.
   b. Bearing weight
      i. The patient stands with most of his weight on the uninjured leg. He then slowly shifts his weight back and forth between the uninjured and injured legs, while progressively bearing more weight on the injured leg.
      ii. When he can bear his full body weight on the injured leg, progress to the next step.

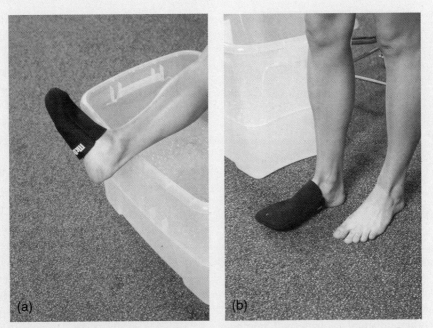

FIGURE 13.5 Begin cryokinetic exercising with **(a)** non-weight-bearing active range-of-motion exercises. Progress to **(b)** weight-bearing ROM exercises with crouching and toe raises.

c. Weight-bearing ROM
   i. With his weight on both legs (Fig. 13.5b), perform plantar flexion and dorsiflexion on the ankle by alternatively crouching and raising up on the toes.
   ii. If dorsiflexion is difficult or extremely limited, have him perform Achilles tendon (heel cord) stretches (Fig. 13.6) as part of each subsequent treatment session.[8]

d. Walking
   i. Begin with short steps (heel to toe) and walk straight ahead, gradually lengthening the steps (Fig. 13.7). Once normal stride length is achieved, walk in gentle arcs or large circles. Progress to making sharper cuts on turns.
   ii. Do not allow the patient to limp.
      (a) Limping is subconscious, and simply telling him not to limp will not help. You must

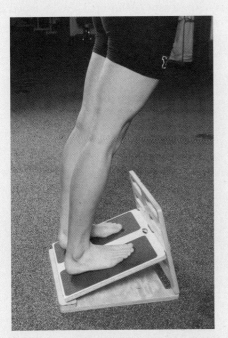

FIGURE 13.6 Achilles tendon (heel cord) stretching is indicated if the patient lacks dorsiflexion.

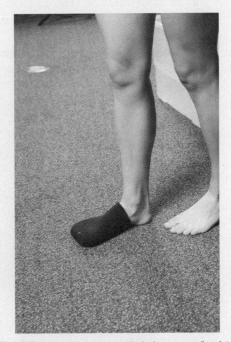

FIGURE 13.7 Walking begins with baby steps (heel to toe as shown below) and progresses to medium-length steps and then to large steps.

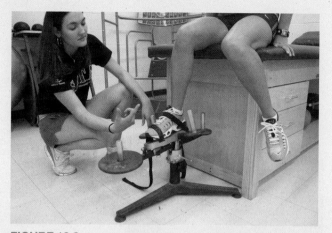

FIGURE 13.8 Resistive ankle strengthening begins as soon as the patient can walk. Ankle strengthening is done without numbness, after a cryokinetic session.

constantly supervise the walking (and subsequent running), looking for limping or any other unnatural gait pattern. If limping persists, work with him to eliminate it.

(b) If the limb is sufficiently numbed, pain during walking or running, he is not ready for this level of activity and should return to a former activity level (short-step walking or weight-bearing ROM).

(c) Limping can also occur if the patient has one shoe on and one off; be sure both shoes are off before the patient begins to walk.

e. Strengthening the ankle muscles

  i. Perform inversion, eversion, and dorsiflexion on an ankle machine (Fig. 13.8) or with a weighted boot, using the daily adjustable pro-

gressive resistive exercise (DAPRE) technique.[9,10] Plantar flexion exercises on a weight machine are not necessary. Walking and normal toe raises are adequate to develop plantar flexion strength.

  ii. Perform the muscle strengthening exercises once a day, after one of the cryokinetic sessions. Cold applications prior to or during weight training are unnecessary.

f. Jogging

  i. Once the patient can walk briskly, with turns and without pain or limping, gradually increase speed until he is jogging. Initial jogging should be slow and straight ahead. As tolerance increases, progress to jogging in a lazy S or figure-eight pattern, then in a sharp Z pattern.

  ii. A hallway is a convenient location for jogging. The patient can begin the S pattern jogging with large sweeps from side to side in the hallway (Fig. 13.9). The S is gradually tightened until the pattern is a sharp Z. Progress to sprinting, hopping, and jogging.

g. Hopping and jumping (performed simultaneously with sprinting)

  i. Any type of hopping and jumping is acceptable, as long as it is pain free. We like the *four-square program*[11] because it provides excellent guidelines for progressing through hopping and jumping with increasing complexity (Fig. 13.10). Place a large + on the floor with adhesive tape. Instruct (and demonstrate if necessary) the patient to jump from square to square (delineated by the taped cross) in

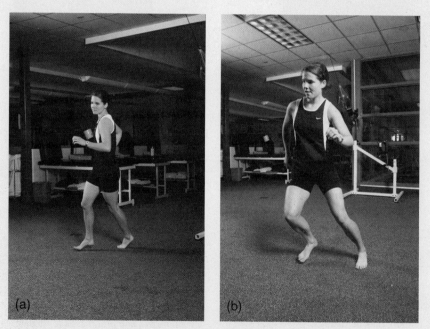

(a)   (b)

FIGURE 13.9 Jogging begins slowly and straight ahead. It progresses to **(a)** lazy S and **(b)** sharp Z patterns. Speed increases until the patient is jogging.

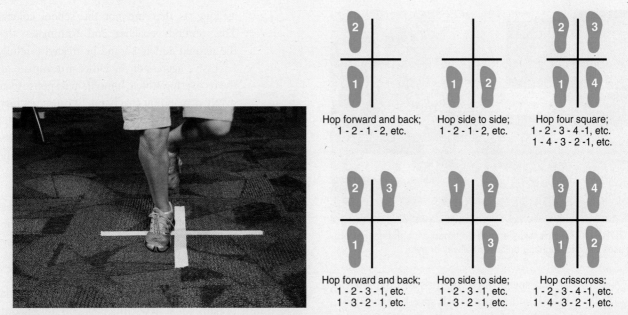

Hop forward and back;
1 - 2 - 1 - 2, etc.

Hop side to side;
1 - 2 - 1 - 2, etc.

Hop four square;
1 - 2 - 3 - 4 -1, etc.
1 - 4 - 3 - 2 -1, etc.

Hop forward and back;
1 - 2 - 3 - 1, etc.
1 - 3 - 2 - 1, etc.

Hop side to side;
1 - 2 - 3 - 1, etc.
1 - 3 - 2 - 1, etc.

Hop crisscross:
1 - 2 - 3 - 4 -1, etc.
1 - 4 - 3 - 2 -1, etc.

FIGURE 13.10 Four-square hopping exercises include hopping forward and back, side to side, in a square, and diagonally—first using both feet and then using only the injured foot. Perform the exercises in the order below, mastering each exercise before performing the next exercise.

the following progression, as tolerated: both feet forward and back, side to side, then diagonally; one foot (injured) forward and back, side to side, then diagonally. Progress also from short shallow hops to long high hops.

ii. After the patient has mastered the four-square program, have him hop on the injured foot back and forth across a crack or imaginary line in the floor while progressing forward across the room (Fig. 13.11).

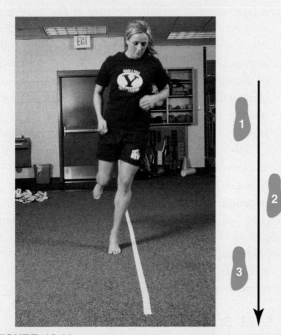

FIGURE 13.11 A line-hopping exercise involves hopping back and forth across a center line, on the injured foot, while progressing forward.

h. Sprinting (performed simultaneously with hopping and jumping)
  i. Begin with short (5–10 yard) straight-ahead, slow sprints. Start and stop slowly at first, then progress gradually to distinct starts and stops (e.g., an explosive push-off and "stopping on a dime").
  ii. Progress to sprinting in a lazy S or figure-eight pattern, then in a sharp Z pattern.

i. Hopping and sprinting without ice numbing
  Gradually increase the duration of hopping, jumping, and sprinting beyond the period of numbing until the patient can perform these activities without the aid of numbing.

j. Ankle taping
  i. The ankle should be taped during the following phases of team drills and practices (Fig. 13.12). During earlier phases of cryokinetic exercising, the ankle need not—in fact, should not—be taped. The earlier exercises are performed indoors, on a smooth surface (such as a hall floor) where there is little chance of reinjury.
  ii. Taping is unnecessary; in fact, it will interfere with treatment. If you tape the ankle prior to numbing, the tape will insulate the ankle and thereby reduce the effects of the ice. If you tape the ankle after numbing it, you will waste valuable exercising time. You only have 2–3 minutes of numbness to work with.

k. Team drills
  i. Team drills are a natural progression from hopping, jumping, and sprinting. Begin them

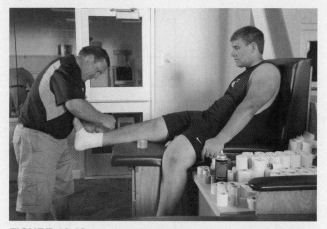

FIGURE 13.12 The injury should be taped once the patient progresses beyond sprinting drills in a hallway or gym.

at half speed, then progress to three-quarter speed, and finally to full speed (Fig. 13.13).

ii. As with all aspects of cryokinetics, pay particular attention during team drills and practice to how the patient performs. All activities must be performed with proper mechanics. Any pain, hesitancy, or irregular movement indicates she is not ready for the complexity of the activity. In that case, have her perform at a lower level for a while.

iii. Patients who are not fully rehabilitated must be protected while performing reduced-intensity team drills. One way of doing so is to have them wear an "off-color" jersey so they are easily distinguished by coaches and teammates. (Red or green jerseys are good colors to use,

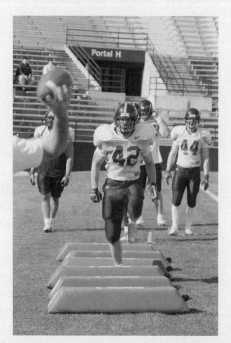

FIGURE 13.13 Individual drills with the team help patients progress beyond running and improve their mental state.

as long as they are not the school colors.) This reminds coaches and teammates that the injured athlete should be treated carefully. Excessive aggression by either a teammate, or the recovering athlete himself, in response to an overly demanding coach, might cause reinjury.

    l. Team practice.
       Begin at reduced speed and intensity the first day, and progress to full speed, complexity, and intensity as quickly as possible.

9. A complete cryokinetic session consists of:
   a. 10–20 minutes ice application for initial numbness
   b. Five exercise bouts with numbness in between
   c. Each exercise bout consists of active exercises during the numbness (about 3 minutes).

B. Dosage
   1. Exercise as vigorously as possible but within the limits of pain. Most new clinicians will not encourage their patients to progress as rapidly as possible.
C. Length of application
   1. Five exercise bouts per treatment session
D. Frequency of application
   1. Two or three times per day
E. Duration of therapy
   1. Until patient returns to full, unhindered activity

4 STEP 4: POSTAPPLICATION TASKS

A. Instructions to the patient
   1. Instruct the patient to use whatever supportive devices (elastic wrap, crutches, sling, etc.) were used before the treatment. Many patients will have a false sense of security because of the numbing; they may feel no pain during activities of daily living during the treatment, but once the joint fully rewarms, such activities may be painful. Our rule of thumb is: Leave with the same joint support you came with. If after a few hours, the support is not needed, the patient can discontinue using it.
   2. Instruct the patient about the level of activity and/or self-treatment prior to the next formal treatment.
   3. Explain that the patient might feel pain in 4–8 hours. If so, apply an ice pack for 30 minutes.
   4. Schedule the next treatment.
B. Record of treatment, including unique patient responses
C. Area cleanup
   1. Put away the ice container, towel, etc.
   2. Wipe up any water from the floor.

5 STEP 5: MAINTENANCE

A. Replace the slush container when it cracks.
B. Sew the sides of the toe caps if they rip.

5 STEPS Application of Cryostretch for Muscle Injuries

1 STEP 1: FOUNDATION

A. Definition. **Cryostretch** includes three techniques: cold application, static stretching, and the hold relax technique of PNF.[12] It is used following muscle strains to increase flexibility by decreasing muscle spasm (Fig. 13.14).

B. Effects
1. Ice decreases pain and muscle spasm.
2. Static stretching overcomes the stretch reflex, thereby reducing muscle spasm.
3. A muscle or muscle group will often relax following a near-maximal contraction to a state of relaxation greater than it was prior to the contraction.

C. Advantages
1. Combining the three techniques (icing, static stretching, and contraction/relaxing) in one procedure is more effective than applying any of the techniques independently.
2. Ice is inexpensive, and exercise is free.

D. Disadvantages
1. Ice is sometimes painful to some people, but the techniques used with cryostretch (ice massage and ice bag) are not as painful as ice immersion, which is preferred with cryokinetics.
2. Melting ice can be messy.

E. Indications
1. Any muscle with residual, low-grade, muscle spasm
2. Any first-degree muscle strain
3. A muscle that is stiff from prolonged disuse (immobilization). Do not confuse this with decreased range of motion due to connective tissue contractures. Cryostretch is contraindicated for the latter.

F. Contraindications
1. Any exercise or activity that causes pain
2. Use of ice on a person who is hypersensitive to cold (see Chapter 6)

3. Decreased range of motion due to connective tissue contractures

G. Precautions
1. Pain must be used as a guideline. The patient should not consciously or willfully overcome or "gut out" the pain.
2. There may be an increase in pain 4–8 hours after treatment.
3. Tearing or pulling a muscle is a possibility if the static exercise begins too quickly or suddenly. It must be a gradual buildup to a maximal contraction.

2 STEP 2: PREAPPLICATION TASKS

Same as cryokinetic preapplication tasks (see above)

3 STEP 3: APPLICATION PARAMETERS

A. Procedures
1. Apply ice to the injured muscle(s) by:
   a. Ice massage (with 6–8 oz ice cubes or popsicle) (see Figs. 13.2 and 13.3)
   b. Ice bag (crushed ice in a plastic bag)
   c. Ice pack (commercial gel pack)
2. Continue the ice application until the body part is numb (10–20 minutes). *Note*: The goal is numbness, not 10–20 minutes of application. Some people, however, cannot judge when they are numb. Therefore, stop the application after 20 minutes, whether or not the patient reports numbness.
3. Stretch the muscle(s), as explained below, for as long as numbness remains (about 3 minutes).
4. Reapply the ice until numbness is again reached (about 3–5 minutes).
5. A complete treatment consists of three bouts of stretching alternating with ice and numbness. Each stretching bout consists of two 60-seconds sets of stretching (Box 13.1).

BOX 13.1 A SUMMARIZED CRYOSTRETCH EXERCISE SET

20-second static stretch
5-second isometric contraction
10-second static stretch
5-second isometric contraction
10-second static stretch
5-second isometric contraction
10-second static stretch

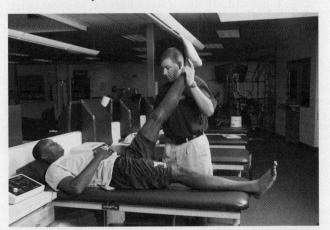

FIGURE 13.14 A hamstring is statically stretched as part of a cryostretch treatment.

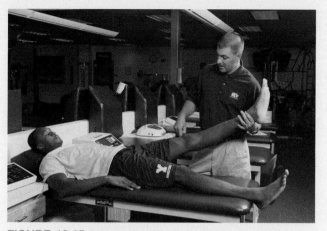

FIGURE 13.15 Prior to the first exercise bout, the patient must learn to contract the proper muscle.

6. Both stretching and the ice result in muscle relaxation, but the stretching is more important than the ice.

7. Each set of stretching consists of passive stretching and static contraction of the muscle(s) needing to be relaxed as follows:

a. (Part of the first bout only.) Help the patient get the feel of using the affected muscle by actively contacting it and moving the appropriate joint through as great a range of motion as possible (Fig. 13.15). Offer no resistance—this is demonstration only. Repeat the motion two or three times, making sure the affected muscle performs the majority of the work.

b. Passively stretch the muscle by moving the affected limb until the patient begins to feel tightness and/or pain. If pain is felt, back off just slightly.

c. Hold the position for 20 seconds.

d. Explain to the patient that in a few moments you will tell him to contract the muscle. At this time:

  i. He attempts to perform the same motion that he practiced earlier.

  ii. Explain that no motion will be possible, however, because you will be holding the limb/body part so as to resist motion.

  iii. State: "Do not contract the muscle quickly or suddenly." Emphasize that the contraction must start slowly and build up to a maximal contraction.

e. The patient contracts the affected muscle for 5 seconds, beginning slowly and building up to a maximal contraction while you resist the movement (it should be an isometric contraction).

f. The patient relaxes the contraction. You then move the limb until he feels tightness and/or pain. (The range of motion should be greater than in step b.) Hold this passive stretch for 10 seconds.

g. Repeat steps d–f twice more.

h. Return the limb to the anatomical position and rest for 20 seconds.

i. Perform the second bout of stretching by repeating steps b–g.

8. A complete cryostretch session consists of:

a. 10–20 minutes of ice application for initial numbness

b. Three exercise bouts with numbness in between (see Box 13.1)

c. Each exercise bout consists of two 65-seconds sets of passive stretch/isometric contractions, with a 20-seconds rest between sets.

B. Dosage

1. Stretch as much as possible but within the limits of pain.

C. Length of application

1. Three exercise bouts per treatment session

D. Frequency of application

1. Two or three times per day

E. Duration of therapy

1. Until the muscle spasm or tightness diminishes. At that points, transition into a combination of cryostretch and cryokinetics

4 | STEP 4: POSTAPPLICATION TASKS

A. Instructions to the patient

1. Instruct the patient to use whatever supportive devices (elastic wrap, crutches, sling, etc.) as were used before the treatment. Many patients will have a false sense of security because of the numbing; they may feel no pain during activities of daily living during the treatment, but once the joint fully rewarms, such activities may be painful. Our rule of thumb is: Leave with the same joint support you came with. If after a few hours the support is not needed, you can discontinue using it.

2. Instruct the patient about the level of activity and/or self-treatment prior to the next formal treatment.

3. Explain that the patient might feel pain in 4–8 hours. If so, apply an ice pack for 30 minutes.

4. Schedule the next treatment.

B. Record of treatment, including unique patient responses

C. Area cleanup

1. Put away the ice container, towel, etc.

2. Wipe up any water from the floor.

5 | STEP 5: MAINTENANCE: NONE

Application of Combined Cryostretch and Cryokinetics

A. This combination of modalities is used to treat muscle strains once spasm is relieved and joint ROM is within 90% of normal.

B. Administer the same as for cryostretch except:
1. During the second set of the first stretching bout, after the initial 20-second stretch, the patient performs 6–10 repetitions of full ROM contraction against manual resistance.
2. The patient performs only one set during each of the second and third exercise bouts. This set is the same as the second set of the first bout, that is, a 20-second passive stretch followed by 6–10 full ROM repetitions against manual resistance.

C. Encourage the patient to work hard during the muscle contraction, especially at the end of the ROM.

D. Once the strength begins to return (2–4 days), switch the patient to some type of isotonic weight lifting, preferably using the DAPRE technique.[9,10]

Application of Connective Tissue Stretch

STEP 1: FOUNDATION

A. Definition. The **connective tissue stretch** is a combination of heat application, long-term passive stretch, and cold applications (Fig. 13.16). It is used to increase joint flexibility following prolonged immobilization during which connective tissue contractures have developed.

B. Effects
1. Heat causes collagen fibers to relax.
2. Stretch lengthens the collagen fibers.
3. Cold causes the collagen fibers to reattach in a lengthened position if the stretch is held.[12]

C. Advantages
1. Heat applications minimize collagen tearing by inducing fiber relaxation.
2. Cold applications cause the fiber to reform in a lengthened position, thus preserving the gains made during stretching.
3. Minimal equipment needed

D. Disadvantages
1. 30 minutes of stretching is boring.

E. Indications
1. Reduced joint flexibility due to immobilization

F. Contraindications
1. Any exercise or activity that causes pain
2. Use of ice on a person who is hypersensitive to cold

G. Precautions
1. Avoid pain during stretching. It usually occurs because resistance is too great.

H. Alternatives
1. Thermal ultrasound or diathermy and mobilization (see Chapters 14 and 15)

STEP 2: PREAPPLICATION TASKS

A. Same as cryokinetics preapplication tasks (see above)

STEP 3: APPLICATION PARAMETERS

A. Procedures
1. Heat the injured joint for 10–30 minutes (depending upon the modality used):
   a. Shortwave pulsed diathermy is preferred for heating large areas.
   b. Use moist hot packs if diathermy is unavailable.
      i. Apply the hot packs to both sides, if it is a large joint.
      ii. Change the hot packs after 15 minutes to compensate for their cooling.
2. Stretch the joint with a low-level continuous passive force for 15 minutes.
   a. Begin stretching after 15 minutes of heating (Fig. 13.17).

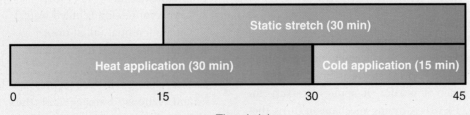

FIGURE 13.16 An outline of the connective tissue stretch, illustrating the timing, length of, and interaction between the three elements: heating, static stretch, and cooling.

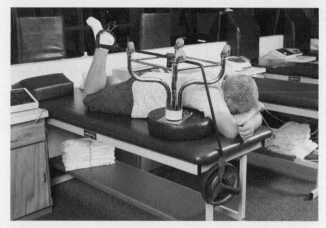

FIGURE 13.17 The hamstring is statically stretched during a connective tissue stretch treatment.

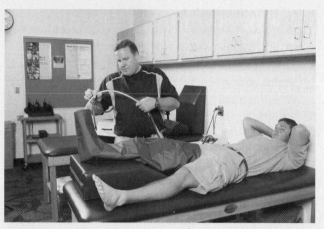

FIGURE 13.18 A lymphedema pump helps reduce swelling by forcing tissue debris from the injured tissue via the lymphatic system.

b. Use an external force such as 3–15 lb of weight. Manual resistance is unacceptable because it ties up a clinician for 15 minutes, because it is quite tiring for the clinician, and because a clinician will not be able to provide consistent constant pressure.

c. There is not a specific way to apply the resistance. Use your ingenuity. Attach one end of a rope or cord to the limb and the other end to the weight. Then place the rope over a fulcrum so the weight hangs down (see Fig. 13.18).

3. Discontinue heating and begin cooling the joint while maintaining the stretch. The collagen fibers that detached during the heating will reattach during cooling. If the joint is held in the stretched position during reattachment, the fibers will reattach in a lengthened position.

B. Dosage
1. Use as much resistance as is comfortable.

C. Length of application
1. 45 minutes
D. Frequency of application
1. Daily
E. Duration of therapy
1. 1–2 weeks

4 STEP 4: POSTAPPLICATION TASKS

A. Instructions to the patient
1. Schedule the next treatment.
2. Instruct the patient about the level of activity and/or self-treatment prior to the next formal treatment.
B. Record of treatment, including unique patient responses
C. Equipment removal

5 STEP 5: MAINTENANCE: NONE

5 STEPS Application of Lymphedema Pumps

1 STEP 1: FOUNDATION

A. Definition. **Lymphedema pumps** (known formerly as *intermittent compression pumps, cold compression devices, pneumatic compression pumps,* and *intermittent compression devices*) are pumps attached to a boot or sleeve that forces air or water (usually chilled water) into the sleeve. The boot or sleeve is fitted around a joint so that when it inflates, it applies pressure to the joint (Fig. 13.18). A timing mechanism turns the pump on and off so the sleeve alternates inflating and

deflating, thus providing intermittent compression. Classified as:
1. Pneumatic (air)
2. Cryocompression (chilled water)
3. Circumferential (all at once)
4. Sequential (distal to proximal)
B. Effects
1. The changes in sleeve pressure force lymphatic and venous drainage and thus reduce edema. Permanent reduction of edema occurs only after free protein from cellular debris is removed from

the tissue and capillary filtration pressure is normalized (see Chapter 5).

  2. Both the lymphatic system and the venous system contain one-way valves that allow contents to move proximally but block distal movement.

C. Advantages

  1. Requires minimal clinician time

D. Disadvantages

  1. The slow rate of boot/sleeve inflation. The rate of compression is much faster with either active exercise or massage.

E. Indications

  1. Post-traumatic edema
  2. Postoperative edema
  3. Chronic edema; primary and secondary lymphedema
  4. Venous stasis ulcers
  5. Persistent swelling caused by venous insufficiency

F. Contraindications. Intermittent compression should not be applied to a patient suffering from the following conditions (it could aggravate the condition):

  1. Compartment syndrome
  2. Peripheral vascular disease
  3. Arteriosclerosis
  4. Deep vein thrombosis
  5. Local superficial infection
  6. Edema secondary to congestive heart failure
  7. Ischemic vascular disease
  8. Gangrene
  9. Dermatitis
  10. Acute pulmonary edema
  11. Displaced fractures

G. Precautions

  1. Pain must be used as a guideline.

H. Alternatives

  1. Active muscle activity
  2. Massage

2 STEP 2: PREAPPLICATION TASKS

A. Same as cryokinetic preapplication tasks (see above)

3 STEP 3: APPLICATION PARAMETERS

A. Procedures

  1. Apply the sleeve or boot to the extremity and tighten it so it is snug but doesn't apply pressure to the limb.
  2. Attach the sleeve tube to the pump.
  3. If using a water device, fill the water container with ice and water.
  4. Select on/off times.
  5. Turn on the device.

B. Dosage

  1. Inflation pressure
     a. 40–60 mm Hg for upper extremity
     b. 60–100 mm Hg for lower extremity, but no greater than the patient's diastolic pressure
  2. On/off time sequence (45–15 seconds; 3:1 duty cycle)

C. Length of application

  1. 20 minutes

D. Frequency of application

  1. Two or three times per day

E. Duration of therapy

  1. Until the condition is resolved

4 STEP 4: POSTAPPLICATION TASKS

A. Instructions to the patient

  1. Schedule the next treatment.
  2. Instruct the patient about the level of activity and/or self-treatment prior to the next formal treatment.

B. Record of treatment, including unique patient responses

C. Area cleanup

  a. Equipment removal
  b. Clean the inside of the cuff or boot with a disinfectant.

5 STEP 5: MAINTENANCE

1. Periodically check hoses, valves, boots, and sleeves for leaks.

CLOSING SCENE

You're attempting to use cryokinetics on Andrew 48 hours after an ankle sprain. Since this is his first time receiving ice immersion, you gently immerse his ankle in the water. Within about 5 seconds, he pulls his leg from the water and yells, "This is too cold!" You now know some strategies to use to help him complete the treatment:

1. Use a toe cap.
2. Explain that using cryokinetics will get him back in 2–4 days (several times faster than using traditional heat treatments).
3. Assure him that subsequent treatments will be much less painful.
4. Explain that he will soon adapt to the cold.
5. Talk to him about anything to take his mind off of the pain, such as asking him about his family or his studies.

Andrew places his ankle back in the slush, and after about 18 minutes, he informs you that his ankle feels numb. He then goes through several sessions of weight bearing, gentle walking, and renumbing. He returns twice a day for cryokinetics and a week later plays in a basketball game, where he scores the winning basket. He thanks you for your wisdom and gives you the game ball.

Chapter Reflections

Now that you have read this chapter,

1. Read and ponder each of the following points. Do you feel you have a clear understanding of each concept? If not, reread the appropriate section of the chapter.

   • Discuss the use of ice water immersion in transitional acute care. Explain how it is different from crushed ice packs and why this is important to this stage of rehabilitation.

   • Explain when and how ice massage is used in transitional acute care.

   • Discuss the use of cryokinetics for joint sprain rehabilitation, including what it is, why it is used, and a brief overview of how to apply the therapy.

   • Discuss the use of cryostretch for muscle injury rehabilitation, including what it is, why it is used, and a brief overview of how to apply the therapy.

   • Why and when do you use combined cryostretch and cryokinetics?

   • Discuss the use of connective tissue stretch in rehabilitation, including what kinds of injuries would you use this technique with and how would you apply it.

   • Discuss why, when, and how you would use intermittent compression during rehabilitation.

2. Write three to five questions to discuss with your class instructor, clinical instructor, classmates, and clinical colleagues.

3. Get together with classmates and quiz each other on the concepts of this chapter. Use the points in reflection no. 1 and questions you wrote for reflection no. 2 as a beginning. Explaining concepts out loud to others requires a deeper grasp of the material than feeling you understand it as you read.

4. Once you feel you understand the principles of application, practice applying cryokinetics, cryostretch, connective tissue stretch, and intermittent compression treatments, using the five-step approach, with a classmate or clinical colleague. Alternate applying each modality to each other. When it is being applied to you, listen and observe carefully to determine whether your classmate is using proper application. Consult your notes when the modality is applied to you, and during the first few times you apply the modality to another person. Continue practicing the application until you can do so without using your notes.

REFERENCES

1. Jutte LS, Konz S, Knight KL. A 15 min immersion in 1°C water produces greater numbness than immersion in 4°C Or 10°C water. *J Athl Train*. 2012; In review.
2. Carman KW, Knight KL. Habituation to cold-pain during repeated cryokinetic sessions. *J Athl Train*. 1992;27:223–230.
3. Tovell J. Ice immersion toe cap. *Athl Train*. 1980;15:33.
4. Nimchick PSR, Knight KL. Effects of wearing a toe cap or a sock on temperature and perceived pain during ice water immersion. *Athl Train*. 1983;18:144–147.
5. Streator SS, Ingersoll CD, Knight KL. The effects of sensory information on the perception of cold-induced pain. *J Athl Train*. 1995;30:293–296.
6. Rogers J. *Increased Pressure of Application during Ice Massage Results in an Increase in Calf Skin Numbing*. [Masters]. Provo, UT: Physical Education, Brigham Young University; 2000.
7. Knight KL. Ankle Rehabilitation with Cryotherapy. *Phys Sportsmed*. 1979;7(11):133.
8. McClusky GM, Blackburn TA Jr, Lewis T. A treatment for ankle sprains. *Am J Sports Med*. 1976;4:158–161.
9. Knight KL. Knee rehabilitation by the daily adjustable progressive resistive exercise technique. *Am J Sports Med*. 1979;7(6):336–337.
10. Knight KL. Quadriceps strengthening with the DAPRE technique: case studies with neurological implications. *Med Sci Sports Exerc*. 1985;17:646–650.
11. Toomey SJ. Four-square ankle rehabilitation exercises. *Phys Sportsmed*. 1986;14(3):81.
12. Knight KL. Cryostretch for muscle injuries. *Phys Sportsmed*. 1980;8(4):126.

Therapeutic Ultrasound

OPENING SCENE

During a clinical rotation, Keira, an athletic training student, overhears some patients talking about previous ultrasound treatments they experienced. One says, "I don't think ultrasound works—I mean, I never feel anything." Another responds, "You're not supposed to feel anything during an ultrasound treatment, at least that's what I've heard." The third replies, "I feel some heat when my knee tendon is treated, but not when my low back is treated." They see Nancy and direct their questions to her. What should she tell them?

Introducing Therapeutic Ultrasound

Ultrasound is one of the most commonly used modalities by athletic trainers, typically employed to bring about deep heating (Fig. 14.1). It is one of the most misunderstood and, therefore, one of the most misused modalities. When placed in the hands of a competent clinician, it can provide positive outcomes; however, when used improperly, there are few benefits from this modality.

ORIGINS AND USE IN MEDICAL PRACTICE

Prior to World War II, German scientists were experimenting with sonar in submarines. Sound was emitted from the vessel to detect objects in the surrounding water. The scientists noticed that fish were destroyed in the process. Thus, the idea of ultrasound producing biological effects was born.

In the health professions, ultrasound is used for a number of different purposes, including the destruction of tissue, fetal development diagnosis, and as a therapeutic agent. Ultrasound has been used to destroy tumors in the breast, liver, kidney, pancreas, abdomen, pelvis, uterus, and lung (some treatments use a combination of chemotherapy and ultrasound).[1] Ultrasound has been used during surgery as recently as 2002 to seal air leaks in lungs, destroy blood clots, obliterate kidney stones, and seal blood vessels. Experiments are under way in using ultrasound for male sterilization[2] and treating some brain disorders.[3] In pregnant women, diagnostic ultrasound can be used to monitor the development of the fetus and determine its gender. Ultrasound is also used in plastic surgery, to heat and soften fat pockets under the eyes and chin prior to liposuction.[4] These various applications use ultrasound with very different characteristics; in this chapter, we are only concerned with ultrasound for treating musculoskeletal injuries.

Clinical Therapeutic Ultrasound

Therapeutic **ultrasound** is inaudible, acoustic vibrations of high frequency that produce thermal and/or nonthermal physiologic effects. It is not a form of electromagnetic energy. It is a valuable tool in the rehabilitation of many different injuries, primarily for the purpose of

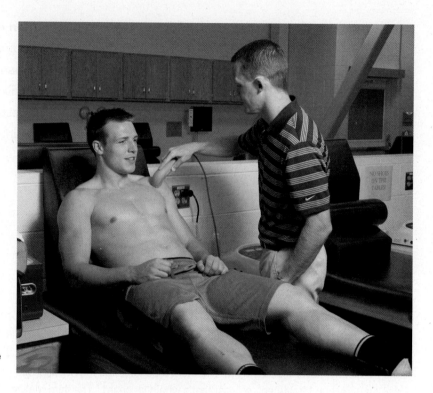

FIGURE 14.1 Ultrasound treatment of the biceps muscle.

stimulating the repair of soft tissue injuries and relieving pain.[5] Although ultrasound has effects on both normal and damaged tissues, damaged tissue may be more responsive to ultrasound than normal tissue.[6]

The primary advantage of ultrasound over other nonacoustic heating modalities is that tissues high in collagen—such as tendons, muscles, ligaments, joint capsules, joint menisci, intermuscular interfaces, nerve roots, periosteum, and cortical bone—as well as other deep tissues may be selectively heated to a therapeutic range without causing a significant tissue temperature increase in skin or fat.[7,8]

! Modality Myth

WHIRLPOOL, PARAFFIN BATHS, OR HOT PACKS ARE JUST AS EFFECTIVE FOR HEAT TREATMENTS AS ULTRASOUND

Warm whirlpools, paraffin baths, and silica gel hot packs all produce therapeutic heat, but their depth of penetration is superficial—at best only 1–2 cm.[9] At 1 cm below the fat surface, a 4-minute warm whirlpool (105°F, or 40.6°C) raises the temperature 2.0°F (1.1°C).[10] At this same depth, 3 MHz (megahertz) ultrasound increases the temperature over 10.8°F (6°C).[10,11] For deep heating, use an ultrasound device.

Components of an Ultrasound Device

An ultrasound device is made up of four main parts: a generator, a crystal, a soundhead, and an applicator.

THE GENERATOR

The largest part of an ultrasound device is the generator. It is typically a rectangular box consisting of a high-frequency electrical generator linked through an oscillator circuit and a transformer. The oscillator circuit produces a specific frequency electrical current at the frequency requirements of the crystal. A coaxial cable connects the generator to the crystal, which is housed in an insulated applicator handle.

The generator also houses a control panel with buttons or switches that regulate the following parameters: on/off; power; time; intensity; duty cycle; continuous or pulsed modes; 1 or 3 MHz frequency; automatic shut-off in case the crystal overheats.

THE CRYSTAL

The crystal is a thin (2–3 mm thick) synthetic ceramic, usually made of lead zirconate or titanate. Decades ago, most ultrasound crystals were made of quartz, but quartz was expensive, and it did not produce a uniform beam. Thus, the crystals used today are ceramic.

The **crystal** is a transducer that converts electrical energy to acoustic energy through mechanical deformation of the crystal. When an alternating electrical current is passed

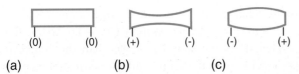

FIGURE 14.2 The contraction or expansion of a crystal is caused by passing an alternating current through it. **(a)** With no current flow, the crystal is normally shaped. **(b)** Current flow in one direction causes the crystal to become concave. **(c)** Current flow in the opposite direction causes the crystal to become convex.

through the crystal, it expands and contracts, creating what is referred to as the **piezoelectric effect**. There are two forms:

1. *Direct piezoelectric effect:* the creation of an electrical voltage across the crystal as it is compressed or expanded.
2. *Reverse piezoelectric effect:* an effect created from an alternating current running through a crystal, resulting in compression or expansion of the crystal (Fig. 14.2).

The expansion and contraction of the crystal creates a vibration at the frequency of the electrical oscillation received from the generator. The vibration of the crystal causes the soundhead to vibrate and results in the mechanical production of high-frequency sound waves.

THE SOUNDHEAD

The soundhead transfers the acoustic energy (sound waves) from the crystal to the tissues where it causes the tissue to vibrate. It is a ceramic, aluminum, or stainless steel plate attached to the crystal. Stainless steel soundheads last longer than aluminum or ceramic, and are therefore one of the features of higher quality ultrasound devices. Imagine the beating that the soundhead takes as a crystal expands and contracts at a speed of 1–3 million times per second.

Soundheads and crystals are manufactured to be matched to a particular generator, so they are generally not interchangeable between generators (Fig. 14.3). Recently, however, dual frequency crystals and soundheads have become standard equipment on ultrasound devices, so clinicians have a greater choice of treatment parameters.

⊙ Modality Myth

THE SOUNDHEAD IS A TRANSDUCER

Many clinicians, scientists, and marketing people refer to the soundhead as a transducer. This is incorrect, since a **transducer** is a device that converts variations in a physical quantity (such as pressure or brightness) into an electrical signal, or vice versa. So the crystal is a transducer that converts electricity to acoustic energy and the soundhead is a transmitter that transfers the acoustic energy to the body.

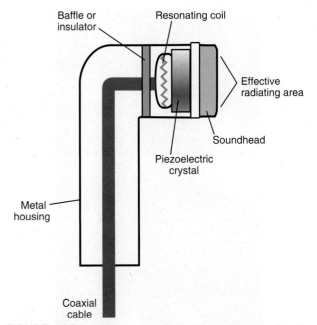

FIGURE 14.3 A typical ultrasound applicator. (Source: Prentice WE. *Therapeutic Modalities for Sports Medicine and Athletic Training*, 5th ed. New York: McGraw Hill, 2003:300.)

THE APPLICATOR

The applicator, which is the housing for the crystal and soundhead, is a device that facilitates application of the ultrasound to patients. The soundhead must be in constant motion during treatment, so the design of the applicator is important. It should allow the clinician to keep the wrist and hand in a neutral position, to avoid a repetitive injury, especially since clinicians often give several ultrasound treatments a day (see Box 14.1).

The applicator is usually made of a hard, insulated plastic. Some newer applicators also have controls on them so

BOX 14.1 A USER-FRIENDLY APPLICATOR

Since some ultrasound treatments may take more than 10 minutes, it is important that the applicator fits comfortably in your hand. Ergonomics is very important, and some manufacturers of ultrasound devices have hired design engineers to create a user-friendly applicator for clinicians. The result is a transducer with a 360° rotating soundhead so that the wrist can always be held in a neutral position. Figure 14.4 shows an ultrasound applicator with a rotating soundhead and control buttons on the handle. This makes it possible for the clinician to increase or decrease the intensity without having to look over to the generator switches and lose eye contact with the treatment area.

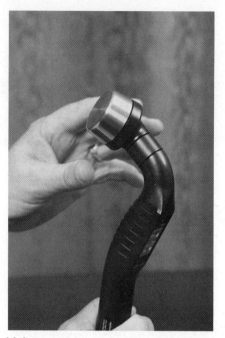

FIGURE 14.4 An applicator with a 360° rotating soundhead enables the clinician to hold the wrist in a neutral position. Notice the convenient location of the control buttons on the handle.

the clinician can vary the treatment characteristics during the treatment.

The Physics of Ultrasound

Now that you have been introduced to the components of an ultrasound device, let's explore the physics behind how ultrasound works.

WHAT IS SOUND?

Solids and liquids are made of molecules held together by forces that act like rubber bands, connecting each molecule to its next-door neighbor. When a force acts upon one molecule, it causes it to vibrate back and forth a small distance from its original position. This movement causes the molecule next door to vibrate, and eventually the whole neighborhood is set in motion. This vibrational energy travels over millions of molecules in the tissue. This transfer or spreading of vibrational motion is basically what sound is. Unlike electromagnetic energy that travels most effectively through a vacuum, acoustic energy is transmitted by molecules bumping against each other. As stated earlier, ultrasound is a mechanical wave in which energy is passed by the vibrations of the molecules of a biological medium through which the wave is traveling.

The human ear can hear sound waves that vibrate 16,000–20,000 times per second. Sound waves that vibrate faster than the human ear can hear are termed "ultra"

sound. Therapeutic ultrasound ranges from 750,000 to 3 million vibrations per second (0.75–3.0 MHz). If the wavelength of the sound is larger than the source that produced it, then the sound will spread in all directions.[12] Such is the case with audible sound, thus explaining why it is possible for a person behind you to hear your voice almost as well as a person in front of you. In the case of therapeutic ultrasound, the sound is less divergent, and energy is concentrated in a limited area.

TYPES OF WAVES

Imagine you are at the beach and decide to go for a swim in the ocean. As you swim out from the shore, waves crash against you and push you back. Ultrasound has a similar effect on tissues as the sound waves travel through them.

Waves travel through solids in two ways, as longitudinal and transverse waves. In a **longitudinal wave**, molecular displacement or vibration is along the direction in which the wave travels (somewhat like a stretched bungee cord); in a **transverse wave**, the molecules are transferred, or vibrate, in a direction perpendicular to that in which the wave is traveling.

Within a longitudinal wave pathway, there are regions of:

- **Compressions**: areas of high molecular density and high pressure as the molecules are squeezed together
- **Rarefactions**: areas of lower molecular density as the molecules are pulled apart (Fig. 14.5)

While longitudinal waves travel in solids and liquids, transverse waves travel only in solids. Ultrasound travels as a longitudinal wave through soft tissue. It becomes a transverse wave as it bounces back or rebounds when it hits bone. The compressions and rarefactions are similar to the squeezing together and pulling apart of a Slinky toy.

WAVE TRANSMISSION FREQUENCY

The higher the frequency of the sound waves emitted from a sound source, the less the sound will diverge (spread out), and thus a more focused beam of sound is produced. Therapeutic ultrasound produces a very focused or **collimated beam**, but not as focused as a laser beam, which has little divergence (see Chapter 19).

Whether or not an ultrasound wave is absorbed locally or transmitted to deeper tissues is also a function of sound frequency. In tissues of the body, ultrasound energy absorption increases as the frequency increases, thus less energy is transmitted to the deeper tissues. For example, most 3 MHz ultrasound waves are absorbed superficially and transmitted about 2–3 cm deep. This amount of absorption occurs in one-third the time of 1 MHz. On the other hand, 1 MHz ultrasound is absorbed deeper than 3 MHz and is transmitted up to 6 cm deep.

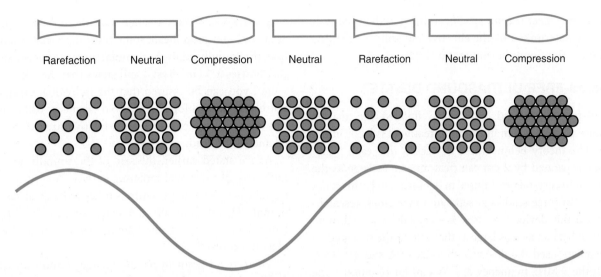

FIGURE 14.5 Ultrasound travels through soft tissue as a longitudinal wave, with alternating regions of high molecular density and pressure called compressions and regions of low molecular density called rarefactions. Thus, the molecules are squeezed together and pulled apart.

The majority of therapeutic ultrasound devices have a frequency between 0.75 and 3.0 MHz. Recently low-frequency or long-wave ultrasound (45 and 90 kHz) has been introduced. It is used for deep muscle heating and for phonophoresis (a technique that is discussed later in the chapter). It is thought that this frequency will provide the greatest depth of penetration in biological tissues, possibly up to 10 cm.

ATTENUATION

Ultrasound transducers produce a sound wave at a preset frequency. As this sound wave passes through various tissues, **attenuation**, or a decrease in energy, occurs as a result of absorption, reflection, and refraction of the wave (Fig. 14.6). Some of the energy is absorbed in the tissues. The remaining energy passes through tissues to deeper layers where it is later absorbed, or else it bounces off tissues. This bouncing off the tissues is known as *dispersion* and *scattering* of the sound wave. When a sound wave encounters a boundary or an interface between different tissues (e.g., fascia), some of the energy will also scatter.

The ability of acoustic energy to penetrate or be transmitted to deeper tissues depends, in part, on the type of tissue being treated. In the case of therapeutic ultrasound, the following tissue types have these responses:

- Tissue that is high in water content: Energy penetrates easily.
- Fat: Energy is absorbed very little and is transmitted to deeper tissues.
- Dense tissue that is high in protein: Energy is absorbed well.
- Muscle: Energy is absorbed in high amounts.

- Peripheral nerves: Energy is absorbed at twice the rate as muscle.
- Superficial bone: Energy is absorbed more efficiently than any other type of tissues.

CRYSTAL CHARACTERISTICS

Another factor that determines how well ultrasound will penetrate tissues is the crystal quality. Some manufacturers of ultrasound devices purchase hundreds of crystals, scan each one, and throw away three out of every four

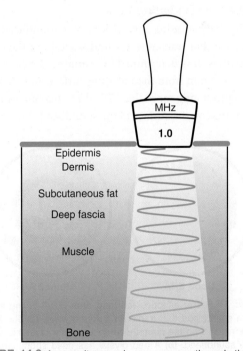

FIGURE 14.6 As an ultrasound wave passes through tissues, a decrease in energy, known as attenuation, results from the absorption, reflection, and refraction of energy. (Adapted with permission from Castel, D. International Academy of Physio Therapeutics. Clip Art.)

that do not meet certain specifications. Crystal quality is partially determined by the effective radiating area (ERA) and the beam nonuniformity ratio (BNR).

HANDS-FREE ULTRASOUND DEVICES

Hands-free ultrasound units have flooded the market because performing an ultrasound treatment is labor intensive. The theory behind these devices is that each 5 cm^2 crystal separated by 2 cm can treat an area as large as the well that the crystals are housed in. Unfortunately, this is not true.[13,14] In three studies at separate universities, researchers used this device that uses 3–4 crystals in a well in an effort to heat an area as large as the well. In the first study,[13] researchers used the device with a 2.9 ERA and 4.4 BNR. With the 3 MHz frequency at 1 W/cm^2 for 8 minutes, the peak heating was only 1.8°C. An Omnisound with the same-sized crystal heated tissue to 3.2°C or over 40% higher. In the second study,[14] a similar unit at 3 MHz, 1.5 W/cm^2, for 10 minutes resulted in a peak temperature of 2.02°C. Two manual technique devices, with similar parameters resulted in 3.38°C and 4.53°C peak temperatures, 33% and 55% greater. The proposed reason for these results is that there is a time delay from one crystal to the next and that there is no heating under the dead space where no crystal exists. Based upon this, we suggest that stationary ultrasound machines not be used for ultrasound purposes, not even for nonthermal effects, as this will compromise the effect of the molecular events from lower joule output.

The Effective Radiating Area

The **effective radiating area (ERA)** of a soundhead is its surface area that transmits a sound wave from the crystal to the tissues. It is determined by scanning the crystal at a distance of 5 mm from the radiating surface and recording all areas producing more than 5% of the maximum power output found on the surface of the soundhead (Fig. 14.7).[12]

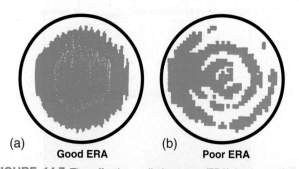

(a) Good ERA **(b) Poor ERA**

FIGURE 14.7 The effective radiating area (ERA) is the surface area of a soundhead that transmits a sound wave. **(a)** The ERA is always smaller than the soundhead because the crystal is smaller than the soundhead. **(b)** A bad crystal has dead spots, where no sound is transmitted, so its ERA is much smaller than the ERA of an equal-sized good crystal. (Adapted with permission from Castel, D. International Academy of Physio Therapeutics. Clip Art.)

The ERA is always smaller than the crystal (typically >0.5 cm^2) and soundhead; sometimes significantly smaller than the soundhead. If the manufacturer produces a device that houses a 5-cm^2 crystal and states that the ERA is also 5 cm^2, you can be assured that the individual crystal has not been scanned for quality.[15] No crystal is 100% active; this is not as big a concern as the relative sizes of the crystal and soundhead.

As we stated earlier, the size of the soundhead is not indicative of the actual radiating surface. A very common mistake is to assume the entire surface radiates ultrasound output. This is generally not true, particularly with the larger 10-cm^2 soundheads (slightly smaller than the size of a doorknob).[16]

There is no point in having a large soundhead with a small radiating surface because it mechanically limits the treatment in smaller areas. The ERA should match the total size of the crystal and soundhead surface as closely as possible for ease of application to various body surfaces, in order to maintain the most effective contact (Fig. 14.8).

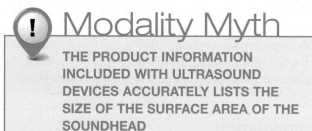

Modality Myth

THE PRODUCT INFORMATION INCLUDED WITH ULTRASOUND DEVICES ACCURATELY LISTS THE SIZE OF THE SURFACE AREA OF THE SOUNDHEAD

Unfortunately, this is a gray area in ultrasound advertising. The majority of ultrasound devices are reported as having a 5-cm^2 soundhead; however, this is the size of the crystal inside the soundhead. Soundheads listed as 5 cm^2 have been found to have surface areas between 7 and 11 cm^2.[16] Thus, if a soundhead surface is twice the size of the crystal, the clinician might think a larger area is being treated than actually is. We suggest that in the future, ultrasound manufacturers list the size of the surface area of the soundhead and the size of the crystal (Fig. 14.9).

CONCEPT CHECK 14.1. You are visiting another clinic and notice that the clinician is treating a patient who has a chronic hamstring strain. He is applying ultrasound to his entire leg. Is this the best treatment choice for heating?

The Beam Nonuniformity Ratio

Ultrasound beams are not completely uniform; they have small peaks and valleys on them. Some points are of higher intensity (peaks) than others away from the

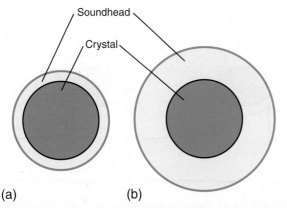

(a)   (b)

FIGURE 14.8 The relationship between soundhead and crystal is illustrated here. In **(a)** the crystal is almost as big as the soundhead, so most of the tissue under the soundhead is treated. But in **(b)** the crystal is much smaller than the soundhead, so much of the tissue under the soundhead is untreated. For best treatments, select an ultrasound machine in which the soundhead and crystal are close to the same size.

soundhead surface. The **beam nonuniformity ratio (BNR)** is an indicator of the variability of intensity within an ultrasound beam. The BNR is the ratio of the **spacial peak intensity**, highest intensity in the beam, to the **spacial average intensity (SAI)**, the average intensity across the beam, both of which are measured with an underwater microphone. For example, a BNR of 5:1 means when the average output intensity is 1 W/cm^2, the highest intensity of the beam is 5 W. Figure 14.10 shows the peaks and valleys of a beam scan of a high and low BNR.

An optimal BNR is 1:1 (a smooth line with no peaks and valleys); however, this is not possible. The BNR should fall between 2 and 5. The lower the BNR, the more uniform the output and therefore the lower the chance of developing hot spots. A **hot spot** is an area at tissue interfaces that may become overheated from too much energy being concentrated in one area. Hot spots often result in pain, and they can damage tissues. A low BNR allows the clinician to deliver ultrasound at a higher energy level without causing discomfort to the patient.

The U.S. Food and Drug Administration (FDA) Center for Devices and Radiological Health requires that the BNR be indicated on all ultrasound devices. Manufacturers do not have to report the BNR of individual crystals, so the BNR of the soundhead being used may be different from that indicated on the label. The FDA allows companies to randomly sample their crystals and report the maximum BNR.[17] Thus, a company might label their crystals as 6:1 BNR Max. If a 6:1 BNR is used at an intensity of 1.5 W/cm^2, tissue damage could occur, since peak intensities of only 8 W have been shown to damage tissue.

The high peak intensities associated with high BNRs cause much of the discomfort often associated with ultrasound treatment.[17] From personal experience, this feels like a dull ache on the outer layer of the bone (*periosteal pain*). Therefore, the higher the BNR, the more important it is to use lower intensities, or to move the soundhead faster during treatment to avoid hot spots and areas of tissue damage.

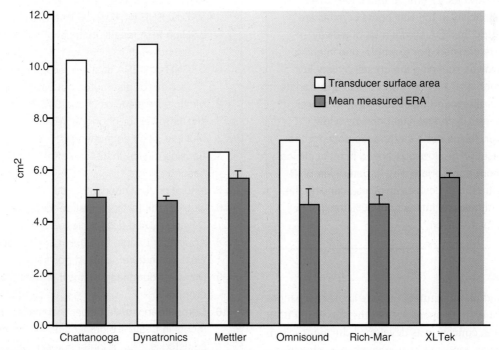

FIGURE 14.9 This graph illustrates the variability that exists between ultrasound manufacturers. Note how the effective radiating area (ERA) of the crystal is <50% the size of the surface of the soundhead in the first two devices. The ERA size should be closer to the transducer surface size, such as the four devices on the right. (Adapted with permission from Johns et al.[16])

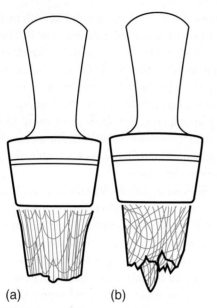

FIGURE 14.10 The BNR represented on a beam scan. The amount of intensity variability within the ultrasound beam is indicated by the BNR. **(a)** A low BNR of 2:1. **(b)** A high BNR of 6:1. (Adapted with permission from Castel, D. International Academy of Physio Therapeutics. Clip Art.)

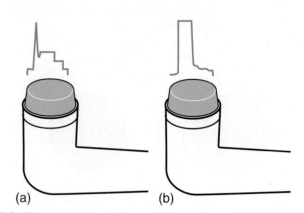

FIGURE 14.11 The peak area of the maximum BNR (PAMBNR) represents the size of the peak intensity. **(a)** Small PAMBNR = small, if any, hot spot. **(b)** Large BNR = large hot spot.

(!) Modality Myth

BNR IS AN OVERRATED CHARACTERISTIC FOR ULTRASOUND UNITS

Some clinicians believe that BNR is not that important to ultrasound devices.[18] Perhaps that's why there is so much variability in the way some crystals are scanned. In fact, the FDA allows a lot of leeway in how BNR is determined. For example, one imaging technique involves scanning the crystal at very low intensities, such as 0.1 W/cm^2, and this is appropriate for diagnostic ultrasound that uses very low power. At this low power, a crystal might display a low BNR. However, this is not a therapeutic dose for the thermal application of ultrasound used in most clinical settings. A more appropriate way to determine BNR for thermal ultrasound devices involves scanning the crystal at an ultrasound intensity of 50% maximum output or about 1.0 W/cm^2.

The PAMBNR

Some ultrasound manufacturers include another aspect to the definition of BNR: the **peak area of the maximum BNR (PAMBNR)**. This concept was developed during research in which subjects reported that one of two ultrasound devices with identical BNRs (2.35:1) was more comfortable than the other. Why? The scientists concluded that

peak intensity is only half the equation. The other half is the area of the crystal that produces the peak intensity, or the beam profile. Thus, one crystal with a BNR of 7:1 over only 1 mm of the crystal will cause less discomfort than a crystal with a BNR of 7:1 over 5 mm of the crystal. This conclusion led to the acronym PAMBNR (Fig. 14.11).[18,19]

As you can see, crystal quality is an important factor for ultrasound, but it is not the only factor. Box 14.2 lists the components of an optimal ultrasound device, and crystal quality is only one of them. Of course, having a good

BOX 14.2 TEN COMPONENTS OF A STATE-OF-THE-ART ULTRASOUND DEVICE

1. High-quality synthetic crystal:
   a. Low BNR ≤4:1); small PAMBNR
   b. High ERA (nearly matches the size of the soundhead)
   c. BNR and ERA scans provided by the manufacturer or distributor, not estimates
2. Multiple frequencies (1 and 3 MHz; possibly 90 kHz or lower for phonophoresis)
3. Multiple-sized soundheads
4. Sensing device that shuts off the unit when overheating occurs
5. Insulation for underwater use
6. Output jack for combination therapy
7. Several pulsed duty cycles
8. Applicator handle that maintains the operator's wrist in a natural, relaxed position
9. Durable soundhead that will protect the crystal if dropped
10. Computer-controlled timer that makes adjustments in treatment duration as the intensity is adjusted (similar to iontophoresis, where the treatment time adjusts according to the dose applied)

ultrasound device is of no value unless you use it properly, so you need to understand the correct treatment parameters.

Treatment Parameters

Can you imagine how ineffective an ice pack treatment would be if applied for only 1–2 minutes immediately following an acute injury? No therapeutic modality is "therapeutic" unless correct treatment parameters are used. Essential treatment parameters for therapeutic ultrasound include:

- Mode
- Frequency
- Intensity
- Treatment length
- Treatment area size

MODE

Practically all therapeutic ultrasound devices can produce either continuous or pulsed ultrasound. With **continuous ultrasound**, the sound energy remains constant throughout the treatment; that is, the ultrasound energy is produced 100% of the time (Fig. 14.12a). With **pulsed ultrasound**, the energy is periodically interrupted with no ultrasound energy being produced during the off period (Fig. 14.12b). Pulsed ultrasound reduces the average

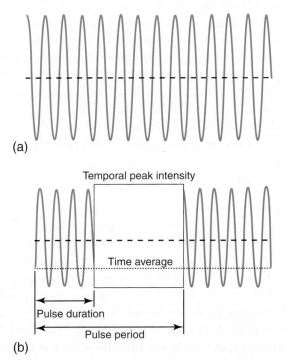

(a)

(b)

FIGURE 14.12 Ultrasound can be delivered in either **(a)** continuous mode or **(b)** pulsed mode. The temporal peak intensity is the same in both **(a)** and **(b)**, but the average intensity is less in **(b)**. (Adapted with permission from Castel, D. International Academy of Physio Therapeutics. Clip Art.)

intensity of the output over time. The term **temporal average intensity (TAI)** is used to describe the power of ultrasonic energy over a given period of time. The percentage of time that ultrasound is generated (pulse duration) over one pulse period is referred to as the **duty cycle**:

$$\text{Duty cycle} = \frac{\text{Pulse duration (on-time)} \times 100}{\text{Pulse period (on-time + off-time)}}$$

For example, if the pulse duration is 10 msec and the total pulse period is 40 msec, the duty cycle would be 25%. Therefore, the total amount of energy delivered to the tissues would be only 25% of the energy delivered if a continuous wave was used.

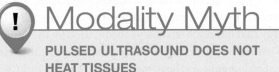

CONCEPT CHECK 14.2. What would be the duty cycle if the pulse duration is 20 msec and the total pulse period is 40 msec?

Many ultrasound devices have preset duty cycles at either 20% or 50%. Some provide several optional duty cycles. Continuous ultrasound is most commonly used when thermal effects are desired, whereas pulsed ultrasound is typically used when nonthermal effects are desired. Thus, pulsed ultrasound typically results in a reduced average heating of the tissues.

Modality Myth

PULSED ULTRASOUND DOES NOT HEAT TISSUES

Some clinicians think that pulsed ultrasound does not produce heat. This is too simplistic, however, since heating is a function of the total energy delivered to the tissue, which in turn is a function of intensity, mode, and ERA. For example, applying the same intensity continuously over an area four times the soundhead surface area, and pulsed at a 50% duty cycle to an area one-half this size will impart the same energy. Also keeping treatment area constant, application of ultrasound at 0.5 W/cm² continuously and application of ultrasound at 1 W/cm² pulsed 50% impart the same energy: about 5.4°F (3°C).[20] Thus, pulsed ultrasound can produce heat when the average intensity is 0.5 W/cm².

FREQUENCY

Therapeutic ultrasound has a frequency range of 0.75–3.0 MHz. Most therapeutic ultrasound devices produced before 1990 were set at a frequency of 1 MHz. After 1990, several manufacturers added a 3 MHz. A generator that can be set between 1 and 3 MHz provides the greatest treatment flexibility because ultrasound frequency determines the depth of tissue penetration and the rate of tissue heating.

⚠ Modality Myth

INCREASING THE ULTRASOUND POWER INCREASES THE DEPTH OF TISSUE PENETRATION

The frequency of the ultrasound determines the depth of penetration into the body's tissues, not the amount of power. Turning up the power (intensity) simply sends more energy to the same depth.[15]

Depth of Tissue Penetration

The depth of ultrasound penetration is described in terms of the *half-value layer,* the depth by which 50% of the ultrasound beam is absorbed in tissue. Temperature effects are expected to be highest at the half-value layer and less at greater depths.[21] Thus, when it is stated that 1 MHz ultrasound will go as deep as 6 cm into the tissue, according to the half-value layer principle, theoretically it will have a higher temperature at half that depth (3 cm).

When a high ultrasound frequency (such as 3 MHz) enters the tissues, some of it is absorbed superficially. The energy that has not been absorbed and used by the superficial tissues will penetrate to deeper tissues. Scientists have measured significant heat increases at 2.5 cm in human muscle.[21] Thus, 3 MHz is ideal for treating superficial conditions such as plantar fasciitis, Achilles tendinitis, and epicondylitis (tennis elbow).[21]

Ultrasound energy generated at 1 MHz is transmitted through the more superficial tissues and absorbed primarily in the deeper tissues at depths of 2–6 cm.[10] A 1-MHz frequency is most useful in patients with a high percentage of cutaneous body fat, and whenever desired effects are in the deeper structures, such as the soleus, piriformis, and hip adductor muscles.[10] Recently low-frequency ultrasound (45 and 90 kHz) has been introduced as a possible modality in orthopedic medicine. The very low frequencies will provide the greatest depth of penetration in body tissues, possibly generating ultrasound energy to deep bone (Fig. 14.13).

 CONCEPT CHECK 14.3. A patient is complaining of pain at the tendon just below the kneecap and has been diagnosed with chronic patellar tendinitis. Which frequency of ultrasound should you use to treat this condition—1 or 3 MHz?

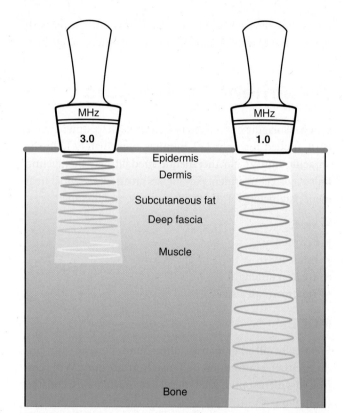

FIGURE 14.13 The depth of tissue penetration is determined by ultrasound frequency. The effects of 3 MHz occur more superficially (2.5 cm deep) than 1 MHz (6 cm deep). (Adapted with permission from Castel, D. International Academy of Physio Therapeutics. Clip Art.)

Rate of Heating

The rate of absorption, and therefore attenuation, increases as the frequency of the ultrasound increases.[22] The 3-MHz frequency is not only absorbed more superficially, it is also absorbed three times faster than 1 MHz ultrasound.[10] This faster rate of absorption results in faster peak heating in tissues. Both 45 and 90 KHz ultrasound are absorbed so slowly that little or no heating occurs; therefore, these lower frequencies are used primarily for nonthermal effects.

INTENSITY

Power is a function of both pulse width and pulse frequency, measured in W. **Intensity** is the rate at which energy is being delivered per unit area. Ultrasound power and intensity are usually expressed in watts per square centimeter. Intensity is also referred to as spatial average intensity (SAI), the intensity of the ultrasound beam averaged over the area of the soundhead. It usually occurs in the central third of the ERA. SAI is calculated by dividing the power output in watts by the total ERA of the soundhead in square centimeters:

$$SAI = \frac{Total\ watts\ (W)}{Effective\ radiating\ area\ (cm^2)} = W/cm^2$$

If ultrasound is produced at a power of 8 W and the ERA of the soundhead is 4 cm², the SAI would be 2.0 W/cm². On many ultrasound devices, both the power in watts and the SAI in W/cm² are displayed. If the power output is constant, increasing the size of the soundhead surface will decrease the SAI.

According to the World Health Organization's guidelines, an SAI of 3.0 W/cm² is the safe limit for therapeutic treatment. Intensities above 10 W/cm² are used to surgically destroy tissue, whereas intensities below 0.1 W/cm² are used for diagnostic purposes.

There are no definitive guidelines for selecting specific ultrasound intensities during treatment; however, if the intensity is too high, tissue damage can occur.[10] We suggest that you use the lowest intensity possible to achieve a desired therapeutic effect.

Modality Myth

PATIENTS DO NOT FEEL ANYTHING DURING ULTRASOUND TREATMENTS

Only when nonthermal ultrasound is being delivered with a low-duty cycle and/or low intensity (low SAI) will patients not feel a thing. Thermal ultrasound treatments should feel slightly warm. Remember that each person's tolerance to heat is different, so ultrasound intensity should always be adjusted to patient tolerance.[15] At the beginning of the treatment, turn the intensity to the point at which the patient feels deep warmth, and then lower the intensity slightly until gentle heating is felt.[15,21] During the treatment, ask the patient for feedback, and make the necessary intensity adjustments. If the patient complains that the soundhead feels hot at the skin surface, the crystal has been damaged, the soundhead is overheating, or there isn't enough ultrasound gel between the skin and soundhead to conduct the energy into the tissues.

The goal of continuous ultrasound treatments should be a specified temperature increase. Thermal ultrasound is used in order to bring about certain therapeutic effects, and tissues respond according to the amount of heat they receive.[22] Therefore, any significant adjustment in the intensity should be countered with an adjustment in the treatment time. It is possible that ultrasound treatments in the future will be like iontophoresis, in which the treatment time depends on the dosage delivered (or the amount of heat absorbed by the tissues). For this reason, one manufacturer of ultrasound devices places a microchip in

TABLE 14.1 TEMPERATURE INCREASES THEORIZED TO BRING ABOUT DESIRED EFFECTS IN TISSUES

TEMPERATURE INCREASE	EFFECT
1.8°F (1°C) (mild heat)	Increases metabolism, reduces mild inflammation
3.6–5.4°F (2–3°C) (moderate heat)	Reduces pain and muscle spasm, increases blood flow
7.2°F (4°C) (vigorous heat)	Increases ROM and tissue extensibility*

*This works best when heat and stretch or heat and mobilization are used in combination.

the generator that makes adjustments in treatment time corresponding to the operator's thermal goals of a 1.8, 3.6, or 7.2°F (1, 2, or 4°C) increase (based on research means). If the intensity is increased, treatment time is reduced; if intensity is reduced, treatment time is increased. Table 14.1 shows treatment goals based on temperature increases.

TREATMENT LENGTH

In the 1980s, most textbooks stated that an ultrasound treatment should last 5–10 minutes. In 2006, many insurance companies would deny payment for ultrasound treatments lasting <8 minutes. It is a mistake to use a predetermined length for all ultrasound treatments. Setting a specific treatment length for all thermal ultrasound treatments would be as ridiculous as saying it takes exactly 3 hours to fly from Salt Lake City to Chicago. Just as travel time from city to city depends on several factors (speed, tailwind, route, size of plane), ultrasound treatment length also depends on several factors.

The length of the treatment is made according to the size of the area to be treated, the ultrasound frequency, the intensity in W/cm², and the desired temperature increase.[15] We suggest that ultrasound be administered in an area two to three times the ERA (roughly twice the size of the soundhead surface). If you desire deep thermal effects in an area larger than this, obviously the treatment time needs to be increased, or use shortwave diathermy (see Chapter 15).

As stated earlier, higher ultrasound frequencies require a shorter treatment length than lower frequencies. Ultrasound at 3 MHz consistently heats tissues three times faster than 1 MHz, thus reducing the required treatment length by one third.[10,11] The lower the intensity, the longer the treatment time, and vice versa. It does not make sense to treat one patient at 1 W/cm² and another at 2 W/cm² for *identical treatment lengths* when both patients require vigorous heating. In this scenario, the second patient will produce tissue temperature increases of twice that of the first one.

TABLE 14.2 RATES OF MUSCLE HEATING USING ULTRASOUND, PER MINUTE*

INTENSITY (W/CM²)	FREQUENCY: 1 MHZ	FREQUENCY: 3 MHZ
0.5	0.07°F (0.04°C)	0.54°F (0.3°C)
1.0	0.36°F (0.2°C)	1.08°F (0.6°C)
1.5	0.54°F (0.3°C)	1.62°F (0.9°C)
2.0	0.72°F (0.4°C)	2.52°F (1.4°C)

*Data were obtained with Omnisound ultrasound devices, Accelerated Care Plus, Reno, NV.

Source: Draper et al.,[11] Wells and Draper,[25] and Anderson et al.[28]

Temperature Increase

The desired temperature increase is also a factor in determining the length of an ultrasound treatment. Table 14.2 shows research results on the rate of muscle temperature increases at various intensities and frequencies.[10] These are average temperature increases recorded for hundreds of subjects using what many consider to be the best ultrasound device available. Such data are difficult to obtain with many ultrasound devices; therefore the table should be used only as a rough estimate.[10,15]

✔ **APPLICATION TIP**

USE ONE OF THESE TWO METHODS TO DETERMINE ULTRASOUND TREATMENT LENGTH

Method A. Based on the information in Table 14.2, you can "guesstimate" the appropriate duration of an ultrasound treatment. For example, if a patient has tennis elbow and chronic pain in the wrist extensor group, you may want to heat the area prior to some massage or stretching. An appropriate goal would be to vigorously heat the muscle/tendon junction (an increase of 7.2°F or 4°C). If 3 MHz ultrasound were used at an intensity of 1 W/cm², the 7.2°F (4°C) increase would take about 7 minutes (1 W = 0.6°C/min × 7 minutes = 7.6°F or 4.2°C). If at 5 minutes into the treatment, however, the patient complains that the treatment is too hot, decrease the intensity until it is comfortable. And since you have decreased the total dosage, it would be wise to counter this by adding a minute or so to the treatment time, if possible. Now you are ready to massage the muscle or perform the passive stretch. Although this tip might not apply to your device, it can be used as an estimate for setting treatment goals with a desired temperature increase, instead of giving a 5-minute treatment all the time.

Method B. Use the heating sensation reported by patients as a guide for peak heating. Experimental subjects reported discomfort from ultrasound as the intramuscular temperature reached 40°C. Therefore, this should signal the end of the treatment. Note that a device with a poor PAMBNR will cause discomfort long before peak heating is reached.

✔ **APPLICATION TIP**

IF ULTRASOUND DOESN'T SEEM TO BE WORKING, TRY SOMETHING ELSE

Some clinicians will give an unlimited number of ultrasound treatments to a patient. The usual recommendation is to limit ultrasound to 14 treatments, because more than 14 can reduce both red and white blood cell counts. After 14 treatments, it is advisable to avoid ultrasound use for 2 weeks.[23] If no improvement is noted following four or five treatments, discontinue the ultrasound, or use different treatment parameters.

TREATMENT AREA SIZE

It is not uncommon to see ultrasound used on large areas such as the hamstrings or low-back muscles. The nonthermal effects may benefit the patient, but research has shown that no heating will occur on this large an area.[24] Scientists have tested the heating capacity of ultrasound over areas of six and four times the size of the soundhead.[25,26] Although the temperature increased 2.3°F (1.3°C) and 3.6°F (2°C), respectively, this is only mild to moderate heating. The appropriate size of the area to be treated using ultrasound is two or three times the size of the ERA of the crystal,[27,28] or twice the size of the soundhead surface (Fig. 14.14a). Thus, ultrasound is most effectively used for treating small areas. Hot packs, whirlpools, and shortwave diathermy have an advantage over ultrasound in that they can be used to heat much larger areas.[24,29]

✔ **APPLICATION TIP**

FOR OPTIMAL HEATING, DIVIDE AND CONQUER

If you have an area four times the size of the soundhead, treat half of the area first, and then treat the second half. For example, when treating a wrist prior to joint mobilization, treat the ventral side first and rest it on a hot pack while treating the dorsal side (Fig. 14.15). If you need to heat much larger areas, consider using whirlpools or hot packs if your target is superficial or pulsed shortwave diathermy if the target tissue is deeper than 1–2 cm.

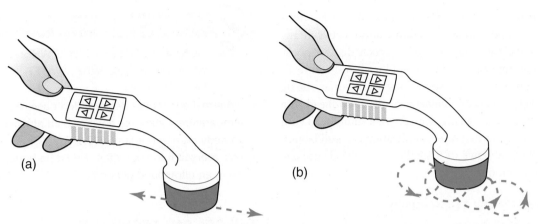

FIGURE 14.14 Ultrasound can be applied in either **(a)** a longitudinal or **(b)** a circular motion. In either case, if heating is desired, the total area covered should not be more than twice the size of the soundhead.

Application Techniques

While administering an ultrasound treatment, it is important to keep the soundhead's surface flat with the surface you are treating at all times. The greatest amount of reflection of ultrasonic energy occurs at the air-tissue interface. If you lift the soundhead from the skin at an angle of more than 15°, a large percentage of the energy will be reflected, and the treatment effects will be minimal.

COUPLING MEDIA

Ultrasound beams are not transmitted through the air, but require a medium to send the energy from the soundhead to the patient.[30] A substance that facilitates the transmission of ultrasound energy by decreasing impedance at the air-skin interface is referred to as a **coupling medium**, or *couplant*. There are three main types of ultrasound coupling media:

- Gels, for direct application
- Water, for the immersion technique
- Gel pads, for use over bony prominences

The most commonly used coupling medium is ultrasound gel. It is composed mainly of distilled water and an inert, nonreflective material that increases the viscosity of the mixture. A thin layer of coupling medium or gel between the skin and the soundhead has two purposes:

1. It allows ultrasonic energy to enter the target tissue at the desired intensity by minimizing the air between the soundhead surface and the tissue.
2. It serves as a lubricant.

A common practice is to mix ultrasound gel with an analgesic cream for use as an ultrasound couplant. Although petroleum-based creams will actually impede the transmission of the sound energy, water-based creams can be beneficial. In 1995, a 50/50 mixture of Flex-All was compared with 100% ultrasound gel as a coupling medium; the study concluded that ultrasound gel was the best couplant.[31] In 2004, the study was repeated, and this time 100% ultrasound gel was compared to a 25% Flex-All/75% ultrasound gel mixture.[32,33] The muscle temperatures reached during treatment were nearly identical. Thus, this commonly used sports cream was found to be an excellent couplant when mixed with ultrasound gel at a 1:3 ratio.

DIRECT CONTACT APPLICATION

The majority of ultrasound treatments are direct applications, in which the soundhead comes in contact with the skin (with a thin film of couplant in between). A layer of

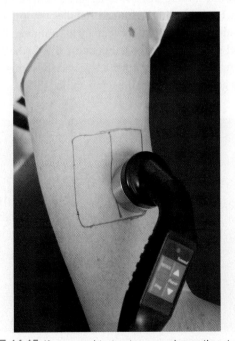

FIGURE 14.15 If you need to treat an area larger than two times the size of the soundhead, outline areas twice the size of the soundhead, and treat each area separately.

gel is applied to the treatment area in sufficient amounts to maintain good contact and lubrication between the soundhead and the skin, but not so much that air pockets form from movement of the soundhead. A direct technique of exposure may be used as long as the surface being treated is larger than the diameter of the soundhead. If a smaller surface area is being treated, use a soundhead with a smaller surface so that direct application can still be performed. In the absence of a smaller soundhead, use the immersion technique.

THE IMMERSION TECHNIQUE

Water is a great coupling medium, but it is not suited for surface application because it will not stay in one place, like gel. There are, however, some instances where you might want to use the underwater technique. The immersion technique is recommended if the area to be treated is smaller than the diameter of the available soundhead, or if the treatment area is irregular with bony prominences (Fig. 14.16).

Use a plastic, ceramic, or rubber basin; a metal basin or whirlpool will reflect some of the ultrasound, thereby increasing the intensity near the basin walls. Tap water seems to be just as effective as degassed water as a coupling medium for the immersion technique and less likely to produce surface heating than mineral oil or glycerin. The soundhead should be moved parallel to the surface being treated at a distance of 0.5–1 cm. If air bubbles accumulate on the soundhead or over the treatment area, wipe them away quickly during the treatment. It is important to use body temperature water, not room temperature water. If room temperature water is used, the area to be treated will chill and the ultrasound will have to work through that.

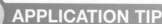

APPLICATION TIP

CONSIDER THESE POINTS WHEN ADMINISTERING UNDERWATER ULTRASOUND

- If thermal effects are desired, don't use room temperature water; use a water bath at least as warm as body core temperature 98.6°F (37°C).
- Ask yourself if the condition would be better served by using an ultrasound gel pad.

THE GEL PAD TECHNIQUE

If the treatment area is irregular but cannot be immersed in water, you can use a gel pad as a medium. Companies have recently been manufacturing ultrasound gel packs, which consist of gel housed in a thin plastic envelope, or gel pads, which resemble gel-filled clear hockey pucks.

A few studies have been performed on the efficacy of gel pads. Two studies suggest that ultrasound gel pads are as effective as ultrasound gel.[34,35] When the gel pad is used over bony prominences, such as the lateral malleolus of the ankle or the knuckles of the hand, you need to apply a thin layer of ultrasound gel on both sides of the gel pad.[35] The bottom layer ensures that no air is trapped between the bony prominences and the gel pad, and the top layer helps the soundhead glide smoothly on the gel pad (Fig. 14.17).

In another study, two thicknesses of gel pads were tested.[36] The regular 2-cm pad was tested against a 1-cm pad to determine if there was any difference in ultrasound transmission 1 cm deep in the human Achilles tendon. We used the parameters of 3 MHz, 1 W/cm² for 10 minutes. The 2-cm thick gel pad increased the temperature 6.5°C; the 1-cm gel pad increased the temperature 9.3°C; and the ultrasound gel with no gel pad increased the temperature 13.3°C.

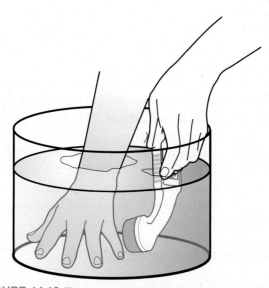

FIGURE 14.16 The immersion technique is recommended if the area to be treated is smaller than the diameter of the soundhead, or if the treatment area is irregular with bony prominences.

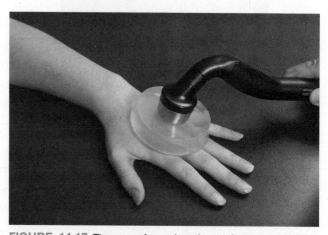

FIGURE 14.17 The use of a gel pad over bony prominences requires a layer of gel on both sides of the pad, to avoid trapping air and to lubricate the soundhead.

CONCEPT CHECK 14.4. A patient reports to you for ultrasound treatment 5 days after getting a cast taken off her hand. You can see that it will be difficult to apply ultrasound over her knuckles and maintain good direct contact over the treatment area. What alternative coupling techniques could you use?

SOUNDHEAD MOVEMENT

The ultrasound soundhead is usually moved on the skin in small, overlapping circular motions, or back and forth strokes (see Fig. 14.14b). The movement is slow, about 3–4 cm/sec.[15] If the patient starts to experience pain during the treatment, move the soundhead faster to avoid periosteal irritation or overheating of the tissue.[15] Turn the intensity down, and then resume the speed of 3–4 cm/sec.

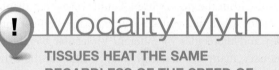

Modality Myth

TISSUES HEAT THE SAME REGARDLESS OF THE SPEED OF SOUNDHEAD MOVEMENT

This statement is true if you can limit the treatment size to a small area.[12] For example, you can use a template to keep the treatment size at 2–3 ERA. Moving the soundhead slowly enables you to control the treatment area. If you move it too rapidly (>4 cm/sec), you run the risk of slipping into treating too large an area (especially if you are carrying on a conversation during treatment), and the desired temperatures might not be attained.

Recording Treatment Parameters

Record the specific treatment parameters whenever you use ultrasound or any other therapeutic modality. There have been several malpractice cases involving the alleged misuse of ultrasound (personal experience as expert witnesses). During the discovery deposition in one such case, the clinician was asked to provide the treatment records of the claimant. Under ultrasound treatment, all that was listed was "10 minutes of ultrasound application." This is irresponsible record keeping. We recommend that you report or record the specific parameters used in an ultrasound treatment to ensure that:

• The treatment can be reproduced.
• The treatment can be adapted to the patient's needs.
• The records can stand alone when challenged.

The parameters that should be recorded include frequency, intensity, mode, duty cycle (if pulsed), type of coupling medium, area treated, treatment length, and the number of treatments per week. For example, a typical treatment might be recorded as 3 MHz, at 1.2 W/cm², continuous, 2–3 ERA (lateral elbow), ultrasound gel, 6 minutes.

Thermal Effects

In orthopedic medicine, ultrasound is primarily used to produce a tissue temperature increase. The clinical effects of thermal ultrasound include, but are not limited to[37]:

• Increased extensibility of collagen fibers in tendons and joint capsules
• Reduced viscosity of fluid elements in the tissues
• Decreased joint stiffness
• Reduced muscle spasm
• Diminished pain perception
• Increased metabolism
• Increased blood flow

As previously mentioned, the primary advantage of ultrasound over nonacoustic heating modalities is that collagen-rich tissues such as tendons, muscles, ligaments, joint capsules, joint menisci, intermuscular interfaces, nerve roots, periosteum, and cortical bone, as well as other deep tissues, can be selectively heated to the therapeutic range without causing a significant tissue temperature increase in skin or fat.[7] Ultrasound will penetrate skin and fat with little attenuation.[38]

OPTIMAL HEATING

One source indicates that tissue temperature must be raised to a level of 104–113°F (40–45°C) for a minimum of 5 minutes in order for most thermal effects to occur.[39] Temperatures above 113°F (45°C) can cause tissue damage, and 113°F (45°C) is a very high temperature. In our 17 years of laboratory experience with ultrasound, we have never raised human muscle temperature higher than 109.4°F (43°C). Our research subjects usually start to experience mild pain at temperatures above 104–105.8°F (40–41°C) even when a unit with a low BNR is used.[10] This agrees with the published recommendation of Merrick et al.[40]

Others are of the opinion that absolute temperatures are not the key, but rather how much the temperature rises above baseline.[10,15,37] They suggest that tissue temperature increases of 1.8°F (1°C) over baseline increase metabolism and healing, increases of 3.6–5.4°F (2–3°C) decrease pain and muscle spasm, and increases of 7.2°F (4°C) or greater increase the extensibility of collagen and decrease joint stiffness (see Table 14.1).[25,39]

In human muscle, which is quite vascular, 1 MHz and 3 MHz ultrasound at 1 W/cm^2 increased the temperature, on average, 0.36°F (0.2°C) and 1.08°F (0.6°C) per minute, respectively.[10] If the intensity is <0.2 W/cm^2, the intensity is too low to produce a tissue temperature increase, and only nonthermal effects will occur.[10]

In tissues with a poor vascular supply, ultrasound at 1 MHz with an intensity of 1 W/cm^2 has been reported to raise soft tissue temperature by as much as 1.5°F (0.86°C) per minute.[13] Caution must be used in evaluating the results of one tendon study (ultrasound at 3 MHz and 1 W/cm^2 intensity) that raised patellar tendon temperatures 3.6°F (2°C) per minute.[41] This increase could have been due to some of the sound energy rebounding off the tibia. Tendon heats faster than muscle, but more research, perhaps in deeper tendons, needs to be performed to better explain the rate of ultrasound heating in tendon.

Nonthermal Effects

Regardless of whether or not thermal effects are produced with ultrasound, nonthermal changes do occur.[42] The nonthermal effects of therapeutic ultrasound in the treatment of injured tissues may be as important if not more important than, the thermal effects. They include[43,44]:

- Increased histamine release
- Calcium ion influx
- Increased phagocytic activity of macrophages
- Increased protein synthesis
- Increased capillary density of ischemic tissue
- Tissue regeneration
- Wound healing
- Cell membrane alteration
- Attraction of immune cells to the injured area
- Increased fibroblasts
- Vascular regeneration

These nonthermal or mechanical effects of therapeutic ultrasound are thought to originate at the cell membrane. As the ultrasound wave exerts pressure against the cell wall, the membrane deforms slightly. This cell deformation, often referred to as "micromassage," occurs from processes known as cavitation and microstreaming. **Cavitation** is the formation of gas-filled bubbles that expand and contract due to ultrasonically induced pressures in tissue fluids.[42] As the sound waves propagate through the medium, the characteristic compressions and rarefactions cause microscopic gas bubbles in the tissue fluid to contract and expand.

Cavitation can produce both positive and negative effects. Positive effects occur from *stable cavitation*, where the bubbles expand and contract in response to regularly repeated pressure changes over many acoustic cycles. Negative effects are produced when unstable cavitation occurs. With *unstable or transient cavitation*, tissue can be damaged from increased bubble volume, implosion, and collapse. Apparently the rapid changes in pressure in and around the cell can result in cell damage caused by the leading and lagging edges of the sound wave. Considerable injury to the cell can occur when gas bubbles expand then collapse rapidly, resulting in a "microexplosion." The pulsation of gas bubbles can disrupt cell activity, thereby altering the function of the cell; however, true microexplosions apparently do not occur at therapeutic levels.[43] One example of cavitation is blisters on the skin over the anterior aspect of the tibia when treatment was applied to the posterior aspect of the tibia.

Acoustic microstreaming is the unidirectional movement of fluids along the boundaries of cell membranes. It results from the pressures of sound waves that displace ions and small molecules.[42] While many cellular organelles and molecules of different molecular weights are stationary, many are also free floating and can be driven to move around the stationary structures. The mechanical pressure from ultrasound waves produces unidirectional movement of fluid along and/or around the cell membrane. Microstreaming produces stresses that can alter the cell membrane's structure and function, thereby affecting the healing process. As long as the cell membrane is not damaged, acoustic microstreaming can be of therapeutic value in accelerating healing.[43,45]

Clinical Applications of Therapeutic Ultrasound

As with many medical devices, research on ultrasound began and continues to be performed on animal models. Results from animal studies have driven much of our human applications for ultrasound. There are a few studies and case reports on humans that continue to point to the efficacy of this modality. We cannot predict what evidence-based research will demonstrate about the future use of therapeutic ultrasound. Yet we can tell you what we know now, and in what direction the research is pointing.

Therapeutic ultrasound research has been an ongoing process since the 1960s. Although there was little research during the 1970s and 1980s, it picked up somewhat in the 1990s. This is important because the ultrasound devices manufactured in the 1990s are of much higher quality than previous ones. We now have a vast amount of information regarding heating rates and treatment parameters for using continuous ultrasound. What is lacking, however, is recent research on the healing effects of ultrasound. Thus, many of the decisions about how ultrasound should be used are based on personal experience and opinion. In this section, we summarize the various clinical applications of therapeutic ultrasound based upon research findings of others and ourselves.

AIDING THE INFLAMMATORY RESPONSE TO INJURY

There is nothing mysterious about ultrasound—it isn't a magic wand. It is theorized that it stimulates bodily functions to perform better. When an injury occurs, some biological mechanisms shut down, and apparently ultrasound can stimulate normal functioning.[45,46]

Scientists have shown that ultrasound stimulated collagen synthesis and cellular proliferation.[46] Macrophages, the main cell type present in wounds 4 or 5 days after injury, secrete substances that stimulate fibroblast proliferation. Using a culture model, Young and Dyson[47] showed that when macrophages were treated with ultrasound, they had a positive effect on fibroblast proliferation.

Ultrasound has been shown to stimulate the release of histamine from mast cells.[48] Histamine is one of the primary initiators of the acute-phase inflammatory response. Histamine attracts leukocytes, which "clean up" debris from the injured area. Histamine also draws monocytes into the area to release agents that stimulate fibroblasts and endothelial cells to form a collagen-rich, well-vascularized tissue for the development of new connective tissue. Thus, ultrasound can be effective in facilitating inflammation and healing.[42,46,49] Scientists suggest that the best parameters to use include pulsed ultrasound at a 20% duty cycle, at 0.5 W/cm², for 5 minutes, or continuous ultrasound at 0.1 W/cm² for 5 minutes.[38]

Johns[43] reports that 1 MHz, 3 MHz, and 45 kHz ultrasound stimulate cellular and molecular effects that are centrally involved in the inflammatory and healing processes. However, he concludes that no clear protocols exist for optimum times and parameters for administration during healing.

✔ APPLICATION TIP

BEGIN NONTHERMAL ULTRASOUND SOON AFTER AN INJURY

To maximize the effects on the healing process, ultrasound treatments, in a nonthermal mode, can begin as soon as possible following an injury, ideally within hours but definitely within 72 hours.[50] Acute conditions may be treated using nonthermal ultrasound once or even twice daily until acute symptoms, such as pain and swelling, subside.

SUPERFICIAL WOUND HEALING

During the healing process, a connective tissue matrix forms into which new blood vessels will grow. Fibroblasts are the main formative component of connective tissue. Fibroblasts exposed to therapeutic ultrasound are stimulated to produce more collagen, which gives connective tissue most of its strength.[51] Rat incisions treated with ultrasound displayed more new blood vessel development than areas not treated with ultrasound.[52]

Research has shown increased strength of incisional wounds and collagen deposition when ultrasound is applied.[53] Ultrasound increases smooth muscle cell activity, which is thought to enhance wound contraction.[54] Contraction is an advantage in tissue repair because it means less scar tissue is required to fill the wound gap. The centralizing tug on healthy collagen fibers at the edge of the lesion pulls the wound together. This process is attributed to myofibroblast activity.

CONNECTIVE TISSUE HEALING

Like many studies, the majority of research of ultrasound on connective tissue healing has been performed on animals. Low-intensity ultrasound has been used to stimulate articular cartilage for healing induced arthritis in animals.[55,56] Muscles of injured rats have shown more healing and force production after ultrasound treatments compared to no treatment.[57,58] When rabbits and rats with surgically induced Achilles tendon tears were treated with ultrasound, they displayed more parallel collagen orientation, and greater strength, compared to controls.[57,58] Ultrasound was used on dogs with ruptured Achilles tendons. They showed more advanced healing, and a faster return to normal gait, than dogs not treated with ultrasound.[59] Turner and Powell[60] studied the effects of ultrasound treatment on torn, then repaired, tendons of chickens. There was no difference in tendon strength between the group treated with ultrasound and the control group.

Scientists have used rats to study ultrasound effects on healing of either cut or crushed sciatic nerves.[61,62] In both cases, rats treated with ultrasound showed improvements over the control group. In one study, quantity and diameter of regenerating nerve fibers increased, and in the other study function of the foot increased, due to the healing of the sciatic nerve.

Torn medial collateral ligaments of rats showed superior healing when ultrasound was used.[63] Unfortunately, there was no improvement noted when ultrasound applications were given to humans with ankle sprains.[64] We point out, however, that no human studies are reported in the literature where low-intensity ultrasound has been used on acute tendon and ligament injury. Thus more evidence-based research on humans is needed in this area.

BONE HEALING

Bone goes through basically the same stages of healing as other soft tissues. Over the past decade, low-intensity pulsed ultrasound to assist fracture healing has increased in orthopedic medicine. Using a 1-MHz therapeutic ultrasound device commonly used by therapists and clinicians, Da Cunha et al.[65] treated damaged rat Achilles tendons, and found superior healing when the pulsed mode was used (20% duty cycle, 0.5 W/cm², 5 minutes, 12 days). Pulsed low-intensity ultrasound using similar parameters has been shown to assist bone healing in patients with non-union fractures who failed previous treatments.[66,67] Compared to controls, rat femur fractures treated with diagnostic ultrasound (7.5 MHz, 11.8, mW/cm², 10 minutes) responded well (between treatments 3–8).[55]

BONE GROWTH STIMULATORS

Ultrasonic bone stimulation produces an ultrasonic wave which delivers mechanical pressure to the bone at the fracture site. Although the mechanism by which the low intensity pulsed ultrasound (LIPUS) device accelerates bone healing is uncertain, it is thought to promote bone formation in a manner comparable to bone responses to mechanical stress.[68,69] The LIPUS bone stimulators accelerate healing of fresh fractures, fusions, or delayed unions at either of the following high-risk sites:

- Fresh fractures
- Fusions
- Delayed unions

LIPUS is mainly used on the tibia shaft, on the scaphoid, and for Colle's fractures. Fractures on these sites are hard to heal because of poor blood supply.[65]

LIPUS has been shown to significantly accelerate the time to clinical healing of fractures of the distal diaphysis and stress fractures.[65,66] Other evidence of the effectiveness of LIPUS for non-unions includes a registry of prescription use of LIPUS for non-unions in the United States that showed a heal rate of 82% of 429 completed cases, and a retrospective study of non-unions that showed a heal rate of 90% of 30 completed cases.[65]

LIPUS is widely used today[67–69] and is probably producing the best evidence that ultrasound is effective.[70,71]

Bear in mind that most of the bone healing performed is with bone growth stimulators, not the typical ultrasound device (Fig. 14.18). Most LIPUS devices use the following parameters for bone growth stimulation:

- Duty cycle: 20%
- Frequency: 1.5 MHz
- Intensity: 30 mW/cm²
- Time: 20 minutes

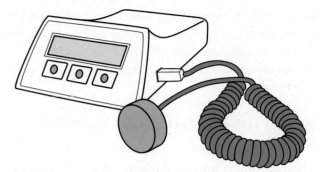

FIGURE 14.18 A low-intensity pulsed ultrasound stimulator for the acceleration of fracture healing.

Animal Studies

There have been several animal studies with positive outcomes when the SAFHS was used at these parameters. Scientists reported a faster healing rate and stronger bones compared to the opposite limb when the SAFHS was used on surgically induced femur fractures in rats.[68,69] Rabbit fibula fractures treated with the SAFHS healed faster when compared to sham treatments on the opposite limb.[72]

Human Studies

The SAFHS has also had success in stimulating bone growth in human patients. Tibial shaft fractures have shown a 38% reduction in healing time.[70] Distal radius fractures treated with the SAFHS have also healed 38% faster than normal.[71,73] Compared to a control group, scaphoid fractures treated with the SAFHS had accelerated healing by 31%.[72] Evidence indicates that bone growth stimulators promote healing of non-union fractures, yet more research is needed in this area. Bone growth stimulators are different than conventional therapeutic ultrasound devices found in many clinics and are the preferred modality to use in bone healing. Some theorize that conventional ultrasound can be used for fracture healing when it is pulsed at a very low intensity, but research in humans is too sparse to support this premise (Table 14.3).

TABLE 14.3 COMPARABLE PARAMETERS OF A BONE STIMULATOR AND A CONVENTIONAL ULTRASOUND DEVICE

PARAMETER	SAFHS (EXOGEN 2000)	OMNISOUND 3000C
Duty cycle	20%	20%
Frequency	1.5 MHz	1 MHz
BNR	3:1	3:1
ERA	3.88 cm²	4.2 cm²
Intensity	0.161 W/cm²	0.15 W/cm²
Treatment length	20 min	20 min

Source: Adapted from Michlovitz and Nolan.[12]

Growth Plates

One area of concern is whether or not it is safe to use ultrasound over epiphyseal plates. In the 1950s, scientists studied the use of ultrasound over growing bone epiphyses in animals. Treatments resulted in premature closure of the epiphysis, epiphyseal displacement, and bone shortening. However, high intensities up to 3.0 W/cm² were used. More recently, some scientists have stated that using ultrasound, at clinically applicable doses, over an epiphysis is no longer a contraindication, and can be used with caution.[12] Therefore, it is not an outright contraindication to use ultrasound over epiphyses at low intensities.

No documented evidence exists that ultrasound treatment can cause the reabsorption of calcium deposits. However, it has been suggested that ultrasound may help reduce inflammation surrounding a calcium deposit, thus reducing pain and improving function.

ASSESSING STRESS FRACTURES

For years, clinicians have used tuning forks to help determine the presence of a stress fracture. If a tuning fork vibrates 16,000 times per second, imagine what an ultrasound crystal can do as it vibrates 1,000,000 times per second on the periosteum! Think of ultrasound, then, as a high-frequency tuning fork. The use of ultrasound as a technique for identifying stress fractures has been recommended for some time.[74]

✔ APPLICATION TIP

USE ULTRASOUND FOR ASSESSING STRESS FRACTURES

Following are the steps for using ultrasound to determine the presence of a stress fracture:

- Ask the patient where the tender area is.
- Apply coupling gel to the same site on the opposite limb.
- Set the ultrasound device on 1 MHz and at a continuous setting.
- Apply ultrasound to a small area over the tender point (keep moving the soundhead).
- Slowly increase the intensity to the point that it is uncomfortable.
- Record the peak intensity in W/cm².
- Repeat this same process on the affected limb and tender area
- Record the peak intensity in W/cm².
- If the intensity in the injured limb is considerably lower than the nonaffected limb, there is a good chance a stress fracture exists (e.g., 0.8 W/cm² compared to 1.5 W/cm²).
- Refer to physician for other diagnostic tests (e.g., x-ray).

PITTING EDEMA

We have found ultrasound to be a valuable tool for the absorption of pitting edema.[15] This condition can be treated with continuous 3-MHz ultrasound at intensities of 1.0–1.5 W/cm². The heat seems to liquefy the gel-like cellular debris. You can then elevate the limb, massage it, or apply an electrical current to pump and push the fluid and promote lymphatic drainage.

REDUCING MUSCLE SPASM

One of the main uses of therapeutic ultrasound is pain reduction. The pain-spasm-pain cycle was introduced in Chapter 10. Heat derived from an ultrasound treatment helps bring fresh blood into the injured area. In turn, the fresh blood aids in washing away chemical irritants, increases the delivery of oxygen, alters nerve conduction speed, and ultimately relaxes muscular tension. As the muscles relax, the pain decreases and the muscle spasm will resolve.

REDUCING PAIN

Ultrasound is often prescribed for other purposes than pain reduction; however, many scientists have reported the added benefit of reduced pain from ultrasound application. Why might ultrasound reduce pain? As previously stated, ultrasound application increases blood flow that may wash away chemical irritants that cause pain. The heat produced by ultrasound in large-diameter myelinated alpha and beta nerve fibers may reduce pain, according to the gate control theory.[9] Thermal ultrasound may also increase nerve conduction speed in normal nerves, creating a counterirritant effect.[75]

RESTORING ROM LOST FROM SCAR TISSUE AND/OR JOINT CONTRACTURE

During the remodeling phase of the healing process, collagen fibers are realigned along lines of tensile stresses and strains. Over the course of months or even years, the injury develops scar tissue. In scar tissue, collagen never achieves the same pattern and remains weaker and less elastic than normal tissue prior to injury. Scar tissue in tendons, ligaments, and capsules surrounding joints can produce joint contractures that limit range of motion (ROM). Some clinicians, including ourselves, theorize that increased tissue temperatures during ultrasound treatment decrease the viscosity of collagen fibers while increasing their elasticity. In this case, ultrasound is the treatment modality of choice, because the deeper tissues surrounding the joints that most often restrict ROM are rich in collagen.

Ultrasound has increased mobility in cases of mature scaring. A greater residual increase in tissue length with less potential damage is produced through preheating with ultrasound prior to stretching or mobilizations.[15,76–79] Tissue extensibility increases when continuous ultrasound is applied at higher intensities, causing a vigorous heating of tissues. Periarticular structures and scar tissues become significantly more extensible following treatment with ultrasound involving thermal effects at intensities of 1.2–2.0 W/cm^2.[10,79] Scar tissue can be softened if treated early with ultrasound.[79]

APPLICATION TIP

USE SEVERAL TECHNIQUES TO RESTORE ROM

Just as ice alone is not adequate for treating acute injuries (you need RICES), ultrasound alone is not sufficient for increasing ROM. Heat and stretch (or stress) are also needed.

STRETCHING CONNECTIVE TISSUE

If you were to take a plastic spoon and dip it in hot water, it would become soft. By pulling on the ends, you would be able to stretch it and bend it. Yet, as the plastic spoon cools, it hardens and is no longer able to be stretched. Like plastic, collagenous tissue is fairly rigid when stressed, yet it yields somewhat when heated.[76] The blend of heat and stretch results in a residual lengthening of connective tissue, which increases according to the force applied by the clinician.

It is a good idea to apply ultrasound prior to exercise, warm-up, stretching, or joint mobilizations. Unfortunately, heating followed by stretching is frequently interrupted with team meetings or other circumstances beyond the clinician's control. Still, it is important to stretch the tissue while it is still warm. The idea that increased muscle temperature from the ultrasound treatment will last 10 minutes or longer is incorrect.

The time period (or window of opportunity) of vigorous heating when tissues will undergo the greatest extensibility and elongation is referred to as the **stretching window** (Fig. 14.19).[10,15,77] If tissue is heated vigorously, it becomes more pliable, yet as it cools, it resists stretching and can actually be damaged if the force applied is too great. The rate of tissue cooling following continuous ultrasound has been studied at both 1- and 3-MHz frequencies.[11,77] For our purposes here, we suggest that stretching, friction massage, or joint mobilization be performed immediately following ultrasound, since this stretching window stays open for only 5–10 minutes after an ultrasound treatment. To increase the duration of the stretching window, you can put the joint on stretch during the last 2–3 minutes of ultrasound application.

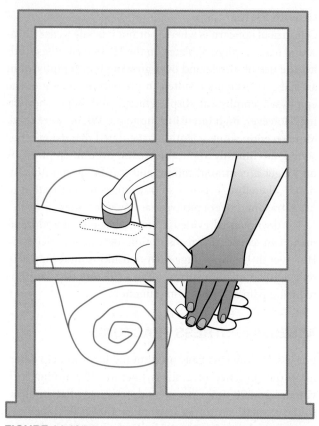

FIGURE 14.19 The stretching window. This is the period of vigorous heating, when tissues undergo the greatest degree of extensibility and elongation.

The stretching window varies according to the type and depth of the tissue heated. Since tendon is much less vascular than muscle, tendon heated with ultrasound cools at a slower rate than muscle. Also, deeper muscle cools at a slower rate than superficial muscle, because the added tissue serves as a barrier to escaping heat. Case 14.1 describes the results of two patients we have treated with ultrasound followed by joint mobilizations.[79]

CONCEPT CHECK 14.5. A patient is recovering successfully from knee surgery, except that his patella isn't moving well. The physician prescribes patellar mobilizations. How could you use ultrasound to assist in obtaining normal ROM of the patella?

TREATING CHRONIC INFLAMMATION

One of the biggest challenges for any clinician is treating chronic injuries that just don't want to go away. Two key ingredients in treating chronic conditions are increased blood flow and decreased pain, both of which result from continuous ultrasound.[80] It might prove beneficial to heat the area with ultrasound and then perform cross-friction

CASE 14.1 ULTRASOUND FOR SEVERE WRIST INJURIES

Case 14-1a:

A 22-year-old soccer goalie had bone graft surgery to help repair a 3-year episode of avascular necrosis of the scaphoid. After being immobilized for 12 weeks in a cast, he had very little wrist ROM. The athletic trainer performed passive stretch for several weeks with some improvement, but was unable to restore the last 30° of extension (Fig. 14.20a). Nearly normal wrist extension was restored after just three treatments (every other day for 1 week) of 3 MHz ultrasound, followed by joint mobilizations (Fig. 14.20b). With subsequent treatments, he gained even more ROM and has maintained it.

Case 14-1b:

While trying to extract a ganglion cyst, the surgeon accidently severed three extensor tendons of a 19-year-old male patient. The patient had the tendons repaired by another surgeon, but could not regain normal wrist flexion. Three years later, the patient reported to our clinic. He lacked 31° of wrist flexion. Ultrasound (3 MHz) at 1.5 W/cm² for 4–5 minutes was applied to the ventral then dorsal side of the wrist, immediately followed by joint mobilizations. After just three treatments (every other day for 1 week), his wrist flexion returned to normal and remained that way.

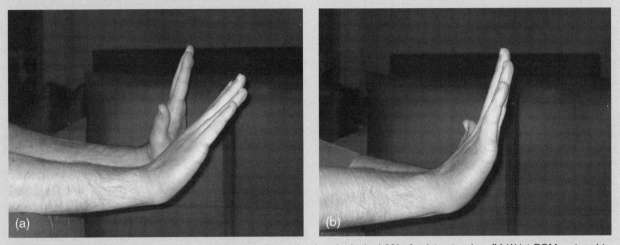

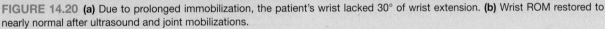

FIGURE 14.20 (a) Due to prolonged immobilization, the patient's wrist lacked 30° of wrist extension. **(b)** Wrist ROM restored to nearly normal after ultrasound and joint mobilizations.

massage to break up the adhesions and allow the tendon to glide more smoothly on the surrounding structures. There are few clinical or experimental studies that discuss the effects of therapeutic ultrasound on chronic inflammation (i.e., tendinitis, bursitis, epicondylitis), and the results are mixed. Ultrasound treatments have proven to be beneficial for treating tibial periostitis[81] and epicondilytis.[82]

A technique that one of us (KK) has used a dozen or so times for treating thrower elbow epicondylitis is to treat the tendon over the epicondyle for about 5 minutes twice a day for 10 or so days. Compliance is crucial. Missing even two treatments seems to invalidate the success (see Case 14.2).

Phonophoresis

Phonophoresis is the use of ultrasound to help move a topical medication into the tissues. The theory is that ultrasound enhances transdermal drug delivery by dilating

CASE 14.2 MEDIAL EPICONDYLITIS IN A BASEBALL PITCHER

A baseball pitcher with increasing medial elbow pain of 2–3 weeks duration decided to seek treatment. The diagnosis was epicondylitis; the plan was to treat with 5 minutes of 1 MHz continuous ultrasound @ 1.5 cm² twice daily for 10 days—with no exceptions. After 9 days, there was little progress, so he and his coach sought consultation with the head AT. During the consultation, the athlete claimed that he had followed the prescribed treatment regimen, although his records revealed he had missed a treatment on Wednesday morning and Friday afternoon. "I had an exam on Wednesday and had to study." "We had a double header in Evansville Friday afternoon and had to leave before noon." After a 4-day rest, the twice-daily US regimen was repeated and led to resolution of the injury.

hair follicles and sweat glands, increasing circulation and kinetic energy of the local cells.[83] Many think that ultrasound drives the medicine into the tissues, but this is not correct. In ultrasound, **sonoporation** occurs, in which the sound waves increase cell membrane permeability, thereby facilitating the delivery of molecules to precise locations in the body.[84,85] The successful delivery of the medication is limited by the inability of the molecules to cross biological barriers like the cell membrane. An advantage of phonophoresis is that medication can be delivered via a safe, painless, noninvasive technique.

DRUG AND MODE DECISIONS

Which medications work well during phonophoresis still remains somewhat of a mystery. Scientists have found that hydrocortisone gels and many salicylate preparations actually block ultrasound wave transmission, while other gels and creams serve as good ultrasound transmitters.[86–88] For treating orthopedic injuries, the most commonly used medications in phonophoresis are either anti-inflammatories, such as cortisol, salicylates, and dexamethasone, or anagelsics, such as lidocaine. With phonophoresis, it is important to select the appropriate drug for the condition. Since phonophoresis can increase drug penetration, it could also increase the clinical benefits as well as the risks of topical drug application.[89,90]

Both pulsed ultrasound and continuous ultrasound have been used in phonophoresis. Strapp et al.[87] reported greater levels of dexamethasone sodium phosphate in the bloodstream following continuous ultrasound application of that medication. However, continuous ultrasound at an intensity great enough to produce thermal effects may induce a pro-inflammatory response.[5] If the goal is to decrease inflammation, phonophoresis using pulsed ultrasound at a low intensity might be the best choice.[23]

TOPICAL PREPARATIONS

Earlier we discussed the ability of various coupling media to actually penetrate the skin barrier. Adding an active ingredient into the coupling medium is common practice; however, topical pharmacologic products are usually not formulated to optimize their efficiency as ultrasound coupling media.[91] For example, 1% or 10% hydrocortisone usually comes in a thick white cream base, which is a poor ultrasound couplant. Clinicians have tried mixing this preparation with ultrasound gel without improvement in transmission capabilities.

The use of topical preparations with poor transmission capabilities may decrease the effectiveness of ultrasound therapy. Unfortunately only a few suitable products are available, and there is clearly a need for appropriate active ingredients in gel form. Since research has shown some of these

medications to impede the sound,[88] we recommend applying the medication and gel separately. This is done by rubbing the medication into the skin and then applying an ultrasound gel couplant, followed by an ultrasound treatment.

EFFECTIVENESS OF PHONOPHORESIS

The effectiveness of phonophoresis is inconclusive, especially at the frequencies commonly used in orthopedic medicine (1 and 3 MHz). Evidence indicates that little medication actually reaches the target tissue. The answer might not come from clinicians who work in physical medicine and rehabilitation, but from chemical engineering where phonophoresis is being used on animals and humans with some positive results.[89–93]

In chemical engineering, the positive results for phonophoresis are being obtained at low frequencies, such as 45 and 20 kHz. Scientists measured the ability of both 1 MHz and 20 kHz ultrasound to facilitate the delivery of butanol, corticosterone, salicylic acid, and sucrose across human cadaver skin.[92] The result: 20 kHz increased skin permeability a thousand fold over that of 1 MHz. Scientists have also been successful at transdermal transport of corticosterone, insulin, interferon, and erythropoietin across human skin using 20 kHz ultrasound.[93] These results indicate that lower frequencies might be useful in treating orthopedic injuries.[91]

Using Ultrasound and Other Modalities Collectively

In an orthopedic setting, it is not uncommon to combine modalities to accomplish a specific treatment goal. Although you want to avoid the shotgun approach, ultrasound is frequently used with other modalities, including hot packs and electrical stimulating currents. Unfortunately, there is very little documented evidence to substantiate the effectiveness of ultrasound and electrical currents; however, studies of heating or cooling the area prior to ultrasound application have produced interesting results.[94–96]

HOT PACKS

Hot packs, like continuous or high-intensity ultrasound, are used primarily for their thermal effects. Heat is effective in reducing muscle spasm and muscle guarding and useful in relieving pain. For these reasons, heat and ultrasound in combination can be effective for accomplishing these treatment goals. In one study, a 15-minute hot pack application prior to ultrasound had an additive heating effect.[96] Based on this finding, we recommend that the ultrasound treatment duration can be decreased by 3–5 minutes when tissues are preheated with hot packs.

APPLYING COLD BEFORE ULTRASOUND ENHANCES HEATING

Although the theory sounds good, this approach doesn't work. According to this premise, applying a cold pack to the tissues initiates physiological responses such as vasoconstriction and decreased blood flow. Thus, cooling the area not only results in decreased local temperature, it may temporarily increase the density of the tissue to be heated. This occurs by decreasing superficial attenuation and facilitating transmission to deeper tissues, thereby enhancing the thermal effects of ultrasound. But studies refute such claims. Applying an ice pack for 5 minutes prior to ultrasound caused the temperature to drop so much that the ultrasound failed to raise the muscle temperature to even 50% of that of subjects who did not receive an ice application prior to ultrasound.[94] Applying an ice pack for 15 minutes prior to ultrasound caused the temperature to drop so much that the ultrasound failed to raise the muscle temperature back to the previous baseline temperature.[95] It just doesn't make sense to cool something that you immediately want to heat.[24]

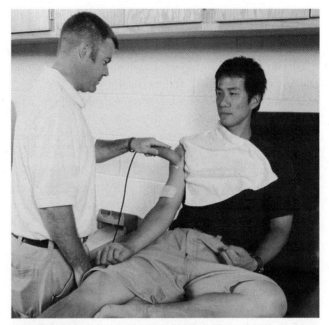

FIGURE 14.21 Ultrasound is frequently used in combination with electrotherapy. The ultrasound head serves as one electrode. Note the second electrode attached to the bicep.

ULTRASOUND AND ELECTROTHERAPY

Ultrasound and electrotherapy techniques, also known as combination therapy, are frequently used (Fig. 14.21). Understand that when combination therapy is used, the ultrasound soundhead acts as an electrode. The muscles will be stimulated to contract, but there will be little, if any, heating. The electrical stimulating currents will cause analgesia and muscle contraction. Combination therapy has been recommended in the treatment of myofascial trigger points.[96] We have had success in treating iliotibial band tightness with combination therapy. Both modalities provide analgesic effects, and both have been shown to be effective in reducing the pain-spasm-pain cycle, although the underlying mechanisms are not clearly understood.

Treatment Precautions and Concerns

As with all therapeutic modalities, specific safety precautions must be observed when using ultrasound:

- Avoid using thermal ultrasound whenever a tissue temperature rise is contraindicated.

- Avoid using high-intensity continuous ultrasound in acute and post–acute conditions because of the associated thermal effects.
- Use caution when treating areas of decreased sensation, particularly when the patient has difficulty perceiving pain and temperature.
- Exercise caution in areas of decreased circulation, because excessive heat buildup can potentially damage tissues.
- Individuals with vascular problems involving thrombophlebitis should not receive ultrasound because of the possibility of dislodging a clot and creating an embolus.
- Ultrasound should not be applied around the eyes where heat is not dissipated well; the lens and retina can be damaged.
- Do not apply ultrasound over reproductive organs, especially the testes; temporary sterility can result. Although the ovaries are fairly deep and well protected, use caution (lower intensities and 3 MHz) when treating the female abdominal region during the reproductive years or immediately following menstruation.
- The use of ultrasound to the abdominal region or lower back is contraindicated during pregnancy because of potential damage to the fetus. Diagnostic ultrasound for tracking maturation of the fetus is delivered in doses <0.1 W/cm² 2.5 MHz, and as such, is safe.
- Use precaution when treating areas around the heart, because of potential changes in EKG activity.
- Avoid using ultrasound below the ribs, directed toward the heart.

- Ultrasound can interfere with the normal functioning of a pacemaker, and should not be applied directly over the device.
- Do not use ultrasound over malignant tissue; it could cause cell detachment and metastasis.
- Do not apply ultrasound over an active infection, as it may cause it to spread.
- Use caution when applying ultrasound over epiphyseal areas in young children. It appears that low-intensity treatment (<1 W/cm^2) can be used, but only for a few treatment sessions. Ultrasound can be used relatively safely over metal implants. According to theory, there is little increase in the temperature of tissue adjacent to the implant because metal has high thermal conductivity, so heat is removed from the area faster than it can be absorbed. However, metal reflects about 90% of ultrasound energy, and adjacent tissues can absorb some of the reflected waves. Regardless, when performing ultrasound on an area with metal implants (or any area for that matter), if the patient complains of pain, reduce the intensity. Be aware that in cases of total joint replacement, the cement used (methyl methacrylate) absorbs heat rapidly, and overheating can damage surrounding soft tissues.

Challenges to the Efficacy of Therapeutic Ultrasound

Some clinicians believe that ultrasound has no therapeutic value. For example, in two articles, Robertson and Baker[97,98] reviewed 35 ultrasound studies performed between 1975 and 1999. Using a model to determine whether the original scientists were rigorous enough in the original research design, the authors eliminated studies because of one or more of the following factors: small sample size; nonclinical condition; inadequate controls; no comparison to placebo; and nonblinding of observers, subjects, or scientists. In all, 25 studies did not match up to this model—leaving just 10 studies to examine. In eight of these, active ultrasound performed no better than placebo ultrasound. From this, the authors concluded that active ultrasound is no more effective than placebo or sham ultrasound.

We analyzed these eight articles in depth and found several research errors from which the authors drew their conclusion. In fact, many of the original scientists made the same mistakes therapists and ATs make in everyday use of this often-misunderstood modality.[15,99,100] These errors included:

- Treating too large an area for thermal goals (four studies). The area should be no more than twice the size of the soundhead[101]
- Using the wrong frequency for superficial tissues (one study). Superficial tissues require 3 MHz[102]
- Inadequate treatment duration (five studies)[103]

It appears that the papers from which Robertson and Baker drew their conclusions were flawed; they mistakenly compared placebo ultrasound with placebo ultrasound. In other words, a study is flawed to begin with if the research doesn't use correct treatment parameters. The authors' impressions that ultrasound is not effective is based on less than adequate research.[12] Until more controlled studies using correct parameters are performed, we cannot rule out ultrasound as a therapeutic modality. Although it can't do everything, when used correctly, it can be a valuable tool for you and your patients.

A 2009 meta-analysis by Jewel et al.[104] also did some damage to the reliability of ultrasound. In her manuscript, "Interventions associated with an increased or decreased likelihood of pain reduction and improved function in patients with adhesive capsulitis: a retrospective cohort study," she found that ultrasound was not helpful in relieving pain or restoring function. Data were mined from studies of 2370 patients. The problem with the study is that a shoulder is much too large to be treated with US. Had the clinicians used a deep heating treatment such as diathermy, we believe their results would have been different.

An evidence-based report by Alexander et al.[105] gives credence to the use of thermal ultrasound. In her meta-analysis, she determined that lower powers (an average of 2019 J) produced no effect, whereas higher joules (an average of 4228 J) produced positive results.

This just makes plain sense. In order for ultrasound to be effective, it must provide sufficient power. An automobile will not arrive at a certain destination on time, unless the accelerator is depressed enough to power the car at a certain speed.

5 STEPS · Application of Therapeutic Ultrasound

1 STEP 1: FOUNDATION

A. Definition. Therapeutic ultrasound is inaudible, acoustic vibrations of high frequency that produce either thermal or nonthermal physiologic effects in tissues.

B. Effects
1. Thermal effects include:
   a. Diminished pain perception
   b. Increased metabolism
   c. Increased blood flow
2. Nonthermal effects include:
   a. Tissue regeneration
   b. Wound healing
   c. Cell membrane alteration

C. Advantages
1. Can heat deep tissues without overheating the surface
2. Heats the deepest of all modalities (except diathermy)

D. Disadvantages
1. Can only heat small areas approximately twice the size of the soundhead surface
2. Variability in the quality of ultrasound devices

E. Indications
1. Acute and post–acute conditions (ultrasound with nonthermal effects)
2. Soft tissue healing and repair
3. Scar tissue
4. Joint contracture
5. Chronic inflammation
6. Increase extensibility of collagen
7. Reduction of muscle spasm
8. Pain modulation
9. Increase blood flow
10. Soft tissue repair
11. Increase protein synthesis
12. Tissue regeneration
13. Bone healing
14. Repair of non-union fractures
15. Inflammation associated with myositis ossificans
16. Plantar warts
17. Myofascial trigger points

F. Contraindications
1. Acute and post–acute conditions (ultrasound with thermal effects)
2. Vascular insufficiency
3. Thrombophlebitis
4. Eyes
5. Reproductive organs
6. Pelvis immediately following menstruation
7. Pregnancy
8. Pacemaker
9. Malignancy
10. Infection

G. Precautions
1. Epiphyseal areas in young children
2. Metal implants
3. Areas of decreased temperature sensation
4. Areas of decreased circulation
5. Total joint replacements

2 STEP 2: PREAPPLICATION TASKS

A. Make sure ultrasound is the proper modality for this situation.
1. Reevaluate the injury/problem. Make sure you understand the patient's condition.
2. If ultrasound was applied previously, review the patient's response to the previous treatment.
3. Confirm that the objectives of therapy are compatible with ultrasound.
4. Make sure ultrasound is not contraindicated in this situation.

B. Equipment preparation. Prepare the equipment before preparing the patient.
1. Make sure the soundhead is clean.
2. Make sure you have enough coupling medium available for treatment.

C. Preparing the patient psychologically
1. Explain the procedure.
   a. Sound waves generated into the body cause an increased movement of molecules, which results in heat, or a type of micromassage of the tissues.
   b. Gentle warmth should be felt during the treatment (unless it is a nonthermal treatment).
   c. Demonstrate the procedure on yourself if the patient is apprehensive.
2. Check for, and warn the patient about, precautions.
   a. If the treatment starts to feel too warm, ask the patient to let you know.

D. Preparing the patient physically
1. Remove any metal or jewelry from the part to be treated.
2. Inspect the area to be treated for rashes or open wounds.
3. Position the patient in a manner that will be comfortable, yet allow accessibility to the ultrasound device.

STEP 3: APPLICATION PARAMETERS

A. Procedures
 1. Obtain the appropriate soundhead size.
 2. Apply the coupling medium to the area.
B. Dosage
 1. Determine the appropriate frequency.
  a. 1 MHz for deep to moderate
  b. 3 MHz for moderate to superficial
 2. Set the duty cycle (choose either continuous or pulsed setting).
 3. Set the treatment duration (vigorous heat: 10–15 minutes at 1 MHz; 3–7 minutes at 3 MHz).
  a. Maintain contact between the skin and the applicator.
  b. Move at a rate of 4 cm/s for 2–3 ERA.
 4. Adjust the intensity to the patient's perception of heat.
  a. If it gets too hot, move the applicator slightly faster as you turn down the intensity.
 5. If the treatment goal is increased joint ROM, put the body part on stretch for the last 2–3 minutes of the ultrasound application, and maintain stretch or friction massage for 5 minutes after the ultrasound application.
C. Length of application
 1. Varies according to treatment goals
D. Frequency of application
 1. One or two times daily
E. Duration of therapy
 1. 14 treatments

STEP 4: POSTAPPLICATION TASKS

A. Equipment removal; patient cleanup
 1. When the timer shuts off, or the patient can no longer tolerate the treatment even at low intensity, remove the soundhead and clean it off. Wipe any ultrasound gel off the patient.
B. Instructions to the patient
 1. Schedule the next treatment.
 2. Instruct the patient about the level of activity and/or self-treatment prior to the next formal treatment.
 3. Instruct the patient about what he/she should feel following treatment.
C. Record of treatment, including unique patient responses
D. Equipment replacement
 1. Towels
 2. Coupling medium

STEP 5: MAINTENANCE

A. Clean the equipment regularly.
B. An ultrasound device that is used daily should be calibrated every 6 months.

CLOSING SCENE

Recall from the chapter opening scene that several patients asked Keira some difficult questions about ultrasound. She told them that there are two types of ultrasound, thermal and nonthermal. A patient should feel gentle warmth during a thermal treatment, but nothing during a nonthermal treatment. As for the patient who could feel an ultrasound treatment on his patellar tendon but not on his back, Nancy informed him that ultrasound is correctly used to heat small areas. That's why he felt the gentle heat on his knee but couldn't feel it on his low back—an area too large to benefit from ultrasound. Hot packs, whirlpools, or, even better, pulsed shortwave diathermy should be used to heat his back. Nancy seems to know her stuff about ultrasound.

Chapter Reflections

1. Read and ponder each of the following points. Do you feel you have a clear understanding of each concept? If not, reread the appropriate section of the chapter.
   - Name the key components of an ultrasound device.
   - What happens when ultrasound enters the body's tissues?
   - Explain the thermal effects of therapeutic ultrasound.
   - Discuss the nonthermal effects of therapeutic ultrasound.
   - Describe the different techniques of ultrasound application.
   - List several parameters associated with ultrasound use.
   - Itemize the contraindications and precautions of using therapeutic ultrasound.
   - Compare and contrast ultrasound with other heating agents.
   - What is the stretching window? Explain how it would be most effectively used with ultrasound.

2. Write three to five questions for discussion with your class instructor, clinical instructor, classmates, and clinical colleagues.

3. Get together with classmates and quiz each other on the concepts of this chapter. Use the points in reflection no. 1 and questions you wrote for reflection no. 2 as a beginning. Explaining concepts out loud to others requires a deeper grasp of the material than feeling you understand it as you read.

4. Once you feel you understand the principles of application, practice applying ultrasound treatments using the five-step approach, to a classmate or a clinical colleague. Once you have applied it, allow the classmate to apply the modality to you, listening and observing carefully to determine if your classmate is applying it properly. You should use your notes when the modality is applied to you and during the first few times you apply the modality. Continue practicing the application until you can do so without your notes.

Concept Check Responses

CONCEPT CHECK 14.1

In this case, the best treatment choice is not to use ultrasound at all. A better decision would be to use either hydrocollator packs or shortwave diathermy, both of which are more useful in treating larger areas. If depth of penetration is a concern, then shortwave diathermy would be the treatment modality of choice.

CONCEPT CHECK 14.2

The duty cycle would be 50%. Duty cycle = total pulse period divided by pulse duration, or 40 msec/20 msec = 50%.

CONCEPT CHECK 14.3

The higher the frequency, the more the energy is absorbed in the superficial tissues. The majority of the sound waves generated from the 3-MHz treatment would be absorbed in

the tendon, whereas 1 MHz goes much deeper and might rebound off of the bone, causing some discomfort.

CONCEPT CHECK 14.4

When using a large soundhead over bony prominences, the immersion technique done in a plastic or rubber tub can be effective. Also, the gel pad technique could be used to ensure that there is consistent contact between the soundhead and the coupling medium. Remember to have a small amount of gel on both sides of the pad.

CONCEPT CHECK 14.5

Application of 3 MHz ultrasound to patient tolerance for 4–5 minutes on the lateral side and 4–5 minutes on the medial side. Immediately apply patellar glides in all directions.

REFERENCES

1. Andrew MA, Crum LA, Vaezy S. *2nd International Symposium on Therapeutic Ultrasound.* Vol 2. Seattle, WA: Center for Industrial and Medical Ultrasound Applied Physics Laboratory: University of Washington, 2002.

2. Fried NM, Roberts WW, Wright EJ, Solomon SB. Noninvasive male sterilization: thermal occlusion of the vas deferens and epididymis in a canine model using a therapeutic focused ultrasound clip. Paper presented at 2nd International Symposium on Therapeutic Ultrasound, Seattle, WA, 2002.

3. Mourad PD, Nemecek A, Mesiwala A, et al. Ultrasound treatment of brain disorders. Paper presented at 2nd International Symposium on Therapeutic Ultrasound, Seattle, WA, 2002.

4. Draper D, Abergel P, Castel J. Rate of temperature change in human fat during external ultrasound: Implications for liposuction. *Am J Cosmet Surg.* 1998;15(4):361–367.

5. Dyson M. The use of ultrasound in sports physiotherapy. In: Grisogono V, ed. *Sports Injuries (International Perspectives in Physiotherapy).* Edinburgh: Churchill Livingstone, 1989.

6. Dyson M, Luke DA. Induction of mast cell degranulation in skin by ultrasound. *IEEE Trans Ultrasonics Ferroelectrics Frequency Control.* 1986;33:194.

7. ter Haar G. Basic physics of therapeutic ultrasound. *Physiotherapy.* 1987;64(4):100–103.

8. Draper D, Sunderland S. Examination of the law of Grotthus-Draper: does ultrasound penetrate subcutaneous fat in humans? *J Athl Train.* 1993;28:246–250.

9. Myrer JW, Draper DO, Durrant E. Contrast therapy and intramuscular temperature in the human leg. *J Athl Train.* 1994;29:318–322.

10. Draper DO, Castel JC, Castel D. Rate of temperature increase in human muscle during 1 MHz and 3 MHz continuous ultrasound. *J Orthop Sports Phys Ther.* 1995;22(4):142–150.

11. Draper DO, Ricard MD. Rate of temperature decay in human muscle following 3 MHz ultrasound: the stretching window revealed. *J Athl Train.* 1995;30:304–307.

12. Michlovitz SL, Nolan TP. *Modalities for Therapeutic Intervention.* 4th ed. Philadelphia, PA: F.A. Davis, 2005.

13. McCutchan ED, Demchak TJ, Brucker JB. A comparison of the heating efficacy of the Autosound with traditional ultrasound methods. *J Athl Train.* 2008;42:s41.

14. Fincher AL, Trowbridge CA Ricard MD. A comparison of the hands free and manual therapeutic ultrasound techniques. *J Athl Train.* 2008;42(2):s41.

15. Draper D. Ten mistakes commonly made with ultrasound use: current research sheds light on myths. *Athl Train Sports Health Care Perspect.* 1996;2:95–107.

16. Johns LD, Straub SJ, Howard SM. Variability in effective radiating area and power output of new ultrasound transducers at 3 MHz. *J Athl Train.* 2007;42(3):22–28.

17. Ferguson BA. A practitioners' guide to ultrasonic therapy equipment standard. *US Dept. HHS, PHS, FDA.* 1985; 35 pp.

18. Draper D. A breakthrough on comfortable ultrasound treatments: Beam non-uniformity ratio is only half of the equation. Paper presented at National Athletic Trainers' Association Annual Symposium; Kansas City, MO, June 18, 1999.

19. Johns LD, Straub SJ, LeDet EG. Ultrasound beam profiling: Comparative analysis of 4 new ultrasound heads a both 1 and 3.3 MHz variability within a manufacturer. *J Athl Train.* 2004;39:S-26.

20. Gallo JA, Draper DO, Thein-Body L, Fellingham GW. Continuous and pulsed ultrasound produce similar increases in human muscle temperature when equivalent temporal average intensities are used. *J Orthop Sports Phys Ther.* 2004;34:339–401.

21. Stewart H. Ultrasound therapy. In: Repacholi M, Benwell D, eds. *Essentials of Medical Ultrasound.* Clifton, NJ: Humana Press; 1982:196.

22. Hecox B, Mehreteax TA, Weisberg J. *Physical Agents.* Norwalk, CT: Appleton & Lange; 1984.

23. Gann N. Ultrasound: current concepts. *Clin Manage.* 1991;11(4):64–69.

24. Garrett CL, Draper DO, Knight KL. Heat Distribution in the Lower Leg from Pulsed Short-Wave Diathermy and ultrasound Treatments. *J Athl Train.* 2000;35(1):13–22.

25. Chudleigh D, Schulthies S, Draper D, Myrer J. Muscle temperature rise during 1 MHz ultrasound treatments of two and six times the effective radiating areas of the transducer. *J Athl Train.* 1998;33(2):s-11.

26. Demchak T, Meyer L, Stemmans C, Brucker J. Therapeutic benefits of ultrasound can be achieved and maintained with a 20-minutes 1 MHz, 4-ERA ultrasound treatment. *J Athl Train.* 2006;41(2):s-42.

27. Castel D. *Electrotherapy and Ultrasound Update.* 2nd ed. Reno, NV: International Academy of Physio Therapeutics, 1996.

28. Reid DC, Cummings GE. Factors in selection the dosage of ultrasound with particular reference to the use of various coupling agents. *Physiother Can.* 1973;63:255.

29. Draper DO, Harris ST, Schulthies SS, et al. Hotpack and 1 MHz ultrasound treatments have an additive effect on muscle temperature increase. *J Athl Train.* 1998;33:21–24.

30. Williams R. Production and transmission of ultrasound. *Physiotherapy.* 1987;73(3):113–116.

31. Ashton DF, Draper DO, Myer JW. Temperature rise in human muscle during ultrasound treatments using flex-all as a coupling agent. *J Athl Train.* 1998;33:136–140.

32. Anderson M, Eggett D, Draper D. Combining topical analgesics and ultrasound, Part 2. *Athl Ther Today.* 2005;10(2):45–47.

33. Draper D, Anderson M. Combining topical analgesics and ultrasound, Part 1. *Athl Ther Today.* 2005;10(1):26–27.

34. Klucinec B, Scheidler M, Denegar C, Domholt E, Burgess S. Transmissivity of common coupling agents used to deliver ultrasound through indirect methods. *JOSPT.* 2000;30:263–269.

35. Merrick MA, Mihalyov MR, Roethemeier JL, Cordova ML, Ingersoll CD. A comparison of intramuscular temperatures during ultrasound treatments with coupling gel or gel pads. *J Orthop Sports Phys Ther.* May 2002;32(5):216–220.

36. Draper DO, Edvalson CG, Knight KL, Eggett DE, Shurtz J. Temperature increases in the human Achilles tendon during ultrasound treatments with commercial ultrasound gel and full-thickness and half-thickness gel pads. *J Athl Train.* 2010;45(3):333–337.

37. Lehmann JF. *Therapeutic Heat and Cold.* 4th ed. Baltimore, MD: Williams & Wilkins, 1990.

38. Draper DO, Abergel PR, Castel JC. Rate of temperature change in human fat during external ultrasound: implications for liposuction. *Am J Cosmetic Surg.* 1998;15(4):361–367.

39. Weaver SL, Demchak TJ, Stone MB, Brucker JB, Burr PO. Effect of transducer velocity on intramuscular temperature during a 1-MHz ultrasound treatment. *J Orthop Sports Phys Ther.* 2006;36(5):320–325.

40. Merrick MA, Bernard KD, Devor ST, Williams MJ. Identical 3-MHz ultrasound treatments with different devices produce different intramuscular temperatures. *J Orthop Sports Phys Ther.* 2003;33(7):379–385.

41. Chan AK, Myrer JW, Measom GJ, Draper DO. Temperature changes in human patellar tendon in response to therapeutic ultrasound. *J Athl Train.* 1998.

42. Dyson M. Therapeutic application of ultrasound. In: Nyborg WL, Ziskin MC, eds. *Biological Effects of Ultrasound.* Edinburgh: Churchill Livingstone, 1985.

43. Johns LD. Nonthermal effects of therapeutic ultrasound: the frequency resonance hypothesis. *J Athl Train.* 2002;37(3).

44. Kimmel E, Dines M, Elad D, Einav S, Rav D. Shear-like response of endothelial cells to therapeutic ultrasound. Paper presented at 2nd International Symposium on Therapeutic Ultrasound, Seattle, WA, 2002.

45. Watson T. Therapeutic ultrasound. Available at: www.electrotherapy.org

46. Draper D, Karns P, Sokolowski M. Chronic ankle and foot injuries in professional ice hockey players: Jump-starting inflammation to re-direct healing. *J Athl Train.* 2001;38(2):s-95.

47. Young S, Dyson M. Macrophage responsiveness to therapeutic ultrasound. *Ultrasound Med Biol.* 1990;16:326–332.

48. Hashish I, Harvey W, Harris M. Anti-inflammatory effects of ultrasound therapy: evidence for a major placebo effect. *Br J Rheumatol.* 1986;25(1):77–81.

49. Ramirez A, Schwane JA, McFarland C, Starcher B. The effect of ultrasound on collagen synthesis and fibroblast proliferation in vitro. *Med Sci Sports Exerc.* 1997;29:326–332.

50. Fyfe MC, Chahl LA. The effect of single or repeated applications of "therapeutic" ultrasound on plasma extravasation during silver nitrate induced inflammation of the rat hindpaw ankle joint in vivo. *Ultrasound Med Biol.* 1985;11(2):273–283.

51. Harvey W, Dyson M, Pond JB, Grahame R. The stimulation of protein synthesis in human fibroblasts by therapeutic ultrasound. *Rheumatol Rehabil.* 1975;14(4):237.

52. Young S, Dyson M. The effect of therapeutic ultrasound on angiogenesis. *Ultrasound Med Biol.* 1990;16:261–269.

53. Byl NN, McKenzie A, Wong T, West J, Hunt TK. Incisional wound healing: a controlled study of low and high dose ultrasound. *J Orthop Sports Phys Ther.* 1993;18(5):619–628.

54. Behrens BJ, Michlovitz SL. *Physical Agents: Theory and Practice for the Physical Therapist Assistant.* Philadelphia, PA: FA Davis; 1996.

55. Heybeli N, Yesildag A, Oyar O, et al. Diagnostic ultrasound treatment increases the bone fracture-healing rate in an internally fixed rat femoral osteotomy model. *J Ultrasound Med.* 2002;21(12):1357–1363.

56. Huang MH, Ding HJ, Chai CY, Huang YF, Yang RC. Effects of sonication on articular cartilage in experimental osteoarthritis. *J Rheumatol.* 1997;24(10):1978–1984.

57. Jackson BA, Schwane JA, Starcher BC. Effect of ultrasound therapy on the repair of achilles tendon injuries in rats. *Med Sci Sports Exerc.* 1991;23:171–176.

58. Enwemeka CS, Rodriguez O, Mendosa S. The biomechanical effects of low-intensity ultrasound on healing tendons. *Ultrasound Med Biol.* 1990;16(8):801–807.

59. Saini NS, Roy KS, Bansal PS, Singh B, Simran PS. A preliminary study on the effect of ultrasound therapy on the healing of surgically severed achilles tendons in five dogs. *J Vet Med A Physiol Pathol Clin Med.* 2002;49(6):321–328.

60. Turner SM, Powell ES, Ng CS. The effect of ultrasound on the healing of repaired cockeral tendon: is collagen cross-linking a factor? *J Hand Surg [Br].* 1989;14:428–433.

61. Crisci A, Ferreira A. Low-intensity pulsed ultrasound accelerates the regeneration of the sciatic nerve after neurotomy in rats. *Ultrasound Med Biol.* 2002;28:1335–1341.

62. Mourad P, Lazar D, Curra F, et al. Ultrasound accelerates functional recovery after peripheral nerve damage. *Neurosurgery.* 2001;48:1136–1140.

63. Takakura Y, Matsui N, Yoshiya S, et al. Low-intensity pulsed ultrasound enhances early healing of medial collateral ligament injuries in rats. *J Ultrasound Med.* 2002;21(3):283–288.

64. Van Der Windt DA, Van Der Heijden GJ, Van Den Berg SG, et al. Ultrasound therapy for acute ankle sprains. *Cochrane Database Syst Rev.* 2002(1):CD001250.

65. da Cunha A, Parizotto NA, Vidal Bde C. The effect of therapeutic ultrasound on repair of the achilles tendon (tendo calcaneus) of the rat. *Ultrasound Med Biol.* 2001;27(12):1691–1696.

66. Nolte PA, van der Krans A, Patka P, et al. Low-intensity pulsed ultrasound in the treatment of nonunions. *J Trauma.* 2001;51(4):693–702; discussion 702–693.

67. Mayr E, Frankel V, Ruter A. Ultrasound—an alternative healing method for nonunions? *Arch Orthop Trauma Surg.* 2000;120(1–2):1–8.

68. Azuma Y, Ito M, Harada Y, et al. Low-intensity pulsed ultrasound accelerates rat femoral fracture healing by acting on the various cellular reactions in the fracture callus. *J Bone Miner Res.* 2001;16(4):671–680.

69. Wang SJ, Lewallen DG, Bolander ME, et al. Low intensity ultrasound treatment increases strength in a rat femoral fracture model. *J Orthop Res.* 1994;12(1):40–47.

70. Pilla AA, Mont MA, Nasser PR, et al. Non-invasive low-intensity pulsed ultrasound accelerates bone healing in the rabbit. *J Orthop Trauma.* 1990;4(3):246–253.

71. Heckman JD, Ryaby JP, McCabe J, Frey JJ, Kilcoyne RF. Acceleration of tibial fracture-healing by non-invasive, low-intensity pulsed ultrasound. *J Bone Joint Surg Am.* 1994;76(1):26–34.

72. Mayr E, Rudzki MM, Rudzki M, et al. Does low intensity, pulsed ultrasound speed healing of scaphoid fractures? *Handchir Mikrochir Plast Chir.* 2000;32(2):115–122.

73. Kristiansen TK, Ryaby JP, McCabe J, Frey JJ, Roe LR. Accelerated healing of distal radial fractures with the use of specific, low-intensity ultrasound. A multicenter, prospective, randomized, double-blind, placebo-controlled study. *J Bone Joint Surg Am.* 1997;79(7):961–973.

74. Lowden A. Application of ultrasound to assess stress fractures. *Physiotherapy.* 1986;72(3):160–161.

75. Kitchen S, Partridge C. A review of therapeutic ultrasound: Part 1, Background and physiological effects. *Physiotherapy.* 1990;79(10):593–594.

76. Lehmann JF, Masock AJ, Warren CG, Koblanski JN. Effect of therapeutic temperatures on tendon extensibility. *Archiv Phys Med Rehabil.* 1970;51:481–487.

77. Rose S, Draper DO, Schulthies SS, Durrant E. The stretching window part two: rate of thermal decay in deep muscle following 1-MHz ultrasound. *J Athl Train.* 1996;31:139–143.

78. Oates D, Draper D. Retoring wrist range of motion using ultrasound and mobilization: a case study. *Athl Ther Today.* 2006;11(1):57–59.

79. Draper DO. Ultrasound and joint mobilizations for achieving normal wrist range of motion after injury or surgery: a case series. *J Athl Train.* 2010; 45(5).

80. Ziskin M, McDiarmid T, Michlovitz S. Therapeutic ultrasound. In: Michlovitz S, ed. *Thermal Agents in Rehabilitation.* Philadelphia, PA: F. A. Davis; 1996.

81. Smith W, Winn F, Parette R. Comparative study using four modalities in shinsplint treatments. *J Orthop Sports Phys Ther.* 1986;8:77–80.

82. Davidson JH, Vandervoort AA, Lessard LA, Miller L. The effect of acupuncture versus ultrasound on pain level, grip strength and disability in individuals with lateral epicondylitis: A pilot study. *Physiother Can.* 2001;53:195–202.

83. Byl NN. The use of ultrasound as an enhancer for transcutaneous drug delivery: phonophoresis. *Phys Ther.* 1995;75(6):539–553.

84. van Wamel A, Bouakaz A, ten Cate F, de Jong N, Houtgraaf J. Effects of diagnostic ultrasound parameters on molecular uptake and cell viability. Paper presented at 2nd International Symposium on Therapeutic Ultrasound, Seattle, WA, 2002.

85. Darrow H, Schulthies S, Draper D, Ricard M, Measom GJ. Serum dexamethasone levels after decadron phonophoresis. *J Athl Train.* 1999;34(4).

86. Cameron MH, Monroe LG. Relative transmission of ultrasound by media customarily used for phonophoresis. *Phys Ther.* 1992;72:142–148.

87. Strapp EJ, Guskiewicz KM, Hirth C, Saliba S, Hackney AC. The cumulative effect of multiple phonophoresis treatments on Dexamethasone and cortisol concentrations in the blood. *J Athl Train.* 2002;35:S-47.

88. Benson HAE, McElnay IC. Transmission of ultrasound energy through topical pharmaceutical products. *Physiotherapy.* 1988;74:587.

89. Draper DO, Ashton DF, Cosgrove C, Myrer JW, Durrant E. Comparison of Flex-all 4554 and Biofreeze as ultrasound couplants. Paper presented at Annual Symposium of the NATA; Orlando, FL, June 14, 1996.

90. Le L, Kost J, Mitragotri S. Combined effect of low-frequency ultrasound and iontophoresis: applications for transdermal heparin delivery. *Pharm Res.* 2000;17(9):1151–1154.

91. Mitragotri S, Blankschtein D, Langer R. Transdermal drug delivery using low-frequency sonophoresis. *Pharm Res.* 1996;13(3):411–420.

92. Tang H, Mitragotri S, Blankschtein D, Langer R. Theoretical description of transdermal transport of hydrophilic permeants: application to low-frequency sonophoresis. *J Pharm Sci.* 2001;90(5):545–568.

93. Tang H, Wang CC, Blankschtein D, Langer R. An investigation of the role of cavitation in low-frequency ultrasound-mediated transdermal drug transport. *Pharm Res.* 2002;19(8):1160–1169.

94. Mitragotri S, Blankschtein D, Langer R. Ultrasound-mediated transdermal protein delivery. *Science.* 1995;269(5225):850–853.

95. Mitragotri S, Kost J. Low-frequency sonophoresis: a review. *Adv Drug Deliv Rev.* 2004;56(5):589–601.

96. Draper DO, Schulthies S, Sorvisto P, Hautala A-M. Temperature changes in deep muscles of humans during ice and ultrasound therapies: an in vivo study. *J Orthop Sports Phys Ther.* 1995;21(3): 153–157.

97. Rimington SJ, Draper DO, Durrant E, Fellingham G. Temperature changes during therapeutic ultrasound in the precooled human gastrocnemius muscle. *J Athl Train.* 1994;29:325–327.

98. Smith K. *The effect of silicate gel hot packs on human muscle temperature* [Masters Thesis, Draper DO, advisor] Provo, UT: Physical Education, Brigham Young University; 1994 abstracted in *J Athl Train.* 1995;30:S-33.

99. Baker KG, Robertson VJ, Duck FA. A review of therapeutic ultrasound: biophysical effects. *Phys Ther.* 2001;81(7):1351–1358.

100. Robertson VJ, Baker KG. A review of therapeutic ultrasound: effectiveness studies. *Phys Ther.* 2001;81(7):1339–1350.

101. McLachlan Z. Ultrasound treatment for breast engorgement: a randomized double blind trial. *Aust J Physiother.* 1991;37:23–28.

102. Lundeberg T, Abrahamsson P, Haker E. A comparative study of continuous ultrasound, placebo ultrasound and rest in epicondylalgia. *Scand J Rehabil Med.* 1988;20(3):99–101.

103. Falconer J, Hayes KW, Chang RW. Effect of ultrasound on mobility in osteoarthritis of the knee. A randomized clinical trial. *Arthritis Care Res.* 1992;5(1):29–35.

104. Jewell DV, Riddle DL, Thacker LR. Interventions associated with an increased or decreased likelihood of pain reduction and improved function in patients with adhesive capsulitis: A retrospective study. *Phys Ther.* 2009;(5) 419–429.

105. Alexander LD, Gilman DRD, Brown DR, Brown JL, Houghton PE. Exposure to low amounts of ultrasound energy does not improve soft tissue pathology: a systematic review. *Phys Ther.* 2010;90, 14–25.

15

Diathermy

Chapter Outline

OPENING SCENE

A cross-country skier reports to Kaitlyn, your clinical supervisor, with pain in the buttocks. When she questions him about his recent skiing regimen, he states that he has been doing a lot of uphill work. Katelyn performs an evaluation. Since she knows that this type of activity stresses the external rotators of the hip, and through other diagnostic measures, she determines that he has piriformis syndrome. Her treatment regimen involves a heat-and-stretch routine of the piriformis. Which modality would be most appropriate to heat this area prior to or during stretching of the piriformis muscle? Why?

Introducing Diathermy

The word *diathermy* means "through heat" (*dia* and *therm*). **Diathermy** is therapeutically defined as a modality that uses high-frequency electromagnetic waves to heat deep tissues. Heat is produced by the resistance of tissue to the passage of the energy.[1,2]

UNPOPULARITY OF DIATHERMY

Diathermy is used frequently in the United Kingdom, but has fallen out of favor among health care professionals in other parts of the world. Surveys of physical therapists in Australia[3] and more recently in Canada[4] indicate that ultrasound was used daily by 93% and 94%, respectively, yet diathermy was used daily by only 8% and 0.6% of them. Informal surveys by one of us (DD, who speaks frequently to regional and national meetings) indicate similar use of these modalities by athletic trainers and physical therapists in the United States.

Diathermy is used infrequently in the United States for several reasons:

- Expense
- Infamous folklore and misinformation
- Outdated research

Shortwave diathermy units are expensive, ranging from $3,000 to $25,000. Their high cost is prohibitive for many situations, especially a high school, college, or university on a limited budget. For those in private practice, there is a risk that the device will not pay for itself. Many insurance claim forms do not include billing codes for diathermy treatment.

> ## ✔ APPLICATION TIP
>
> ### TRY LEASING
>
> If the price of a diathermy device is out of your price range, you might consider leasing. Some manufacturers will lease on a per-use billing. A timer is placed in the device to keep track of how many minutes the unit is used each month, and the clinician is billed by the minute.

Another reason for limited diathermy use is rumor and folklore. Many of the contraindications regarding diathermy use are untested; they have been based on speculation and shallow research. For example, authors of a 1993 paper concluded that a possible reason physical therapists were having miscarriages was proximity to their patients being treated with diathermy.[5] Rumors spread that if a pregnant woman was even in the same room as an operating diathermy unit, she risked losing her baby. All of those surveyed, however, who reported having miscarried worked in an office where microwave diathermy was in use, not the safer shortwave diathermy. But more importantly, the rate of miscarriages among respondents to this survey was the same as the national average.

There has also been speculation concerning the leak of electromagnetic energy during diathermy use. Whether or not this is true, manufacturers responded in the 1990s by improving the design and safety of the equipment. These improvements include shielding from electromagnetic waves, which not only protects the patient but also safeguards the clinician.[6,7]

Reliance on outdated diathermy research has also contributed to ignorance about this modality. Many of the diathermy studies were performed prior to 1970 on equipment that was inferior to currently produced units. The latest research, performed on updated and improved equipment, indicates that concerns with older equipment do not apply to current equipment.[8–16]

Types of Diathermy

There are two main classifications of diathermy: medical, for therapeutic purposes, and surgical, for cauterizing or burning tissue. The three types of medical or therapeutic diathermy including their common frequencies are:

- Longwave (1 MHz or 300 m). The oldest method of diathermy, but is no longer used. We will not discuss it further.
- Shortwave (27.12 MHz or 11 m). The wave is identical to shortwave radio; therefore, it is regulated by the government to specific frequencies. Shortwave diathermy forms mainly magnetic fields in the tissues.[2]
- Microwave (2450 MHz or 0.12 m). Similar to radar; it mainly produces electrical fields in the tissues.[2] It is seldom used in the United States, partly because of its many contraindications[5] (Fig. 15.1).

MICROWAVE DIATHERMY

Microwave diathermy (MWD) uses high-frequency (300 MHz–300 GHz) electromagnetic waves to heat tissues. A 1984 survey by the U.S. Food and Drug Administration (FDA) indicated that clinics were using shortwave diathermy (SWD) fewer than 6 hours/week, and microwave even less. Here are a few reasons why MWD is so rarely used:

- Metals in the vicinity. Just as with microwave ovens, most metals in contact with MWD reflect the rays. When this occurs outside the body, these rays may reflect back to the *director* (the part of the device that emits the waves),

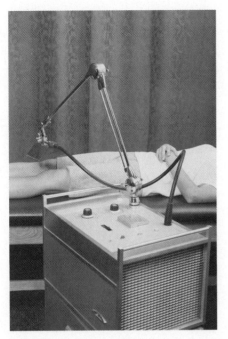

FIGURE 15.1 A microwave diathermy device, rarely used today in the United States.

the patient, or the clinician—thereby resulting in burns. When metal implants are within the body, the reflected rays may overheat adjacent tissues. It is recommended that no metal be any closer than 4 ft during MWD use.

• Skin burning. The higher frequency that MWD uses results in more absorption of the electromagnetic energy in the shallow, fatty tissues. This may result in overheating and superficial burning of the skin and underlying tissues.

• Overheating of superficial tissues. The most common frequency used with MWD is 2450 MHz. This higher frequency easily heats fat and skin, but doesn't heat muscle very well, only about one third as much as SWD. Microwave diathermy at 915 MHz appears to be capable of deeper heating. However, since it is similar to the frequency of cellular phones (840–880 MHz), the risk of tumors has not been ruled out.

• Increased reflection at tissue interfaces. As MWD energy enters the tissues, much of the energy is reflected at tissue interfaces, creating a standing wave (concentrated area of energy) that might lead to hot spots and burning.

• Lost effects. At 2450 MHz, the wave director is placed a certain distance from the body part it is treating, so some of the energy is emitted into the surrounding environment. Thus, some of the therapeutic effects could be lost. The power must be high enough to heat the tissues, but low enough so that skin and fat are not overheated. These calculations can be complicated.

• Hot spots. Little MWD energy is reflected at the bone's surface, which can lead to hot spots.

Ongoing work is being done on producing a lower frequency (750 MHz) microwave diathermy that might heat deep tissues as well as SWD. However, since the majority of treatments in the United States and Europe include SWD, and most of the recent research has been performed on SWD, we will focus on SWD in this chapter. Table 15.1 compares microwave and SWD as used in a clinical setting.

SHORTWAVE DIATHERMY

Shortwave diathermy (SWD) uses high-frequency (10–100 MHz) electromagnetic waves, similar to radio waves, to heat deep tissues; it basically is a radio transmitter. Three frequencies have been assigned to SWD devices by the U.S. Federal Communications Commission (FCC): 13.56, 40.68, and the most common 27.12 MHz, which has a wavelength of 11 m.

Components of a Shortwave Diathermy Device

An SWD device has two main parts (Fig. 15.2):

• Generator—A box-shaped unit (about the size of a miniature refrigerator) contains all of the electrical components of the machine which generate the

TABLE 15.1	SHORTWAVE AND MICROWAVE DIATHERMY COMPARED
SHORTWAVE (SWD)	**MICROWAVE (MWD)**
10–50 MHz frequency	2456–915 MHz frequency
Heating mainly due to magnetic fields	Heating mainly due to electrical fields
Penetrates fat layer easily	Difficult penetration of fat (If fat layer is >0.5 cm, penetration is only one third of SWD)
Unlikely to create hot spots	Can create hot spots
Can apply directly to skin	Spacing required between skin and applicator
Does not heat metal as much as MWD	No metal can be within 4 ft of applicators
Most commonly used in orthopedics	Becoming obsolete

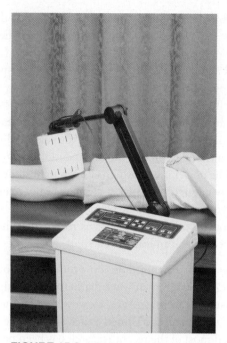

FIGURE 15.2 A SWD generator and drum.

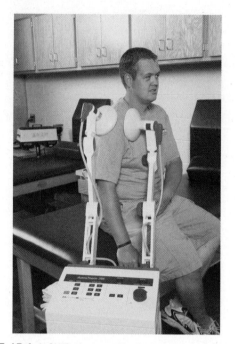

FIGURE 15.4 A SWD device with dual drums can treat a larger area than conventional one-drum units. They can also be used to treat two patients at a time.

electromagnetic waves. A control panel usually sits on the top of the generator. It houses buttons, knobs, and switches for operating the machine.

• Drum (or applicator)—One or more flat spiral copper coils, rigidly fixed inside a hard plastic housing (Fig. 15.3). Its surface area, which varies between manufacturers, is about 200 cm². Some manufacturers

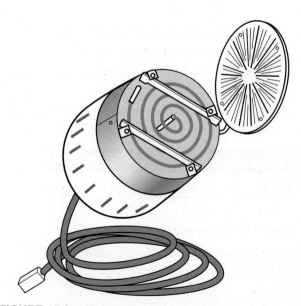

FIGURE 15.3 A SWD drum includes a specifically designed coil of wire through which an electrical current flows, creating a magnetic field that causes an induction field in the tissues to which the drum is applied. (Source: Adapted with permission from Castel, D. International Academy of Physio Therapeutics. Clip Art.)

of SWD produce a device with two drums attached on a hinged arm for treating large or contoured areas (Fig. 15.4).

A diathermy drum serves the same purpose as an ultrasound transducer soundhead; it delivers energy to the tissues. In the past, SWD devices interfaced with several types of applicators, including air space plates, pad electrodes, and cable electrodes. Many of these are now outdated. By far, the most common type of SWD drum currently in use is the induction drum, and as such will be emphasized in this chapter.

An alternative application method, in which the coils are imbedded in a garment, was introduced in 2007 by ReBound (Fig. 15.5). There are separate garment applicators for legs, arms, shoulders, and the back. The idea is to deliver diathermy to a larger area than a drum does.

Despite its larger delivery area, however, the ReBound generator does not produce as much power as drum-type units, and therefore appears to not heat as much as traditional drum type diathermy units. In one case study, it was effective in heating muscle prior to join mobolization.[17] In the only published comparative studies, the Megapulse II PSWD produced 2.4 times more heating than the ReBound at 3.0 cm into the triceps surae muscle group after 20 minutes of application.[18] At a more superficial level (0.7 cm deep), a hot pack heated tissue about the same as the ReBound unit.[19] More research will clarify these points.

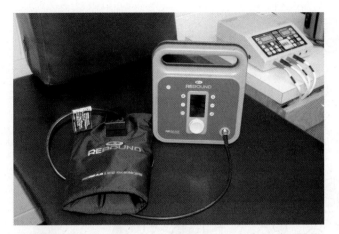

FIGURE 15.5 Diathermy is delivered to the body through this knee garment in which diathermy coils are imbedded. The advantage to this is the entire limb is heated, not just the area that the drum or applicator is over.

How Shortwave Diathermy Works

An SWD device runs on 110 V, 60 Hz AC electricity from a wall outlet. The generator converts the 60 Hz electricity to a radio frequency, usually at 27.12 MHz, and passes it into the spiral copper coil housed in the drum. As the current passes through the coil, it generates a fluctuating, or alternating, magnetic field around the coil. This external magnetic field creates small currents in the tissue next to the drum, known as *eddy currents* (Fig. 15.6). The creation of eddy currents in the tissues differs from electrical nerve and muscle stimulation in that the electrical current of the diathermy drum does not pass through the tissues (see Chapter 16).

The alternating tissue eddy currents cause dipoles, especially water molecules, to rotate (Fig. 15.7). A *dipole* is a pair of equal and opposite electric charges separated by a small distance. A water molecule is a dipole because it is triangularly shaped, and the oxygen molecule has a stronger attraction for the electrons of the two hydrogen atoms than the hydrogen does. Thus, the oxygen side of the molecule becomes slightly negatively charged, and the hydrogen side becomes positively charged (note the individual molecules in Fig. 15.7).

As the dipole (water molecule) rotates due to the changing polarity of the eddy currents, the tissue kinetic energy increases. This increased kinetic energy is known as the nonthermal effects of diathermy. Friction between the rotating dipoles results in an additional increase in kinetic energy, which is manifested in an increase in tissue temperature, or the thermal effect. Thus, diathermy affects tissues that are high in water content (muscle) more than tissues with less water (skin, tendon, bone) (Fig. 15.8).

Current Flow

The greatest current flow is through the tissues with the smallest resistance. When SWD produces a magnetic field, adipose tissue (fat) does not provide much resistance to the flow of energy, but it will heat up to some extent.[20] Thus, tissues that are high in water (i.e., muscle and blood) respond best to a magnetic field and produce heat[21] (see Fig. 15.8).

Continuous and Pulsed Shortwave Diathermy

SWD can be applied in either continuous or pulsed mode. *Continuous shortwave diathermy (CSWD)*, where a continuous current is generated, has been used in the treatment of a variety of conditions for some time. In the 1930s, it was used in the United States for treating infections, but its use declined in the 1950s with the introduction of antibiotics to fight infection, and with concerns about safety of the device. CSWD is rarely used today because it causes too rapid, and too much, heating in the patient and can be quite uncomfortable. It has been replaced by pulsed SWD.

Pulsed shortwave diathermy (PSWD) transmits a series of high-frequency (10–100 MHz) electromagnetic pulse trains of waves to produce nonthermal and thermal effects in deep tissues. The modality was first developed in 1940.[7] Although its use has declined, PSWD has recently been the subject of renewed interest, and research documenting its clinical efficacy continues to grow.[6,8,9,14,16]

The electromagnetic waves create a sine wave current that is interrupted (pulsed) at regular intervals. Each

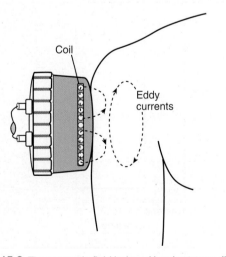

FIGURE 15.6 The magnetic field induced by shortwave diathermy creates small eddy currents in the body tissues, resulting in heat.

Coil

Eddy currents

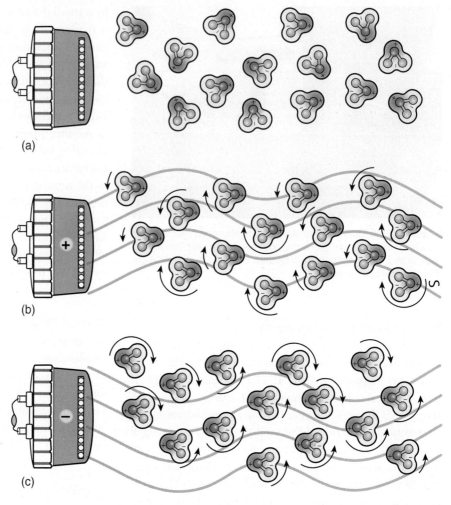

FIGURE 15.7 Dipole response. **(a)** Dipoles (water molecules) in untreated tissue, **(b)** dipoles rotate varying amounts to line up parallel to eddy current lines of force after diathermy is applied to surface of tissue, **(c)** dipoles rotate as the diathermy current alternates.

series of *pulses, or pulse trains,* similar to those used in electricity (see Chapter 17), can be adjusted to where nonthermal or thermal effects are generated in the tissues. In much the same way that a pulsed electrical current is created by periodically interrupting continuous current flow, PSWD is created by interrupting CSWD at consistent intervals. Thus, PSWD has distinct on and off times (Fig. 15.9).

Three factors determine how much heat a PSWD device produces: pulse width, pulse rate, and power, which is a function of pulse width and pulse rate.

• **Pulse width,** also known as *pulse duration,* is the on time, the time required for each pulse to complete its cycle. The interval between pulses is the off time. A wide pulse generates more tissue energy than a narrow pulse. Pulse widths are very short, 20–400 microseconds (μs; millionths of

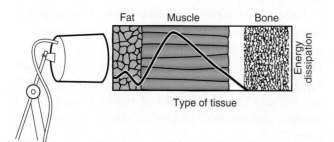

FIGURE 15.8 The greatest amount of SWD heating is in tissues with low impedance, especially muscle.

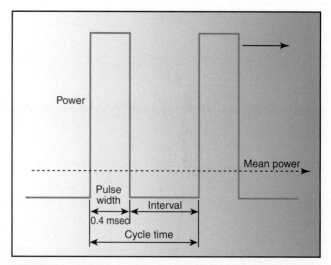

FIGURE 15.9 Pulsed shortwave diathermy (PSWD results from interrupting CSWD).

a second). Each manufacturer provides several preset options. For example, the Megapulse II has pulse widths of 20, 40, 65, 100, 200, and 400 µs. The Curapulse 403 offers pulse widths of 65, 82, 110, 150, 200, 300, and 400 µs.

- **Pulse rate**, or pulse repetition rate, is the number of pulses delivered per second (pps, in Hz). The greater the number of pulses per second, the more energy produced. Pulse rate ranges from 1 to 7000 Hz. Each manufacturer provides several preset options. For example, the Megapulse II has pulse rates of 100, 200, 400, 600, and 800 pps; the Curapulse 403 offers pulse rates of 26. 35, 46, 62, 82, 110, 150, 200, 300, and 400 pps.

- **Power**, also referred to as *intensity*, is measured in watts (W). It is the power delivered from the machine, and is a function of both pulse width and pulse frequency. SWD with a long pulse width and a high pulse frequency generates more power than a short pulse width and low pulse frequency.

With PSWD, energy is transmitted to the tissues in a series of high-frequency pulse trains. Pulse width is generally short, ranging from 20 to 400 µs with an intensity of up to 1000 W per pulse. For example, if PSWD is used at 400 Hz with a pulse duration of 400 µs, the machine is on about 0.16 sec or 16% of the time.

The pulse repetition rate is chosen using the pulse-frequency button on the generator control panel.[7,22] Typically, the on time is shorter than the off time. This has led many to believe that even if heat is produced during the on time, the long off-time interval allows blood flow to enter the area causing the heat to disperse, thereby reducing the likelihood of any significant tissue temperature increase. This assumption is not correct because researchers have found significant temperature increases of over 104°F (40°C) in human muscle when PSWD was applied at 400 and 800 Hz (or just 48 W average power).[8,10,14]

When PSWD is used at intensities that create an increase in tissue temperature, its effects are no different from those of CSWD. Successful treatments have largely resulted from the application of higher intensities and longer treatment times. In order to increase temperature in tissues, the average intensity needs to be above 12 W. In general, PSWD produces lower intensities than CSWD (80–120 W).

Table 15.2 lists the common pulse width and pulse rate settings available on many PSWD devices. Note that we often refer to 48 W average power in this chapter. It is simply the 7.2°F (4°C) increase in muscle temperature that we have repeatedly obtained in 15–20 minutes using the parameters of 400 µs and 800 pps.

Physiological Effects of Diathermy

The physiological effects of SWD are categorized as thermal and nonthermal. Whenever diathermy is applied, nonthermal effects occur. When enough energy is absorbed by the tissue, both nonthermal and thermal effects occur.

Mild heating can occur with an average power of just 10.88 W.[23] In our experience, 12 W PSWD produces a mild temperature increase of 1.8°F (1°C). For nonthermal effects, we suggest using an average power of 10 W or less when the effects of heat are not desired (i.e., acute swelling), but when mechanical effects are desired for the treatment of soft tissue injuries.[7,24]

NONTHERMAL EFFECTS

To put it simply, when a patient has an injury, cells are affected. The cells that are unable to perform their normal function are referred to as "sick cells." Basically

DOSE	TEMPERATURE SENSATION	INDICATIONS	PULSE WIDTH	PULSE RATE	AVERAGE WATTS
n/a	Nonthermal	Acute trauma, not noticeable inflammation, edema reduction, cell repolarization and repair	65 µs	100–200 pps	n/a
1°C	Mild warmth	Subacute inflammation	100 µs 200 µs	800 pps *or* 400 pps	12
2°C	Moderate warmth	Pain reduction, muscle spasm, chronic inflammation	200 µs 400 µs	800 pps *or* 400 pps	24
4°C	Vigorous heating	Stretching collagen-rich tissues	400 µs	800 pps	48

TABLE 15.2 PSWD PARAMETERS BASED ON TREATMENT GOALS

electromagnetic energy from PSWD helps sick cells to get better and return to their normal function.

The nonthermal effects of PSWD appear to be at the cell membrane level. They are caused by changes in the way ions bind to the cell membrane, as well as changes in cell function caused by the electromagnetic waves.[25] The nonthermal effects include:

- Repolarization of damaged cells, enabling them to return to normal function.[26] Although the mechanism behind this is not well understood, some speculate that it has to do with cell membrane potential.[27] Injured cells experience depolarization, which may cause the cell to lose its ability to divide, multiply, and regenerate. It is thought that both PSWD and ultrasound can stimulate increased macrophage activity.
- Acceleration of cell growth and division when it is too slow, and inhibition of cell growth when it is too fast[28]
- Reestablishment of the sodium pump. During injury, energy deficiencies occur in the cell, and the sodium pump slows down (see Chapter 5). Thus, an excess of sodium is deposited in the cell, producing a negatively charged environment. When a magnetic field is induced, the sodium pump speeds up, thereby allowing the cell to regain normal ionic balance.[29]
- Increased microvascular perfusion.[30,31] This increase in local circulation can increase oxygen uptake in local tissues, increase nutrient availability, and promote phagocytosis.
- Improved cell function. A cell involved in the inflammatory process demonstrates a reduced cell membrane potential; thus, cell function is disturbed. The altered potential affects ion transport across the membrane, and the resulting ionic balance alters cellular osmotic pressures often resulting in pain and edema. Apparently, application of PSWD to these cells restores cell membrane potential to their normal values and also restores normal membrane transport and ionic balance.
- Increased number of white cells in a wound[23]

THERMAL EFFECTS

PSWD can cause significant temperature increases up to 4–5 cm deep in the muscle when the drum is placed directly on the skin.[8,10,14] The physiological effects of PSWD at ≥12 W average power are primarily thermal and include:

- Tissue temperature rise[6,10,14,32–36]
- Increased blood flow[32–35]
- Vasodilation[37]
- Relaxation[37]

- Decreased joint stiffness[38–40]
- Increased membrane filtration and diffusion
- Increased tissue metabolic rate
- Changes in some enzyme reactions[41]
- Alterations in the physical properties of fibrous tissues (tendons, joints, and scars)[42]
- Muscle relaxation[42]
- Pain reduction[32–34,38,43–45]
- Reduction of knee synovitis in arthritic patients[43]
- Reduction of the inflammatory process[23,43]
- Encouragement of collagen layering at an early stage[23]
- Hematoma absorption[23]

Optimal Tissue Temperatures

Views regarding the temperature required to bring about the various physiological effects are diverse. Some are of the opinion that a 7.2°F (4°C) increase above baseline produces optimal thermal effects[22] (see Table 15.1). Others believe that the temperature must reach 100.4–104°F (38–40°C).[44] Most researchers believe the temperature of deep tissues with a baseline temperature of 98.6°F (37°C) should be raised as close as possible to 104°F (40°C) for diathermy to reach its optimal therapeutic effectiveness.[8,46,47] Too rapid or too great a temperature increase can be detrimental. As temperature rises past 113°F (45°C), it alters the structural characteristics of protein, as it does when burned.[1]

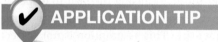

✔ APPLICATION TIP

As with all modalities, you should experience for yourself the effects of thermal PSWD. Compare them to the sensation of other heating devices, such as hot packs, whirlpools, ultrasound, and even paraffin baths.

Treatment Time

Vigorous heating (104°F, or 40°C, from a baseline temperature of 98.6°F, or 37°C) 3–5 cm deep in the lower leg can be reached in as little as 15–20 minutes when treated with PSWD at 48 W average power.[8,10] A 20-minute treatment for one body area is probably all that is necessary to reach maximum physiological effects. In fact, in two studies, the temperature actually started to drop slightly 0.54°F (0.3°C) during the last 5 minutes of a 20-minute treatment.[8,48] Apparently as the tissue temperatures reach 104–105.8°F (40–41°C), the thermoregulatory aspect of the cerebral cortex responds to this high localized temperature, and

BOX 15.1 A USER-FRIENDLY PSWD DEVICE

In Chapter 14, we described an ultrasound device that enabled the clinician to use temperature increases for treatment goals, instead of a clock to measure treatment time. A PSWD device has been developed in much the same way. The research involved measuring temperature in the leg muscles of over 50 subjects to determine the pulse rate and pulse width required to raise muscle temperature 1.8°F, or 1°C (mild heat); 3.6°F, or 2°C (moderate heat); and 7.2°F, or 4°C (vigorous heat). Based on this research, a diathermy device was equipped with a keypad that included these three levels of heat (Fig. 15.10). After setting up the device over the area to be treated, the clinician selects the heating level that best achieves the treatment goal. The device automatically tunes

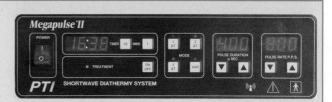

FIGURE 15.10 The control panel on a typical PSWD device.

into the preprogrammed settings (pulse width, pulse rate) to reach that goal. The device shuts off when the desired temperature is theoretically reached (theoretical because the device does not measure the current patient's temperature, but is based on the means of 50 previous subjects).

blood flow increases to the area in an attempt to cool the tissues.[46] Increased blood flow is one of the benefits of using any thermal modality.[34]

Trying to determine the correct parameters such as time, pulse frequency, and duration to reach specific treatment goals can be overwhelming. Box 15.1 shows the control panel of a user-friendly PSWD machine.

Clinical Applications of Shortwave Diathermy

There are several situations in which PSWD is considered appropriate or in some cases optimal:

- The skin or some underlying soft tissue is very sensitive and will not bear the pressure of a moist heat pack or the jet from a whirlpool.
- A tissue temperature rise is desired in tissues deeper than 1–2 cm beneath the skin.
- Nonthermal effects are desired in tissues deeper than 1–2 cm beneath the skin.
- The treatment goal is to increase deep tissue temperatures over a large area (approximately the size of the drum), such as the shoulder girdle, low back, or the hamstring or triceps surae muscle belly.
- Nonthermal effects are desired in deep tissue over a large area.
- Over irregular or uneven surfaces, such as the hand or foot
- Prior to passive stretch or joint mobilizations of any joint larger than the wrist

 CONCEPT CHECK 15.1. A lean patient comes to you with some muscular back pain over a large area. He can pinpoint two or three silver dollar-sized tender areas, but the rest of his back is generally sore. Unfortunately you don't have a PSWD device. What can you do to heat the area?

HEATING JOINT CAPSULES PRIOR TO STRETCHING OR MOBILIZATIONS

Some of the most promising uses of PSWD have been with stretching or joint mobilizations to increase range of motion (ROM).[11,16,38,39,49,50] A heat-and-stretch regimen using PSWD increases the flexibility of subjects with tight muscles,[11] and limited ankle dorsiflexion.[49] This effect probably results from:
- Local relaxation by decreasing muscle guarding and pain[46]
- Decreased stiffness of tissues[27]
- Increased extensibility of the collagen fibers and the resilience of contracted soft tissues[27,38,49]

✔ APPLICATION TIP

USE PSWD PRIOR TO STRETCHING

If you have a patient with joint capsule adhesions that won't allow normal ROM, use PSWD prior to stretching. Case 15.1 provides an example of how this can be accomplished.

CASE 15.1 REGIMEN OF PSWD AND STRETCHING RESTORES ROM TO ANKLE

In 1995, 34-year-old Brian rolled his jeep and was stabbed in the calf by the knobless gear-shift shaft, which caused significant muscle damage and a fractured tibia. Following surgery and some physical therapy, he had 0° dorsiflexion range of motion. Four years later (1999), he was treated with a regimen of 20-minute PSWD at 800 Hz, at a pulse width of 400 μs (48 W average power). Ten minutes into the heat treatment, stretch was applied for 10 minutes. By the seventh treatment, he reached 16° of dorsiflexion (20° is normal). Seven years after his treatments (2006), he still had all the ROM he gained from the diathermy and stretching regimen (Fig. 15.11).

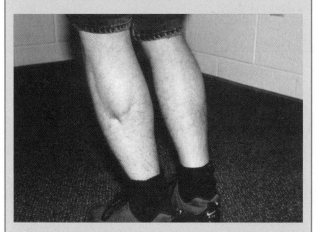

FIGURE 15.11 Dorsiflexion was restored in the left ankle with PSWD and stretching 4 years after an accident that caused significant muscle damage and a fractured tibia. (Note the divot in the calf, a residual of the accident.)

Joint mobilizations should always be preceded by some form of heat.[49] Heated tissue stretches more easily, thus increasing the efficacy of mobilization, and is more comfortable for the patient. Cases 15.2–15.5 illustrate the application of PSWD with joint mobilization to restore ROM in patients with a frozen joint.[36] In most of these cases, traditional interventions had failed to restore ROM.

 CONCEPT CHECK 15.2. While visiting another clinic, you notice a clinician using ultrasound in an attempt to heat the entire knee on a patient. In the corner, you see a PSWD device, and ask why it is not being used instead. The clinician replies, "Diathermy is dangerous and could overheat the patient and cause stray electromagnetic rays to effect other modalities and computers in the clinic." How would you respond?

CASE 15.2 PSWD AND JOINT MOBILIZATIONS TO RESTORE ELBOW ROM

Brittany experienced a fracture/dislocation 2 years prior to reporting to our lab. She underwent three surgeries to repair her elbow, during one of which a radial head prosthesis was inserted in her elbow (Fig. 15.12a). Figure 15.12b (before) and 15.12c (after) show her ROM progress during 5 PSWD and joint mobilization treatments.

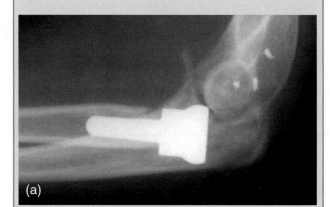
(a)

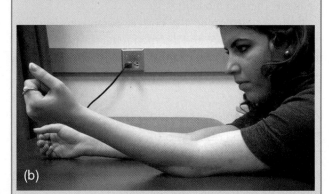
(b)

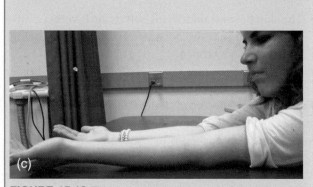
(c)

FIGURE 15.12 This patient was able to gain full elbow range of motion when a regimen of PSWD and joint mobilizations was followed.

USE PSWD PRIOR TO JOINT MOBILIZATIONS

We agree with joint mobilization specialist Kaltenborn[40] that joint mobilizations should be preceded by some form of heat. Then why not deep heat aimed right at the source? PSWD for 15–20 minutes prior to joint mobilizations will not only help heat the tissues to be stressed, but it will reduce the discomfort patients often experience during mobilizations.

Diathermy Treatment Contraindications and Precautions

There are more precautions and contraindications for the use of microwave diathermy than for that of SWD. In addition, there are apparently more treatment precautions and contraindications for the use of PSWD than any of the other physical modalities used clinically. However, don't let this discourage you from using it. Many prescription medications have a long list of contraindications, but when used appropriately, the benefits far outweigh the risks. This same approach should be taken with SWD. It is a powerful tool when used correctly.

Remember that the power meter on a diathermy device does not indicate the actual amount of energy that is being absorbed in the tissues. Thus, you must rely on the sensation of pain for a warning that the patient's tolerance level has been exceeded.

CONTRAINDICATIONS

The contraindications of PSWD include:

- Implanted pacemaker, neurostimulator, or defibrillator.[51] The lead wires can act as antennas and provide intensely focused fields at the tissue-lead junction, causing significant tissue damage that could lead to serious injury or death. Application of PSWD should be limited to below the waistline.
- Some surgically implanted metals. Don't use PSWD over metal implants that form closed loops such as might occur with wires used for fixating rods and plates in surgical fracture repairs. The current can flow in the wire loops, resulting in excessive heating.[2]
- Pregnancy. Avoid treating the abdomen, pelvis, or back, in view of the probable effect that PSWD might have on embryonic tissue and the placenta.[46]

- Over tumors. Some physicians use very high-power PSWD to destroy cancerous cells; however, due to the possibility that PSWD increases the activity of tumor cells, this is beyond the scope of the athletic trainer or therapist.[46,52]
- Fever. PSWD can cause the temperature to increase even more.[52]
- Infection. PSWD can increase metabolism, thereby causing the infection to spread.
- Growth plates. Although this has not been tested in humans, we surmise that a rapid increase in temperature may damage epiphyseal plates.
- Testes. A rapid increase in temperature might lead to sterility.
- On or near the eyes or contact lenses for any prolonged period of time
- Joint effusion
- Protruded nucleus pulposus[52]

! Modality Myth

PSWD CANNOT BE USED NEAR METAL

Metal is highly conductive when an electrical current is applied, and it is thought to become very hot when diathermy is applied. This is true with MWD and CSWD, but not true for PSWD. We list it as a precaution with PSWD.

In the past, it was considered unsafe to treat a patient with PSWD on a wooden table or a plastic chair if it had been constructed with metal screws.[2] But it is safe. The energy will not heat up the screws, nor will it be transmitted to the patient.

PRECAUTIONS

Care should be taken when using PSWD:

- For conditions where increased temperature is not desired
- Over traumatic musculoskeletal injuries with acute bleeding
- For acute inflammatory conditions[46]
- On areas with reduced blood supply
- Over areas with reduced sensitivity to temperature or pain[53]
- Over fluid-filled areas or organs
- During menstruation. PSWD applied to the abdomen, pelvis, or low back could increase bleeding.[54]

CASE 15.3 PSWD AND JOINT MOBILIZATIONS TO RESTORE SHOULDER ROM FROM ADHESIVE CAPSULITIS

Frank, a 45-year-old, suffered from adhesive capsulitis in his right shoulder, due to insidious onset. Entry and discharge ROM in degrees were:

- Flexion 126/146
- Extension 13/47
- Internal Rotation 20/51
- External Rotation 10/52
- Abduction 95/155

Treatments of PSWD, ultrasound (of the vertebral boarder of the scapula), and joint mobilizations were given once a day for 6 days. He finished equal to, or within, 90% of the opposite limb in all actions. Figure 15.13a and 15.13b illustrate abduction and flexion before treatment; Figure 15.13c and 15.13d illustrate abduction and flexion after treatment.

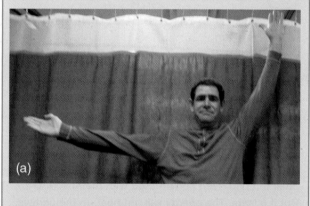

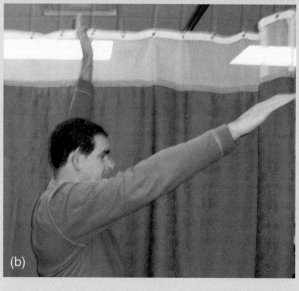

CASE 15.3 PSWD AND JOINT MOBILIZATIONS TO RESTORE SHOULDER ROM FROM ADHESIVE CAPSULITIS (*Continued*)

FIGURE 15.13 This physical therapy assistant was able to have the majority of his shoulder range of motion restored when a regimen of PSWD and joint mobilizations was followed.

- Over wet or infected wound dressings. If the wound is dry and not infected, PSWD is safe.
- Over some implanted metals.[51] PSWD can be used to treat soft tissue adjacent to most metal implants that don't form a loop, without much increase in the temperature of the metal. Before treating any patient with metal implants, be aware of what type of implant is involved. If you do proceed with a treatment, and the patient complains of too much heat, turn the machine off.
- Near other equipment. Some of the newer PSWD devices are shielded from emitting stray electromagnetic waves and are probably safe to use around other equipment. If your unit was manufactured prior to 1993, it may be wise to use it at a safe distance from other types of medical electrical devices or equipment that is transistorized. Transcutaneous electrical nerve stimulation (TENS) units and other low-frequency current units often have transistor-type circuits, and these can be damaged by the reflected or stray radiation that might be produced by PSWD devices.

Modality Myth

PSWD CANNOT BE USED OVER ANY METAL

Many are of the opinion that PSWD can't be used on a patient with braces in his/her mouth. This is safe, unless the face is being treated. For treating TMJ, we suggest ultrasound.

Several authors[1,2,7,46,55] claim that PSWD is contraindicated on a patient with surgically implanted pins, rods, or screws. Not true, at least for the Megapulse II (Accelerated Care Plus, Reno, NV) at 48 W, as long as the metal implant is not a circular wire or loop.[2,16,52] Other units may be safe as well, but have not yet been tested.

PSWD USE ON PATIENTS WITH SURGICALLY IMPLANTED METAL

Perhaps the greatest controversy regarding the use of SWD is treating an area with surgically implanted metal plates, screws, and pins.[56] It is thought that the shunting of the radio frequency field through a metal implant may increase the current density around the implant and cause a greater local temperature increase than in tissue without metal implants.[6,14,16,57] Neither microwave diathermy nor CSWD should be applied over tissue with implanted metal. Such patients can be safely treated with PSWD at 48 W, however.[16,54] Cases 15.4 and 15.5 describe two of the many patients with implanted metal treated in our laboratory.

CONCEPT CHECK 15.3. You begin a PSWD treatment on a padded table that has a metal frame. Your superior comes in, calls you "ignorant," and immediately turns the machine off. Why did this happen? What can you do to rectify it?

Modality Myth

A FOLDED TOWEL MUST BE PLACED BETWEEN THE DIATHERMY DRUM AND THE PATIENT

In the past, clinicians placed a single layer of toweling between the drum and the skin to absorb perspiration. With the newer developments with PSWD, this practice is necessary only in humid climates or when the tissue temperature becomes a little uncomfortable for the patient. Also, toweling might be used in areas of the body where moisture accumulates (such as the axillas or gluteal cleft). The results are best when the drum is placed directly on the skin, but the area treated must remain dry.

Clinicians also used to think it was important to remove clothing from the treatment area. While this is true with synthetic fabrics that do not allow moisture to evaporate, SWD can safely be applied over cotton clothing. This is a great advantage for modest patients.

CASE 15.4 LAUREL'S LONG ROAD TO RECOVERY[12]

In 2002, Laurel fractured her elbow in several places during an automobile accident. During two surgeries, physicians installed plates, pins, and screws to repair her arm (Fig. 15.14a). After 10 weeks of immobilization, she started physical therapy. Within several months, some of the ROM was restored. However, during the next 2 months, little progress was made, and she lacked the last 12° of flexion and 28° of extension (Fig. 15.14b). She reported to our lab where PSWD (48 W) and joint mobilizations were applied to her elbow. She gained 5° flexion and 7° extension on the first visit. By her fourth visit, all of her flexion had returned, and by her sixth visit, she had regained all but 3° of extension (Fig. 15.14c). Upon evaluation a few months later, she had full active elbow extension. Three years later (2006), she still had full ROM.

CASE 15.4 LAUREL'S LONG ROAD TO RECOVERY[12] (Continued)

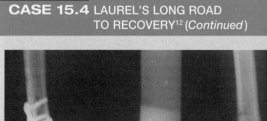

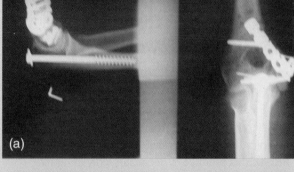

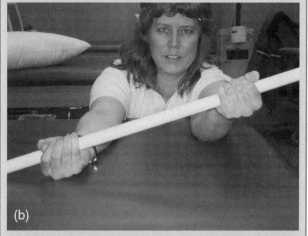

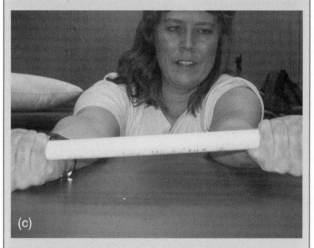

FIGURE 15.14 This high school English teacher was able to have her elbow range of motion restored when a regimen of PSWD and joint mobilizations was performed. (Note the metal plates and screws in her elbow).

CASE 15.5 PSWD AND JOINT MOBILIZATIONS TO RESTORE ANKLE ROM

Figure 15.15a is an x-ray of the leg of a 48-year-old woman who suffered a severe automobile accident. The injury was so bad that the physician suggested amputation. Instead, surgery was performed using extensive metal plates, pins, and screws to repair the leg. One year later, she reported to our lab with very little ROM in the ankle. After several treatments of PSWD (Fig. 15.15b) and joint mobilizations, she returned to pain-free gait and improved her dorsiflexion 15°. Note that the entire ankle was heated with two units, one on each side. A dual-drum unit could also be used.

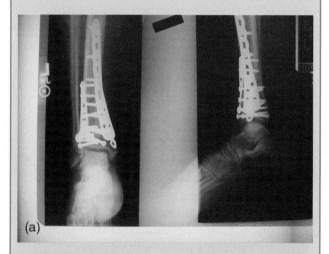

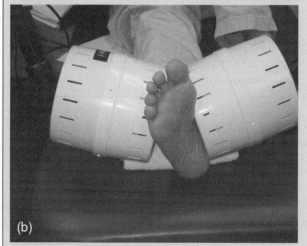

FIGURE 15.15 This patient was able to obtain full range of motion in dorsiflexion and plantar flexion restored following a regimen of PSWD and joint mobilizations. (Note the metal implants in her tibia).

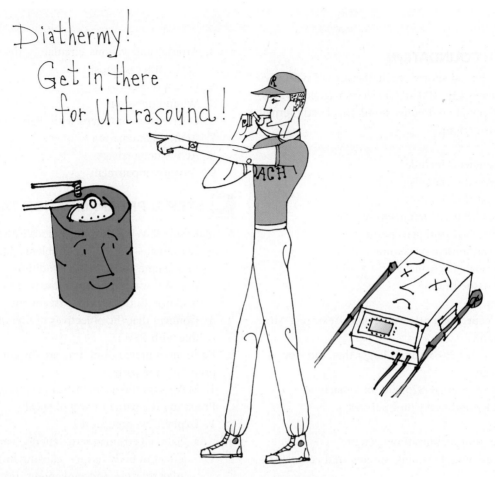

FIGURE 15.16 PSWD is more effective for large areas than ultrasound.

Advantages of PSWD over Ultrasound

There are several advantages of using PSWD instead of ultrasound (Fig. 15.16):

- A larger area is heated. The surface of a diathermy drum is about the size of a small salad plate, whereas the ultrasound treatment size is about the size of a tablespoon. Thus, the diathermy drum is often 25–30 times larger than the treatment area for ultrasound (50–60 times larger if a two-drum applicator is used).
- The energy is more uniform in a diathermy drum than in an ultrasound head (see discussion of BNR and hot spots in Chapter 14). Therefore, a PSWD drum remains stationary during the treatment, freeing the clinician to work on other patients.

- The heat provided by diathermy lasts two or three times longer than that provided by ultrasound, enabling the clinician to perform low-load, long-duration stretching for 10–15 minutes while the tissue is still warm.
- No messy gels or couplants are required.
- The treatment can be applied over some clothing.
- Ultrasound application requires a clinician or aide to be present during the entire treatment; PSWD application requires only periodic monitoring by the clinician or aid, so the clinician is free to work with multiple patients simultaneously.

 CONCEPT CHECK 15.4. Now you have read both the ultrasound and diathermy chapters, and have just finished reading about some of the advantages of PSWD use over ultrasound. Can you think of some advantages of ultrasound use over PSWD?

Application of Diathermy

STEP 1: FOUNDATION

A. Definition. Pulsed shortwave diathermy (PSWD) uses high-frequency (10–100 MHz) electromagnetic waves, in a pulsed mode, to produce nonthermal and thermal effects in deep tissues.

B. Effects
   1. Thermal effects include:
      a. Increased metabolism
      b. Increased blood flow
      c. Increased tissue temperature
      d. Diminished pain perception
      e. General muscle relaxation
   2. Nonthermal effects include:
      a. Soft tissue healing

C. Advantages
   1. Heats deeper than other modalities (except 1 MHz ultrasound)
   2. Heats an area 25–30 times larger than ultrasound

D. Disadvantages
   1. Expensive ($3,000–$25,000 for a machine)
   2. Big, bulky, and heavy; not portable

E. Indications
   1. Prior to joint mobilization exercise
   2. Post acute muscle strains, sprains, and contusions
   3. Pain
   4. Tendinitis
   5. Tenosynovitis
   6. Bursitis
   7. Myofascial trigger points
   8. Joint contracture

F. Contraindications
   1. General heat contraindications
   2. Cardiac pacemaker
   3. Pregnancy
   4. Malignant tumor
   5. Fever
   6. Ischemic areas
   7. Peripheral vascular disease
   8. Tuberculosis
   9. Sites of infection
   10. Eyes
   11. Genitals
   12. Epiphyseal plates in children
   13. Protruded nucleus pulposus

G. Precautions
   1. Surgically implanted metals (especially circular, or loops)
   2. Pelvic or lumbar exposure during menstruation

   3. Arterial and venous circulatory disorders (thrombosis, atherosclerosis, etc.)
   4. Osteoporosis
   5. Wound dressings
   6. Over tissues or organs with high fluid volume
   7. Acute inflammation
   8. Active hemorrhage
   9. Sensory impairment

STEP 2: PREAPPLICATION TASKS

A. Make sure PSWD is the proper modality for this situation.
   1. Reevaluate the injury/problem. Make sure you understand the patient's condition.
   2. If PSWD was applied previously, review the patient's response to the previous treatment.
   3. Confirm that the objectives of therapy are compatible with PSWD.

B. Equipment preparation. Prepare the equipment before preparing the patient.
   1. Make sure the drum is clean and dry.

C. Preparing the patient psychologically
   1. Explain the procedure.
      a. Safe electromagnetic energy causes a dipole effect in body tissues, causing increased molecular rotation and movement, resulting in heat.
      b. Gentle warmth should be felt during the treatment (unless it is a nonthermal treatment).
      c. Demonstrate the procedure on yourself if the patient is apprehensive.
   2. Check for, and warn the patient about, precautions.
      a. If the treatment starts to feel too warm, ask the patient to let you know.

D. Preparing the patient physically
   1. Remove any metal or jewelry from the part to be treated.
   2. Remove any synthetic fabrics that might trap heat in the area to be treated.
   3. Position the patient in a comfortable yet modest position, while allowing accessibility to the diathermy device.
   4. Inspect the area to be treated. If there are rashes or moist open wounds, do not proceed.

STEP 3: APPLICATION PARAMETERS

A. Procedures
   1. Place the drum on the treatment area (place a towel between the drum and the skin if desired).
   2. Turn the device on.

B. Dosage
1. Set the pulse duration (low for acute, nonthermal; high for thermal).
2. Set the pulse frequency (low for acute, nonthermal; high for thermal).
3. Set the treatment time (15–30 minutes).
4. Depress the start button.
5. Adjust the intensity according to the patient's comfort. Recheck in 4–5 minutes as the tissues heat up.

C. Length of application
1. 15–30 minutes

D. Frequency of application
1. 1–2 times daily

E. Duration of therapy
1. Until treatment goals are reached

4 STEP 4: POSTAPPLICATION TASKS

A. Equipment removal and replacement
1. When the timer shuts off signaling the end of the treatment, make sure all knobs/buttons are at zero.

B. Instructions to the patient
1. Schedule the next treatment.
2. Instruct the patient about level of activity and/or self-treatment prior to the next formal treatment.
3. Instruct the patient about what he/she should feel following treatment.

C. Record of treatment, including unique patient responses

D. Equipment cleaning and replacement
1. Clean off the table, removing any sweat or moisture.
2. If you used a towel, replace it with a clean one.

5 STEP 5: MAINTENANCE

A. Clean the equipment regularly.
B. Make sure all cables and connections are in good repair.

CLOSING SCENE

Recall from the chapter opening scene that Katelyn was presented a case of a cross-country skier who had piriformis syndrome. In preparation for applying a heat-and-stretch routine to the piriformis, she considered which modality would be most appropriate to heat this area and why. After reading this and previous chapters, you know that hot packs and whirlpools, though convenient, can penetrate only the superficial structures from 1–2 cm deep. In order to penetrate the gluteal muscles to get at the source of the problem (piriformis), she must use a deep-heating modality. Although ultrasound is a deep-heating modality, is not appropriate in this situation because it only heats a small area.[14] Diathermy heats deep tissues and heats an area as large as the applicator drum, so PSWD is the modality of choice in this situation.[10,14]

Chapter Reflections

1. Read and ponder each of the following points. Do you feel you have a clear understanding of each concept? If not, reread the appropriate section of the chapter.
   - What is diathermy?
   - Name two types of diathermy.
   - Identify the most popular type of diathermy in the United States and explain the reasons for its popularity.
   - List the effects of diathermy.
   - Describe the indications of diathermy.
   - List several contraindications of diathermy.
   - Compare and contrast diathermy with ultrasound.
   - Discuss some diathermy myths.
2. Write three to five questions to discuss with your class instructor, clinical instructor, classmates, and clinical colleagues.

3. Get together with classmates and quiz each other on the concepts of this chapter. Use the points in reflection no. 1 and questions you wrote for reflection no. 2 as a beginning. Explaining concepts out loud to others requires a deeper grasp of the material than feeling you understand it as you read.
4. Once you feel you understand the principles of application, practice applying PSWD treatments using the 5-step approach to a classmate or a clinical colleague. Once you have applied it, allow the classmate to apply the modality to you, listening and observing carefully to determine if your classmate is applying it properly. You should use your notes when the modality is applied to you, and during the first few times you apply the modality. Continue practicing the application until you can do so without your notes.

Concept Check Responses

CONCEPT CHECK 15.1

The key here is that the patient is lean, so you can apply hot packs to the general sore areas. On the silver dollar-sized tender areas, consider using ultrasound. The treatment size is perfect, and the 1 MHz setting will penetrate deep enough to get at the problem.

CONCEPT CHECK 15.2

Explain that ultrasound ideally will heat structures about two times the size of the soundhead, whereas PSWD will heat an area as large as the applicator (drum of coil; ~20–25 times larger than a US applicator), making it ideal for knees and much larger areas. As far as safety goes, the clinician must have PSWD confused with microwave diathermy, which currently is not approved by the FDA. The newer PSWD devices do not emit stray electromagnetic waves and therefore are save for the patient, others, and surrounding equipment.

CONCEPT CHECK 15.3

Actually it is your superior who is ignorant. She is confusing this with microwave diathermy which is no longer approved by the FDA in the United States. PSWD with low watts (100) will not heat metal. Try to explain this to her and even demonstrate it by using it on yourself over a ring or chain.

CONCEPT CHECK 15.4

Therapeutic ultrasound has the following advantages over SWD:

- It is less expensive.
- There are fewer contraindications.
- The devise is smaller and portable.
- It has variable frequencies for treating various tissue depths.
- It can be used under water.
- It can provide phonophoresis.
- Servicing is easier (there are more distributors).

REFERENCES

1. Michlovitz SL, Sparrow KJ. Therapeutic ultrasound. In: Michlovitz SL, Nolan TP, Bellew JW, eds. *Modalities for Therapeutic Intervention.* 5th ed. Philadelphia, PA: F.A. Davis Co., 2011:85–134.

2. Cameron MH. *Physical Agents in Rehabilitation; From Research to Practice.* 2nd ed. Philadelphia, PA: WB Saunders, 2003.

3. Lindsay DM, Dearness J, Richardson C, Chapman A, Cuskelly G. A survey of electromodality usage in private physiotherapy practices. *Aust J Physiother.* 1990;36(4):249–256.

4. Lindsay DM, Dearness J, McGinley CC. Electrotherapy usage trends in private physiotherapy practice in Alberta. *Physiother Can.* 1995;47(1):30–34.

5. Hellstrom RO, Stewart WF. Miscarriages among female physical therapists who report using radio- and microwave-frequency electromagnetic fields. *Am J Epidemiol.* 1993;138(10):775–785.

6. Draper DO. Interest in diathermy heats up again. *Biomech anics.* 2001;8(9):77–83.

7. Kitchen S, Partridge C. Review of shortwave diathermy continuous and pulsed patterns. *Physiotherapy.* 1992;78(4):243–252.

8. Draper DO, Knight KL, Fujiwara T, Castel JC. Temperature change in human muscle during and after pulsed short-wave diathermy. *J Orthop Sports Phys Ther.* 1999;29(1):13–18; discussion 19–22.

9. Draper DO, Abergel PA, Castel JC, Schlaak C. Pulsed shortwave diathermy restricts swelling and bruising of liposuction patients. *Am J Cosmet Surg.* 2000;17(1):17–22.

10. Draper DO, Garrett C. Pulsed shortwave diathermy heats a considerably larger area than 1 MHz ultrasound treatments. *Am Athl Train.* 1999;34(2):21–23.

11. Draper DO, Castro J, Feland JB, Schulthies SS, Eggett D. Shortwave diathermy and prolonged stretching increase flexibility more than prolonged stretching alone. *J Orthop Sports Phys Ther.* 2003;34(1):13–20.

12. Draper DO, Castel JC, Castel D. Low-watt pulsed shortwave diathermy and metal-plate fixation of the elbow. *Athl Ther Today.* 2004;9(5):27–31.

13. Draper DO. Shortwave diathermy in the athletic training room. Paper presented at: Annual Symposium of the NATA; Los Angeles, CA, June 2001.

14. Garrett CL, Draper DO, Knight KL. Heat distribution in the lower leg from pulsed short-wave diathermy and ultrasound treatments. *J Athl Train.* 2000;35(1):13–22.

15. Peres S, Draper DO, Knight KL, Ricard MD, Durrant E. Pulsed short-wave diathermy used prior to stretch increases flexibility more than stretch alone. *J Athl Train.* 2000;37(1):43–50.

16. Seiger C, Draper D. Use of pulsed shortwave diathermy and joint mobilization to increase ankle range of motion in the presence of surgical implanted metal: A case series. *J Orthop Sports Phys Ther.* 2006;36(9):669–677.

17. Draper DO. Shortwave diathermy and joint mobilizations for postsurgical restoration of knee motion. *Athl Ther Today.* 2010;15(1):38–40.

18. Draper D, Hawkes A, Johnson A, Diede M, Rigby J. The Megapulse II shortwave diathermy heats muscle better than the ReBound diathermy. *J Athl Train.* 2012 (in press).

19. Draper D, Hawkes A, Johnson A, Diede M, Rigby J. The Rebound shortwave diathermy has a greater heating capacity over moist hot packs at superficial depths. *J Athl Train.* 2012 (in press).

20. Abergel RP, Meeker CA, Lam TS, et al. Control of connective tissue metabolism by lasers: recent developments and future prospects. *J Am Acad Dermatol.* 1984;11:1142–1150.

21. Van der Esch M, Hoogland R. *Pulsed Shortwave Diathermy with the Curapuls 419.* Delft, The Netherlands: Delft Instruments Physical Medicine BV, 1990.

22. Castel D. *Electrotherapy and Ultrasound Update.* 2nd ed. Reno, NV: International Academy of Physio Therapeutics, 1996.

23. Bricknell R, Watson T. The thermal effects of pulsed shortwave therapy. *Br J Ther Rehabil.* 1995;2:430–434.

24. Brown M, Baker RD. Effect of pulsed short wave diathermy on skeletal muscle injury in rabbits. *Phys Ther.* 1987;67(2):208–214.

25. Pilla AA, Mont MA, Nasser PR, et al. Non-invasive low-intensity pulsed ultrasound accelerates bone healing in the rabbit. *J Orthop Trauma.* 1990;4(3):246–253.

26. Low JL. Dosage of some pulsed shortwave clinical trial. *Physiotherapy.* 1995;81(10):611–616.

27. Kloth L, Ziskin M. Diathermy and pulsed electromagnetic fields. In: Michlovitz SL, ed. *Thermal Agents in Rehabilitation.* 2nd ed. Philadelphia, PA: F.A. Davis, 1990.

28. Canaday D, Lee R. Scientific basis for clinical application of electric fields in soft tissue repair. In: Brighton C, Pollack S, eds. *Electromagnetics in Biology Medicine.* San Francisco, CA: San Francisco Press, 1991.

29. Sanseverino EG. Membrane phenomena and cellular processes under the action of pulsating magnetic fields. Presented at the 2nd International Congress of Magneto Medicine. Rome, Italy. 1980.

30. Mayrovitz H, Larson P. A preliminary study to evaluate the effect of pulsed radio frequency field treatment on lower extremity peri-ulcer skin microcirculation of diabetic patients. *Wounds.* 1995;7(3):90–93.

31. Mayrovitz H, Larson P. Effects of pulsed electro-magnetic fields on skin microvascular blood perfusion. *Wounds.* 1992;4(5):197–202.

32. Svarcova J, Trnavsky K, Zvarova J. The influence of ultrasound, galvanic currents and shortwave diathermy on pain intensity in patients with osteoarthritis. *Scand J Rheumatol.* 1987;67:83–85.

33. Jan M, Chai H, Wang C, Lin Y, Tsai L. Effects of repetitive shortwave diathermy for reducing synovitis in patients with knee osteoarthritis: An ultrasonographic study. *Phys Ther.* 2006;86:236–244.

34. Jan M, Lip P, Lin K. Change of arterial blood flow and skin temperature after direct and indirect shortwave heating on knee. *Formosan J Phys Ther.* 1993;18:64–71.

35. Jan M, Lin Y. Clinical heat effect of shortwave diathermy on knee joint. *Formosan J Phys Ther.* 1990;15:7–13.

36. Draper DO. Induction cable diathermy and joint mobilization restore range of motion in a post-operative ACL patient. *Athl Ther Today.* 2010;15(1):36.

37. McMeeken J, Bell C. Effects of selective blood and tissue heating on blood flow in the dog hindlimb. *Exp Physiol.* 1990;23(2):359–366.

38. Goats G. Continuous short-wave (radio-frequency) diathermy. *Br J Sports Med.* 1989;23(2):123–127.

39. Brucker JB, Knight K, Rubley M, Draper D. Effect of an 18-day stretching regimen, with or without PSWD on ankle dorsiflexion and 3 weeks. *J Athl Train.* 2005;40(4):104–108.

40. Kaltenborn FM. *Manual Mobilization of the Joints.* Minneapolis, MN: OPTP, 2002.

41. Wright GG. Treatment of soft-tissue and ligamentous injuries in professional footballers. *Physiotherapy.* 1973;59(12):385–387.

42. McCray RE, Patton NJ. Pain relief at trigger points: comparison of moist heat and shortwave diathermy. *J Orthop Sports Phys Ther.* 1984;5:175–178.

43. Lehmann JF, de Lateur BJ. Therapeutic heat. In: Lehmann JF, ed. *Therapeutic Heat and Cold.* 4th ed. Baltimore, MD: Williams & Wilkins, 1990:417–581.

44. Behrens BJ, Michlovitz SL. *Physical Agents: Theory and Practice for the Physical Therapist Assistant.* 2nd ed. Philadelphia, PA: FA Davis, 2008.

45. Lowe J, Reed A. *Electrotherapy Explained; Principles and Practice.* Boston, MA: Butterworth & Hynman, 1994.

46. Lehmann JF. *Therapeutic Heat and Cold.* 4th ed. Baltimore, MD: Williams & Wilkins, 1990.

47. Berne R, Levy MN. *Cardiovascular Physiology.* 3rd ed. St. Louis, MO: CV Mosby, 1993.

48. Miner L, Draper DO, Knight KL, Ricard RM. Pulsed short-wave diathermy application prior to stretching, does not appear to aid hamstring flexibility. *J Athl Train.* 2000;35(2):S48.

49. Peres SE, Draper DO, Knight KL, Ricard MD. Pulsed shortwave diathermy and prolonged long-duration stretching increase dorsiflexion range of motion more than identical stretching without diathermy. *J Athl Train.* 2002;37(1):43–50.

50. Draper D, Miner L, Knight K, Ricard M. The carry-over effects of diathermy and stretching in developing hamstring flexibility. *J Athl Train.* 2002;37(1):37–42.

51. Smyth H. The pacemaker patient and the electromagnetic environment. *JAMA.* 1974;227:1412.

52. van den Bouwhuijsen F, Maassen V, Meijer M, van Zutphen H. *Pulsed and Continuous Short-Wave Diathermy.* Delft, The Netherlands: B.V. Enraf-Nonius Delft, 1985.

53. Kloth LC, Cummings JP. Section on Clinical Electrophysiology and the American Physical Therapy Association. *Electrotherapeutic Terminology in Physical Therapy.* Alexandria, VA: American Physical Therapy Association, 1990.

54. Draper DO, Castel JC, Castel D. Rate of temperature increase in human muscle during 1 MHz and 3 MHz continuous ultrasound. *J Orthop Sports Phys Ther.* 1995;22(4):142–150.

55. Shields N, Gormley J, O'Hare N. Short-wave diathermy: current clinical and safety practices. *Physiother Res Int.* 2002;7(4):191–202.

56. Physiotherapy CSo. *Guidelines for Safe Use of Microwave Therapy Equipment.* London: Chartered Society of Physiotherapy, 1994.

57. Draper D, Trowbridge C. Continuous low-level therapy; What works and what doesn't. *Athl Ther Today.* 2003;8(5):46–48.

Chapter 10

1. The process that occurs when two objects of uneven temperatures come into contact with each other is defined as _____.
   a. conduction
   b. convection
   c. conversion
   d. radiation
   e. evaporation

2. The process that occurs when a form of energy other than heat is converted to heat within the body is known as _____.
   a. conduction
   b. convection
   c. conversion
   d. evaporation
   e. none of the above

3. The transfer of heat to an object by the passage of a fluid or air past its surface is known as _____.
   a. conduction
   b. convection
   c. conversion
   d. radiation
   e. evaporation

4. What is the most commonly used form of heat distribution in physical medicine?
   a. conduction
   b. convection
   c. conversion
   d. radiation
   e. evaporation

5. An example of heating by convection is _____.
   a. whirlpool
   b. hot pack
   c. ultrasound
   d. paraffin bath
   e. analgesic balm

6. An example of heating by conduction is _____.
   a. diathermy
   b. hot pack
   c. ultrasound
   d. paraffin bath
   e. both b and d

7. An example of heating by conversion is _____.
   a. whirlpool
   b. hot pack
   c. ultrasound
   d. paraffin bath
   e. analgesic balm

8. All substances with a temperature above absolute zero radiate heat to a lower temperature substance through _____.
   a. conduction
   b. convection
   c. conversion
   d. electromagnetic waves
   e. evaporation

9. The physiological effects of heat application include all of the following *except* _____.
   a. increased circulation: 3.5–4 times normal resting blood flow
   b. increased metabolism
   c. decreased pain
   d. decreased muscle spasm
   e. decreased tissue stiffness

10. General contraindications of heat application include all of the following *except* _____.
    a. within the first 12–72 hours of injury
    b. area with compromised circulation
    c. area with compromised sensation
    d. over the spine
    e. none of the above

Chapter 11

1. Which of the following is the most common type of superficial heat used in an athletic training clinic?
   a. whirlpool
   b. hot pack
   c. paraffin bath
   d. infrared lamp
   e. ultraviolet light

2. Which of the following is a disadvantage of a paraffin bath?
   a. It doesn't allow for range of motion during treatment.
   b. It feels too hot.
   c. The mineral oil can irritate the skin.
   d. It is messy.
   e. both a and d

3. Which of the following is a disadvantage of whirlpool?
   a. can treat the whole body
   b. provides irregular surfaces with total contact
   c. loses (or gains) heat very slowly
   d. can provide multiple treatments simultaneously
   e. difficult to keep the treatment area clean and sanitary

4. Which of the following is essential to have when using a whirlpool?
   a. IFC
   b. GFI
   c. RICES
   d. DC
   e. rubber duck

5. Which of the following is not an advantage of hot packs?
   a. easy to apply
   b. relatively expensive
   c. can treat over an open wound without fear of spreading germs to others
   d. durable
   e. portable

6. Which of the following is an advantage of topical heat wraps, such as the ThermaCare wrap?
   a. easy to apply
   b. difficult to keep the treatment area clean and sanitary
   c. heat lasts for only 15 minutes
   d. portable
   e. both a and d

7. The appropriate water temperature for treating a limb in a warm whirlpool is _____.
   a. 100–108°F (37.7–42.2°C)
   b. 105–112°F (40.5–44.4°C)
   c. 95–100°F (35–38°C)
   d. 112–117°F (44.4–47.2°C)
   e. none of the above

8. The appropriate water temperature for treating a full body in a warm whirlpool is _____.
   a. 100–108°F (37.7–42.2°C)
   b. 105–112°F (40.5–44.4°C)
   c. 95–100°F (35–38°C)
   d. 112–117°F (44.4–47.2°C)
   e. none of the above

Chapter 12

1. Which of the following is not a physiological effect of cold application?
   a. decreased temperature
   b. increased metabolism
   c. decreased or increased pain
   d. decreased muscle spasm
   e. increased tissue stiffness

2. Which of the following are not suggested hot-to-cold ratios (in minutes) for contrast therapy?
   a. 4:1
   b. 3:1
   c. 3:2
   d. 5:5
   e. All of the above have been suggested.

3. A sudden, intense, painful, tetanic muscle contraction that is short-lived, usually lasting 20 seconds, is called a _____.
   a. muscle spasm
   b. muscle cramp
   c. charley horse
   d. muscle strain
   e. two of the above

4. A gradual onset of tightness in a muscle, usually not particularly painful, is known as a _____.
   a. muscle spasm
   b. muscle cramp
   c. charley horse
   d. muscle strain
   e. two of the above

5. The increase in vascular circumference of blood vessels as a result of cold applications is known as _____.
   a. cryostretch
   b. cryotherapy
   c. cold-induced vasodilation
   d. cold-induced vasoconstriction
   e. the Lewis effect

6. Cryokinetics refers to _____.
   a. alternating of cold applications to numb an area, followed by active graded exercise
   b. three techniques for reducing muscle spasm: cold application, static stretching, and isometric contraction (the hold-relax technique of PNF)
   c. a combination of heat application, long-term passive stretch, and then cold applications, used to increase joint flexibility after prolonged immobilization
   d. a therapeutic agent that uses a pump attached to a boot or sleeve that intermittently forces air or chilled water into the sleeve for the purpose of decreasing lymphedema
   e. alternating immersion of the injured body part in hot and cold water baths

7. Which of the following is the best to use to increase joint flexibility after prolonged immobilization during which connective tissue contractures have developed?
   a. cryostretch
   b. connective tissue stretch
   c. lymphedema pump
   d. contrast bath stretch
   e. cryokinetics

8. Which of the following is the best to use to increase joint flexibility following an acute muscle strain?
   a. cryostretch
   b. connective tissue stretch
   c. lymphedema pump
   d. contrast bath stretch
   e. cryokinetics

Chapter 13

1. During ice massage, numbness can be increased by _____.
   a. applying more pressure with the ice
   b. moving the ice faster
   c. using an ice bag
   d. heating the area with ultrasound before icing
   e. applying a compression wrap

2. A toe cap is used during the application of which modality?
   a. RICES
   b. ice bag
   c. ice massage
   d. ice water immersion
   e. hot whirlpool

3. Which of the following is *not* a beneficial effect of cryokinetics?
   a. decreased pain, thus allowing exercise
   b. exercise increases blood flow
   c. exercise reestablishes neuromuscular functioning
   d. decreased metabolism
   e. none of the above; all are beneficial

4. Which of the following is *not* a contraindication for intermittent compression pumps?
   a. compartment syndrome
   b. peripheral vascular disease
   c. arteriosclerosis
   d. lymphedema
   e. local superficial infection

5. Which of the following is the reason an ice pack is used after connective tissue stretch?
   a. Ice causes collagen fibers to relax.
   b. Ice lengthens the collagen fibers.
   c. Ice causes the collagen fibers to reattach in a lengthened position.
   d. Ice helps cause plastic elongation.
   e. two of the above

6. Which of the following includes five sets of exercise?
   a. cryostretch
   b. cryokinetics
   c. lymphedema pump
   d. ice massage
   e. two of the above

Chapter 14

1. Within ultrasound waves are regions of high molecular density called _____ and regions of low molecular density called _____.
   a. compressions; reflections
   b. compressions; refractions
   c. refractions; compressions
   d. absorptions; transmissions
   e. none of the above

2. Which of the following would be the best crystal BNR?
   a. 3:1
   b. 1:3
   c. 4:1
   d. 1:4
   e. 6:1

3. Spatial average intensity is the amount of energy passing through a specified area, such as an ultrasound transducer soundhead. If 8 W are being delivered through a 5 cm soundhead, the SAI is _____.
   a. 2 W/cm^2
   b. 1.8 W/cm^2
   c. 1.6 W/cm^2
   d. 1.4 W/cm^2
   e. 0.62 W/cm^2

4. Which of the following is *true* with respect to temporal average intensity?
   a. It is the amount of energy passing through a specified area.
   b. It is the power of ultrasonic energy over a given period of time.
   c. It refers to continuous ultrasound.
   d. two of the above
   e. none of the above

5. A low PAMBNR provides for _____.
   a. a more comfortable treatment
   b. more even heating of tissue layers
   c. greater depth of penetration
   d. all of the above
   e. two of the above

6. During the ultrasound application, unstable cavitation can occur from _____.
   a. moving the soundhead too slow
   b. moving the soundhead too fast
   c. using a high intensity
   d. using a poor conducting medium
   e. both a and c
   f. both b and d

7. When reading your ultrasound manual, it says that during the pulsed mode, your unit has a 1:5 duty cycle. This means that the current is _____.
   a. off 80% of the time
   b. off 75% of the time
   c. on 30% of the time
   d. on 25% of the time
   e. none of the above

8. Which of the following is the least effective ultrasound couplant?
   a. water
   b. ultrasound gel pad
   c. ultrasound gel
   d. massage lotion
   e. petroleum jelly

9. The abbreviation W refers to the _____.
   a. power or intensity of the treatment
   b. pulse duration (width)
   c. number of pulses per second
   d. type of current (alternating or direct)
   e. stretching window

10. The decrease of energy contained within a sound wave as it travels through tissue is known as _____.
    a. the Ardnt-Schultz principle
    b. the law of Grotthus-Draper
    c. attenuation
    d. the piezoelectric effect
    e. rarefaction

11. According to the text, a state-of-the-art ultrasound device would contain which of the following?
    a. a high-quality natural crystal
    b. a pause button
    c. a high BNR
    d. a high ERA
    e. a gel warmer

12. Which of the following is a contraindication for ultrasound?
    a. pain
    b. skin anesthesia
    c. muscle spasm
    d. heat before stretching
    e. orthopedic implanted metal

Chapter 15

1. Which of the following is true with respect to microwave diathermy?
   a. If fat is 1 cm, it can penetrate up to 5 cm.
   b. Spacing is required between the applicator and the skin.
   c. It heats by the production of magnetic fields.
   d. all of the above
   e. both a and b

2. Which of the following is true with respect to short-wave diathermy?
   a. It heats fat more than muscle.
   b. Spacing is required between the applicator and the skin.
   c. It heats by the production of magnetic fields.
   d. all of the above
   e. both a and b

3. Which of the following is not part of a SWD machine?
   a. generator
   b. copper coil
   c. drum
   d. power switch
   e. transducer

4. The term *diathermy* means _____.
   a. excessive fluid in cells
   b. changing from one energy form into another
   c. loss of sensation
   d. heat loss or gain through direct contact
   e. to heat through

5. Which is the most common type of diathermy applicator?
   a. induction coil
   b. drum
   c. pad
   d. pancake cable
   e. air space plates

6. Which of the following is a contraindication for PSWD?
   a. myofascial trigger points
   b. pain
   c. removal of the byproducts of the inflammatory process
   d. joint contracture
   e. cardiac pacemaker

7. Which of the following pulsed SWD treatments would provide the most heat?
   a. 400 pps; 200 s
   b. 200 pps; 400 s
   c. 600 pps; 200 s
   d. 800 pps; 100 s
   e. All of the above produce the same amount of heat.

8. Which of the following has the greatest effect on increasing ROM in a contracted joint?
   a. diathermy
   b. ultrasound
   c. diathermy and passive stretch
   d. ultrasound and passive stretch
   e. diathermy and joint mobilizations

9. What is the most commonly used frequency for microwave diathermy?
   a. 2450 MHz
   b. 27.12 MHz
   c. 915 MHz
   d. 40.68 MHz
   e. 11 MHz

10. What is the most commonly used frequency for shortwave diathermy?
   a. 2450 MHz
   b. 27.12 MHz
   c. 915 MHz
   d. 40.68 MHz
   e. 11 MHz

Part V

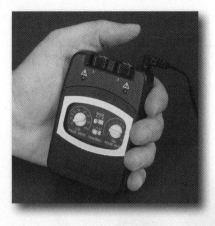

Electrotherapy

For many students and clinicians, understanding electricity and how to use it therapeutically is difficult, partly because in many cases, their background in chemistry and physics (the basis of electricity) is not as strong as their background in anatomy and physiology. In addition, not all clinicians and manufacturers of electrotherapy devices use the same vocabulary to explain how various electrotherapy devices work.

Chapter 16 is a review of the basic science of electricity. We review basic chemistry and physics and then discuss the principles and characteristics of electricity that are necessary for understanding electrotherapy. We then discuss various current characteristics, how these characteristics are manipulated to produce different output forms, and how the output form is transmitted from the device to the patient. Last, we present general principles of electrotherapy application for achieving various therapeutic goals. In Chapter 17, we present specific application techniques for achieving the most common electrotherapeutic goals.

16

Principles of Electricity for Electrotherapy

OPENING SCENE

While visiting his uncle's dairy farm, a young city boy was invited to play a game of tag with some neighboring farm children. As he chased the other children, he noticed they took the long way around a wire fence through a gate and out across a field. Sensing an opportunity to take a short-cut and catch up, he grabbed ahold of the wire fence to pull it down low enough to step across it. Whap—he felt a jolt as he touched the wire and quickly let go. The other kids heard his painful cry and began laughing and joking about the city slicker who thought he could outsmart them. You see, the boy's uncle had installed an electric fence around the field to remind the cows to stay in the field. The boy learned a few things about electricity that day, and he learned to respect it.

A Common Language

The therapeutic value of electrical currents is centuries old.[1,2] Your great grandparents could have purchased an "electrical stimulator" from their Sears, Roebuck catalog, or many other vendors.[3] But the claims of its efficacy were so outlandish that the use of electrical modalities waned. The discovery of silicon resistors and microcircuits during space exploration led to the introduction of high-volt and *Russian current* stimulators in the 1980s; and a rebirth occurred.

Many types of electrical stimulators followed. To be competitive, manufacturers developed variations, with a plethora of electrical current characteristics, and they used arbitrary terms to differentiate these characteristics.[1] In an effort to sell their products, they made unfounded claims about effectiveness. The combination of the variety of electrical current characteristics and the inconsistent terminology for describing them led to confusion. It seemed as though each manufacturer spoke a different language.

In 1990, the Section on Electrophysiology of the American Physical Therapy Association published a common language for electrotherapy. The use of these common terms by educators, clinicians, and manufacturers has helped minimize confusion.

Clinicians must understand and use a common language for two important reasons. First, they need to be able to use electrical stimulation intelligently. Decision-making professionals must understand why as well as how to use electrical stimulation so they can provide the most benefit to patients. Second, they need to be capable of intelligently discussing the features of various electrical simulators with sales personnel, and thus make informed purchasing decisions when the need arises.

The Basics of Electricity

Numerous definitions of electricity can be found. Here are four definitions, all correct, each one emphasizing a different aspect of electricity:

- A property of certain fundamental particles of all matter that have a force field associated with them, manifested by either an accumulation of, or an absence of, electrons on an atom or body.[4]
- A form of energy associated with the existence and interaction of electrical charge, manifested by the accumulation of, or absence of, electrons on an atom or body. It exhibits magnetic (electromagnetic), chemical (electrokinetic), and thermal properties.

- A form of energy that exhibits magnetic, chemical, mechanical, and thermal effects; formed from the interaction of positive (+) and negative (–) charges.[5]
- The physical phenomena associated with the existence and interaction of electrical charge, either static charges (electrostatics) or moving streams of charge (current).[6]

STATIC AND CURRENT ELECTRICITY

There are two types of electricity; static and current. **Static electricity** is frictional electricity, created by rubbing two objects together. In the process, one object gains electrons, the other object loses electrons. Examples are rubbing your shoes on carpet, running a comb through dry hair, and rubbing a balloon on hair.

Static electricity can be stored in an insulated conductor in which the charges are in a state of tension, ready to flow. The discharge is often a single discharge into the ground or through something else and into the ground. The body of the earth is considered an electrical "sink," which means it can accept or supply any reasonable amount of charge without changing its electrical characteristics.

Current electricity is characterized by a stream of loose electrons passing along a conductor. Current passes in one of two ways, and therefore is named after its method of moving along the conductor:

- *Direct current (DC)*: A steady, or continuous, unidirectional flow of electrons between the anode and cathode of a battery; also known as *galvanic current* (Fig. 16.1).
- *Alternating current (AC)*: A continuous flow of electrons that rhythmically changes direction. It occurs because the two terminals of its generator (source) alternatively change from positive to negative (see Fig. 16.1).

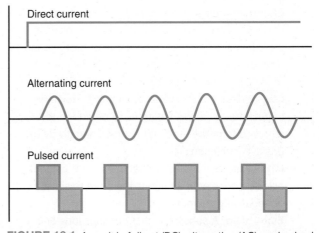

FIGURE 16.1 A model of direct (DC), alternating (AC), and pulsed current flow.

Electrotherapy often uses modulated, or modified, electrical currents. The most common form is **pulsed current**, wherein AC current is modulated (modified) including being interrupted or discontinuous (see Fig. 16.1).

A BRIEF REVIEW OF CHEMISTRY AND PHYSICS

Box 16.1 contains a brief review of chemistry and physics as they apply to electricity. Understanding these definitions, concepts, and principles is essential to understanding electrotherapy. Make sure you have a firm understanding of this material. For further elaboration, consult any introductory chemistry or physics text.

CURRENT FLOW AND OHM'S LAW

Current flow is the result of the interaction of force (voltage) and resistance (ohm). The relationship between current, force, and resistance is defined by **Ohm's law**, which is:

$$current = force/resistance$$

or

$$amp(A) = volt(V)/ohm(S)$$

BOX 16.1 A REVIEW OF BASIC CHEMISTRY AND PHYSICS

Essential Terms

- **Matter**: Anything that has weight and occupies space
- **Element**: The primary substance of matter (e.g., oxygen, copper, carbon)
- **Atom**: A single unit of an element; composed of protons, electrons, neutrons, and other smaller substances
- **Molecule**: Two or more atoms held together in a chemical bond. The atoms can be the same (O_2) or different (H_2O).
- **Proton**: A subunit of an atom, located in the nucleus, with a mass of 1 and an electrical charge of +1
- **Neutron**: A subunit of an atom, located in the nucleus, with a mass of 1 and an electrical charge of 0
- **Electron**: A subunit of an atom, orbiting the nucleus, with a negligible mass and an electrical charge of –1.
- **Electrical charge**: The net sum of the charges of electrons and protons in an atom or molecule; the difference between the number of protons and electrons. Normally, an atom has an equal number of electrons and protons and is, therefore, electrically neutral. If a chemical, mechanical, solar, or thermal force causes electrons to be added to or removed from the atom, it becomes negatively or positively charged.
- **Ion**: An atom or molecule that has lost or gained one or more electrons and is therefore positively or negatively charged
- **Electrolyte**: A substance that contains ions and can therefore conduct electricity

Current Flow

- **Current flow:** The flow of electrical charge (electrons) from one point to another, from an area of higher electron concentration (the negative pole or cathode) to an area lacking electrons (the positive pole or anode)
- **Direction of current flow**: Electrons flow, but by convention, current is said to flow from the positive pole to the negative pole. At one time people thought there was a positive particle whose flow caused electrical current. Although we now know this is not true, the idea that current flows from the positive to the negative has remained.
- **Conductor:** A substance that can transport electrical charge (or current) from one point to another. It must have free electrons that can be pushed along. Thus, metals are the best conductors because their atoms have weak bonds with their outer electrons, and thus can give them up easily. Water, with minerals or electrolytes, is a good conductor (e.g., salt or NaCl, in water becomes Na^+ and Cl^-). Good conductors of electricity are usually also good conductors of heat. Electrical conductors allow electricity to flow yet still provide some resistance.
- **Insulator:** A nonconductor; something that resists the flow of electrons, such as glass, rubber, oil, paraffin, and pure distilled water. Insulators have no free electrons to move.
- **Semiconductor:** A substance whose conductivity is poor at low temperatures but increases when small amounts of certain other substances are added to it, or by the application of heat, light, or voltage. Used to regulate the flow of electricity.

BOX 16.1 A REVIEW OF BASIC CHEMISTRY AND PHYSICS (*Continued*)

Carbon, silicone, and germanium are common semiconductors.

- **Partial conductor:** A substance that allows some flow of electricity under certain conditions, such as dry wood, paper, tap water, moist air, and kerosene.

Quantifying Electricity

- **Coulomb:** The basic unit of charge, produced by 6.28×10^{18} displaced electrons (6280 quadrillion).
- **Voltage:** The force created by an accumulation of extra electrons (electrical charge) at one point in a circuit, usually corresponding to a deficit of electrons at another point in the circuit. If the two points are connected by a suitable conductor, the difference in electron population will cause electrons to move from the area of higher concentration to the area of deficit.
- **Volt**: A unit of force required to push a current of 1 amp through a resistance of 1 ohm. It can come from a storage battery or from a generator. The voltage from a generator is called electromagnetic force (emf). Commercial emf is 110 or 220 volts (V). High-power transmission lines are 220 V. Storm clouds carry several million volts.

- **Ampere (amp, A):** A unit of current flow, equal to the passage of 1 coulomb per second (i.e., 6.28×10^{18} electrons passing per second). Several hundred amperes are needed for lights and motors, for example. Electromedical work requires much less. Some therapeutic devices use 0.1–1 mA, others use 500–1500 mA.
- **Ohm:** A unit of resistance or opposition to the flow of DC. One ohm (Ω) is equal to the resistance caused by a column of mercury that is 1 mm^2 in cross-sectional area, 106 cm high, and at a temperature of 0°C (32°F). It is equal to 1 V/A.
- **Resistance:** The opposing of the flow of electricity, caused by the conductor. Resistance is determined by the type of material of the conductor, the cross-sectional area of the conductor, the conductor length and conductor temperature. Electricity will always flow via the path of least resistance.
- **Impedance:** Resistance or opposition to the flow of AC. It results from a combination of factors, but for our purposes it can be thought of as simply resistance.

If you know two, the third can be calculated. For example, if you have 6 V of force and 6000 Σ of resistance, what is the amperage? Substituting the values of volts and ohms in the second definition gives: A = 6V/6000 Σ = 0.001 A or 1 milliamp (mA).

A helpful analogy for understanding the flow of electricity through a circuit is the flow of water through a city (Table 16.1). Both require a volume of material to flow, a force to cause the material to flow, and other factors to control and regulate the flow. There is resistance to the flow, and each factor is defined as a rate of flow past a certain point.

 CONCEPT CHECK 16.1. (a) If you had a 100 V electrical stimulator applied to a muscle that was providing 20,000 Ω resistance, how much current would flow through the muscle? (b) What would the current flow be if you decreased skin/muscle resistance to 10,000 Ω?

 CONCEPT CHECK 16.2. Ohm's law tells us there are two ways of increasing current in a circuit. What are they?

A magnetic field always develops around electricity, whether it be static or current electricity. This causes particles with like charges to repel each other and particles with opposite charges to attract each other. This relationship is essential to the generation of AC, and is a factor in some therapeutic applications, such as wound healing and iontophoresis.

Electrical Equipment

In this section, we provide definitions of basic equipment used to deliver therapeutic doses of electricity to the body.

THE GENERATOR

The term **generator** is used to describe two very different devices:

- A device that converts some other types of energy into AC current electricity, such as a power plant or a small gas power generator that you might take on a camping trip.
- A medical device that converts an input electrical current (AC or DC) into various output currents (AC, DC, or pulsed); for example, an electrical muscle stimulator.

TABLE 16.1   WATER-ELECTRICITY FLOW ANALOGY

FACTOR	WATER	ELECTRICITY
Volume	Gallons	Coulombs
Force, to cause flow	Water pressure, caused by gravity and difference in water level	Voltage, caused by difference in free electron level
Resistance, to control the flow	Friction in pipe	Resistance in conductor
Rate of flow past a certain point	Gallons/second	Coulombs/second or amps
Requirements for flow:	Gallons of water	Coulombs of electrical charge.
	Water pressure that is greater than resistance	Voltage that is greater than resistance
Method of flow	By displacing air, so it can flow into open space, but you have no control over it.	By displacing electrons that must be accepted by something else; therefore must have a complete circuit. However, it can flow into the ground, which is a huge electron sink, but you have no control over it.
Methods of controlling the flow	A closed system of pipes in which to carry the water (if you want to control the flow)	A closed system (circuit) of conductors
	Valves or faucets to help direct the flow to different places in the system. (The faucet is said to be open when it allows flow.)	Switches to help direct the flow (The switch is said to be closed when it allows flow)
	Different sizes of pipe to provide resistance and help control the volume of flow	Different sizes of resistors to provide resistance and help control the volume of flow

- A **terminal (pole)** is the output device of a battery or generator. Two terminals must be paired in order to complete the circuit. The terminals are generally attached by wires to electrodes, which are attached to the body. Terminals are classified in one of two ways:
- **Positive**: The terminal from which the current leaves the battery or generator to enter the body.
- **Negative**: The terminal into which the current enters the battery or generator from the body.

An **electrical circuit** is a system of conductors that allows electrons to move between the two poles of a generator or battery. One example of an electrical circuit is a battery, with a wire connecting one of its terminals to one side of a light bulb, and a wire connecting the other side of the light bulb to the second terminal of the battery. Electrical circuits are either open or closed:

- **Closed circuit**: A complete circuit, allowing flow; there are no breaks in the circuit.
- **Open circuit**: An interrupted or broken circuit; flow ceases.

MEDICAL DEVICES

There are two classes of electrotherapy devices used in rehabilitation: those that stimulate muscles and those that stimulate nerves. A muscle stimulator—**neuromuscular electrical stimulator (NMES)**—is a therapeutic device that delivers current to the body to cause sensory and motor nerve depolarization. Its purpose is to cause muscle contraction.

A nerve stimulator—**transcutaneous electrical nerve stimulator (TENS)**—is a therapeutic device that delivers current to the body to cause sensory nerve depolarization. Its purpose is to stimulate sensory nerves to modulate pain. Although some muscle contraction may occur, this is not the purpose of, or necessary for, TENS stimulation.

SAFETY DEVICES

A **circuit breaker** is a safety device that protects equipment and body structures against excess current by opening the circuit when it is overloaded—that is, when so much current is flowing through the circuit that it will damage

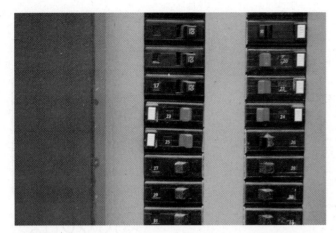

FIGURE 16.2 The panel of a circuit breaker in an athletic training clinic. Each breaker controls a specific electrical circuit. Circuit breakers "trip" or open the circuit if the current flow exceeds the specific rating of the circuit breaker. The six white-labeled breakers contain GFIs. (Courtesy of Jody Brucker.)

the wiring or devices of the circuit (Fig. 16.2). Circuit breakers are manufactured to respond to specific amounts of current flow, such as 10, 30 A, and so on. When current exceeds the specific rating of the breaker, it "trips" or opens the circuit, thus interrupting the current flow, and protecting the associated devices.

A **ground-fault interrupter (GFI)** is similar to a circuit breaker in that it interrupts current flow, but it works very differently (Fig. 16.3). Whereas a circuit breaker senses total current and trips when total current exceeds its rating, a GFI senses very small, abrupt increases in current (ground-fault currents) such as current flowing through the body of

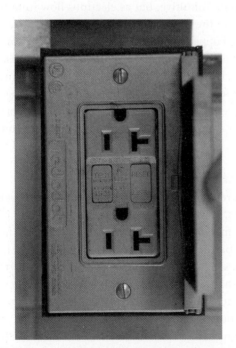

FIGURE 16.3 A ground fault interrupter (GFI) in a wall outlet.

a person standing on damp ground while touching a hot AC line wire. The GFI acts in as little as 0.025 seconds to trip (interrupt) the circuit, thereby limiting the total energy flow through the human body to a safe value.

A typical trip current setting for GFIs in homes is 5 mA. Electrocution occurs when a current as small as 200 mA flows through the heart for 1–3 seconds. GFIs are used chiefly for wall outlet circuits into which potentially dangerous appliances might be plugged. They may be in an individual outlet (see Fig. 16.3) or integrated with the circuit breaker so they protect the outlets of the whole circuit (see white-labeled circuit breakers in Fig. 16.2). Larger versions are used in power stations.

The Generation of Electricity

The generation of electricity is a process of converting another form of energy into electrical energy. Most electricity is converted from thermal, chemical, mechanical, or solar energy. The processes of converting chemical and mechanical energy to electricity are presented in this section. Understanding these processes will help you understand current flow and the therapeutic use of electrical currents. Chemical generation illustrates DC and mechanical generation illustrates AC.

CHEMICAL GENERATION

The most common device for the chemical generation of electricity is a battery. Two different metal plates are placed in a solution. A chemical reaction occurs, causing electrons to be liberated from one plate and accumulate on the other plate. If a wire is attached between the two metal plates, electrons will flow from the plate with an accumulation of electrons, through the wire and into the plate that lost electrons.

 CONCEPT CHECK 16.3. In the above descriptions, what type of current is generated? How do you know? (Review the definition of current flow.)

The key to chemical generation of electricity is dissociation of molecules into ions. When certain substances are placed in a solution, they dissociate into free ions or groups of ions with an electrical charge. Electrons leave one molecule and attach to the other, leaving one negatively charged and the other positively charged. For example, when table salt (NaCl) is added to water, part of the salt dissociates into Na^{2+} and Cl^{2-}. (These dissociated ions are known as electrolytes.)

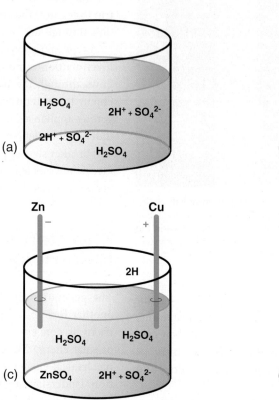

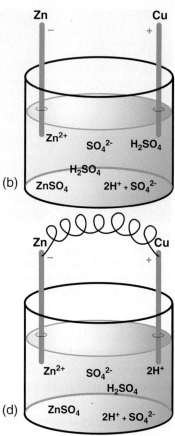

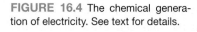

(a)

(b)

(c)

(d)

FIGURE 16.4 The chemical generation of electricity. See text for details.

Chemical generation is illustrated in Figure 16.4, and explanatory details are given in the text.

1. A dilute solution of sulfuric acid will partially dissociate, meaning that some of the sulfuric acid dissociates into hydrogen and sulfate ions. The electrons lost by the hydrogen attach to the sulfate. $H_2SO_4 \rightarrow 2H^+ + SO_4^{2-}$ (Fig. 16.4a).

2. Adding plates of zinc and copper into the solution causes zinc ions (Zn^{2+}) to be attracted by the sulfate (SO_4^{2-}), leaving the zinc plate negatively charged. The Zn^{2+} and SO_4^{2-} combine to form zinc sulfate ($ZnSO_4$), which then precipitates to the bottom of the battery (Fig. 16.4b).

3. The two dissociated hydrogen ions (H^+) are attracted to the copper plate. There they each attract an electron from a copper molecule, become free hydrogen, and bubble to the surface and into the airs. This causes the copper plate to become positively charged (Cu^{2+}) (Fig. 16.4c).

4. As the processes in steps 2, 3, and 4 continue, a difference in potential (the accumulation of charge or voltage) develops between the negatively charged zinc plate and the positively charged copper plate.

5. If the two charged plates are attached via a wire, some of the accumulated electrons will travel from the zinc plate to the copper plate, thus producing electrical current (Fig. 16.4d). And since the electrons always flow from one pole to the other, this is called direct current.

It is counter-intuitive, but as electrons flow from the zinc (–) pole to the copper (+) pole, we say that current flows from the copper (+) pole to the zinc (–) pole. Don't try to reason this out, because it doesn't make sense. Just accept it. Logic is the bedrock of science, but this is an exception. An erroneous concept hundreds of years ago—that electricity involved the movement of positive particles—influenced the naming of current flow, and the terminology remains.

Types of Batteries

There are two main types of batteries: wet cells and dry cells. A **wet cell**, also called a *galvanic cell*, consists of two metals and an electrolyte solution. The zinc-copper battery described earlier, and car batteries, are examples of a wet cell. **Dry cells** use electrolyte paste rather than a solution. One example is a zinc-carbon battery in which a zinc tube is filled with electrolyte paste and a carbon rod is inserted into the middle. Flashlight batteries are dry cells. Both wet and dry cells produce DC current.

A storage battery is one in which an electrical current causes the chemical reactions to go in reverse, thus rejuvenating or restoring the solution, H_2SO_4 in the above example. Thus, the battery is recharged. Storage batteries can be either wet or dry cells. A car battery and a rechargeable flashlight battery are examples of storage batteries.

MECHANICAL POWER GENERATION

Mechanical power generation is based on the relationship between electricity and magnetism. Most people think of magnetism in terms of a magnet that attracts iron or steel, or of a compass that lines up so that it points to the magnetic north pole. There's more. A force develops when a critical number of a substance's ionized molecules polarize, or line up so the positive end of the molecules points in one direction and the negative end points in the opposite direction (Fig. 16.5). The substance is then said to have poles. The force field that develops between the two poles is called a **magnetic field**.

Like poles repel, and unlike poles attract. The Earth is a big magnet. The magnetic field around the Earth causes a smaller magnet, such as one on a compass, to line up parallel to the lines of force between the Earth's north and south poles.

Electromagnetic Induction
In 1831, Faraday discovered that when a coil of insulated wire is moved toward or away from a magnet, electricity flows in the wire. Conversely, when electricity passes through a wire, a magnetic field is created. This principle is known as **electromagnetic induction**. It is the basis for converting mechanical power into electrical power (electrical generator) and for converting electrical power into mechanical power (electrical motor).

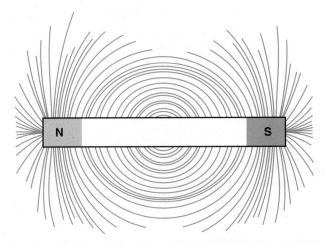

FIGURE 16.5 A metal bar becomes a magnet when its molecules polarize or line up with their positive ends facing in the same direction. Lines of force develop between the two poles of the magnet.

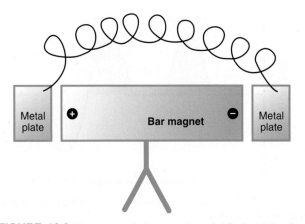

FIGURE 16.6 The mechanical generation of AC electricity. See text for details.

Generating Alternating Current, Simplified
In its most simplified form, an electrical generator consists of the following:

- A bar magnet mounted on a rotating pedestal (Fig. 16.6).
- Two metal plates positioned at the end of the magnet and connected with a large loop of wire
- A source of mechanical energy to keep the bar magnet spinning in a circle

Common mechanical sources are water power from water falling over a dam and steam power from burning coal or a nuclear reaction.

When the magnet is in its starting position, its positive pole attracts the electrons to the plate next to it, and its negative pole repels electrons from the metal plate next to it. Because the two plates are attached with a wire, electrons flow from the plate next to the magnet's negative pole and toward the plate next to the positive pole. The magnet is then rotated 180°, reversing the poles. This causes the electrons to reverse and move in the opposite direction. Continue rotating the magnet and the electrons will move back and forth in the metal plates and wire, which by definition is alternating current (AC). As long as the mechanical power keeps the magnet turning, AC current will flow.

An Electrical Motor Versus an Electrical Generator
An electrical motor is conceptually the same as a generator; they consist of the same basic components, but they have opposite processes. A generator converts mechanical power to electrical power, whereas an electrical motor converts electrical power to mechanical power.

Alternating Current Terms
A graph of AC flow versus time appears as a sine wave as the current flows in one direction and then the other (Fig. 16.7). The following terms define AC flow, and are

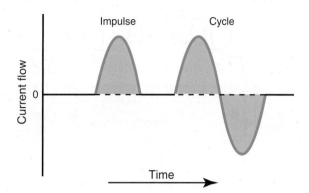

FIGURE 16.7 Impulse and cycle are shown in this graph of current flow versus time.

essential to understanding the use of electrical currents in therapy:

- **Impulse**: AC flows in a single direction. In Figure 16.7, it appears as a half-circle (or egg); the portion of the graph representing current flowing from the baseline to the maximum in one direction and back to the baseline. In the example above of generating AC, it represents electron flow during the time the magnet rotates 180°.
- **Cycle**: Two impulses. The portion of the graph representing current flowing from the baseline to the maximum in one direction, back across the baseline to the maximum in the opposite direction, and back to the baseline. In the example above of generating AC, it represents electron flow during the time the magnet rotates 360°.
- **Frequency**: The rate of passage of cycles of AC; expressed as cycles per second (cps). Ordinary electricity in the United States is 60 cps; in Europe and parts of Asia it is 50 cps. Low-frequency current is under 1000 cps; high-frequency current is over 1,000,000 cps.

Devices for measuring and regulating electricity are described in Box 16.2

Output Current Characteristics

Therapeutic medical devices operate on (are powered by) either AC or DC, which is called the input current. The device then sends either "pure" current (AC or DC) or a modulated (manipulated) pulsed current to the body. These three basic forms of output current, in order of increasing complexity, are (see Fig. 16.1):

- *DC*: Continuous flow of electrons in a single direction
- *AC*: Continuous flow of electrons; defined by frequency or cycles per second. AC can be turned off and on to create bursts of current
- *Pulsed current*: Interrupted electron flow

BOX 16.2 DEVICES FOR MEASURING AND REGULATING ELECTRICITY

Measurement instruments are based on the electromagnetic effects of current. In the most simple case, they include a permanent magnet and an electromagnet that can rotate. When the electromagnet is charged, the two magnets repel each other, causing the electromagnet to rotate away from the permanent magnet. The amount of repulsion is proportional to the strength of the electromagnet, which is proportional to the amount of current flowing through it. Adding a display and calibrating it creates a measuring device. The generic device is called a **galvanometer** (Fig. 16.8). With additional circuitry it can be configured to become an **ampmeter** (ampere meter), which measures the flow rate of current (most are actually milliampmeters); a **voltmeter**, which measures voltage; or an **ohmmeter**, which measures resistance to current flow.

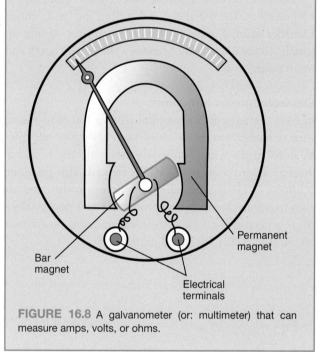

FIGURE 16.8 A galvanometer (or: multimeter) that can measure amps, volts, or ohms.

The simplest form of interrupting current flow is turning the switch on and off. The process is much more complicated, however, as the input current is manipulated, regulated, and adjusted in numerous ways to create a variety of output current wave forms.

CURRENT MODULATION

Current modulation is the process of varying one or more properties of basic electrical waveforms (AC or DC) to create additional specific waveforms. It includes all the manipulating, regulating, and adjusting of the input current to create a variety of specific output waveforms.

Electrotherapy devices (stimulators) are derived by modulating three key parameters: current flow, timing, and amplitude

Current flow is the movement of charged particles through the tissues. It is described by **phase** and **pulse** characteristics. Those most commonly used in electrotherapy are explained and illustrated in Box 16.3.

A second way that input currents are modulated is the timing of the current flow. The basic unit of timing is **phase duration**, the time during which current flows in a single direction. This and other aspects of current timing modulation are explained and illustrated in Box 16.4.

Amplitude (*intensity, output*) is measured in one of two ways: voltage delivered to the electrodes, or current flowing through the circuit (which includes the body part being treated). Current amplitude modulation is explained and illustrated in Box 16.5.

A **waveform** is the shape of an output electrical current, manifested when current flow is graphed with amplitude on the vertical axis and time on the horizontal axis.

BOX 16.3 PHASE AND PULSE CHARACTERISTICS

Phase and pulse characteristics are defined by the following:

- A **Phase** is a period of unidirectional charged particle movement (current flow) (Fig. 16.9). It is similar to an AC impulse, but can be modulated from either AC or DC input current and can be in one of many shapes.
- **Phase shape**: The shape of an output current after being modulated. The phase shapes that are most commonly used therapeutically are rectangular, spike, triangular, and sawtooth.
- **Phase charge**: The total electrical charge of a single phase, expressed as coulombs (microcoulombs for NMES). It is the time integral (area under the curve); the result of both amplitude and duration.
- A **pulse** is a finite period of charged particle movement, separated from other pulses for a limited time during which no current flows (see Fig. 16.9). A pulse consists of one or more phases, and named accordingly:
  - **Monophasic**: One phase; therefore, current flows in one direction only.

- **Biphasic**: Two phases; current flows in both directions.
- **Triphasic**: Three phases
- **Polyphasic**: Many phases
- **Pulse charge**: The amount of electrical charge of a single pulse; the sum of phases charges
- **Pulse Symmetry**: The relationship between the shapes of the two phases of a biphasic pulse (Fig. 16.10):
  - *Symmetrical pulse*: A pulse with identical phases
  - *Asymmetrical pulse*: A pulse with differing phases
- **Pulse charge balance**: The relationship between the charges of two phases of a biphasic pulse, independent of whether or not the phases are symmetrical (see Fig. 16.10):
  - *Balanced*: A pulse containing equal phase charges
  - *Unbalanced*: A pulse containing unequal phase charges
- **AC Train:** A continuous repetitive series of pulses at a fixed frequency; a segment of AC. It could also be called a continuous unmodulated AC polyphasic pulse.
- **Burst:** A finite series of pulses (or a finite interval of AC at a specific frequency) flowing for a limited time, followed by no current flow. Think of it as turning a pulse train or AC on and off (Fig. 16.11).
  - *Burst interval*: The time during which burst occurs, usually in milliseconds
  - *Interburst interval*: The time between bursts, usually in milliseconds

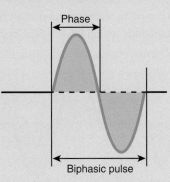

FIGURE 16.9 Two continuous phases form a biphasic pulse.

BOX 16.3 PHASE AND PULSE CHARACTERISTICS (*Continued*)

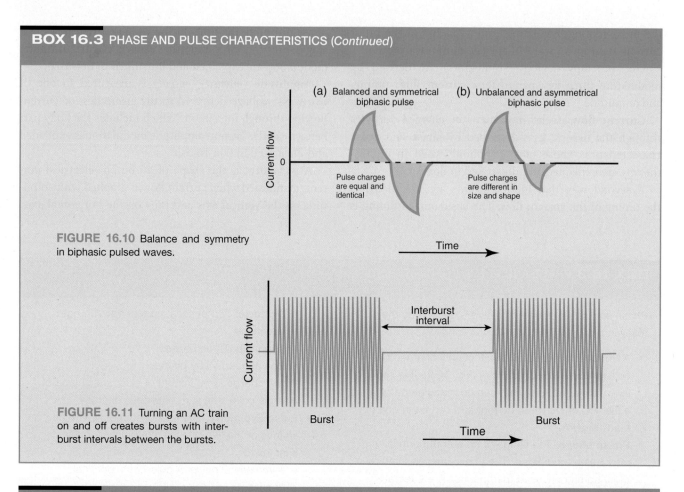

FIGURE 16.10 Balance and symmetry in biphasic pulsed waves.

(a) Balanced and symmetrical biphasic pulse — Pulse charges are equal and identical

(b) Unbalanced and asymmetrical biphasic pulse — Pulse charges are different in size and shape

FIGURE 16.11 Turning an AC train on and off creates bursts with interburst intervals between the bursts.

BOX 16.4 CURRENT TIMING MODULATION

Phase Duration and the timing of current flow are defined by the following (Fig. 16.12):

- **Rise time**: The time from the beginning of a phase until it reaches maximal amplitude
- **Decay time**: The time from maximal amplitude to the end of a phase
- **Pulse duration** (pulse width): The time required for each pulse to complete its cycle, usually reported in microseconds or milliseconds
  - *Short pulse duration*: A pulse that lasts <150 μsec
  - *Long pulse duration*: A pulse that lasts >200 μsec

- **Interpulse interval**: The time between successive pulses
- **Pulse Period**: The beginning of the pulse to the beginning of the subsequent pulse; pulse duration plus interpulse interval
- **Pulse rate** (pulse frequency): The rate at which pulses are repeated; usually expressed as pps, similar to AC input cps
- **Duty cycle:** The ratio of time on versus total time, expressed as a percentage. Thus, current with an on time of 10 milliseconds and an off time of 40 milliseconds would have a 20% duty cycle.

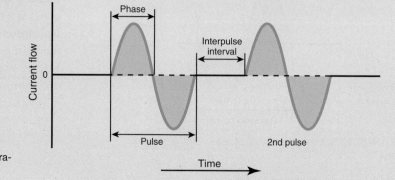

FIGURE 16.12 Pulse and phase duration characteristics.

BOX 16.5 CURRENT AMPLITUDE MODULATION

Current amplitude is characterized by the following (Fig. 16.13):

- **Peak current**: The highest magnitude of the pulse
- **Average current**: The average magnitude of a pulse. It is computed in one of two ways: the average current during the pulse or the average current during the period. The second method includes the off time between pulses.
- **Stimulation pattern:** The structure of the pulses used in the current
- **Constant stimulation**: Stimulation in which amplitude of successive pulses (or cycles) is the same
- **Surged stimulation**: Stimulation in which amplitude of successive pulses (or cycles) gradually

increase from zero to a maximum preset intensity (Fig. 16.14)

- Surge characteristics:
- *Ramp up*: The time during which the intensity of an electrical charge increases
- *Plateau*: The time during which pulses remain at maximum preset intensity
  - *Ramp down*: The time during which the intensity of an electrical charge decreases
  - *Time on*: The time during which current flows from the beginning to the end of a surge
  - *Time off*: The time during which current does not flow; the time between surges

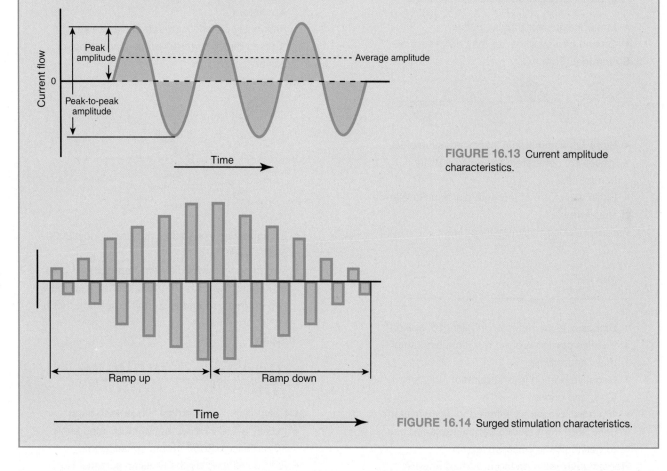

FIGURE 16.13 Current amplitude characteristics.

FIGURE 16.14 Surged stimulation characteristics.

The modulation of DC and AC produces a variety of output waveforms. The most commonly used therapeutic waveforms are described and illustrated in Box 16.6. Originally, electrical simulators output a single waveform. Manufacturers vigorously argued the merits of their specific waveform, claiming it was superior to the others. In time, however, as technology advanced, they began to develop generators with a variety of waveforms.

Tissue Responses to Electrical Stimulation

Therapeutic electrical applications cause four types of responses in the tissue: thermal, chemical, magnetic, and kinetic. Thermal effects are discussed in Chapter 16 on diathermy. Aspects of the other three are presented below.

BOX 16.6 COMMONLY USED WAVEFORMS

Following are nine frequently used electrotherapy waveforms with their descriptions:

1. **Direct (galvanic)**: Pure DC, used for iontophoresis

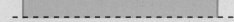

- Monophasic, rectangular current
- Previously called a square wave, but is rectangular rather than square

2. **Interrupted DC**: Unidirectional flow caused by rapid and repeated turning the current on and off. Similar to the modified square wave

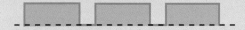

- Monophasic, rectangular, pulsed
- On and off times may or may not be equal.

3. **Sinusoidal**: Pure AC.

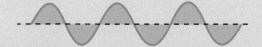

- Biphasic, symmetrical, balanced, sinusoidal.
- Waveform generated and sold by utility companies.
- Basic waveform of Interferential and Russian waveforms.

4. **Faradic**: Induced asymmetrical AC

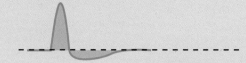

- Biphasic, asymmetrical, unbalanced, spiked
- Positive portion is short duration, high amplitude, and spiked.
- Negative portion is long duration, low amplitude, and curved.
- "Faradic" previously referred to any waveform generated from an AC, but the preferred use is to define this specific waveform.

5. **Rectangular (also called modified square)**: Similar to the interrupted DC, but modulated from AC input current

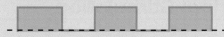

- Monophasic, rectangular, pulsed

6. **Biphasic**

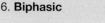
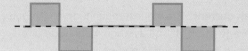

- Biphasic, symmetrical, balanced, rectangular, pulsed

7. **Twin pulse**

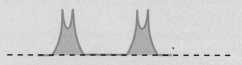

- Monophasic, pulsed, twin spiked
- Common waveform of high-volt muscle simulators
- Previously called "high-volt galvanic" and "pulsed direct current," but it is not direct or galvanic current.

8. **Interferential**

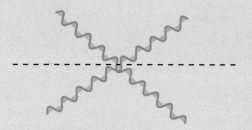

- Symmetrical, sinusoidal, high-frequency (2000–5000 Hz) AC
- Two channels, with different frequencies, used simultaneously. The interference between the two currents causes a current amplitude modulation in the tissue.

9. **Russian**

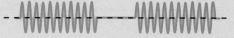

- Polyphasic, symmetrical, sinusoidal, burst
- Initially a 2500 Hz AC burst, modulated every 10 milliseconds (50 bursts per second)
- First developed by the Russian scientist Kots, hence its name.

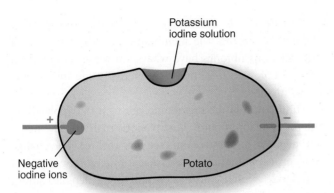

FIGURE 16.15 The chemical effects of electrical stimulation: LeDuc's potato experiment. As a direct current was passed through a potato containing a small pool of potassium iodine solution, negative iodine ions migrated to the end of the potato with a positive pole. Analysis was easy. The iodine interacted with the starch near the positive pole to form blue starch iodine, visible with the naked eye.

CHEMICAL EFFECTS

The chemical effect of electrical stimulation involves driving ions of medication into the body. When a direct electrical current is passed through the solution, the ions wander or move:

- Positively charged ions move to the negative pole, the cathode
- Negatively charged ions move to the positive pole, the anode

This effect is illustrated by two classic, simple experiments performed by LeDuc in the 1890s.[2]

LeDuc's Experiments

In his first experiment, LeDuc cut a hole in a potato and filled it with a potassium iodine solution, which was partially dissociated into positive potassium ions and negative iodine ions (Fig. 16.15). He then stuck wires into either end of the potato and attached them to a battery. As the DC passed through the potato, the ions were attracted to the poles: the positive potassium ion to the negative pole and the negative iodine ion to the positive pole.

In the second experiment, LeDuc placed two rabbits in series in an electrical circuit so that the current passed through both animals, as illustrated and described in Figure 16.16.

 CONCEPT CHECK 16.14. In LeDuc's rabbit experiment, when electrode A was negative and electrode B was positive, the current passed through the rabbits with little external effect. When the electrodes were reversed, however, both rabbits died, one of strychnine poisoning and the other of cyanide poisoning. Why?

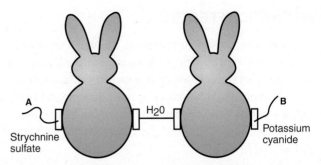

FIGURE 16.16 The chemical effects of electrical stimulation: LeDuc's rabbit experiment. Two rabbits are placed in series in an electrical circuit, with an electrode soaked in a strychnine sulfate solution attached to one rabbit and an electrode soaked in potassium cyanide attached to the other. The electrodes attached to the wire between the rabbits were soaked in plain water (H_2O). **(a)** The battery was attached so that electrode A was negative and electrode B was positive, so the current passed through the rabbits without harming them. **(b)** When the battery was reversed, both rabbits died, the first from strychnine poisoning and the second from cyanide poisoning. The positive A pole repelled the positive strychnine and caused it to enter the first rabbit. The negative B pole repelled the negative cyanide and caused it to enter the second rabbit.

LeDuc's two experiments clearly illustrated that direct current can drive ionized molecules into the skin. This concept is the basis of iontophoresis, discussed later in this chapter.

Requirements for Ion Migration

Continuous monophasic DC electron flow is necessary for ion migration. The process moves electrons against a gradient, so if the electron flow is discontinuous, the electrons will diffuse back to their starting position during the "no flow" time. It is like pushing a car up a hill; if you push for a while and then move away from the car, it will roll back down to the starting position.

In the 1980s, there was a misconception that high-volt twin-pulsed simulators created a chemical effect.[7,8] In fact, they were once called "high-volt galvanic simulators." They do produce a monophasic waveform, but they are pulsed, so they do not produce the continuous electron flow necessary to cause a chemical effect. The confusion occurred because of an incomplete understanding of the chemical effect of electricity.

Iontophoresis

Iontophoresis is application of mild DC current for transporting positively or negatively charged ions from a drug solution on the skin into the underlying tissues.[9–11] It requires long-term flow (5–10 minutes) of a pure DC. The medication must ionize in solution and be placed under the appropriate electrode so that the active ion is driven into the tissue.

MAGNETIC EFFECTS

Any time an electrical current flows through a conductor, it causes a magnetic field to form around the conductor (the body part through which therapeutic electrical stimulation is applied). Although the specific responses of tissue to this magnetic field are poorly understood, there is much speculation. Some claim that the responses promote bone and wound healing.[12,13]

KINETIC EFFECTS

Kinetic effects include sensation and muscle contraction, which result from the stimulation of sensory and motor nerves, respectively. Muscle contraction can be either a single contraction, called a *twitch*, or multiple contractions fused together into a continuous or sustained contraction, called a *tetanic contraction*.

Polarization and Action Potentials

In the absence of intervention, cell membranes would be unpolarized, meaning, the number of positive ions would be equal on either side of the membrane and the number of negative ions would be equal on either side (Fig. 16.17a). Neural stimulation requires a polarized neuron membrane, which occurs when ion distribution between the inside and outside of the membrane is unequal—that is, there are more positive ions than negative ions on the outside of the membrane and more negative ions than positive ions on the inside of the membrane (Fig. 16.17b).

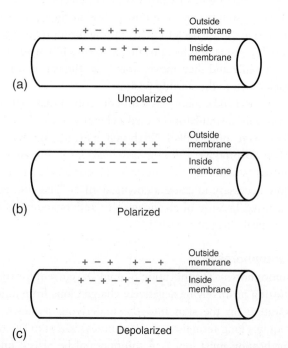

(a) Unpolarized

(b) Polarized

(c) Depolarized

FIGURE 16.17 Positive (+) and negative (–) ion distribution outside and inside of a neuron membrane during three states: when the membrane is **(a)** unpolarized, **(b)** polarized, and **(c)** depolarized.

Polarization is accomplished by active transport of sodium ions across the membrane (see Fig. 5.6). When polarized, membranes have what's known as an electrical potential of –70 to –90 mV between the inside and outside of the membrane.

Stimulation of the membrane causes it to depolarize at the point of stimulation. Positive ions rush into the nerve and negative ones move out (see Fig. 16.17c). The change in electrical potential causes adjacent membrane tissue to depolarize, which causes adjacent tissue depolarization, and so on. This spreading of depolarization down the axon of a nerve cell (neuron) is called an **action potential**. An action potential is also described as a wave of depolarization sweeping along the nerve.

Action potentials on a single fiber are essentially the same. Altering the intensity or duration of the stimulus has no effect on the amplitude or speed of the generated action potential. A stimulus that just reaches threshold causes the same action potential that a stimulus a thousand times greater causes.

Action potentials occur in both nerve cells and muscle cells. They are called nerve action potentials and muscle action potentials, respectively.

Once an action potential reaches the axon terminal (see Fig. 8.3), it crosses the synapse and stimulates the postsynaptic nerve or muscle cell. The axon branches of a single motor nerve synapse with multiple muscle fibers (thousands, in some muscles). A motor nerve and all the muscle fibers it synapses with are known as a **motor unit**.

All the muscle fibers of a motor unit contract in response to a single action potential in its nerve, a principle known as the *all-or-none law*. Gradation of a contraction comes from the number of motor units stimulated, not by the strength of stimulation of individual motor units. If the stimulation is great enough to cause an action potential, it will cause all associated muscle fibers to contract.

Once an action potential sweeps down a membrane, the nerve is unexcitable to further stimulation until it repolarizes. The time during which the membrane repolarizes is known as the **refractory period** (Fig. 16.18). The refractory period is divided into two phases, the relative and absolute refractory periods. During the absolute refractory period, nothing can be done to make the membrane fire (generate an action potential). During the relative refractory period, the membrane can fire, but it requires a much greater stimulus.

Nerve tissue depolarizes quickly.[6,14] Absolute refractory periods last about the same time as the action potential; they vary from 0.4 to 2 milliseconds, depending on the specific nerve.

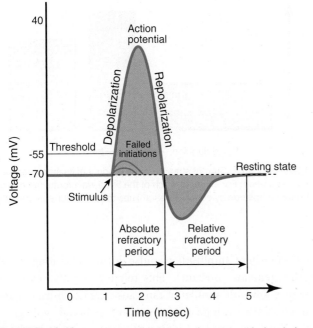

FIGURE 16.18 Absolute and relative refractory periods, during which subsequent stimulation is impossible or requires a greater stimulus, respectively. Note also the two failed initiations that resulted from subthreshold stimulation

Mixed Nerves

Our discussion thus far about the kinetic effects of electrical stimulation has focused on stimulating an individual, isolated nerve fiber. In patients, however, therapeutic electrical stimulation treatments stimulate mixed nerves. *Mixed nerves* are the nerves you learned in anatomy, such as the median nerve and sciatic nerve; they are composed of numerous nerve fibers of differing sizes and functions. Although they are more accurately called peripheral nerves, for simplicity we usually just refer to them as nerves.

Nerves are categorized into three main types: A, B, and C fibers (see Table 8.1):

- **A fibers** are the largest (1–22 μm in diameter), and conduct action potentials the most rapidly (5–120 m/sec). Some A fibers are sensory; others have a motor function.
- **B fibers** are between A and C fibers in size (1–3 μm) and in rate of conduction (3–14 m/sec). They are autonomic motor nerves.
- **C fibers** are the smallest (<1 μm) and slowest (<2 m/sec). They are sensory nerves.

In general, a nerve's response to excitation is a function of its size (diameter). And larger fibers generally have these characteristics:

- More rapidly conducting action potentials
- Greater recorded electrical response
- A lower threshold of excitability to electrical stimulation
- A shorter duration of response
- A shorter refractory period

Nerve Excitability and Stimulation Parameters

Stimulating a single isolated nerve in a laboratory is very different from stimulating part or all of a mixed nerve located within other tissue in the body. In both cases, once the stimulus reaches threshold, it generates an action potential, which then travels down the nerve. The amount of electrical current applied to the surface necessary to elicit an action potential in a specific nerve is known as **nerve excitability**. Following are factors that influence nerve excitability.

Nerve Size and Depth. All other things being the same, the larger a nerve is, the more easily it can be stimulated, and the more superficial it is, the more easily it can be stimulated (Fig. 16.19). In a practical sense, this means that large sensory nerve fibers (A fibers) are more excitable than motor nerves, and motor nerves are more excitable than pain fibers.

Tissue Resistance. Whether or not a nerve is stimulated by a given electrical stimulus depends to some degree on the resistance of the tissue. Technically, resistance depends on tissue impedance, which is a combination of

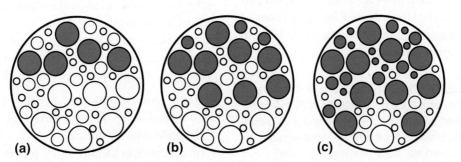

FIGURE 16.19 The influence of nerve size and depth on nerve fiber excitability in a mixed nerve. *Solid circles* represent stimulated neurons. **(a)** A current that is just strong enough to reach threshold will stimulate only the largest and most superficial fibers. **(b)** A more intense current will also stimulate medium-sized superficial fibers and large fibers in the middle of the nerve bundle. **(c)** A still larger current will also stimulate small superficial fibers, medium-sized fibers in the middle, and large fibers deep in the nerve.

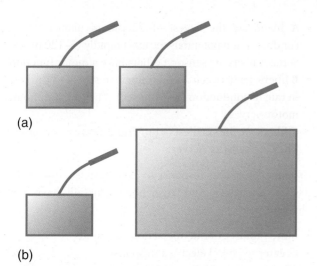

(a)

(b)

FIGURE 16.20 Current density is a measure of the quantity of charged ions moving through a particular cross-sectional area of an electrode. **(a)** If the electrodes through which the current flows are of equal size, the current density underneath the electrodes will be equal. **(b)** If one of the electrodes is bigger than the other, the bigger electrode will have less current density.

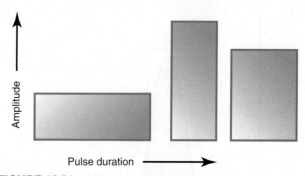

FIGURE 16.21 Current strength is the product of its amplitude and pulse duration. For example, each of the three waveforms (graphs of current amplitude by current strength) has the same current strength.

resistance, capacitance, and inductance, but for our purposes, think of it as resistance. The outer layer of the skin (*stratum corium* or *horny layer*) consists mainly of dead or peeling cells and therefore is a good insulator. Hair and oils add to the insulation. One purpose of a **coupling medium** (*or couplant*), such as electrosonic gel or water, between the electrode and the patient's skin, is to decrease skin resistance and therefore increase transmission. In some cases, such as with *electromyography (EMG)* or *electrocardiography (EKG)*, the skin is scraped to remove as much of the outer layer as possible. This is rarely necessary for orthopedic injury rehabilitation.

Current Density. **Current density** is a measure of the quantity of charged ions moving through a particular cross-sectional area of an electrode and the skin beneath the electrode (Fig. 16.20). For example, a current of a 500 mA applied through a 25 cm² electrode would have a current density of 20 mA/cm². If the two electrodes through which the current flows are of equal size, the current density beneath the electrodes will be equal. If one of the electrodes is bigger than the other, the tissue beneath it will have less current density.

 CONCEPT CHECK 16.5. (a) If the current density under a 2 × 2 cm electrode is 80 mA/cm², what would the current density be under its paired electrode, which is 8 × 8 cm? (b) What would it be under a paired electrode that was 2 × 2 cm?

Interaction of Current Amplitude and Pulse Duration. Current strength is a product of its amplitude and pulse duration (Fig. 16.21). Thus, average current (and fiber recruitment) can be increased by increasing

either current amplitude or pulse duration (as long as the other remains constant). This relationship also explains why a low-volt simulator can cause greater muscle contraction than a high-volt simulator. Although voltage is five times greater in the high-volt simulator, its pulse duration is much less than five times shorter, so the average current is lower.

Frequency of Stimulation. Frequency of stimulation has no effect on the stimulation threshold of individual muscle fibers, however, the force of whole muscle contraction and muscle fatigue increase. As the frequency of stimulation increases, muscle fibers don't have time to relax between stimuli (action potentials), so the contraction becomes steady, as opposed to a series of individual twitches. This is known as a **tetanic contraction**, and the point at which it begins is known as **tetany**. Tetany occurs when the stimulation frequency exceeds 20–30 pps, depending on the type of muscle fiber.

Electrode Orientation. Muscle conducts electricity four times better longitudinally than transversely.[6] Therefore, electrodes should be applied parallel to muscle fibers rather than perpendicular to them.

Motor Point. The point where the motor nerve enters the muscle is called the **motor point.** It is usually located at the beginning of the muscle belly. Its significance is that a given amount of current will elicit greater muscular contraction at the motor point than any other place in the muscle. Be aware of the following:

• Motor points are located by trial and error, by looking for a good sharp muscle contraction while moving the electrode over the muscle.
• Charts can help identify motor points, but there is a certain amount of anatomical variation in location.
• Motor points should not be confused with trigger points. A trigger point is a localized area of the body that is extremely sensitive to palpation, electrical stimulation, or ultrasound.

ELECTRODES

Electrodes are devices attached to the terminals of a generator or electrical stimulator through which current enters and leaves the body. Electrodes come in a variety of sizes, shapes, and materials, and are named according to their function. The three most popular electrode systems over the years have been:

- *Metal-sponge electrodes.* A thin metal plate is attached to the wire from the terminal. A wet sponge is placed between the metal plate and the skin to increase the conductivity between the plate and skin. These are held in place with a flexible rubber belt or with a sand bag.
- *Carbon- or silicon-impregnated rubber electrodes with sponge, paper towel, or conductive gel interface.* Carbon or silicon is added to the rubber, which is an insulator, so that it becomes a conductor. A wet sponge, a wet paper towel, or conductive gel is placed between the rubber plate and the skin to increase the conductivity between the two. These are held in place with a flexible rubber belt or with a sand bag.
- *Adhesive-backed carbon- or silicon-impregnated rubber electrodes.* Adhesive is used in place of the sponge or paper towel and the rubber belt or sand bag. These are quicker and easier to apply, but more expensive than other systems. They were intended to be single-use disposable electrodes, but many people reuse them multiple times until the adhesive loses its stickiness.

Recently, companies have begun to distribute inexpensive, one-use electrodes (Fig. 16.22). These electrodes resemble a roll of stickers or stamps. You simply remove the electrode from the roll and stick it on the treatment site. After the treatment, the electrode is removed and thrown into a trash receptacle. Manufacturers claim these electrodes deliver current to the body as effectively as adhesive reusable electrodes.

Physical Characteristics

The shape of an electrode is not important. Most of them are round, square, or rectangular. However, the size and the material that electrodes are made of are significant.

- *Size*: The size of the electrode, and its placement, determine the number of motor units that are stimulated. A small electrode placed over a single muscle will stimulate only that muscle, whereas a larger electrode can span, and therefore, stimulate two or more muscles. The size of electrodes also has a bearing on the current density under the electrode. The smaller the electrode is, the greater the current density will be, as long as the current output is the same.
- *Material*: The conductivity of the material will affect the amount of current flow. Carbon- or silicon-impregnated rubber electrodes seem to have better conductivity than metal-sponge electrodes, but their useful life is limited. The carbon or silicon will "leach out" with use, reducing the electrode's conductivity.

Cross-Contamination of Reusable Electrodes

Self-adhesive electrodes should only be reused on the same patient. If used on different patients it may transfer bacteria from one patient to the next. Figure 16.23 shows a culture dish with several colonies of bacteria on it. This culture was taken from a randomly selected electrode in a sports medicine and physical therapy clinic. It is important that the area to be treated be cleaned before treatment and not used on several patients; these measures help prevent the cross-contamination and spread of germs among patients. Plus there is no risk of cross-contamination with single-use electrodes, since they are discarded after one use.

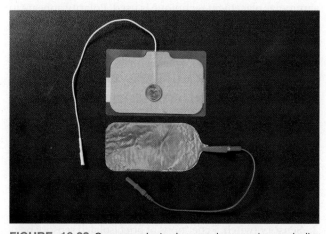

FIGURE 16.22 One-use electrodes are inexpensive and discarded after each use. Note: The dime on the multiple use electrode shows size.

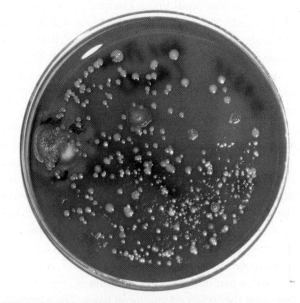

FIGURE 16.23 Bacterial culture from an electrode that had been applied on several patients. Notice the several colonies of bacteria that were growing on the electrode. (Courtesy of Alex Pinto.)

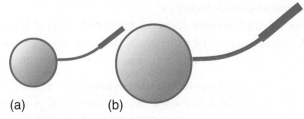

FIGURE 16.24 Electrodes may be active or dispersive depending on their size relative to the opposite electrode of their pair. **(a)** An active electrode is always much smaller than **(b)** a dispersive electrode and therefore has a greater current density.

Electrode Function

An electrode's function—what happens to the tissues under it when stimulated—depends on its relative size in relation to its paired electrode. Electrodes are classified as active or dispersive:

- **Active electrode**: An electrode under which the current density is great enough to elicit the desired response (Fig. 16.24).
- **Dispersive electrode**: (indifferent electrode) An electrode under which the current density is not great enough to elicit the desired response. An electrode is dispersive when it is much larger than the electrode(s) from the opposite terminal. It is used to complete the circuit, and usually is applied to a location remote to the area being treated.

Placement Techniques

There are three basic techniques for placing electrodes. These techniques facilitate different responses in the tissues under them:

- **Bipolar technique**: Electrodes from the two terminals are of equal size, resulting in essentially equal current density under them (Fig. 16.25a). (There will be some difference in current density if there is a difference in tissue resistance under the two electrodes). Both electrodes are, therefore, active. The electrodes are both applied to the treatment area in relative proximity to each other.
- **Unipolar technique**: Electrodes from the two terminals are of unequal size, thus creating active and dispersive electrodes (Fig. 16.25b). There may be multiple active electrodes, all coming from the same generator terminal, as long as their aggregate size is less than the dispersive electrode. The active electrode(s) is (are) applied to the treatment area and the dispersive electrode is applied to a remote location.
- **Quadripolar technique**: Four electrodes of equal size are used, a pair from each of two channels (Fig. 16.25c). Generally, they criss-cross the target tissue. The most popular use of this technique is with interferential stimulation, where two currents of differing frequencies are applied.

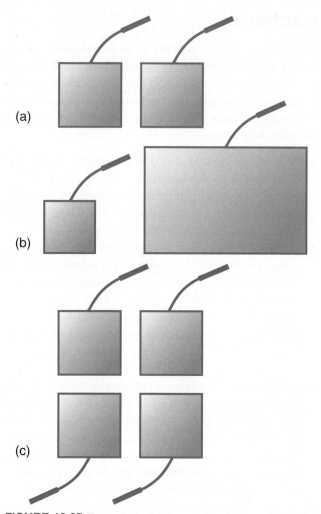

FIGURE 16.25 Three electrode placement techniques: **(a)** bipolar, with a pair of equal sized electrodes; **(b)** unipolar, with a pair of unequal sized electrodes; and **(c)** quadripolar with four electrodes of equal size.

Polarity

Polarity is the positive or negative voltage on the active electrode compared to the voltage on the dispersive electrode. This should not be confused with unipolar and bipolar placement techniques. Polarity only applies when a unipolar placement technique is used. Polarity appears to affect the excitability of nerves, but some people respond better to negative polarity and others to positive polarity.

Therapeutic Uses of Electrical Stimulation

There are five types of tissue responses to electrical stimulation, four of which are evoked by therapeutic stimulation (Table 16.2). The five types of responses are:

1. **Ion migration**: Ions move through the tissue in response to continuous DC stimulation.
2. **Sensory twitch**: Repetitions of brief isolated sensory ticks in response to moderate-amplitude, low-frequency pulsed stimulation. This response is not used therapeutically.

TABLE 16.2   TISSUE RESPONSES TO ELECTRICAL STIMULATION AND TYPES OF STIMULATORS

| TISSUE RESPONSE | CURRENT CHARACTERISTICS | | THERAPEUTIC GOAL | WAVE FORM |
	AMPLITUDE	FREQUENCY		
DC STIMULATORS				
Ion migration	Moderate	None	Iontophoresis	DC
AC STIMULATORS				
Sensory twitch	Low	Low	None known	all but DC
Sensory fused	Low	High	Pain reduction	Interferential
			Wound healing	Twin pulse
			Edema reduction	Twin pulse
Twitch (pulsed) contraction	Moderate	Low	Muscle re-education	Biphasic, Russian
			As part of ultrasound for tendinitis	Twin pulse, biphasic, Russian,
Tetanic contraction (with surge)	High	High	Strength development	Biphasic, Russian
			Spasm reduction	Biphasic, Russian

3. **Fused response**: A sustained sensory response that feels like "pins and needles," in response to moderate-amplitude, high-frequency pulsed, or AC stimulation.

4. **Twitch contraction**: Repetitions of isolated brief muscular contraction followed by relaxation in response to low-frequency, high-amplitude pulsed stimulation. It occurs in individual muscle fibers or in entire muscle groups.

5. **Tetanic contraction**: A sustained muscular contraction in response to repetitive high-frequency, high-amplitude pulsed or AC stimulation of at least 20–30 pps. It occurs in individual muscle fibers or in entire muscle groups.

Specific uses of these types (except sensory twitch) and the applications that invoke them are presented in Chapter 19.

CLOSING SCENE

Recall from the chapter opening scene that a young boy got shocked when he touched an electric fence on his uncle's dairy farm. (This is a true experience of a young DD). After reading this chapter, you can understand that the electrical shock would have been greater if the boy was standing in water, or absent if he had touched the fence while wearing rubber gloves. You now know that the power of electricity can be harnessed and used to decrease pain or elicit a muscle contraction. Our goal for this chapter was to provide you with a basic understanding of electricity and how it relates to therapeutic modalities, as you will appreciate when you use electrical stimulation clinically.

Chapter Reflections

1. Read and ponder each of the following points. Do you feel you have a clear understanding of each concept? If not, reread the appropriate section of the chapter.
   • Why is there confusion about the therapeutic use of electrical currents?

   • What is meant by "a common language" in relation to NMES? Why is this concept important for clinicians, scientists, and manufacturers?
   • What is electricity?
   • What is an electrical charge?

- Differentiate between static and current electricity.
- Give three example of why an understanding of chemistry and physics are essential for understanding electricity.
- Differentiate between AC, DC, and pulsed currents. How is each type of current produced?
- What is Ohm's law?
- Explain the relationship between electricity and magnetism.
- Differentiate between conductor, insulator, semiconductor, and partial conductor.
- Discuss the following aspects of quantifying electricity: coulomb, voltage, ampere, and ohm.
- Compare and contrast electrical current and the flow of water. Include the requirements of each.
- Describe each of the following elements of electrical equipment: generator, terminal, electrical circuit, muscle stimulator, nerve stimulator, circuit breaker, GFI.
- Discuss how electricity is generated and/or converted, including the requirements in each case.
- Compare and contrast an electrical motor and an electrical generator.
- Define each of the following as they apply to electrical stimulation: impulse, cycle, frequency, pulsed current, current modulation, phase, phase duration, phase shape, pulse, monophasic pulse, biphasic pulse, polyphasic pulse, phase charge, pulse charge, pulse symmetry, pulse charge balance, burst, pulse duration (width), interpulse interval, period, pulse rate, duty cycle, amplitude, peak current, average current.
- Differentiate between constant and surged stimulation. When would you use each?
- Define the following: ramp up, plateau, ramp down, time on, time off.
- What is a waveform? Define the most commonly used electrotherapy waveforms.

- Describe LeDuc's experiments, and explain their relevance to electrical stimulation.
- What role do magnetic effects have in tissue rehabilitation?
- Define each of the following and explain the relevance of each to NMES: polarized neuron membrane, action potential, and nerve excitability.
- What is a mixed nerve?
- Differentiate between A fibers, B fibers, and C fibers, including size, speed, and function.
- Explain the effect of the following on nerve excitability: nerve size, nerve depth, and tissue resistance.
- What is current density, and what is its role in NMES?
- Discuss the relationship between pulse duration, current amplitude, and frequency of stimulation on muscle fiber recruitment.
- Explain the difference between a trigger point and a motor point. Describe the role of each in NMES.
- Discuss the role of electrodes in NMES, including physical dimensions, function, and placement techniques.
- Define and differentiate among the following tissue responses to NMES: chemical, thermal, magnetic, and kinetic.
- Define and differentiate the five basic types of tissue responses to electrical stimulation. Include the characteristics of each response, generator settings necessary to evoke each one, and why each is used.

2. Write three to five questions for discussion with your class instructor, clinical instructor, classmates, and clinical colleagues.

3. Get together with classmates and quiz each other on the concepts of this chapter. Use the points in no. 1 and the questions you wrote for no. 2 as a beginning. Explaining concepts out loud to others requires a deeper grasp of the material than feeling you understand it as you read.

Concept Check Responses

CONCEPT CHECK 16.1

(a) 0.005 A or 5 mA; 100 V/20,000 Ω
(b) 0.01 A or 10 mA; 100 V/10,000 Ω.

CONCEPT CHECK 16.2

Increase voltage, and decrease resistance. Yes, cleaning oils from the skin will decrease its resistance and current flow will increase.

CONCEPT CHECK 16.3

The battery generates DC (direct current). We know this because electrons flow from one place to another.

CONCEPT CHECK 16.4

When electrode A was negative and electrode B was positive, negative electrode A attracted the positive strychnine and repelled the negative sulfate. At the same time, positive electrode B attracted the negative cyanide and repelled the positive potassium. Thus, the current passed through the rabbits but the poisons did not.

When electrode A was positive and electrode B was negative, positive electrode A attracted the negative sulfate and repelled the positive strychnine. Simultaneously, negative electrode B attracted the positive potassium and repelled the negative cyanide. Thus, as the current passed through the rabbits, it drove the poisons into them—the strychnine into the first rabbit and the cyanide into the second rabbit.

CONCEPT CHECK 16.5

(a) 5 mA/cm^2. The second electrode is 16 times as big; $2 \times 2 = 4$, $8 \times 8 = 64$, $64/4 = 16$. Did you mistakenly think it was four times as big? Granted, 8 is four times 2, but we are talking about area here, not linear dimensions.

(b) 80 mA/cm^2. The two electrodes are the same size.

REFERENCES

1. Currier DP. *Guide to Electrotherapy Instruments and History of Their American Makers*. West Conshohocken, PA: Infinity Publishing, 2004.
2. Shriber WJ. *A Manual of Electrotherapy*. 4th ed. Philadelphia, PA: Lea & Fibiger, 1975.
3. Behray J. *The Turn of the Century Electrotherapy Museum*. Available at: http://www.electrotherapymuseum.com/Library/ Library2008Quackery.htm. Accessed August, 2012.
4. *Merriam-Webster's Collegiate Dictionary*. 11th ed. Springfield, MA: Merriam-Webster, 2008.
5. Venes D, Biderman A, Fenton BG, Patwell J, Enright AD. *Taber's Cyclopedic Medical Dictionary*. 21st ed. Philadelphia, PA: FA Davis, 2009.
6. Benton LA, Baker LL, Bowman BR, Walters RL. *Functional Electrical Stimulation; A Practical Clinical Guide*. 2nd ed. Downey, CA: Rancho Los Amigos Rehabilitation Engineering Center, Rancho Los Amigos Hospital, 1981.
7. Ralston DJ. High voltaage galvanic stimulation: can there be a "state of the art"? *Athlet Train JNATA*. 1985(20):291–293.
8. Voight M. Reduction of post traumatic ankle edema with high voltage pulsed galvanic stimulation. *Athlet Train JNATA*. 1984;19:278–279, 311.
9. Hasson SM, Wible CL, Barnes WS, Williams JH. Dexamethasone iontophoresis: effect on delayed muscle soreness and muscle function. *Can J Sports Sci*. 1992:8–13.
10. Kahn J. Iontophoresis and ultrasound for postsurgical temporomandibular trismus and paresthesia. *Phys Ther*. 1980;60(3):307–308.
11. Kahn J. Iontophoresis dissected. *Biomechanics*. 1996:81–83.
12. Lunt MJ. Magnetic and electric fields produced during pulsed-magnetic-field therapy for non-union of the tibia. *Med Bil Eng Comput*. 1982;20:501–511.
13. Brighton CT, Pollack SR. Treatment of recalcitrant non-union with a capacitively coupled electrical field. A preliminary report. *J Bone Joint Surg Am*. 1985;67(4):577–585.
14. Guyton AC, Hall JE. *Textbook of Medical Physiology*. 12th ed. Philadelphia, PA: Saunders Elsevier, 2011.

Application Procedures: Electrotherapy

Chapter Outline

OPENING SCENE

Jose, a physical therapy clinic director, is reviewing the day's treatment forms after an unusually busy day. Patients have come in for the treatment of acute and chronic pain, muscle spasms, and acute and chronic edema and for the prevention of postoperative muscle atrophy. In fact, a soccer player has even been in for treatment of a slow-healing strawberry (abrasion) on her thigh caused by sliding on the turf in a game. Jose noticed that when the staff has used electrotherapy for the above conditions, they have often chosen the wrong parameters. He decides it's time for a refresher course on standard operating procedures (SOPs) for electrotherapy modalities.

Electrotherapy Applications: An Overview

There are a variety of electrotherapy devices, each with different current characteristics and resulting in somewhat different responses. The competing claims by various manufacturers have created much confusion. An analogy with vehicles helps cut through this confusion. A subcompact car is excellent for one or two people to commute to work and could serve the needs of a family. A minivan would be a better vehicle for a family, but would not be as economical as the subcompact car for commuting. A family with a large yard, lots of trees, a big vegetable garden, and snow mobiles for winter recreation would find a pickup truck very useful. A mini van could tow the snowmobiles and haul fertilizer to, and waste from the garden and orchards, but it would not be as effective as a pickup truck.

Electrotherapy modalities are similar to the vehicles. One type of electrotherapy modality might be the best tool for a certain indication and be appropriate for several other purposes, but not work as effectively as other electrotherapy modalities. Stated another way, several electrotherapeutic modalities can cause a muscle to contract, but some do it better than others. If you owned just one electrotherapy modality, you would use it to decrease pain, decrease swelling, decrease muscle spasm, increase strength, and increase range of motion. To offer the best care, however, you need to have a variety of electrotherapy modalities and use each one to treat only those conditions for which it is most effective. Modern technology has made it possible to own a variety of devices.

For years, manufacturers argued the merits of the current characteristics of their particular devices. Due to technological advances and clinical and research results, most of them now produce electrotherapy modalities with multiple current forms. It is not uncommon to see transcutaneous electrical nerve stimulation (TENS), interferential current (IFC), neuromuscular electrical stimulation (NMES), high-volt pulsed current (HVPC), and microcurrent with ultrasound or light therapy included on one machine.

Continuing the vehicle analogy, it would be like having push-button controls for converting your vehicle into a subcompact car, a minivan, a pickup truck, or an SUV.

The multicurrent devices strain our vocabulary. What were four to six modalities of 15 years ago are now in a single device. In an effort to avoid confusion, we discuss each of the various current types as separate electrotherapy modalities. As in previous chapters, you need to learn the advantages and disadvantages of each individual modality (or current type) so you can choose the best tool to use to reach specific therapeutic goals.

STANDARD OPERATING PROCEDURES

SOPs for the five most common electrotherapy modalities are presented in this chapter. They are:

1. TENS for pain relief
2. IFC therapy for pain relief
3. NMES for muscle re-education, preventing disuse atrophy, decreasing muscle spasm, and decreasing edema
4. Iontophoresis for transcutaneous drug delivery
5. HVPC stimulation for wound healing and edema control

Key parameters for these modalities are summarized in Table 17.1.

Think of SOPs as a road map. For example, on a road trip, there are several routes you can take to get from one place to another. But you need to determine which route is the best, most efficient one under certain circumstances. As you read this chapter, think of how you can use electrotherapy modalities to reach your treatment goals. Don't fall into the habit of using SOPs inattentively; it might lead to a dead end.

Transcutaneous Electrical Nerve Stimulation for Pain Relief

Transcutaneous electrical nerve stimulation (TENS) is a modality that uses surface electrodes to deliver a pulsed electrical current through the skin to stimulate nerves for the purpose of controlling and relieving pain (Fig. 17.1). The word "transcutaneous" means through the skin, and "nerve stimulation" refers to the current having enough intensity to depolarize sensory nerves.

TABLE 17.1   KEY PARAMETERS FOR ELECTROTHERAPY MODALITIES

	TENS	IFC THERAPY	NMES	IONTOPHORESIS	HVPC STIMULATION
Current type	AC	Two ACs criss-cross, forming one interference current	AC	DC	AC (monophasic)
Wave form	Biphasic	Sine	Russian or biphasic	Rectangular	Twin pulse
Total current flow	1–100 mA	1–100 mA	0–200 mA	1–5 mA	0–500 mA
Frequency	1–150 pps	Carrier: 2500–5000; Beat: 0–299 pps	1–200 pps	NA	1–120 pps
Pulse width	10–500 msec	NA	20–300 msec	NA	13–100 msec
Electrode placement	Directly on pain, dermatome, motor points, trigger points, acupuncture points, nerve root, contiguous, contralateral	Criss-cross with area to be stimulated in center of the X	Bipolar on motor point and on belly of muscle	Monopolar with drug delivery electrode on treatment site	Monopolar; active electrode on area to be treated
Primary indications	Acute and chronic pain	Acute and chronic pain; muscle spasm	Disuse atrophy; muscle re-education; muscle spasm; post-acute edema	Acute and chronic pain; inflammation; arthritis	Acute and chronic edema; wound healing

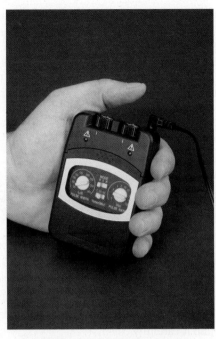

FIGURE 17.1 A portable TENS unit.

A SHORT HISTORY OF TENS

The establishment of TENS for pain relief began in the early 1970s, based mainly on the findings of Canadian psychologist Ronald Melzack and British neuroanatomist Patrick Wall.[1] In 1965, these scientists published their classic paper on the gate control theory of pain (see Chapter 8) and how stimulating afferent nerves could close a gate in the spinal column to pain signals coming from other nerves.[2] Several companies began marketing transcutaneous electrical nerve stimulators. Later, Melzack and Wall revised their theory to include how cognition might affect pain.[3,4]

THE PHYSIOLOGICAL EFFECT OF TENS

The physiological effect of TENS is selective depolarization of afferent nerves. Electrodes are placed on the skin, usually at the site of the pain. By adjusting different parameters on a TENS unit, the clinician can change the patient's perception of acute and chronic pain.

TENS MODES

There are three major modes of TENS, each applied by modulating the intensity and beat frequency (adjustable pulses per second [pps]):

- **Sensory TENS**: Used to treat acute pain by stimulating large-diameter sensory nerves. The beat frequency is high (80–200 pps), and the intensity is adjusted to the point where the patient reports a buzzing or tingling. This is conventional or traditional TENS.

- **Motor TENS**: Used to treat chronic pain by stimulating small-diameter afferent nerves. The beat frequency is low (1–5 pps), and the intensity is higher than sensory TENS (to the patient's tolerance). The patient reports some burning, needling sensation, and a slight muscle twitch.
- **Brief-intense TENS**: Used to treat chronic pain prior to rehabilitation by stimulating C fibers. The beat frequency varies between low and high and changes periodically. The intensity is also higher than sensory TENS (to the patient's tolerance). The patient reports some burning, needling sensation, and twitch and tetanic muscle contractions.

HOW TENS WORKS

There are many theories about how TENS works. Many scientists believe that pain modulation during and after TENS is achieved either through the gate control system or the opiate system (see Chapter 8). The gate control system is typically activated by sensory TENS mode, whereas the opiate system is activated by motor TENS and brief-intense TENS modes.

Evidence supports the opiate system for pain modulation when a particular TENS mode, such as motor or brief-intense TENS, is used. When patients whose pain was being relieved by TENS treatment were given naloxone, an inhibitor of exogenous and endogenous opiates, the pain returned rapidly.[4,5]

RESEARCH ON TENS

Since TENS is used primarily for pain management, research in this area is often difficult to perform. Recall from Chapter 8 that pain varies from one person to the next, and measuring pain and pain relief is very hard to do.

TENS relieves pain associated with osteoarthritis,[6] rheumatoid arthritis,[7] dysmenorrhea,[8,9] and low-back pain.[10,11] Reports of postoperative pain relief with TENS include total knee replacement surgery,[12,13] shoulder surgery,[14] and other orthopedic conditions.[15–17] To date, the results are still mixed on the effectiveness of TENS to produce analgesia postoperatively. TENS has not been effective in relieving myofascial pain.[18]

 CONCEPT CHECK 17.1. What is an advantage of using TENS postoperatively?

MAKING TENS THERAPY MORE EFFECTIVE

To be successful in using TENS, consider the following:

- Do not treat all your patients the same (e.g., don't use a blanket protocol for everyone). Patients are not alike; therefore, parameters, electrode placements, and treatment protocols need to be modified to meet the needs of individual patients.

• Be flexible. Scientists are unclear regarding which TENS mode is more effective under which conditions. It might be best to start with sensory TENS because it is easily tolerated by the patient. If the patient doesn't respond, progress to either motor TENS or brief-intense TENS.

• TENS by itself is not a cure for pain, but it can relieve pain long enough to help a patient complete an exercise session or get a good night's sleep.

Now that you have a little background, you are ready for the five-step application procedure for TENS therapy.

5 STEPS Application of Transcutaneous Electrical Nerve Stimulation

1 STEP 1: FOUNDATION

A. Definition. TENS is a modality that uses surface electrodes to deliver a pulsed electrical current through the skin to stimulate nerves.
B. Effects
  1. Afferent nerve stimulation
  2. Pain relief
  3. Some motor nerve stimulation (and associated muscular contraction) at higher amplitudes
C. Advantages
  1. Portable; can be used while exercising or at work
  2. Self-treatment
  3. Alternative to cold during cryokinetics
  4. Alternative to painkilling medication
D. Disadvantages
  1. Eliminates pain; does not treat the cause of the pain
  2. May mask more serious problems
  3. Inconclusive research results
  4. Sometimes becomes a "cure-all"
E. Indications
  1. Pain of peripheral origin
  2. Acute pain
  3. Chronic pain
F. Contraindications
  1. Do not use with a person who has:
    a. An implanted pacemaker
    b. A history of heart disease
  2. Do not treat the transthoracic area.
  3. Discontinue use if a skin irritation develops.
G. Precautions
  1. Be cautious when using TENS over an area with:
    a. Impaired sensation
    b. Skin lesions (cuts, abrasions, new skin, recent scar tissue, etc.)
  2. A patient should be cautious when using TENS while driving or operating heavy machinery, since reaction time might be hindered.

  3. Remember that a temporary decrease in pain does not mean the cause of the pain has gone (although pain sometimes persists long after its cause has been resolved).
  4. A TENS unit is delicate; instruct the patient to handle it carefully.

2 STEP 2: PREAPPLICATION TASKS

A. Make sure TENS is the proper modality for this situation.
  1. Reevaluate the injury/problem. Make sure you understand the patient's condition.
  2. If TENS was applied previously, review the patient's response to the previous treatment.
  3. Establish (or confirm) treatment goals
  4. Confirm that the objectives of therapy (goals) are compatible with TENS
  5. Make sure TENS is not contraindicated in this situation.
B. Preparing the patient psychologically
  1. Explain the procedure if the patient is being treated for the first time, or if the treatment is being changed.
    a. Describe the expected sensation (e.g., pricking pins and needles).
    b. Only a small amount of current will be used.
    c. TENS will not cause electrocution.
    d. It should not be painful; if it is, ask the patient to let you know, and then lower the intensity.
  2. Demonstrate the procedure on yourself if the patient seems particularly apprehensive.
  3. Check for, and warn the patient about, precautions.
C. Preparing the patient physically
  1. Remove clothing, tape, etc., from the electrode contact area. It is not necessary to remove them from the area between the two contact points.
  2. Position the patient in a comfortable position.

D. Equipment preparation
  1. Make sure the output is at the minimal setting.
  2. Prepare the electrodes.
     a. Attach the electrodes to the leads (cords) and the leads to the TENS unit.
     b. Apply a conducting medium (electrode gel) to the electrode surface (unless self-adhering electrodes are used).
  3. Electrode placement is very important, but most clinicians use trial and error to determine the best placement. The following systems are recommended:
     a. Over acupuncture points
     b. Directly over the pain
     c. Proximal-distal to pain (Fig. 17.2)
     d. Criss-cross over the pain (requires a two-channel unit)
     e. Over a motor point
     f. Along a dermatome
  4. Check the equipment and electrode operation.
     a. If nonadhering electrodes are used, place them on the table and cover the electrodes with your hand (Fig. 17.3). Turn up the intensity until current is felt.
     b. Check the connecting leads, especially for loose-fitting electrode tips, if current is absent or reduced.
  5. Place the electrodes on the patient's skin.
     a. Electrodes must be firmly attached to the body part, while also allowing movement of the body part (especially if worn during athletic activity or at work).

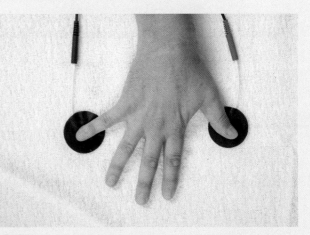

FIGURE 17.3 Testing electrodes to confirm they are functioning properly.

     b. Good contact is essential but sometimes hard to achieve.
     c. If nonadhering electrodes are used, tape them to the skin and/or wrap with an elastic or Velcro strap.

3 STEP 3: APPLICATION PARAMETERS

The following are general procedures for TENS. For parameters for treating specific conditions, (Table 17.2). Also see the specific instructions in the manufacturer's manual of the modality your clinic uses.

A. Procedures
  1. Select the pulse width and rate, according to the manufacturer's guidelines.
  2. Turn the unit on.
  3. Tell the patient you are beginning.
  4. Slowly increase the current intensity.
     a. Ask the patient to tell you when he/she begins to feel pins and needles.
     b. Increase the current until it feels most comfortable to the patient (for sensory TENS).
     c. There should be no muscular contraction (for sensory TENS).
  5. Adjust the pulse width and rate; here are two options:
     a. Go through the entire range and select the most comfortable setting.
     b. Use specific settings for specific problems.
        i. For treating acute pain, set a narrow pulse width (75 μsec) with a high pulse rate of 80–200 pps. (Pain relief is almost immediate but lasts only a few minutes to 1 hour.)

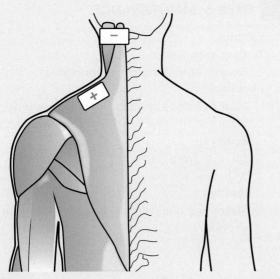

FIGURE 17.2 Electrodes placed distal-proximal of the affected area.

TABLE 17.2   KEY PARAMETERS OF TENS THERAPY FOR VARIOUS CONDITIONS

PARAMETER	ACUTE PAIN (SENSORY TENS)	CHRONIC PAIN (MOTOR TENS)	PAIN REDUCTION PRIOR TO REHABILITATION (BRIEF-INTENSE TENS)
Pulse duration	60–100 μsec	150–250 μsec	>250 μsec
Pulse rate	80–200 pps	1–5 pps	variable
Electrode placement	Directly on painful area; nerve root and dermatome	Motor points, trigger points, acupuncture points	Motor points, trigger points, acupuncture points
Output intensity	Pleasant tingling without contraction	To tolerance; burning needling sensation slight muscle twitch	To tolerance; visible twitch and tetanic muscle contraction
Modulation	Modulated rate	Modulated burst	Modulated amp
Treatment sequence	15–30 min; 1 or 2 times daily	15–30 min; 1 or 2 times daily	10–20 min; 1 or 2 times daily
Onset of relief	<10 min	20–40 min	<15 min
Duration of relief	30 min to 2 h	6–7 h	<30 min
Opioid peptide	dynorphin	Beta-endorphin	Enkephalin
Fiber activation	A-beta	A-delta and C	A-beta, A-delta, and C

ii. For treating chronic pain, set a wide pulse width (200 μsec) with a low pulse rate of 1–5 pps. (Pain relief may take ½ hour, but it may last 6–7 hours.)

6. Show the patient how to increase the intensity and pulse rate. (TENS is often a take-home modality, so it is important that the patient knows how to use it.)

B. Dosage
1. Use the maximal current that is comfortable for the patient.
2. It might be necessary to increase every 17 minutes as the body adapts to the stimulus.

C. Length of application
1. Extremely variable, from 30 to 60 minutes to hours

D. Frequency of application
1. Three or four times a day as needed for pain

E. Duration of therapy
1. Use until TENS is no longer effective.

4 STEP 4: POSTAPPLICATION TASKS

A. Equipment removal
1. Turn off the power.
2. Return all controls to off or the minimum setting.

3. Remove and clean the electrodes.
4. Place the electrodes and TENS unit in proper place, preferably locked up.

B. Instructions to the patient
1. Schedule the next treatment.
2. Instruct the patient about the level of activity and/or self-treatment prior to the next formal treatment.

C. Record of treatment, including unique patient responses

D. Battery recharging (if charging unit is used)

5 STEP 5: MAINTENANCE

A. Batteries
1. Keep a spare set.
2. Keep charged (if charging unit is used).

B. Electrodes
1. Must be kept clean; body oils will accumulate
2. Wash the electrodes with warm water and a mild detergent.
3. Do not wash self-adhering electrodes, as this will cause the adherent and coupling medium to dissolve.
4. Make sure the wire is firmly attached to the electrode post.

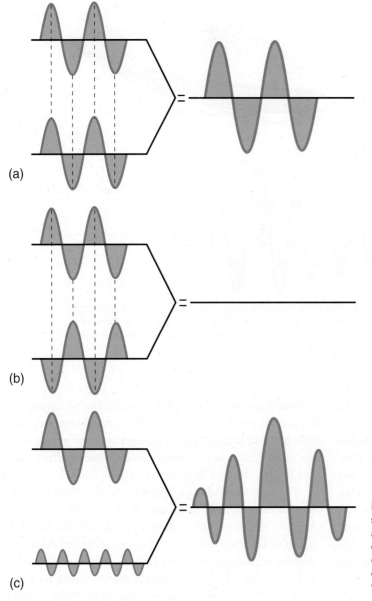

(a)

(b)

(c)

FIGURE 17.4 IFC therapy is based on the concept of two sinusoidal currents (**left**) interacting with each other that create a third current (**right**). **(a)** Two currents of the same frequency and in phase double the amplitude. **(b)** Two currents of the same frequency and 180° out of phase cancel each other. **(c)** Two currents of differing frequency create a current with varying amplitude.

Interferential Current Therapy for Pain Relief

Interferential current (IFC) therapy is the application of two separate medium-frequency sinusoidal currents of different frequencies to the same area.[1,19] The two currents interfere with each other so that their individual effects are increased, diminished, or neutralized (Fig. 17.4). The resulting current is thus different than either of the beginning currents. If you have ever been in a speeding motorboat, you have seen the large wake or waves that are created by the boat. As another boat crosses these waves at a 90° angle, the other boat may fishtail a little, and the mutual action of the bisecting (or interfering) waves causes an agitating, uneven, sometimes bigger wave (Fig. 17.5).

The use of IFC therapy started in Europe in the 1950s and was introduced in the United States and Canada in the early 1980s. This took place about the same time as the publication of several texts on the subject.[20–22] In 1999, it ranked as high as fifth among the most frequently used therapeutic modalities by physical therapists in Ireland[23] and Australia.[24,25]

THE THEORY OF IFC THERAPY

Advocates of IFC therapy claim that you can achieve the stronger physiological effects of low-frequency (<250 pps) electrical stimulation of muscle and nerve tissues without the associated painful and unpleasant side effects of such stimulation.[26] They claim that to produce low-frequency effects at sufficient intensity and depth, most patients

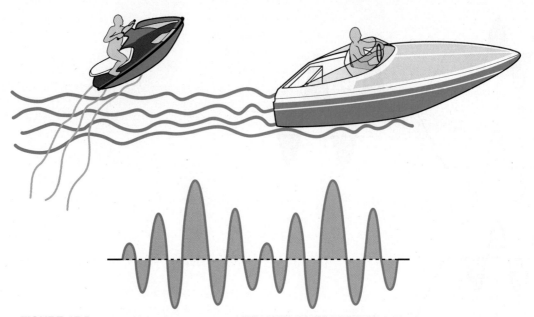

FIGURE 17.5 Interference waves or current. Notice the large waves created by the speeding motorboat. As another boat crosses these waves at a 90° angle, the other boat may fishtail a little; the mutual action of the bisecting (or interfering) waves causes an agitating, uneven, sometimes bigger wave. In essence, this is what happens when electrical currents cross during IFC therapy.

experience considerable discomfort. This is due to the resistance of the skin being inversely proportional to the frequency of the stimulation. The lower the stimulation frequency, the greater the resistance to the passage of the current; thus, more discomfort is experienced. The skin impedance of low-frequency 50 Hz is approximately 3200 Ω, while at medium frequency 4000 Hz, it is reduced to approximately 40 Ω.[26] Thus, a medium frequency current will pass more easily through the skin, requiring less electrical energy input to reach the deeper tissues and giving rise to less discomfort. We note that this concept is not supported by all scientists, as some feel that medium frequency is no more comfortable to the patient than low frequency.

There is no scientific evidence to support or refute this theory. Our experience with NMES (low-frequency stimulation) indicates that the strength of contraction, rather than pain, is the limiting factor to the amount of current a patient can tolerate. Also, clinicians generally use NMES to produce high-intensity muscle contraction.

USING IFC THERAPY

The main use of IFC is for pain relief, although there are protocols for edema control, muscle re-education and bone stimulation.[19] Probably its greatest advantages over traditional TENS therapy are its ability to cover a large area and perhaps to penetrate deeper into the tissues.[19]

Two channels (and four electrodes) are used to deliver IFC. One channel has a set frequency, which is called the carrier frequency. The other channel has an adjustable frequency, which is used to produce a **beat frequency**, the difference between the two frequencies. For example, if the carrier frequency is 5000 Hz and the second frequency is 5200 Hz, the beat frequency would be 200 Hz.

The four electrodes are applied in a criss-cross pattern, so that each channel forms one of the legs of the X. The location where the two currents cross or interfere is called a vector. There are two types of vectors, static and dynamic. A **static vector** does not move but stays centered where the currents cross. A **dynamic vector** moves throughout the treatment field between the four electrodes. This is done by altering the beat frequency (by changing the second current's frequency), a feature known as sweep or scan. The advantages of the vector pattern are that you can treat both localized pain, with a static vector (Fig. 17.6), and poorly defined pain, with a dynamic vector (Fig. 17.7).

Suppose you want to decrease a patient's poorly localized back pain. Your carrier frequency is 5000 Hz and you decide to choose a beat frequency (the frequency that can be adjusted) of 100 Hz. After the patient has "guesstimated" the area of most pain, apply four electrodes on the patient in a criss-cross pattern with the pain centered in the middle. Hook up two electrodes to one channel and two electrodes to another. Then slowly turn up the intensity to where the patient feels tingling without contracting of the muscle. One channel will run the current at 5000 Hz while the other runs it at 5100 Hz. Since the pain is poorly localized, you can use a dynamic vector (or sweep or scan, depending

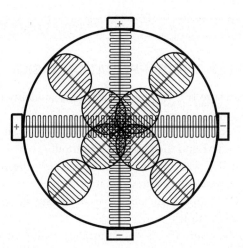

FIGURE 17.6 In IFC therapy, a static vector can be locked on to the area where the pain is easily located. (Adapted from Castel, D. International Academy of Physio Therapeutics. Clip Art, with permission.)

upon the manufacturer's instructions). As the vector moves throughout the back, it stimulates a large area, treating most of the area bracketed by the electrodes (see Fig. 17.7).

There is a setting on most machines that have IFC labeled *premodulated*. This is for treating mainly longitudinal areas where four electrodes can't effectively bracket the treatment area. With this two-pole stimulation, electronic manipulation of the currents results in interference in the machine, not the body.

THE EFFECTIVENESS OF IFC THERAPY

Palmer[27] expressed the opinion that IFC is unlikely to produce physiological and therapeutic effects different from those of a TENS unit. Alon[28] referred to IFC as simply a different, more expensive, redundant approach to

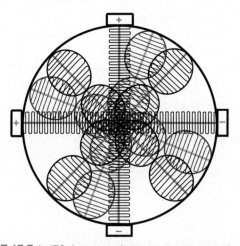

FIGURE 17.7 In IFC therapy, a dynamic vector moves the current throughout a large area to treat pain that is hard to pinpoint. (Adapted from Castel, D. International Academy of Physio Therapeutics. Clip Art, with permission.)

achieving the same effects as other electrical stimulators capable of generating pulsed current wave forms with short pulse duration.

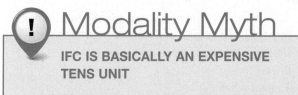

! Modality Myth

IFC IS BASICALLY AN EXPENSIVE TENS UNIT

It is true that the beat frequency of IFC brings about responses similar to a TENS unit. However, due to the medium-frequency generator of IFC and less resistance by the skin, IFC can deliver a total current to the tissues of 70–100 mA greater than TENS.[29]

The differences in opinion about the effectiveness of IFC are probably due to the lack of, and conflicting, clinical research. One group of scientists[30] reported IFC therapy to be effective at increasing blood flow, while others failed to show an increase in circulation with IFC.[31–33] IFC therapy was beneficial for osteoarthritic pain in one study[34] while showing little or no benefit in others.[35,36] Chronic post-traumatic edema was reduced due to the milking of the venous and lymphatic return systems through electrically evoked muscle contractions using IFC.[37]

✔ APPLICATION TIP

When pain reduction is desired, use IFC for large, deep areas and TENS for smaller, superficial areas

The bottom line is, IFC can cover a large area and can stimulate deep tissues. The vector field can be crossed at the joint providing more current density and pain relief to the deeper tissues. TENS is ideal for treating painful conditions, such as trigger points. Most trigger points are superficial and are within the appropriate range to be treated with low-frequency currents (i.e., TENS).

To achieve success in using IFC, review the information earlier in this chapter about how to make TENS treatments more beneficial. Also consider that those who have had success with IFC therapy do the following[19]:

- Correctly position the vector to stimulate the target tissue.
- Use the appropriate size and positioning of the electrodes to stimulate the target tissue.
- Use the appropriate stimulation parameters (frequency, amplitude) for activation of the correct sensory fiber.
- Persevere, if pain relief is not immediately obtained.

Application of Interferential Current Therapy

STEP 1: FOUNDATION

A. Definition. IFC therapy is the interference or super-imposition of at least two separate medium-frequency sinusoidal currents upon one another.
B. Effects
   1. Pain relief
   2. Some motor nerve stimulation (and associated muscular contraction) at higher amplitudes
   3. Muscle spasm reduction
   4. Edema control (perhaps)
C. Advantages
   1. Stimulates tissues deeper than a TENS unit (due to medium carrier frequency)
   2. Larger coverage area than with TENS because of criss-cross pattern of four electrodes surrounding the area of pain
   3. Possibly more comfortable than a TENS unit because of narrow pulse duration and low skin resistance. Medium-frequency currents (IFC) meet with less skin resistance than low-frequency currents (TENS).
D. Disadvantages
   1. Eliminates pain; does not treat the cause of the pain
   2. May mask more serious problems
   3. Few, if any, portable units are available.
   4. Sometimes becomes a panacea
E. Indications
   1. Acute pain
   2. Chronic pain
   3. Pain that covers a large area
   4. Muscle spasm (by decreasing pain)
F. Contraindications
   1. Do not use on a person who has:
      a. An implanted pacemaker
      b. A history of heart disease
   2. Do not treat the transthoracic area.
   3. Discontinue use if a skin irritation develops.
G. Precautions
   1. Be cautious when using IFC over an area with:
      a. Impaired sensation
      b. Skin lesions (cuts, abrasions, new skin, recent scar tissue, etc.)
   2. A patient should be cautious when using IFC while driving or operating heavy machinery.
   3. Remember that a temporary decrease in pain does not mean the cause of the pain has gone (although pain sometimes persists long after its cause has been resolved).

STEP 2: PREAPPLICATION TASKS

A. Make sure IFC therapy is the proper modality for this situation.
   1. Reevaluate the injury/problem. Make sure you understand the patient's condition.
   2. If IFC was applied previously, review the patient's response to the previous treatment.
   3. Confirm that the objectives of therapy are compatible with IFC.
   4. Make sure IFC is not contraindicated in this situation.
B. Preparing the patient psychologically
   1. Explain the procedure if the patient is being treated for the first time, or if the treatment is being changed.
      a. Describe the expected sensation (e.g., pricking pins and needles).
      b. Only a small amount of current will be used.
      c. IFC will not cause electrocution.
      d. It should not be painful; if it is, ask the patient to let you know, then lower the intensity.
   2. Demonstrate the procedure on yourself if the patient seems particularly apprehensive.
   3. Check for, and warn the patient about, precautions.
C. Preparing the patient physically
   1. Remove clothing, tape, etc., from the electrode contact area. It is not necessary to remove them from the area between the two contact points.
   2. Position the patient in a comfortable position, usually sitting or lying.
D. Equipment preparation
   1. Make sure the output is at the minimal setting.
   2. Prepare the electrodes.
      a. Attach four electrodes to the leads and the leads to the IFC unit.
      b. Apply a conducting medium (electrode gel) to the electrode surface (unless self-adhering electrodes are used).
   3. Check the equipment and electrode operation.
      a. If nonadhering electrodes are used, place them on the table and cover them with your hand. Turn up the intensity until current is felt.
      b. Check the connecting leads, especially for loose-fitting electrode tips, if current is absent or reduced.
   4. Determine where to apply the electrodes.
      a. Locate the center of the patient's pain, and make a small mark on that area with an erasable marker.

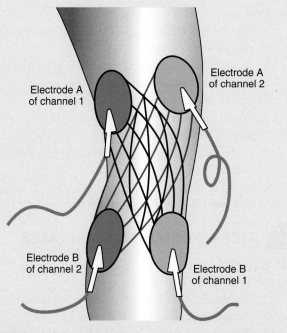

FIGURE 17.8 IFC therapy: Criss-crossing over the painful area. Find out where the patient's pain is, and make a small mark on that area with an erasable marker. Bracket the pain with the electrodes.

Electrode A of channel 1

Electrode A of channel 2

Electrode B of channel 2

Electrode B of channel 1

b. Imagine a clock, where the pain is the center of the clock. The two electrodes from channel 1 are placed at 9 o'clock and 3 o'clock and two electrodes from channel 2 are placed at 12 o'clock and 6 o'clock. Thus, the electrodes criss-cross and the pain is in the center (Fig. 17.8).

5. Attach the electrodes on the patient's skin.

   a. Electrodes must be firmly attached to the body part, while also allowing movement of the body part (especially if worn during athletic activity or at work).

   b. Good contact is essential but sometimes hard to achieve.

   c. If nonadhering electrodes are used, tape them to the skin and/or wrap with an elastic or Velcro strap.

3 | STEP 3: APPLICATION PARAMETERS

The following are general procedures for reducing pain using IFC therapy. For parameters for treating other conditions, see Table 17.3. Also see the specific instructions in the manufacturer's manual of the modality your clinic uses.

TABLE 17.3 KEY PARAMETERS OF IFC THERAPY FOR VARIOUS CONDITIONS

CONDITION	CARRIER FREQUENCY	PULSE RATE	ELECTRODE PLACEMENT	OUTPUT INTENSITY	CTOR	TREATMENT SEQUENCE
Acute pain	4000–5000 Hz	80–150 pps	Criss-cross painful area; dermatome of involved tissue	Pleasant tingling without contraction	Target (specific pain), or sweep to increase treatment area	10–30 min; 3 or 4 times daily
Chronic pain	2500 Hz	1–10 pps	Criss-cross painful area; dermatome of involved tissue	Pleasant tingling with or without mild twitch contraction	Target (specific pain), or sweep to increase treatment area	10–30 min; 1 or 2 times daily
Muscle spasm	2500 Hz	4 pps	Criss-cross local trigger points	Moderate visible muscle contraction	Target (specific spasm), or sweep to increase treatment area	10–30 min; 1 or 2 times daily
Nerve block	4000–5000 Hz	Contin-uous	Over local peripheral nerve(s) innervating the painful area(s)	Pleasant tingling without contraction	Target specific pain	10 min; 1 or 2 times daily
Bone healing	4000–5000 Hz	100 pps	Criss-cross the fracture	Pleasant tingling without contraction	Target specific area	10–20 min; daily
Edema control	4000–5000 Hz	50 pps	Criss-cross the swelling	Strong but comfortable contraction	Sweep to cause pumping action	10–30 min; 3 or 4 times daily

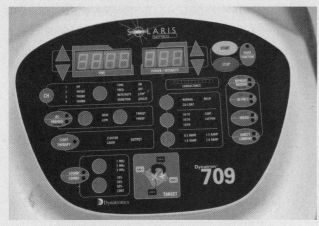

FIGURE 17.9 A typical IFC control panel.

A. Procedures
   1. Turn the unit on.
   2. Tell the patient you are beginning.
   3. Slowly increase the current intensity (Fig. 17.9).
      a. Ask the patient to tell you when he/she begins to feel pins and needles.
      b. Increase the current until it feels most comfortable to the patient.
      c. There should be no muscular contraction.
   4. Adjust the pulse rate settings for specific problems.
      a. For treating acute pain, use a high pulse rate of 80–200 pps. (Pain relief is almost immediate but lasts only a few minutes to 1 hour.)
      b. For treating chronic pain, use a low pulse rate of 1–5 pps. (Pain relief may take ½ hour, but it may last 6–7 hours.)
      c. Target or vector: For pain that is easily identifiable and pinpointed, use the target or vector buttons to move where the current intersects to the area directly over the pain. For pain that is hard to pinpoint, use the dynamic vector (this will continuously move the intersection of the currents throughout the area, thus treating a larger area of pain).

B. Dosage
   1. Use the maximal current that is comfortable for the patient.
   2. It might be necessary to increase every 17 minutes as the body adapts to the stimulus.
C. Length of application
   1. 20–30 minutes
D. Frequency of application
   1. Once or twice daily, as needed for pain (see Table 17.3)
E. Duration of therapy
   1. Use until IFC is no longer effective.

4 STEP 4: POSTAPPLICATION TASKS

A. Equipment removal
   1. Turn off the power.
   2. Return all controls to off or the minimum setting.
   3. Remove and clean the electrodes.
   4. Place the electrodes, leads, and wraps in the proper place, not on top of the unit.
B. Instructions to the patient
   1. Schedule the next treatment.
   2. Instruct the patient about the level of activity and/or self-treatment prior to the next formal treatment.
C. Record of treatment, including unique patient responses
D. Return of the generator cart to the proper place, area cleanup

5 STEP 5: MAINTENANCE

A. Check the fuse in back if the unit will not turn on (also make sure it is plugged in).
B. Electrodes
   1. Must be kept clean; body oils will accumulate
   2. Wash the electrodes with warm water and a mild detergent.
   3. Do not wash self-adhering electrodes, as this will cause the adherent and couplant to dissolve.
   4. Make sure the leads are firmly attached to the electrode post.

 CONCEPT CHECK 17.2. Suppose you want to use IFC with a carrier frequency of 2500 Hz. Your goal is long-lasting pain relief for someone with chronic pain. (a) What would be a good range for your beat frequency? (b) What would be a good range for your carrier frequency?

 CONCEPT CHECK 17.3. You are treating an athlete who has low-back pain. You feel he could benefit from electrical current stimulation for pain control at home, yet your unit that provides IFC is too large. What option do you have?

(?) CONCEPT CHECK 17.4. You are treating an athlete who has pain in her hip. When you ask her to point to the pain, she replies, "It's hard to localize and seems to move around." Which modality would be best to use under these circumstances and why?

Neuromuscular Electrical Stimulation

Neuromuscular electrical stimulation (NMES) refers to eliciting a muscle contraction with electrical currents. In orthopedics and rehabilitation, muscle contractions via NMES therapy are induced for:

- Muscle re-education, that is, reestablishing or strengthening muscle contraction
- Preventing disuse atrophy
- Decreasing muscle spasm
- Decreasing edema

A BRIEF HISTORY OF NMES

NMES has been used for decades. It was first combined with ultrasound, to provide a sensation so patients would feel they were getting something from the ultrasound treatment. However, it was not used aggressively through the 1950s because of a common belief that faradic (alternating current) stimulation was too painful.

The Russians began using NMES to increase muscle strength in trained athletes during the 1970s. In 1977, the Russian physiologist Yakov Kots[38] made some astounding claims and demonstrations at a meeting of Canadian and Soviet scientists.[1] Kots claimed that the use of his "Russian current" could produce the following:

- Up to 30% more force than a voluntary maximal contraction
- Lasting strength gains of up to 40% in healthy athletes
- No sensory discomfort. His treatment was *painless*.[1]

In 1980, a Canadian company started manufacturing these so-called Russian current stimulators. To date, no North American scientist has been able to duplicate Kots' claims of pain-free current flow during high-level muscle contractions. In fact, most subjects in the studies complained of a great amount of pain as the current amplitude tried to replicate the force of a voluntary muscle contraction.[1] Indeed, NMES increases muscle strength; however, it does not appear to be superior to voluntary training.[39–46]

In the 1970s, HVPC was introduced. Advocates claimed that it was more comfortable than traditional low-volt stimulation and that it penetrated deeper and therefore would result in greater muscle contraction than low-volt modified square wave stimulators. Research, however, proved that it did not result in greater muscle contraction.[47] The interest generated by the Russian and HVPC stimulators lead to the development of low-volt pulsed current stimulators.

NMES FOR MUSCLE RE-EDUCATION AND PREVENTION OF DISUSE ATROPHY

If a healthy athlete can generate a stronger voluntary muscle contraction than an electrically induced contraction, why use NMES? The answer is simple. NMES is used on patients who cannot perform a voluntary muscle contraction. These might be patients where peripheral nerve innervation is intact but normal voluntary contraction is weak or limited from muscle atrophy after prolonged immobilization, surgery, or from pain. Scientists have not only found NMES to be of value in maintaining muscle integrity and combating disuse atrophy but NMES has also been effective in promoting early active range of motion in postsurgical and immobilized limbs.[48–51]

The Effect of NMES on Injured Muscle

When a patient suffers a musculoskeletal injury or undergoes surgery, she often loses the ability to fully contract some muscles. NMES can help restore muscle function, following this process:

- Hook up the patient to a NMES device.
- By depolarizing alpha motor neurons, NMES causes muscles to involuntarily contract.
- After several repeated contractions, the CNS receives and processes afferent feedback from the muscle.
- This improves the patient's proprioceptive and visual sense of the motions.
- The patient begins to relearn the motions.
- As the patient gets stronger, he/she needs to isometrically contract his/her muscles as much as possible during the stimulation.[52]

The use of NMES on a muscle with strength deficits increases a patient's awareness of contractile motions by providing proprioceptive, kinesthetic, and sensory input. Treatment goals focus on assisting with motion and on re-educating a muscle toward normal motion so that an active exercise program can begin as soon as possible.[52] For key parameters to use for muscle re-education and the prevention of disuse atrophy, see Table 17.4.

Avoiding Replacing Strength Training with NMES

It is very important that a patient not become too dependent on NMES. Electrical muscle stimulation recruits fibers in the opposite order than a voluntary contraction. For example, when a patient is hooked up to an NMES unit

TABLE 17.4　KEY PARAMETERS OF NMES FOR VARIOUS CONDITIONS

PARAMETER	POST-ACUTE EDEMA	MUSCLE SPASM	MUSCLE RE-EDUCATION (DISUSE ATROPHY)
Carrier frequency	5000 Hz	5000 Hz	2500 Hz
Pulse rate	30–50 pps	50–70 pps	50–70 pps
Electrode placement	Bipolar on muscle group proximal to edema	Bipolar on motor points and muscle spasm	Bipolar on motor points and muscle belly for optimal contraction
Output intensity	Visible muscle contraction	Visible muscle contraction	Visible muscle contraction
Duty cycle	5–10 s on/5–10 s off	10 s on/10 s off	10 s on/50 s off 10 s on/30 s off (later during rehab)
Ramp	Minimum (0.5 s on/0.5 s off) to none	1–2 s on/1–2 s off	2–3 s on/2–3 s off
Patient duty	Elevate part	Try to relax	Contract with "on" cycle
Treatment sequence	10–20 min; twice daily	10–20 min; daily	20 min daily

and allows the machine to produce a passive contraction, the large nerve fibers fire first, followed by the smaller fibers. However, when a patient performs an active voluntary contraction, the small fibers fire first, followed by the larger ones. Thus, the patient needs to move on to more traditional weight training as soon as possible to develop muscle strength appropriately.

ⓘ Modality Myth

EFFORTLESS EXERCISE WITH NMES CREATES WASHBOARD ABDOMINALS

You might have seen some advertisements claiming that muscle stimulation of the abdominal muscles will result in improved muscle tone and strength to this area. This idea is entirely false, for three main reasons:

1. Electrical muscle stimulation cannot cause as strong a muscle contraction as a voluntary muscle contraction can. Also, if it were possible to elicit a strong enough contraction with a machine to produce a "six-pack," or washboard abdominals, the intensity would have to be turned up so high that it would be unbearable.
2. The order of stimulation of muscle fibers is the reverse of normal; large fibers are stimulated first. In a voluntary contraction, small fibers are stimulated first.
3. The exercise is not effortless. It is nonvoluntary, but not effortless. The muscle still contracts, using ATP and all the other metabolic components and mechanisms.

NMES FOR DECREASING MUSCLE SPASM

The exact cause and mechanism of a muscle spasm are not clearly defined. By spasm, we mean a low-grade contraction or tightness as opposed to a muscle cramp, which is a complete, massive, sudden-onset contraction. A spasm can result from microtrauma, macrotrauma, accumulation of chemical irritants, muscle weakness, and pain. Regardless of the original cause, pain and discomfort lead to more pain and a protective muscle spasm. As the spasm puts pressure on sensitive nerve endings, more pain is produced—causing the vicious pain-spasm-pain cycle.

Avoid being overly concerned with what caused the muscle spasm, because the "pain" derived from the spasm is the reason the patient is seeing you. The goals of the treatment should be to break the pain-spasm-pain cycle, while providing normal range of motion to the area of pain.

Tetanic Contraction Stimulation

The goals of tetanic contraction stimulation are to[52]:

- Increase local circulation
- Remove metabolic wastes
- Mechanically stimulate muscle fibers
- Induce some muscle spasm fatigue

See Table 17.4 for key parameters to use for reducing muscle spasm.

NMES FOR DECREASING EDEMA

NMES can produce "cyclic" muscle contractions (twitch contractions) to stimulate lymphatic flow and help remove free protein and edema from the area. If the patient is able, he/she should contract the muscles being treated during the "on" phase of each stimulation to help milk out the edema.

Application of Neuromuscular Electrical Stimulation

STEP 1: FOUNDATION

A. Definition. NMES is the eliciting of muscle contraction by electrical currents.
B. Effects
 1. Muscle contraction, to:
  a. Increase blood flow
  b. Retard atrophy development
  c. Decrease/retard neuromuscular inhibitions
  d. Increase muscle relaxation—decrease spasm
 2. Pain relief, possibly by decreasing muscle spasm
C. Advantages
 1. Can be applied to immobilized body part
 2. Can supplement voluntary muscular contraction
D. Disadvantages
 1. Sometimes becomes a "cure-all"
E. Indications
 1. Residual or chronic muscle spasm
 2. Any time normal neuromuscular function is not possible
 3. Muscle strains
 4. During cast immobilization or disuse atrophy
 5. Pain (due to muscle spasm)
F. Contraindications. Do not use:
 1. On a person with a pacemaker
 2. Over the heart or brain
 3. Over recent or nonunion fractures
 4. Over potential malignancies
G. Precautions. Be cautious when using NMES over an area with:
 1. Impaired sensation
 2. Skin lesions (cuts, abrasions, new skin, recent scar tissue, etc.)
 3. Decreased range of motion
 4. Extensive torn tissue

STEP 2: PREAPPLICATION TASKS

A. Make sure NMES is the proper therapy for this situation.
 1. Reevaluate the injury/problem. Make sure you understand the patient's condition.
 2. If NMES was applied previously, review the patient's response to the previous treatment.
 3. Confirm that the objectives of therapy are compatible with NMES.
 4. Select or review the electrical current characteristics of your NMES units.

5. Make sure NMES is not contraindicated in this situation.
B. Preparing the patient psychologically
 1. Explain the procedure if the patient is being treated for the first time, or if the treatment is being changed.
  a. Describe the expected sensation—moderate, prickling pins and needles progressing to strong contraction.
  b. Explain that:
   i. Electricity will cause the muscle to contract (tell how much).
   ii. Only a small amount of current will be used.
   iii. NMES will not cause electrocution.
   iv. NMES should not be painful; if it is, tell the patient to let you know.
 2. Demonstrate the procedure on yourself if the patient seems particularly apprehensive.
 3. Check for, and warn the patient about, precautions.
  a. Inspect the skin for cuts, abrasions, new skin, etc., and make sure it is clean and free from oils.
  b. If the area to be treated has excess hair, it will need to be shaved to ensure electrode conductivity.
  c. Determine that skin sensation is not impaired by lightly taping or rubbing the skin and asking the patient if and where he/she feels pressure.
  d. Determine that joint range of motion is not impaired by moving the joint though complete range of motion.
C. Preparing the patient physically
 1. Remove clothing, tape, etc., from electrode contact area. It is not necessary to remove them from the area between the two contact points.
 2. Position the patient in a comfortable position.
D. Equipment preparation
 1. Turn the unit on to warm up (necessary only in older units).
  a. Make sure the output is at minimal setting.
  b. Pulse rate (at least 30 Hz) must be displayed in the output window.
 2. Prepare the electrodes.
  a. Attach the electrodes to the leads and the leads to the generator.
  b. No preparation is needed for self-adhering electrodes.
  c. Prepare carbon-rubber electrodes with the proper medium.

i. Carbon-rubber electrodes require either water or a gel-based couplant.

ii. A gel-based couplant is applied directly to the electrode and is placed between the skin and the electrode.

iii. When water is used as a couplant, it is applied to a small sponge that is placed between the skin and the electrode. In that case, wet the sponge; remove excess water but do not squeeze dry.

3. Check the equipment and electrode operation.

a. If nonadhering electrodes are used, place them on the table and span them with your hand. Turn up the intensity until current is felt.

b. Check the connecting leads, especially for loose-fitting electrode tips, if current is absent or reduced. Reduce the current to zero before the next step.

4. Firmly attach bipolar electrodes on the patient's skin.

a. Place one near the center of the muscle belly and the other on the proximal or distal end of the muscle (Fig. 17.10).

i. Good contact is essential.

ii. Remove the adhesive backing for self-adhering electrodes.

iii. For nonadhering electrodes, place a wet sponge, or piece of wet paper towel, between the electrode and skin, and use elastic belts, straps, body weight, sandbags, etc. to hold the electrodes in place.

3 ▪ STEP 3: APPLICATION PARAMETERS

The following are general procedures for conditions requiring muscle contraction. For parameters for treating specific conditions, see Table 17.4. Also see specific instructions in the manufacturer's manual of the modality your clinic uses. Figure 17.11 is a NMES control panel. Refer to it as an example of the various switches and knobs on a NMES unit.

A. Procedures

1. Set the pulse rate:

a. Less than 10 pps for twitch contraction, which is used for:

i. Edema control

ii. Chronic pain

b. Greater than 30 pps for tetanic contraction, which is used for:

i. Spasm reduction

ii. Disuse atrophy

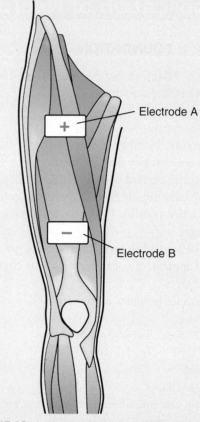

FIGURE 17.10 In NMES therapy, in order to produce a strong muscle contraction, one electrode is applied to the muscle belly and the other electrode is applied at either the distal or proximal end of the muscle.

2. Set the duty cycle (amount of time the current will be on, compared to the amount of time the current will be off).

3. Set the timer.

4. Adjust the surge (ramp) controls as necessary. If you are inducing a tetanic contraction, you must use a surge (ramp).

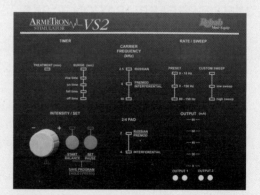

FIGURE 17.11 A typical NMES control panel.

5. Tell the patient that you are beginning the treatment and that he/she must tell you when it is uncomfortable.
6. Slowly increase the current intensity until the patient responds.
   a. Decrease the intensity slightly.
   b. Intensity must be sufficient to cause muscle contraction.
7. Skin resistance may decrease after 5–10 seconds and then intensity may be increased.
8. If treating a motor point, move the electrode around to find the motor point.
   a. Look for the area that causes maximal contraction.
   b. Pause 5–10 seconds in each area to overcome skin resistance.
9. If the patient complains of discomfort, the following might be causes:
   a. Too much current (most probable cause)
   b. Insufficient moistening of sponge
   c. Minor small denuded area (scratches, cuts, abrasions, etc.)
   d. The patient's hypersensitivity
   e. Poor electrode conformity
10. As the patient gets stronger, resistance can be applied during the contraction (Fig. 17.12).
B. Dosage
   1. Use the maximal current that is comfortable for the patient.

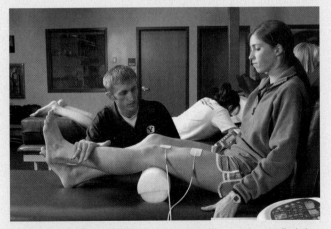

FIGURE 17.12 In NMES therapy, resistance can be applied during the muscle contraction as the patient gets stronger.

C. Length of application
   1. 10–30 minutes
   2. See individual manufacturer instructions.
D. Frequency of application
   1. As often as twice per day if separated by 3–4 hours
E. Duration of therapy
   1. Continue treatment until the goals have been met, which usually means when active exercise is under way.

STEP 4: POSTAPPLICATION TASKS

A. Equipment removal
   1. The timer will stop the current.
   2. Return all controls to off or the minimum setting.
   3. Remove the electrodes.
   4. Place the electrodes and belts in the proper place, not on top of the unit.
B. Instructions to the patient
   1. Schedule the next treatment.
   2. Instruct the patient about the level of activity and/or self-treatment prior to the next formal treatment.
C. Record of treatment, including unique patient responses
D. Return of the generator cart to the proper place; cleanup

STEP 5: MAINTENANCE

A. Check the fuse in back if the unit will not turn on (also make sure it is plugged in).
B. Electrodes
   1. Must be kept clean; body oils will accumulate
   2. Wash sponges or carbon-rubber electrodes with warm water and a mild detergent.
   3. Do not wash self-adhering electrodes, as this will cause the adherent and couplant to dissolve.
   4. Make sure the wire is firmly attached to the electrode post.
   5. The carbon in the electrode will leach out with time. Check the current flow, and assess the need for a new electrode.

CONCEPT CHECK 17.5. If NMES doesn't provide for as strong a muscle contraction as a voluntary contraction, why do clinicians use it postoperatively?

Iontophoresis for Transcutaneous Drug Delivery

Iontophoresis was developed over 50 years ago as a less painful way to deliver medication ions to a specific area via surface electrodes. **Iontophoresis** is the application of a mild direct current (DC) to drive negatively or positively charged ions of a drug solution into a patient's skin and underlying tissues.[65-67] The main barrier to transdermal drug uptake is the most superficial avascular stratum corneum layer of the epidermis. The principle behind iontophoresis involves placing an ionic compound on a like-charged electrode and using electrical repulsion to drive the compound through the skin. Although still contested, it is thought that the pores (especially of the sweat glands) that pass through the skin are used as pathways of the electrical current that the compound follows. The movement of the compound beyond the skin is thought to occur as a result of blood flow and diffusion.[66,69-71] According to Banga, the diffusional resistance of the skin to ions is lowest in the hair follicles and sweat gland regions compared with other regions of the epidermis.[72]

Most iontophoresis devices are small (about the size of a TENS unit). They are portable 9-V battery-operated devices of one or two channels (Fig. 17.13).

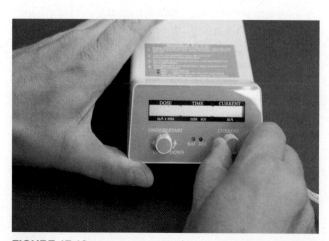

FIGURE 17.13 An iontophoresis unit uses a mild DC to transport negatively or positively charged ions from a drug solution into a patient's skin and underlying tissues.

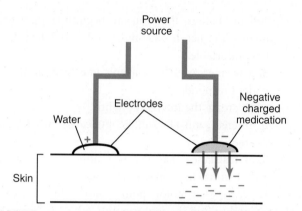

FIGURE 17.14 In iontophoresis, drug ions are repelled or pushed into the skin and surrounding tissues. The positively charged electrode delivers (repels or pushes) positively charged drug ions, or (as shown here) the negatively charged electrode delivers (repels or pushes) negatively charged drug ions.

HOW IONTOPHORESIS WORKS

The underlying principle is that like charges repel each other, so the drug ions are repelled or pushed into the skin and surrounding tissues by DC. Two electrodes—one to deliver the drug and one larger dispersive electrode—are applied to the patient's skin at least 3–6 in. (8–15 cm) apart. The drug delivery electrode can be either positively or negatively charged depending on the charge of the ion to be pushed. Ionized medication is placed in the active electrode reservoir, and its polarity is selected so that it is same as the drug ion (Fig. 17.14).

When a DC is applied:

- The positively charged electrode delivers (repels or pushes) positively charged drug ions into the skin and surrounding tissues.
- The negatively charged electrode delivers (repels or pushes) negatively charged drug ions into the skin and surrounding tissues.

BENEFITS OF IONTOPHORESIS

Iontophoresis has the benefit of delivering medicine, such as anti-inflammatories and painkillers, directly to the area safely without the following disadvantages:

- Painful needle injections
- Risk of infection from nonsterile needle injections
- Systemic effects from taking a pill, such as stomach or intestinal irritation
- Light, mild, or severe side effects from orally ingested drugs

Patients report a mild tingling or warm sensation during treatment, much like the sensation derived from a TENS unit.

Iontophoresis has been effective in reducing pain and inflammation associated with arthritis,[73] plantar fasciitis,[74] temporomandibular joint (TMJ) disorders,[75] and epicondylitis[76] when dexamethasone, lidocaine, or sodium salicylate was used. Unfortunately, little research exists on how much medicine actually enters the tissues and is delivered to the treatment site.

COMMON DRUG IONS USED IN ORTHOPEDIC MEDICINE

Some of the more common drug ions used for iontophoresis in orthopedic medicine, their polarities, and their function are:

- *Dexamethasone (negative ion):* Helps reduce inflammation by inhibiting the biosynthesis of prostaglandins and various other inflammatory substances (possibly the most used in physical medicine and rehabilitation)
- *Acetate (negative ion):* Helps dissolve calcium deposits and scar tissue in soft tissues such as muscles and tendons
- *Hydrocortisone (positive ion):* Helps decrease tissue inflammation by inhibiting the biosynthesis of prostaglandins and various other inflammatory substances
- *Lidocaine (positive ion):* Helps decrease local pain by blocking nerve impulse transmission

Before using a needle to inject children, or even prior to insertion of an IV catheter,[77] pediatricians use iontophoresis to deliver lidocaine and numb the area. This might sound antiproductive because the child needs to get a shot anyway. But children need to be vaccinated against diseases, and if the area can be anesthetized to lessen the pain of the shot, why not give it a try? It requires at least 10 minutes of current stimulation before the skin is anesthetized with a 50% concentration of lidocaine.[78]

NEGATIVE EFFECTS OF USING IONTOPHORESIS

Even though iontophoresis is delivered in small doses (<5 mA), skin irritation can occur from using a DC. The skin under the electrodes may turn light red, from the expansion of small blood vessels in the skin. DC can also cause *mast cells*, which synthesize and store histamines, to release histamine, causing small bumps or red dots to appear at either electrode site. Patients sometimes complain of dry skin or itching around the area. Factors that increase skin reactions include:

- *Skin type:* Fair-skinned people show a tendency toward skin irritation.
- *Skin pigmentation:* In darker-skinned patients, the normal reddening is usually less visible than with lighter-skinned people.

Some patients find out that they are sensitive to DC. Typical symptoms of DC sensitivity are redness and hives resembling small white bumps.

To help reduce the risk of skin irritation:

- Use an alcohol scrub on the skin to clean off any oils or dirt before treatment.
- After the treatment, apply a lotion containing aloe vera gel.
- Increase the size of the anode or cathode to decrease current density.
- Increase the spacing between the electrodes to decrease current intensity.

TYPES OF DELIVERY

Most iontophoresis is delivered via electrodes attached to the power source (see Figs. 17.13 and 17.14). Advances in microcircuitry (using miniaturized components) have led to wireless iontophoresis (Fig. 17.15). A miniature microprocessor and miniature 6-V battery (both disposable) are imbedded in a single patch that holds the two electrodes.

Despite little research on the wireless patches, millions are being sold. One advantage of these patches is that they can be left on the patient for a long time. (Actually the wired electrodes can be left on for an extended time, but typical protocol doesn't call for this.) Manufacturers of patches suggest wearing times for as long as 12–24 hours, to as short as 2.5 hours.[1] It has been suggested that this long passive delivery is probably more important than current amplitude in determining the depth of penetration of the drug.[105] A second advantage of the patches is the freedom of not having to be hooked up to the device.

There are disadvantages to the wireless patches. First, the farther apart the electrodes are, the deeper the current goes. It is suggested that electrodes be as far apart as the diameter of the largest electrode.[1] No patches meet this criteria. Second, is takes at least 6-V for the current to pass through the skin. The traditional programmable stimulator runs on a 9-V battery; however, most patches run on 1.5–3-V batteries. Only one patch runs on a 6-V battery (Activa Patch, ActivaTek, Salt Lake City, UT).

SUCCESS AND FAILURE WITH IONTOPHORESIS

There are conflicting reports of the effectiveness of iontophoresis. It appears to be effective in treating epicondylitis,[106] TMJ,[59] Achilles tendonitis, plantar warts, carpal

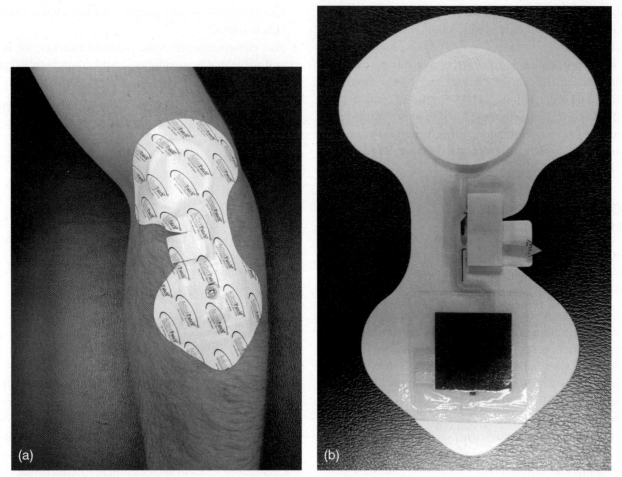

FIGURE 17.15 Wireless iontophoresis patch applied to the elbow **(a)**; note the LED light that provides feedback during operation. Viewing the underside of the patch **(b)** reveals the active drug containment chamber **(top)**, the battery and microprocessor **(middle)**, and an integrated hydrogel dispersive electrode that does not require saline **(bottom)**.

tunnel syndrome, and plantar fasciitis[1] using dexamethasone, sodium diclofenac/salicylate, acetic acid, and lidocaine, but ineffective with hydrocortisone.[1] Lidocane appears to be effective in pain relief.[1] Ciccone[107] reported conflicting results when using acetic acid with iontophoresis to accelerate the resorption of calcium deposits in calcific tendinitis of the shoulder. And a meta-analysis of studies with over 1250 patients concluded it was not helpful in relieving pain or restoring function in patients with shoulder adhesive capsulities.[104]

A common factor in the failures was attempting to treat deep injuries. For example, the shoulder capsule lies deep underneath the rotator cuff and the deltoid muscles and thus is probably too deep for iontophoresis to penetrate. Bicipital brachii tendonitis, however, could be treated with ionotophoresis because this tendon is fairly superficial.

We also would expect that iontphoresis would be effective on plantar fasciitis at the attachment on the calcaneus (a fairly shallow area), but not in the arch since this area is probably too deep for the iontophoresis-driven drug to reach. There is one report of penetration in monkey tissue up to 17 mm deep.[57] It occurred, however, at current densities that were 2½ greater than recommended for humans.[82]

Another factor in the success of iontophoresis is the state of localized blood flow at the site of delivery.[109] If the local cutaneous capillary beds under the active electrode are dilated, drug penetration depth will be reduced. This is illustrated by two studies from our lab. In the first, we reported the presence of lidocaine at 3 mm but not at 5 mm below the skin's surface.[108] In the second, we used epinephrine (a vasoconstrictor) with 2% lidocaine; lidocaine was delivered at 5 mm.[109]

Application of Iontophoresis for Transcutaneous Drug Delivery

5 STEPS

1 STEP 1: FOUNDATION

A. Definition. Iontophoresis is an active transdermal drug delivery process that delivers drug ions through the skin using a DC.

B. Effects. Depends on the drug ion being delivered:
1. Pain relief
2. Anesthesia
3. Decreased inflammation
4. Decrease in size of calcium deposits

C. Advantages
1. Prevents the pain and skin damage that accompanies needle injection of drug medication
2. Avoids the risk of needle injection to clinicians
3. Localized drug delivery; does not have to travel through the entire system like a pill
4. Avoids the GI side effects of NSAIDs (nonsteroidal anti-inflammatory drugs) and COX-II inhibitors
5. Portable; the patient can travel with it.

D. Disadvantages
1. Eliminates pain or inflammation; it does not treat the cause of the pain/inflammation
2. DC runs a slight risk of electrode burns.
3. Some believe transdermal drug delivery is not possible.

E. Indications
1. See Effects above.
2. Delivery of soluble salts and drug ions into the body for medical purposes as an alternative to needle injection or taking a pill.

F. Contraindications
1. Do not use with a person who has:
   a. An implanted pacemaker
   b. Damaged or denuded skin on the treatment area
   c. Drug allergies to medicine to be delivered transdermally
   d. Recent laceration of the treatment area
2. Do not treat the transcranial area.
3. Do not treat the orbital region.

G. Precautions. Be cautious when using iontophoresis over an area with:
1. Impaired sensation
2. Recent scar tissue
3. Exposed metal (it is safe to use over implanted surgical metal, screws, plates, etc.)

2 STEP 2: PREAPPLICATION TASKS

A. Make sure iontophoresis is the proper modality for this situation.
1. Reevaluate the injury/problem. Make sure you understand the patient's condition.
2. If the modality was applied previously, review the patient's response to the previous treatment.
3. Confirm that the objectives of therapy are compatible with iontophoresis.
4. Make sure iontophoresis is not contraindicated in this situation.
5. Above all else, make sure you have a physician's prescription to deliver the medication.

B. Preparing the patient psychologically
1. Explain the procedure if the patient is being treated for the first time, or if the treatment is being changed.
   a. Describe the expected sensation—mild tingling or warm.
   b. Electricity will not cause the muscle to contract.
   c. Only a small amount of current will be used.
   d. Iontophoresis will not cause electrocution.
   e. It should not be painful; if it is, tell the patient to let you know. Decrease the intensity (but the treatment will take a few minutes longer).
2. Demonstrate the procedure on yourself if the patient seems particularly apprehensive. Do a "dry run;" do not use any medication or open any electrode packages.
3. Check for, and warn the patient about, precautions.

C. Preparing the patient physically
1. Position the patient in a comfortable position.
2. Use an alcohol preparation to clean the area where the electrodes are going to be applied.

D. Equipment preparation
1. Remove the electrodes from the pouch or container. Make sure both the delivery electrode and the dispersive electrode appear to be in working order.
2. Prepare the medication:
   a. Fill a syringe or marked eyedropper with the appropriate amount of medication typically used for iontophoresis.
3. Prepare the active (drug delivery) electrode:
   a. Remove the backing on the electrode.

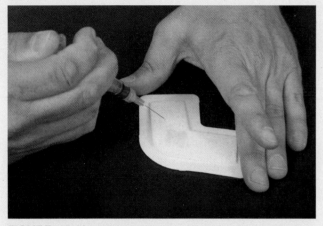

FIGURE 17.16 In iontophoresis, medication that is ionized in solution is placed on the appropriate electrode so that the active ion is driven into the tissue.

b. Place it on a table and saturate the sponge side of the electrode with the medication (Fig. 17.16). Do not overfill; no medication should seep over onto the adhesive backing.

4. Apply the electrodes (note steps 4 and 5 are for wired application—see step 6 for wireless application):

a. Remove the backing on the dispersive pad and attach it on a large muscle belly at least 6 inches (15 cm) away from the active electrode site.

b. Apply the saturated active electrode to the area to which you want the drug ions delivered (Fig. 17.17).

5. Attach the electrodes to the appropriate cords or lead clips. Make sure the leads are connected properly for the polarity of the drug you are delivering (see the specific manufacturer's manual).

6. For wireless application apply the single patch to the treatment area, with the active (medicated) electrode over the injury.

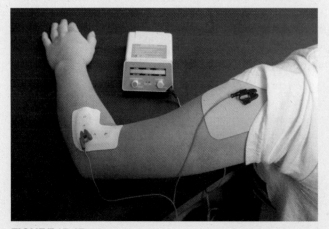

FIGURE 17.17 Iontophoresis application via wired delivery system. See text for details.

STEP 3: APPLICATION PARAMETERS

The following are general procedures for iontophoresis. See specific instructions in the manufacturer's manual of the modality your clinic uses.

A. Procedures
1. Turn the unit on.
2. Tell the patient you are beginning.
3. If the unit has an automatic ramp, the current amplitude will slowly increase to maximize the patient's comfort.
4. If the unit does not have an automatic ramp, you can maximize the patient's comfort by:
   a. Slowly increasing current intensity
   b. Ask the patient to tell you when he/she begins to feel mild tingling or warm under the drug delivery electrode.
5. Adjust the intensity according to the patient's tolerance and dosage.
   a. Many electrodes are operational up to a maximum total delivered dose of 80 mA/min when negative polarity is used and 40 mA/min when positive polarity is used.

B. Dosage
1. Set the unit to deliver the recommended dose of medication (Table 17.5).

C. Length of application.
1. Dose-specific (see Table 17.5)

D. Frequency of application
1. Every other day

E. Duration of therapy
1. Up to 3 weeks

STEP 4: POSTAPPLICATION TASKS

A. Equipment removal
1. Turn off the power.
2. Return all controls to off or the minimum setting.
3. Remove and dispose of the electrodes (the dispersive electrode can be reused, after cleaning).
4. Place unit in the proper place, preferably locked up.
B. Battery recharging, if necessary
C. Instructions to the patient

TABLE 17.5 SAMPLE DOSE DELIVERY FOR IONOTOPHORESIS

TOTAL CHARGE	CURRENT	TIME
40 mA/min	2 mA	20 min
40 mA/min	3 mA	13.5 min
40 mA/min	4 mA	10 min

1. Schedule the next treatment.
2. Instruct the patient about the level of activity and/or self-treatment prior to the next formal treatment.

D. Record of treatment, including unique patient responses
   1. Typical skin reactions that occur from a DC are:
      a. Erythema (redness) under one or both electrodes.
      b. Small bumps
   2. Neither is of any significance and typically disappears in a few hours.

CONCEPT CHECK 17.6. An athlete with fair skin received an iontophoresis treatment. The next day she reports to you that the treatment was uncomfortable. You notice redness on the skin where the treatment occurred. What can you do to help prevent this irritation during the next treatment?

High-Volt Pulsed Current Stimulation for Wound Healing

High-volt pulsed current (HVPC) is a twin-peak, monophasic, pulsed current driven by its characteristically high electromotive force or voltage. High-volt stimulators enable the clinician to use either positive or negative polarity, but because of the low average current and duty cycles, skin injuries caused by changes in skin pH are unlikely.[62] HVPC stimulators are versatile and are used in several treatments, including:

- Wound management
- Edema management
- Muscle re-education and spasm reduction
- Pain modulation

Its major advantage, however, is promoting wound healing. The other functions are more effectively performed by other types of electrical stimulation.

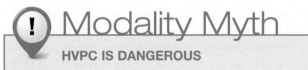

Modality Myth

HVPC IS DANGEROUS

Some people are under the impression that HVPC is dangerous because it uses higher voltages than most electrotherapeutic devices. This is not true; the pulse width is much smaller than other devices, so the average current is less than other devices. Thus, amperage is also less.

STEP 5: MAINTENANCE

A. Batteries
   1. Keep a spare set.
   2. Keep them charged (if a charging unit is used).
B. Electrodes
   1. Keep specific iontophoresis electrode pouches on hand.
   2. Make sure the wire is firmly attached to the electrode post.

CHARACTERISTICS OF HIGH-VOLT STIMULATORS

Electrical stimulators that generate <150 V are termed low-volt. Electrical stimulators that can generate more than 150 V are termed high-volt. An HVPC stimulator uses 150–500 V. Therefore, the chief characteristics of HVPC are high peak voltages with a low average current. HVPC uses a twin-peak monophasic wave form, resembling a double spike with a fast rise followed by a fast decline (see Box 16.6). Its pulse widths are short, in the microsecond range (65–200 µsec), with pulse rates of 1–200 Hz. Box 17.1 lists the typical features of a HVPC stimulator.

BOX 17.1 TYPICAL FEATURES OF HVPC STIMULATION

Current
- Twin peaked, pulsed unidirectional
- Each peak 65–200 µsec wide
- Modified square wave, M wave, or sawtooth

Controls
- Amplitude or amount of current
- Controlled by "output" control knob
- Continuously variable up to 500 V
- Pulse rate
- Controlled by "pulse rate" knob
- 1–120 pps Surge rate or ramp control

Technique
- Can use monopolar or bipolar technique. Monopolar is used for wound healing, or when treatment is directed over a large area (edema reduction, acute pain control). Bipolar technique is used for muscle contraction or chronic pain.

Treatment time
- 15 minutes if pulsed or if the patient is going to engage in vigorous activity following treatment.
- 15–30 minutes if surge mode is used or the patient athlete is not engaging in vigorous activity.

HVPC and Electrode Polarity

Many HVPC stimulators include the option of selecting polarity (either negative or positive). This grew out of an early misconception that HVPC produced galvanic stimulation. Since it does not, we question what changing polarity does. We have observed that uninjured subjects have a definite preference for one or the other when stimulated for a maximal tetanic contraction, although the selection did not change the strength of the contraction. We also note that wound repair protocols include the suggestion that polarity be changed every few days.[63,64]

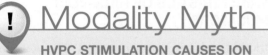

Modality Myth

HVPC STIMULATION CAUSES ION MIGRATION

In the 1980s, there was a misconception that high-volt twin-pulsed simulators created a chemical effect. In fact, they were once called "high-volt galvanic simulators." While it's true that these are monophasic, they are pulsed, so they do not produce the continuous electron flow necessary to cause a chemical effect. Continuous monophasic DC electron flow is required for ion migration. The process is moving electrons against a gradient, so if the electron flow is discontinuous, the electrons will diffuse back to their starting position during the "no flow" time. It's like pushing a car uphill; if you push for a while and then rest, the car will roll back down to the starting position (see Chapter 16).

HVPC FOR WOUND MANAGEMENT

Wound management with HVPC involves high-frequency, low-amplitude stimulation, creating a sustained sensory response that many report as pins and needles. Most of the research on HVPC has been done on wound management of pressure sores (ulcers). Results are as follows:

- HVPC has a greater impact in treating pressure ulcers than whirlpool and HVPC treatments combined.[65]
- Pressure ulcers treated with HVPC for 45 min/d for 5 days each week were completely healed within 7.3 weeks. In the same study, ulcers not treated with HVPC increased in size by 29%.[64]
- Scientists reported that pressure ulcers treated with HVPC (200 V; 100 Hz) 1 hour a day for 20 days decreased by 80%, compared to 52% for a control group.[66]

How HVPC Stimulates Wound Repair

Bioelectrical currents exist in the body's vascular and interstitial tissues. Structures such as blood vessel walls, insulating tissue matrix, extracellular fluid, and intravascular plasma are capable of conducting bioelectricity.[67] When tissues are damaged, an electrical potential is created between the injured and noninjured tissues. The DC potentials of the skin, subcutaneous tissue, and blood vessels may stimulate cellular activity when injured, thereby stimulating tissue regeneration and tissue remodeling. The use of HVPC may speed up healing by promoting the natural healing process, including the development of a difference in potential, referred to as the *injury potential*, between the wound area and the surrounding healthy tissue. The injury potential typically becomes positive 24–48 hours after the injury and becomes negative 8 or 9 days after the injury. As the wound heals, the difference in potential slowly returns to baseline.[68,69] Therefore, HVPC stimulation can be used to enhance the natural process of tissue recovery and healing.[52]

Many clinicians are under the mistaken notion that HVPC outputs a DC, and tissue responses to HVPC are similar to those of DC.[70] There is no question that HVPC stimulates wound healing, and skepticism is probably unfounded. Keep this in mind as you read the next three paragraphs.

Individual cells migrate toward DC electrodes; the direction and speed of migration are influenced by the strength of the field and polarity of the electrodes.[71] Negative polarity increases vascularity and stimulates fibroblastic growth, collagen production, and epidermal cell migration. Negative polarity has also been shown to inhibit bacterial growth. Positive current polarity attracts macrophages and promotes epithelial growth.[72,73]

Most treatments begin with the negative polarity. The negative polarity encourages blood clots to dissolve and increases inflammatory by-products, leading to the healing of damaged tissues.[63] Positive polarity encourages clot formation around the wound and in granulation tissue.[63]

If after a few days of treatment the condition is not improving, switching electrode polarity might help. For example, when Kloth and Feedar[64] used HVPC for would healing of pressure ulcers, they began their study using the positive electrode polarity. When a patient reached a healing plateau, the electrode polarity was switched to the negative side. If a second plateau was reached, electrode polarity was switched again. This technique seemed to be effective for reducing wound size or complete healing. In three animal studies, the best healing results for epithelialization involved using the negative polarity for 3 days and then switching to the positive polarity.[74–76]

HVPC FOR EDEMA MANAGEMENT

HVPC stimulation is used for two purposes in edema management: curbing edema formation and resolving edema once it has formed, although NMES may be a better choice for resolving edema.

Edema is the accumulation of the fluid portion of blood in the tissues (see Chapter 5). To understand how edema accumulates, it is necessary to first understand normal fluid dynamics, the movement of fluid back and forth between capillaries and normal injured tissue. If this balanced movement of fluid is upset so that more fluid flows into the tissue than what is absorbed, the excess fluid is called edema. Thus, edema is simply the result of a normal process that is slightly out of balance. The longer it is out of balance, the greater the edema accumulation and the greater the swelling.

Laboratory results are mixed with respect to the effect that HVPC has on edema management. Michlovitz et al.[77] reported that there was no difference in edema control when HVPC stimulation was included with the application of ice, compression, and elevation in the treatment of acute ankle sprains. Cosgrove et al.[78] studied the effects of HVPC; symmetrical, biphasic pulsed current; and placebo electrical current on edema reduction after blunt trauma to rats. There were no differences in edema reduction among the groups.

The application of HVPC may be effective in curbing post-traumatic edema for 4 hours, yet long-term edema was not significantly reduced.[79,80] Taylor et al.[81] reported that HVPC using either the positive or the negative polarity was effective in decreasing macromolecular leakage from blood vessels in hamster cheek pouches following histamine treatment. Dolan et al.[82] reported that 3 hours of HVPC or a combination of HVPC and cold water immersion was effective at curbing edema formation by 50% in rats. Ideally, the treatment should be applied as soon as possible after the injury, and it should be maintained during the entire time that edema is forming.[82]

HVPC is sometimes confused with DCs and the belief that the negative electrode repels plasma proteins, thus preventing them from moving from the capillary to extracellular spaces and therefore thwarting edema formation. Since HVPC is not a DC, and because of the short duty cycle (1–2%) of HVPC, it is unlikely that it prevents edema formation this way. The physiological mechanism for curbing edema formation seems centered on the ability of HVPC to decrease the permeability of blood vessels. Reed[83] and Taylor et al.[81] suggest that HVPC decreases the leakiness of the vessels, thereby reducing the number of plasma proteins and fluid that leave the vessels and enter the extracellular spaces.

Based on the results of animal studies, two protocols for curbing edema formation with HVPC have been proposed. The first, called the water immersion technique,[84] involves HVPC applied with negative polarity, 120 pps, 90% of visible motor threshold, for 30 minutes every

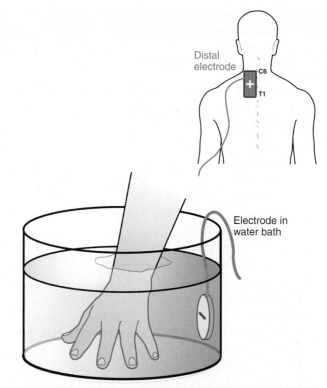

FIGURE 17.18 The water immersion technique using HVPC.

4 hours (Fig. 17.18). They advocate that application begins as soon as possible after the injury and continues as long as the edema is still forming.

The second protocol is similar to the first, but it is applied in a near-continuous format along with RICES.[62] It is based on the concept that HVPC is effective only while it is being applied.[82]

Like NMES, HVPC stimulation can be used in a muscle-pumping action to get rid of edema once it has formed. In this case, the intensity is increased until there is a strong muscle contraction. We prefer NMES, however, because it produces stronger muscle contractions.[85] And better still is active exercise, if possible.

HVPC FOR MUSCLE RE-EDUCATION AND SPASM REDUCTION

Muscle contraction for re-education involves high-frequency, high-amplitude, surged stimulation that generates a tetanic contraction. HVPC is not as effective as NMES for this purpose because its average current is not as high as low-volt stimulators and therefore does not generate as strong a contraction.[85] We recommend that HVPC be used only if NMES is unavailable.

HVPC FOR PAIN MODULATION

HVPC is ineffective in reducing the pain of delayed-onset muscle soreness.[86,87] However, HVPC stimulation appears to help relieve pain due to muscle spasm.[88]

Application of High-Volt Pulsed Current Stimulation

STEP 1: FOUNDATION

A. Definition. HVPC stimulation is the production of a twin-peak monophasic pulsed current driven by a large electromotive force.

B. Effects
  1. Wound healing
  2. Pain relief
     a. Sensory level (acute pain)
     b. Motor level (chronic pain)
  3. Muscle contraction
     a. Disuse atrophy
     b. Spasm reduction
     c. Edema reduction
  4. Edema control (maybe)

C. Advantages
  1. The only electrical stimulator proven to promote wound healing
  2. Can be applied to immobilized body part
  3. Highly versatile in function

D. Disadvantages
  1. Cannot provide as strong a contraction as low-volt stimulators (NMES)
  2. Many units are not portable.
  3. Sometimes trial and error is needed to determine the appropriate electrode polarity for wound healing.

E. Indications
  1. Wound lesions (pressure sores, scarring from incisions)
  2. Pain
  3. Residual or chronic muscle spasm (if a low-volt unit is unavailable)

F. Contraindications
  1. Do not use on a person with a pacemaker.
  2. Do not use in these locations:
     a. Over the heart or brain
     b. Over the lumbar and abdominal area of pregnant women
     c. Over potential malignancies
     d. Over the anterior cervical area

G. Precautions
  1. Be cautious when using HVPC over an area with:
     a. Impaired sensation
     b. Extensive torn tissue
     c. Hemorrhage
  2. Epileptic patients should be monitored during treatment.

STEP 2: PREAPPLICATION TASKS

A. Make sure HVPC is the proper therapy for this situation.
  1. Reevaluate the injury/problem. Make sure you understand the patient's condition.
  2. If HVPC stimulation was used previously, review the patient's response to the previous treatment.
  3. Confirm that the objectives of therapy are compatible with HVPC.
  4. Select or review the electrical current characteristics.
  5. Make sure HVPC is not contraindicated in this situation.

B. Preparing the patient psychologically
  1. Explain the procedure if the patient is being treated for the first time, or if the treatment is being changed.
     a. Describe the expected sensation, depending on treatment goals.
        i. Wound repair or acute edema reduction: moderate, prickling pins and needles over smaller electrode; little sensation over large dispersive electrode
        ii. Sensory level pain (acute pain reduction): moderate, prickling pins and needles
        iii. Conditions requiring muscle contraction: moderate prickling pins and needles progressing to strong contraction
     b. Electricity will cause the muscle to contract, or assist the normal healing of the body.
     c. Only a small amount of current will be used.
     d. HVPC stimulation will not cause electrocution.
     e. It should not be painful; if it is, ask the patient to let you know.
  2. Demonstrate the procedure on yourself if the patient seems particularly apprehensive.
  3. Check for, and warn the patient about, precautions.
     a. Inspect the skin for cuts, abrasions, new skin, etc., and make sure it is clean and free from oils.
     b. If the area to be treated has excess hair, it will need to be shaved to ensure electrode conductivity.
     c. Determine whether skin sensation or joint range of motion is impaired. If the patient lacks sensation in the area, he/she may not be able to determine when the current intensity is painful.

C. Preparing the patient physically
  1. Remove clothing, tape, etc., from the electrode contact area. It is not necessary to remove them from the area between the two contact points.
  2. Position the patient in a comfortable position.
D. Equipment preparation
  1. Turn the unit on.
    a. Make sure the output is at the minimal setting.
    b. Set the pulse rate.
  2. Prepare the electrodes.
    a. Attach the electrodes to the leads and the leads to the generator.
    b. No preparation is needed for self-adhering electrodes.
    c. Prepare carbon-rubber electrodes with the proper medium.
      i. Carbon-rubber electrodes require either water or a gel-based couplant.
      ii. A gel-based couplant is applied directly to the electrode and is placed between the skin and the electrode.
      iii. When water is used as a couplant, it is applied to a small sponge placed between the skin and the electrode. In that case, wet the sponge; remove excess water but do not squeeze dry.
  3. Check the equipment and electrode operation.
    a. If nonadhering electrodes are used, place them on the table and span them with your hand. Turn up the intensity until current is felt.
    b. Check the connecting cords, especially for loose-fitting electrode tips, if current is absent or reduced.
  4. Firmly attach the electrodes on the patient's skin.
    a. Monopolar: active electrode over the injury and the dispersive electrode over a remote site, such as the back, abdomen, or thigh
    b. Bipolar: proximal and distal to the muscle belly
    c. Good contact is essential.
    d. Remove the adhesive backing for self-adhering electrodes.
  e. For nonadhering electrodes, place a wet piece of paper towel between the electrode and skin, and use elastic belts, straps, body weight, sandbags, etc., to hold the electrodes in place.

3 STEP 3: APPLICATION PARAMETERS

The following are general procedures for HVPC stimulation. For parameters for treating specific conditions (Table 17.6). Also see specific instructions in the manufacturer's manual of the modality your clinic uses.
A. Procedures
  1. Set the pulse rate.
    a. Less than 15 pps for individual or twitch contractions
    b. Greater than 50 pps for moderate to tetanic contractions
  2. Set the polarity. Negative over motor point (monopolar).
  3. Set the duty cycle.
  4. Set the timer.
  5. Tell the patient you are beginning the treatment.
  6. Slowly increase the current intensity.
    a. Ask the patient to tell you when it is uncomfortable.
    b. Decrease the intensity slightly.
    c. Intensity must be sufficient to cause muscle contraction.
  7. Skin resistance will decrease after 5–10 seconds, and then the intensity may be increased.
  8. If treating a motor point, move the anode electrode probe around to find the motor point.
    a. Look for the area that causes maximal contraction.
    b. Pause 5–10 seconds in each area to overcome skin resistance.
  9. If the patient complains of discomfort, the following might be causes:
    a. Too much current
    b. Insufficient moistening of sponge

TABLE 17.6	KEY PARAMETERS OF HVPC STIMULATION FOR VARIOUS CONDITIONS			
CONDITION	**POLARITY**	**PULSE SETTING**	**ELECTRODE PLACEMENT**	**OUTPUT**
Edema control	Negative	120 pps	Under water or large surface	90% of visible motor threshold
Wound management	Negative to attract fibroblasts; positive to attract macrophages	100 pps	Active electrode in wound or adjacent to wound edges	Pins and needles; tingle

c. Minor small denuded area (scratches, cuts, abrasions, etc.)

d. The patient's hypersensitivity

B. Dosage

1. Use the maximal current that is comfortable for the patient.

C. Length of application

1. 15 minutes if pulsed or if the patient is going to vigorously exercise following the treatment

2. 15–30 minutes if surge mode is used or the patient is not going to vigorously exercise following the treatment

3. See the individual manufacturer's instructions.

D. Frequency of application

1. As often as three times per day if separated by 3–4 hours.

E. Duration of therapy

1. Continue treatment until goals have been met.

4 STEP 4: POSTAPPLICATION TASKS

A. Equipment removal

1. The timer will stop the current.

2. Return all controls to off or the minimum setting.

3. Remove the electrodes.

4. Place the electrodes and belts in the proper place, not on top of the unit.

B. Instructions to the patient

1. Schedule the next treatment

2. Instruct the patient about the level of activity and/ or self-treatment prior to the next formal treatment.

C. Record of treatment, including unique patient responses.

D. Return of the generator cart to the proper place; area cleanup

5 STEP 5: MAINTENANCE

A. Check the fuse in back if the unit will not turn on (also make sure it is plugged in).

B. Electrodes

1. Must be kept clean; body oils will accumulate.

2. Wash sponges or carbon-rubber electrodes with warm water and a mild detergent.

3. Do not wash self-adhering electrodes, as this will cause the adherent and couplant to dissolve.

4. Make sure the wire is firmly attached to the electrode post.

5. The carbon in the electrode will leach out with time. Check the current flow, and assess the need for a new electrode.

Microcurrent Electrical Nerve Stimulation

Microcurrent electrical nerve stimulation (MENS) is the therapeutic use of constant (DC) and pulsed (interrupted) currents, where the stimulus amplitude is in the microamperage (millionth of an ampere) range. Since microcurrents are a major factor in the control of various body functions, it seems reasonable that treatment with MENS would be effective. The evidence does not support the therapeutic use of this modality. In spite of the lack of evidence, there are many passion adherents of MENS therapy.

THE MANY NAMES FOR MENS

The name MENS does not accurately describe this modality because the current intensity is too low (<1 mA) to cause nerve depolarization.[89] Perhaps this is why the American Physical Therapy Association labeled it low-intensity direct current (LIDC) in 1990.[90]

Other than MENS, this modality has been referred to as[91]:

- Low-intensity direct current
- Low-voltage pulsed microamperage stimulation
- Biostimulation
- Bioelectric therapy
- Low-intensity electrical stimulation
- Microcurrent

Despite the logic of these other names, most people continue to use MENS, so we will also use this name.

THE THEORY BEHIND HOW MENS WORKS

The creation of MENS originated with studies by Becker and Murray[69] on animal soft tissue healing and limb regeneration in the 1960s. According to Becker, after injury or disease, injured cells from skin, nerve, and muscle are theorized to posses their own injury currents in the microamperage range that might play a role in healing the injury. Thus, if human tissue repair is mediated in part by electrical signals, an electrical current applied to the injury site may enhance the injury process.

For example, neutrophils, macrophages, and fibroblasts (key cells involved in wound healing) carry a positive or negative charge. By applying the anode or cathode over the wound, the microcurrent helps in the galvanic attraction of these cells into the wound, thereby promoting wound healing.[1]

The MENS unit is programmed to produce a specific current intensity so low that often the patient cannot feel the current. Manufacturers of microcurrent devices state that a primary characteristic is its ability to generate a fixed current by adjusting the voltage to account for variations in skin resistance. Some scientists doubt that microamperage current can even penetrate the skin.[92] Regardless, many companies are including MENS on their multimodality machines.

The Effectiveness of MENS

There is no clear-cut research supporting the therapeutic use of MENS. Scientists have found it to have a positive effect in treating:

- Pressure ulcers[93]
- Diabetic ulcers[94]
- TMJ disorders[95]

However, other scientists have reported it to have no effect in treating:

- Pressure ulcers[96]
- TMJ pain[97]
- Delayed-onset muscle soreness[87,98–100]
- Coracoacromial arch pain[101]
- Surgically induced wounds[102]

Most of the instances where MENS might play a positive role is in wound healing, an area that is typically outside the practice of athletic trainers. Further research is needed to determine whether this modality has a place in treating orthopedic injuries.

For those who wish to use MENS as a modality, follow the manufacturer's directions. It is safe; however, the same precautions that apply to TENS apply to this modality.

CLOSING SCENE

It has now been 2 weeks since the clinic staff took a refresher course on electrotherapy. The staff is showing improved use of electrotherapy, based on observations of treatments and review of the treatment forms. The staff is using the correct modality and optimal parameters to reach treatment goals, and the patients are responding positively to the treatments. Jose is pleased.

Chapter Reflections

1. Read and ponder each of the following points. Do you feel you have a clear understanding of each concept? If not, reread the appropriate section of the chapter.
   - Define TENS.
   - Explain the theory behind how TENS works.
   - What are the indications/contraindications for using TENS?
   - Describe how a TENS treatment is applied.
   - Define IFC therapy.
   - Explain the theory behind how IFC therapy works.
   - What are the indications/contraindications for using IFC therapy?
   - Describe how an IFC treatment is applied.
   - Define NMES.
   - Explain the theory behind how NMES works.
   - What are the indications/contraindications for using NMES?
   - Describe how an NMES treatment is applied.
   - Define iontophoresis.
   - Explain the theory behind how iontophoresis works.
   - What are the indications/contraindications for using iontophoresis?
   - Describe how an iontophoresis treatment is applied.
   - Define HVPC stimulation.
   - Explain the theory behind how HVPC works.
   - What are the indications/contraindications for using HVPC stimulation?
   - Describe how an HVPC treatment is applied.
   - Define MENS.
   - Explain the theory behind how MENS works.
   - What are the indications/contraindications for using MENS?
2. Write three to five questions for discussion with your class instructor, clinical instructor, classmates, and clinical colleagues.
3. Get together with classmates and quiz each other on the concepts of this chapter. Use the points in no. 1 and questions you wrote for no. 2 as a beginning.

Explaining concepts out loud to others requires a deeper grasp of the material than feeling you understand it as you read.

4. Once you feel you understand the principles of application, practice applying TENS, IFC therapy, NMES, iontophoresis, and HVPC treatments, using the five-step approach, with a classmate or clinical colleague.

Alternate applying each modality to each other. When it is being applied to you, listen and observe carefully to determine whether your classmate is using proper application. Consult your notes when the modality is applied to you, and during the first few times you apply the modality to another person. Continue practicing the application until you can do so without using your notes.

Concept Check Responses

CONCEPT CHECK 17.1

The advantage of using TENS postoperatively is that the patient might require fewer painkilling drugs, thereby negating the possibility for drug dependency.

CONCEPT CHECK 17.2

Settings for long-lasting analgesia:
(a) 1–5 Hz or pps; (b) 2501–2505 Hz

CONCEPT CHECK 17.3

Since your IFC unit is too large, loan the athlete a portable TENS unit, or have the physician write him a prescription for TENS. (Some insurance companies will pay for a TENS unit.)

CONCEPT CHECK 17.4

Since the patient has hip pain that is hard to localize, the best modality would be IFC, because it has a dynamic vector that can move the current to cover a large area for treating pain that is hard to pinpoint.

CONCEPT CHECK 17.5

NMES is often used postoperatively because the muscle is often weak and cannot elicit a strong contraction. NMES is used to assist the patient in contracting the affected muscles.

CONCEPT CHECK 17.6

What can you do to help prevent electrode irritation during an iontophoresis treatment on a fair-skinned patient?

- Use an alcohol scrub on the skin to clean off any oils or dirt prior to treatment.
- Increase the size of the anode or cathode to decrease current density.
- Increase the spacing between electrodes to decrease current intensity.
- After the treatment, apply a lotion containing aloe vera gel.

REFERENCES

1. Belanger AY. *Therapeutic Electrophysical Agents: Evidence Behind Practice.* Baltimore, MD: Lippincott Williams & Wilkins, 2010.
2. Melzack R, Wall PD. Pain mechanisms: a new theory. *Science.* 1965;150:971–979.
3. Wall PD. The gate control theory of pain mechanisms. A re-examination and re-statement. *Brain.* 1978;101(1):1–18.
4. Wall PD. *Textbook of Pain.* 3rd ed. London: Churchill Livingstone, 1994.
5. Mannheimer JS, Lampe GN. *Clinical Transcutaneous Electrical Nerve Stimulation.* Philadelphia, PA: FA Davis Co., 1984.
6. Fargas-Babjak A, Rooney P, Gerecz E. Randomized trial of Codetron for pain control in osteoarthritis of the hip/knee. *Clin J Pain.* 1989;5(2):137–141.
7. Abelson K, Langley GB, Sheppeard H, Vlieg M, Wigley RD. Transcutaneous electrical nerve stimulation in rheumatoid arthritis. *N Z Med J.* 1983;96(727):156–158.
8. Dawood MY, Ramos J. Transcutaneous electrical nerve stimulation (TENS) for the treatment of primary dysmenorrhea: a randomized crossover comparison with placebo TENS and ibuprofen. *Obstet Gynecol.* 1990;75(4):656–660.
9. Lundeberg T, Bondesson L, Lundstrom V. Relief of primary dysmenorrhea by transcutaneous electrical nerve stimulation. *Acta Obstet Gynecol Scand.* 1985;64(6):491–497.
10. Melzack R, Vetere P, Finch L. Transcutaneous electrical nerve stimulation for low back pain. A comparison of TENS and massage for pain and range of motion. *Phys Ther.* 1983;63(4):489–493.
11. Cheing GL, Hui-Chan CW. Transcutaneous electrical nerve stimulation: nonparallel antinociceptive effects on chronic clinical pain and acute experimental pain. *Arch Phys Med Rehabil.* 1999;80(3):305–312.
12. Walker RH, Morris BA, Angulo DL, Schneider J, Colwell CW Jr. Postoperative use of continuous passive motion, transcutaneous electrical nerve stimulation, and continuous cooling pad following total knee arthroplasty. *J Arthroplasty.* 1991;6(2):151–156.
13. Angulo DL, Colwell CW. Use of postoperative TENS and continuous passive motion following total knee replacement. *J Orthop Sports Phys Ther.* 1990;11:599–604.
14. Morgan B, Jones AR, Mulcahy KA, Finlay DB, Collet B. Transcutaneous electric nerve stimulation (TENS) during distension shoulder arthrography: A controlled trial. *Pain.* 1995;64:265–267.
15. Arvidsson J, Eriksson E. Postoperative TENS pain relief after knee surgery: Objective evaluation. *Orthopedics.* 1986;9:1346–1351.

16. Jensen JE, Conn RR, Hazelrigg G, Hewett JE. The use of transcutaneous neural stimulation and isokinetic testing in arthroscopic knee surgery. *Am J Sports Med*. 1985;13(1):27–33.

17. Cornell PE, Lopez AL, Malofsky H. Pain reduction with transcutaneous electrical nerve stimulation after foot surgery. *J Foot Surg*. 1984;23(4):326–333.

18. Kruger LR, van der Linden WJ, Cleaton-Jones PE. Transcutaneous electrical nerve stimulation in the treatment of myofascial pain dysfunction. *S Afr J Surg*. 1998;36(1):35–38.

19. Castel D. *Electrotherapy and Ultrasound Update*. 2nd ed. Reno, NV: International Academy of Physio Therapeutics, 1996.

20. de Domenico G. *Basic Guidelines for Interferential Therapy*. Sydney: Theramed Boors, 1981.

21. de Domenico G. *New Dimensions in Interferential Therapy. A Theoretical and Clinical Guide*. Lindfield: Reid Medical Books, 1987.

22. Savage B. *Interferential Therapy*. London: Faber & Faber, 1984.

23. Foster NE, Thompson KA, Baxter GD, Allen JM. Management of nonspecific low back pain by physiotherapists in Britain and Ireland. A descriptive questionnaire of current clinical practice. *Spine*. 1999;24(13):1332–1342.

24. Lindsay DM, Dearness J, Richardson C, Chapman A, Cuskelly G. A survey of electromodality usage in private physiotherapy practices. *Aust J Physiother*. 1990;36(4):249–256.

25. Lindsay DM, Dearness J, McGinley CC. Electrotherapy usage trends in private physiotherapy practice in Alberta. *Physiother Can*. 1995;47(1):30–34.

26. Watson T. Electrotherapy on the Web. May 2006. Available at: www.Electrotherapy.org.

27. Palmer ST, Martin DJ, Steedman WM, Ravey J. Alteration of interferential current and transcutaneous electrical nerve stimulation frequency: effects on nerve excitation. *Arch Phys Med Rehabil*. 1999;80(9):1065–1071.

28. Alon G. Principles of electrical stimulation. In: Nelson RM, Hayes KW, Currier DP, eds. *Clinical Electrotherapy*. 3rd ed. Stamford, CT: Appleton & Lange, 1999:82–85, 108–109.

29. Kloth LC, Cummings JP. Section on clinical electrophysiology and the American Physical Therapy Association. *Electrotherapeutic Terminology in Physical Therapy*. Alexandria, VA: American Physical Therapy Association, 1990.

30. Noble JG, Henderson G, Cramp AF, Walsh DM, Lowe AS. The effect of interferential therapy upon cutaneous blood flow in humans. *Clin Physiol*. 2000;20:2–7.

31. Nussbaum EL, Rush P, Disenhaus L. The effects of interferential therapy on peripheral blood flow. *Physiotherapy*. 1990;76:803–807.

32. Indergand NJ, Morgan BJ. Effect of interference current on forearm vascular resistance in asymptomatic humans. *Phys Ther*. 1995;75:306–312.

33. Olson SL, Perez JV, Stacks LN, Walsh MH. The effects of TENS and interferential current on cutaneous blood flow in healthy subjects. *Physiother Can*. 1999;51:27–31.

34. Shafshak TS, el-Sheshai AM, Soltan HE. Personality traits in the mechanisms of interferential therapy for osteoarthritic knee pain. *Arch Phys Med Rehabil*. 1991;72(8):579–581.

35. Quirk A, Newham RJ, Newham KJ. An evaluation of interferential therapy, shortwave diathermy, and exercise in the treatment of osteoarthrosis of the knee. *Physiotherapy*. 1985;71:55–57.

36. Hurley DA, Minder PM, McDonough SM, Walsh DM, Moore AP, Baxter DG. Interferential therapy electrode placement technique in acute low back pain: a preliminary investigation. *Arch Phys Med Rehabil*. 2001;82(4):485–493.

37. Hobler C. Case study: Reduction of chronic postraumatic knee edema using interferential stimulation. *Athl Train*. 1991;26:364.

38. Kots YM. Electrostimulation (Lecture Notes). Paper presented at Canadian-Soviet Exchange Symposium on Electrostimulation of Skeletal Muscles, Concordia University, Montreal, December 6–15, 1977.

39. Currier DP, Mann R. Muscular strength development by electrical stimulation in healthy individuals. *Phys Ther*. 1983;63(6):915–921.

40. Wolf SL, Ariel GB, Saar D, Penny MA, Railey P. The effect of muscle stimulation during resistive training on performance parameters. *Am J Sports Med*. 1986;14(1):18–23.

41. Selkowitz DM. Improvement in isometric strength of the quadriceps femoris muscle after training with electrical stimulation. *Phys Ther*. 1985;65:186–195.

42. Laughman RK, Youdas JW, Garrett TR, Chao EY. Strength changes in the normal quadriceps femoris muscle as a result of electrical stimulation. *Phys Ther*. 1983;63(4):494–499.

43. McMiken DF, Todd-Smith M, Thompson C. Strengthening of human quadriceps muscles by cutaneous electrical stimulation. *Scand J Rehabil Med*. 1983;15(1):25–28.

44. Wadey VMR. *The Effects of Daily Adjustable Progressive Resistive Exercise and Electrical Stimulation on Strength*. Terre Haute, IN: Dept of Physical Education, Indiana State University, 1988.

45. Massey BH, Nelson RC, Sharkey BC, Comden T, Otott GC. Effects of high frequency electrical stimulation on the size and strength of skeletal muscle. *J Sports Med Phys Fitness*. 1965;5(3):136–144.

46. Mohr T, Carlson B, Sulentic C, Landry R. Comparison of isometric exercise and high volt galvanic stimulation on quadriceps femoris muscle strength. *Phys Ther*. 1985;65(5):606–612.

47. Wadey VM, Knight KL. Four week training of quadriceps strength with electrical muscle stimulation and the isotonic DAPRE technique. *J Can Athl Therap Assoc*. 1989;16(2):14–20.

48. Knight KL. Electrical muscle stimulation during immobilization. *Phys Sportsmed*. 1980;8(2):147.

49. Eriksson E, Haggmark T. Comparison of isometric muscle training and electrical stimulation supplementing isometric muscle training in the recovery after major knee ligament surgery. A preliminary report. *Am J Sports Med*. 1979;7(3):169–171.

50. Godfrey CM, Jayawardena H. Comparison of electro-stimulation and isometric exercise in strengthening the quadriceps muscle. *Physiother Can*. 1979;31:265–267.

51. Gould N, Donnermeyer D, Gammon GG, Pope M, Ashikaga T. Transcutaneous muscle stimulation to retard disuse atrophy after open meniscectomy. *Clin Orthop*. 1983;178:190–197.

52. Hecox B, Mehreteax TA, Weisberg J. *Physical Agents*. Norwalk, CT: Appleton & Lange, 1994.

53. Hasson SM, Wible CL, Barnes WS, Williams JH. Dexamethasone iontophoresis: effect on delayed muscle soreness and muscle function. *Can J Sport Sci*. 1992;17(1):8–13.

54. Kahn J. Iontophoresis and ultrasound for postsurgical temporomandibular trismus and paresthesia. *Phys Ther*. 1980;60(3):307–308.

55. Kahn J. Iontophoresis Dissected. *Biomechanics*. 1996:81–83.

56. Hasson SH. Exercise training and dexamethasone iontophoresis in rheumatoid arthritis: A case study. *Physiother Can*. 1991;43(11):11–14.

57. Glass JM, Stephen RL, Jacobson SC. The quantity and distribution of radiolabeled dexamethasone delivered to tissue by iontophoresis. *Int J Dermatol*. 1980;19(9):519–525.

58. Gudeman SD, Eisele SA, Heidt RS Jr, Colosimo AJ, Stroupe AL. Treatment of plantar fasciitis by iontophoresis of 0.4% dexamethasone. A randomized, double-blind, placebo-controlled study. *Am J Sports Med*. 1997;25(3):312–316.

59. Schiffman EL, Braun BL, Lindgren BR. Temporomandibular joint iontophoresis: a double-blind randomized clinical trial. *J Orofac Pain*. 1996;10(2):157–165.

60. Demirtas RN, Oner C. The treatment of lateral epicondylitis by iontophoresis of sodium salicylate and sodium diclofenac. *Clin Rehabil*. 1998;12(1):23–29.

61. Oshima T, Kashiki K, Toyooka H, Masuda A, Amaha K. Cutaneous iontophoretic application of condensed lidocaine. *Can J Anaesth*. 1994;41(8):677–679.

62. Dolan MG, Mendel FC. Clinical application of electrotherapy. *Athl Ther Today*. 2004;9(5):11–16.

63. Feedar JA, Kloth LC, Gentzkow GD. Chronic dermal ulcer healing enhanced with monophasic pulsed electrical stimulation. *Phys Ther*. 1991;71(9):639–649.

64. Kloth LC, Feedar JA. Acceleration of wound healing with high voltage, monophasic, pulsed current. *Phys Ther.* 1988;68:503–508.

65. Akers TK, Gabrielson AL. The effect of high voltage galvanic stimulation on the rate of healing of decubitus ulcers. *Biomed Sci Instrum.* 1984;20:99–100.

66. Griffin JW, Tooms RE, Mendius RA, et al. Efficacy of high voltage pulsed current for healing of pressure ulcers in patients with spinal cord injury. *Phys Ther.* 1991;71(6):433–442; discussion 442–434.

67. Nordenstrom BE. *Biologically Closed Electric Circuits: Clinical, Experimental and Theoretical Evidence for an Additional Circulatory System.* Stockholm: Nordic Medical Publishers, 1983.

68. Burr H, Taffel M, Harvey S. An electrometric study of the healing wound in man. *Yale J Biol Med.* 1940;12:483–485.

69. Becker RO, Murray DG. Method of producing cellular dedifferentiation by means of very small electrical current. *Trans NY Acad Sci.* 1967;29:606–615.

70. Ralston DJ. High voltage galvanic stimulation: can there be a "state of the art"? *Athl Train.* 1985;(20):291–293.

71. Mustoe TA, Pierce GF, Thomason A, Gramates P, Sporn MB, Deuel TF. Accelerated healing of incisional wounds in rats induced by transforming growth factor-beta. *Science.* 1987;237(4820):1333–1336.

72. Gentzkow GD, Miller KH. Electrical stimulation for dermal wound healing. *Clin Podiatr Med Surg.* 1991;8(4):827–841.

73. Reich JD, Tarjan PP. Electrical stimulation of skin. *Int J Dermatol.* 1990;29(6):395–400.

74. Fakhri O, Amin MA. The effect of low-voltage electric therapy on the healing of resistant skin burns. *J Burn Care Rehabil.* 1987;8(1):15–18.

75. Brown M, McDonnell MK, Menton DN. Electrical stimulation effects on cutaneous wound healing in rabbits. A follow-up study. *Phys Ther.* 1988;68(6):955–960.

76. Brown M, McDonnell MK, Menton DN. Polarity effects on wound healing using electric stimulation in rabbits. *Arch Phys Med Rehabil.* 1989;70(8):624–627.

77. Michlovitz S, Smith W, Watkins M. Ice and high voltage pulsed stimulation in treatment of acute lateral ankle sprains. *J Orthop Sports Phys Ther.* 1988;9:301–304.

78. Cosgrove KA, Alon G, Bell SF, et al. The electrical effect of two commonly used clinical stimulators on traumatic edema in rats. *Phys Ther.* 1992;72(3):227–233.

79. Taylor K, Fish DR, Mendel FC, Burton HW. Effect of electrically induced muscle contractions on posttraumatic edema formation in frog hind limbs. *Phys Ther.* 1992;72(2):127–132.

80. Mohr TM, Akers TK, Landry RG. Effect of high voltage stimulation on edema reduction in the rat hind limb. *Phys Ther.* 1987;67(11):1703–1707.

81. Taylor K, Mendel FC, Fish DR, Hard R, Burton HW. Effect of high-voltage pulsed current and alternating current on macromolecular leakage in hamster cheek pouch microcirculation. *Phys Ther.* 1997;77(12):1729–1740.

82. Dolan MG, Mychaskiw AM, Mattacola CG, Mendel FC. Effects of cool-water immersion and high-voltage electric stimulation for 3 continuous hours on acute edema in rats. *J Athl Train.* 2003;38(4):325–329.

83. Reed BV. Effect of high voltage pulsed electrical stimulation on microvascular permeability to plasma proteins. A possible mechanism in minimizing edema. *Phys Ther.* 1988;68(4):491–495.

84. Mendel FC, Fish DR. New perspectives in edema control via electrical stimulation. *J Athl Train.* 1993;28(1):63.

85. Rauh JG. *Comparison of Muscular Force Production as a Result of Voluntary Contraction and Three Electrical Stimulators.* Masters Thesis. Terre Haute, IN: Physical Education, Indiana State University, 1982.

86. Butterfield DL. The effects of high-volt pulsed current electrical stimulation on delayed-onset muscle soreness. *J Athl Train.* 1997;32:15.

87. Wolcot C. A comparison of the effects of high volt and microcurrent stimulation on delayed onset muscle soreness. *Phys Ther.* 1991;71:S117.

88. Morris L, Newton RA. Use of high voltage pulsed galvanic stimulation for patients with levator ani syndrome. *Phys Ther.* 1987;67(10):1522–1525.

89. Picker RI. Current trends: low-volt pulsed microamp stimulation, part 1. *Clin Manage.* 1989;9(2):10–14.

90. Jewell DV, Riddle, Thacker. Interventions associated with an increased or decreased likelihood of pain reduction and improved function in patients with adhesive capsulitis: A retrospective cohort study. *Phys Ther.* 2009;89:419–429.

91. Association APT. Section on Clinical Electrophysiology. *Electrotherapeutic Terminology in Physical Therapy.* Alexandria, VA: APTA Publication, 1990.

92. Driban JB. Bone stimulators and microcurrent: clinical bioelectrics. *Athl Ther Today.* 2004;9(5):22–27.

93. Merrick MA. Unconventional modalities: microcurrent. *Athl Ther Today.* 1999;4(5):53–54.

94. Wood JM, Evans PE III, Schallreuter KU, et al. A multicenter study on the use of pulsed low-intensity direct current for healing chronic stage II and stage III decubitus ulcers. *Arch Dermatol.* 1993;129(8):999–1009.

95. Baker LL, Chambers R, DeMuth SK, Villar F. Effects of electrical stimulation on wound healing in patients with diabetic ulcers. *Diabetes Care.* 1997;20(3):405–412.

96. Bertolucci LE, Grey T. Clinical comparative study of microcurrent electrical stimulation to mid-laser and placebo treatment in degenerative joint disease of the temporomandibular joint. *Cranio.* 1995;13(2):116–120.

97. Baker LL, Rubayi S, Villar F, DeMuth SK. Effect of electrical stimulation waveform on healing of ulcers in human beings with spinal cord injury. *Wound Repair Regen.* 1996;4:21–28.

98. Zuim PRJ, Garcia AR, Turcio KHL, Hamata MM. Ealuation of microcurrent electrical nerve stimulation (MENS) effectiveness on muscle pain in temporomandibular disorders patients. *J Appl Oral Sci.* 2006; 14:61–66.

99. Allen JD, Mattacola CG, Perrin DH. Effect of microcurrent stimulation on delayed-onset muscle soreness: a double-blind comparison. *J Athl Train.* 1999;34(4):334–337.

100. Weber MD, Servedio FJ, Woodall WR. The effects of three modalities on delayed onset muscle soreness. *J Orthop Sports Phys Ther.* 1994;20(5):236–242.

101. Denegar C. The effects of low-volt microamperage on delayed onset muscle soreness. *J Sport Rehabil.* 1992;1:95.

102. Sinnreich MJ. Microcurrent electrical nerve stimulation (MENS) and coracoacromial arch pain: The effects after one treatment. *Phys Ther.* 1992;72:S68.

103. Byl NN, McKenzie AL, West JM, et al. Pulsed microamperage stimulation: a controlled study of healing of surgically induced wounds in Yucatan pigs. *Phys Ther.* 1994;74(3):201–213; discussion 213–218.

104. Jewell DV, Riddle DL, Thacker LR. Interventions associated with an increased or decreased likelihood of pain reduction and improved function in patients with adhesive capsulitis: A retrospective cohort study. *Phys Ther.* 2009;89:419–429.

105. Bellew JW. Clinical electrical stimulation: application and techniques. In: Michlovitz SL, Nolan TP, Bellew JW, eds. Modalities for Therapeutic Intervention. 5th ed. Philadelphia, PA: F.A. Davis Co., 2011:241–277.

106. Yarrobinoa TE, Kalbfleisch JH, Ferslew KE, Panus PC. Lidocaine iontophoresis mediates analgesia in lateral epicondylalgia treatment. Physiother Res Int. 2006;11(3):152–160.

107. Ciccone CD. Does acetic acid iontophoresis accelerate the resorption of calcium deposits in calcific tendinitis of the shoulder. Phys Ther. 2003;83(1):68–74.

108. Coglianese M, Draper DO, Shurtz J, Mack G. Microdialysis and delivery of iontophoresis-driven lidocaine into the human gastrocnemius muscle. J Athl Train. 2011;46(3):270–276.

109. Draper DO, Coglianese M, Castel JC. Absorption of iontophoresis-driven 2% lidocaine with epinephrine in the tissues at 5 mm below the surface of the skin. J Athl Train. 2011;46(3):277–281.

Review Questions

Chapter 16

1. What is the resistance found in a 40 V circuit possessing a current flow of 10 A?
   a. 4 Ω
   b. 400 Ω
   c. 0.25 Ω
   d. 30 Ω
   e. 10 Ω

2. Monopolar stimulation involves the use of active and dispersive electrodes. The parameter that determines which pad(s) will be active is the _____.
   a. polarity adjustment
   b. average current
   c. pulse duration
   d. current density
   e. electrode material

3. During NEMS, the A electrode is 10 × 5 in. and electrode B 7 × 7 in. This type of stimulation would be classified as _____.
   a. monopolar
   b. bipolar
   c. quadripolar
   d. polypolar
   e. unipolar

4. The amount of energy required to produce a muscle contraction is _____.
   a. <10 mA
   b. 11–20 mA
   c. >30 mA
   d. 1–15 μA
   e. 15–30 μA

5. Which of the following would provide the most resistance to current flow?
   a. material with many free electrons
   b. material that is short
   c. material of wide cross-sectional size
   d. material of low temperature
   e. both a and d

6. The most common AC wave form is _____.
   a. square
   b. triangular
   c. sine
   d. rectangular
   e. sawtooth

7. To form a closed circuit in the body's tissues, at least one electrode from each of the generator's output leads must _____.
   a. touch the skin
   b. be larger than the other electrode
   c. be saturated in water
   d. be smaller than the other electrode
   e. be made of insulated material

8. What happens when the number of twitch contractions per second rises?
   a. improved lymphatic drainage
   b. relaxation
   c. tetany
   d. pain reduction
   e. all of the above

9. Two equal-size electrodes are placed in the target treatment area and an equal amount of stimulation is felt under each electrode. This is known as _____.
   a. bipolar placement
   b. monopolar placement
   c. quadripolar placement
   d. dual-polar placement
   e. all of the above

10. The large electrode that is used with a unipolar technique is called _____.
    a. alternating
    b. an ampere
    c. the circuit
    d. dispersive
    e. the cathode

11. Any alteration in the magnitude or any variation in the duration of an electrical current is called _____.
    a. frequency
    b. modulation
    c. ohm
    d. adaptation
    e. on-off ratio

12. A unit of measure that indicates the rate at which electrical current is flowing is the _____.
    a. volt
    b. ampere
    c. ohm
    d. watt
    e. joule

Chapter 17

1. Which type of modality uses medium frequency as its carrier frequency?
   a. TENS
   b. MENS
   c. iontophoresis
   d. IFC
   e. HVPC

2. Which type of modality uses a direct current?
   a. TENS
   b. MENS
   c. iontophoresis
   d. IFC
   e. both b and c

3. Which type of modality uses a low-frequency alternating current?
   a. TENS
   b. MENS
   c. iontophoresis
   d. IFC
   e. HVPC

4. Which on-off cycle would be the best for the prevention of atrophy during the early phases of rehabilitation using Russian stimulation?
   a. 10/10
   b. 20/20
   c. 30/10
   d. 10/30
   e. 10/50

5. Which on-off cycle would be the best for reducing a muscle spasm using NMES?
   a. 10/10
   b. 20/20
   c. 30/10
   d. 10/30
   e. 10/50

6. Which type of TENS is used primarily to treat acute pain by stimulating the large-diameter sensory nerves using a frequency of 80–200 pps with the intensity adjusted to the point at which the patient reports a buzzing or tingling?
   a. sensory TENS
   b. motor TENS
   c. brief-intense TENS
   d. opiate TENS
   e. noxious TENS

7. Which type of TENS is used to treat chronic pain by stimulating the small-diameter afferent nerves using a low frequency of 1–5 pps with an intensity that results in a twitch contraction?
   a. sensory TENS
   b. motor TENS
   c. brief-intense TENS
   d. opiate TENS
   e. all of the above

8. Which type of modality uses a twin-peak monophasic pulsed current driven by a large electromotive force?
   a. TENS
   b. MENS
   c. iontophoresis
   d. IFC
   e. HVPC

9. Which of the following modalities is primarily used to modulate pain?
   a. TENS
   b. MENS
   c. IFC
   d. HVPC
   e. a and c

10. Which modality uses DC and pulsed currents with a stimulus amplitude that is imperceptible?
    a. TENS
    b. MENS
    c. iontophoresis
    d. IFC
    e. HVPC

Part VI

Other Modalities

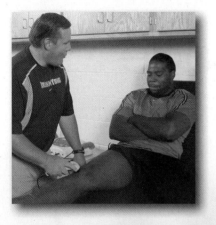

I n part IV we discuss three modalities that don't fit anywhere else. Some authors classify massage and traction, along with intermittent compression, as mechanical modalities. We chose to classify intermittent compression with immediate care, since its primary purpose is removing edema, which is associated with immediate care. Laser and light therapy is in a class of its own.

18

Therapeutic Massage

Chapter Outline

Massage as a Therapeutic Modality

Massage Therapy: What Is It?

Ten Common Massage Techniques for Athletes

Facts and Misconceptions About Massage

The Therapeutic Effects of Massage

Misconceptions About Massage

Indications and Contraindications

Therapeutic Massage Versus a Rubdown

Massage Use and Abuse

Common Massage Strokes Used in Basic (Swedish) Massage

Myofascial Release

Sports Massage

Massage Lubricants

Lotions

Oils

Creams

Powders

Application of Therapeutic Massage

Step 1: Foundation

Step 2: Preapplication Tasks

Step 3: Application Parameters

Step 4: Postapplication Tasks

Step 5: Maintenance

OPENING SCENE

On your first day with Kate, your clinical instructor and the track and field athletic trainer (AT), you ask her what is involved in working with track and field. She chuckles a little and then says, "We do a lot of massage, because the coaches and athletes insist on it. But I try to educate them on the appropriateness of massage—when they need it and when they don't." You think to yourself, "I have had some classroom theory on massage, but I've never given a real sports massage, and I don't even know where to start. It must involve more than giving the athlete's legs a good rubdown." This chapter helps you understand how and when to deliver a therapeutic sports massage.

368

Massage as a Therapeutic Modality

Many people think a therapeutic modality is a black box that you plug into the wall. It has blinking lights and all the "bells and whistles" to help patients think they are being treated with a modern medical device. Massage does not meet these criteria. This might be why some textbooks on therapeutic modalities don't include massage. We are of the opinion that massage is an important modality if used appropriately. But therein lies the rub! (Pun intended.) How often is massage used appropriately in a sports medicine environment? We have worked as ATs in many settings—somewhere massage is rarely used, somewhere it is used appropriately, and somewhere it is overused. Let's face it, massage feels good and can be psychologically relaxing. If you could lay down on a comfortable table for a half hour or so every day and have someone use trained hands to gently (or not so gently) rub your sore, aching muscles, and relieve your stress, would you do it? Most people would. In fact, many people pay $40–$50 for a 30-minute massage.

Currently in North America, massage is considered to be a complementary therapy to conventional medical practice.[1] Elsewhere in the world, and throughout much of medical history, massage has been regarded as an important component of mainstream health care. In fact, many of the greatest proponents of the clinical use of massage include such respected physicians as Cyriax, Mennell, Travell, and Hippocrates,[2] although it could be argued that all Hippocrates had to work with was his hands. Massage is one of the oldest and most widespread healing techniques. It is practiced in most cultures, and there are many variations. It is a skill-based technique that is licensed in many states.

Massage Therapy: What Is It?

The terms therapeutic massage, massage therapy, and manual therapy are often used interchangeably, and are often discussed in relation to bodywork and somatic therapy. And there are more than 250 variations of massage, bodywork, and somatic therapies, many of which are variations of each other.[3] Many practitioners use multiple techniques to accomplish their goals. It is easy to get confused about what massage is, and isn't.

The "massage community" is inclusive of three groups of therapies[3]:

- *Massage:* The application of soft tissue manipulation techniques to the body, generally intended to reduce stress and fatigue while improving circulation. The many variations of massage account for several different techniques.
- *Bodywork:* Various forms of touch therapies that may use manipulation, movement, and/or repatterning to affect structural changes to the body.
- *Somatic:* Meaning "of the body." Many times this term is used to denote a body/mind or whole-body approach as distinguished from a physiology-only or environmental perspective.

Therapeutic massage is the systematic manual manipulation of the body's tissues in order to restore normal function. "In general, therapists press, rub, and otherwise manipulate the muscles and other soft tissues of the body. They most often use their hands and fingers, but may use their forearms, elbows, or feet."[4] But how they do so varies greatly, and has lead to a variety of techniques. There are also differences among practitioners and patients concerning the most viable techniques to use. For example, there were only three common techniques listed on two Web sites listing the 10 most popular massage techniques (Accessed March 2012).[5,6] The following, however, are the ones we feel are most often used by ATs. Although it is beyond the scope of this text to discuss these techniques (other than the first two) in enough detail to allow you to apply them, we feel ATs should understand the basics of these techniques. Access other sources concerning how to apply the other techniques.

TEN COMMON MASSAGE TECHNIQUES FOR ATHLETES

1. *Swedish massage:* Classic, traditional, or basic massage. What most people think of when the word massage is mentioned. Used for both relaxation and injury rehabilitation. It uses a variety of strokes, including effleurage (sliding or gliding strokes) and petrissage (lifting, kneading of soft tissue), friction (nongliding, shearing forces that cause movement between underlying tissues), tapotement (hacking or pounding), and vibration (rapidly shaking a muscle for a few seconds).[1]

2. *Sports massage:* Application of Swedish massage techniques to athletes, and others involved in physical activity.[1] The focus is on preventing and treating injury and enhancing athletic performance. Case series provide little support for the use of massage to aid muscle recovery or performance after intense exercise, whereas randomized clinical trials provide moderate support for its use to facilitate recovery from intense repetitive muscular contractions.[7] Further investigation using standardized protocols and similar outcome variables is necessary to determine the efficacy of sport massage

and the optimal strategy for its implementation to enhance recovery following intense exercise.[7]

3. *Myofascial Release* (MFR): Light sustained pressure applied in opposite directions to gently stretch and release myofascia restrictions that inhibit movement or cause pain.[1,8–11] The technique is preferred over high velocity techniques (manipulation) by a group 171 osteopathic physicians.[12]

4. *Graston*: An instrument-assisted soft tissue mobilization method that requires specific training and certification.[8,13] The stainless steel instruments are designed with a unique curvilinear treatment edge, contoured to fit various shapes of the body.[14]

5. *Rolfing*: (also known as *Structural Integration*) Vigorous deep tissue massage and MFR to restore normal body alignment, structure, and function. A key principle is that fascial contractures result from chronic dysfunctional movement and imbalanced muscular tension, resulting in pain and lessened muscle and joint motion. The body must be released from these learned patters and malaligned structures.[15,16] Fingers, the thumb, fist, and elbow are all used to apply deep pressure. The individual techniques used in Rolfing are not unique to this Rolfing.[16]

6. *Neuromuscular therapy* (NMT): Practitioners address (a) compressed or entrapped nerves by osseous or myofascia structures, (b) trigger points, (c) postural distortion or imbalance, (d) emotional factors, (e) ischemia, and (f) nutritional deficiencies.[17,18] A variety of techniques are used, including trigger point pressure release, cryospray, needling, and myofacial release. Proponents claim it helps improve functioning of the immune system, glands, joints, muscles, and related soft tissues.[6,18]

7. *Shiatsu*: A form of Japanese pressure point therapy, similar to trigger point therapy but concentrating on application of pressure to acupuncture points. *Prenatal/postpartum massage*: Specific strokes and positions used with women to address muscular issues that occur secondary to pregnancy.[1]

8. *Craniosacral therapy* (CST; also known as cranial sacral therapy) is a gentle, hands-on method of enhancing the craniosacral system—the spine and the membranes and cerebrospinal fluid that surround and protect the brain and spinal cord. The idea is to improve the functioning of the central nervous system by releasing restrictions in the craniosacral system. Although this therapy has many supporters,[19–21] its validity has been challenged, and lacks scientific support.[19,22,23]

9. *Trigger Point Therapy*: Repetitive cycles of isolated pressure and release over a trigger point, a painfully tight area in a muscle caused by muscle overuse or injury.

10. *Reflexology*: The application of finger and thumb pressure to specific reflex areas of patients hands and feet that are thought to correspond to all of the glands, organs, and parts of the body. Advocates claim it helps to relieve stress and tension, improve blood supply, promote the unblocking of nerve impulses, and help nature achieve homeostasis.[1]

Facts and Misconceptions About Massage

For decades the physiological effects of massage have been debated. Scientific evidence is limited,[4] The pathophysiological changes that massage causes to occur are unknown and whether massage influences health are uncertain.[4,24] Possible mechanisms have been suggested.[24] Thus it is difficult for clinicians to differentiate between science and tradition in the use of therapeutic massage. There is no doubt massage has a "feel good" effect, but does it do more?

THE THERAPEUTIC EFFECTS OF MASSAGE

Depending on the type, speed, and pressure of the strokes, the benefits of massage have been described as follows:

- Invigorates the body prior to athletic competition[2]
- Promotes relaxation prior to and after competition[2]
- Promotes blood flow in the skin,[25,26] but not to deeper tissues[25,27]
- Decreases pain by interrupting muscle spasm and reducing edema, increasing blood and lymph flow to rid tissue of cellular wastes, and activating cutaneous receptors to close the gate to pain[2] (see Chapter 6)
- Mildly promotes lymph flow, but no greater than active or passive movement of the limbs (in dogs)[28]
- Increases muscle flexibility following a routine of deep effleurage, circular friction, and transverse friction. Massage might aid in short-term flexibility, especially if applied to an area where an accumulation of scar tissue has resulted in lost range of motion (ROM).
- Recovery following intense short duration exercise is unsettled. There are conflicting research reports, in part because of differences in variables measured, subjects, type and duration of exercise, and type of massage (Table 18.1). It appears that 10–20 minutes of Swedish/Sports massage impedes[27] or has no effect on blood lactate,[25,29–31] heart rate (HR),[25,29–31] or arterial blood flow.[25] MFR for 40 minutes, however, reduced HR volume and diastolic blood pressure.[11] Fatigue also appears to benefit from 10 to 20 minutes of petrissage.[30,31]
- Decreases scar tissue in tendintitis.[32,33] Friction massage is often the manual intervention of choice for repetitive strain injuries, such as tendinitis where there is ongoing microtrauma, low-grade inflammation, and pain.

TABLE 18.1   RESEARCH SUMMARY OF THE EFFECTS OF MASSAGE ON RECOVERY AFTER SHORT-TERM, INTENSE EXERCISE

AUTHORS	SUBJECTS	EXERCISE TIME AND REST BETWEEN BOUTS	MASSAGE: TYPE AND TIME	RESULTS
Hinds et al.[25]	13M healthy	3 × 2 min Quad extension@ 240°/s	12 min effleurage and petrassage	No dif: blood lactate, HR, BP, arterial blood flow Diff: skin blood flow
Martin et al.[29]	10M cyclists, competitive	wingate: cycling, 3 × 30 s, w/2 min rest	10 min Swedish, each leg,	No diff: blood lactate
Ogai et al.[31]	11F active	cycling, 8 × 5 s w/15 s rest	10 min petrissage	No diff: blood lactate Diff: muscle stiffness, perceived fatigue, power
Robertson et al.[30]	9M athletes	cycling, 6 × 30 s w/30s active recovery	30 min active + 20 min leg "massage"	No diff: blood lactate, HR, power Diff: fatigue index
Wiltshire et al.[27]	12M "healthy"	2 min isometric hand grip @ 40% MVIC	10 min effleurage and petrissage	Blood flow and lactic acid removal decreased
Arroyo-Morales et al.[11]	37M, 25F active	wingate: cycling 3 × 30 s w/3 min rest	40 min myofascial release	Diff: heart rate volume, and diastolic BP

- Appears to be an effective treatment for persistent low-back pain, providing long-lasting benefits,[34] and chronic pediatric pain[35]
- Appears that a 10-week regimen of weekly massage is beneficial for treating chronic neck pain, at least in the short term.[36] And acupuncture was not beneficial in this clinical trial.
- Blood pressure in normotensive and prehypertensive adults (BP < 150/95) decreased slightly (systolic 1.8 mm Hg) during 30–90 minute Swedish massage, but increased during vigorous or potentially painful massage techniques, such as sports massage and trigger point therapy.[37]

Beneficial in treating cancer, by reducing side affects of chemotherapy and radiation and improving perceived quality of life and overall functioning.[38–40]

✔ APPLICATION TIP

USE FRICTION MASSAGE TO BOOST HEALING

Think of friction massage as rebooting the body's healing computer. In much the same way that rebooting a computer enables the machine to work appropriately, friction massage might help restart the inflammatory process so that the affected tissues can progress normally through the various phases of healing.

MISCONCEPTIONS ABOUT MASSAGE

For a long time, many clinicians used massage thinking it would remove lactic acid from overworked muscles. Today, however, we now know this premise is false.[25,41,42]

Massage has also been used to increase blood flow, and this effect is only partially true. Massage does increase blood flow to the skin, but not to the arteries.[25,43,44] In a muscle recovering from a bout of exercise, massage could thus be problematic. If massage increases skin blood flow but not arterial blood flow, the blood might be rerouted to the skin from the skeletal muscles, thereby hindering the recovery process.[25]

Massage also carries with it a large placebo effect, so it is difficult to differentiate between physiological and psychological effects. Here is a list of other effects that massage does not have on the body, as shown through research:

- No effect on stride frequency or length in sprinters[45]
- Muscular fatigue is unaffected by massage between bouts (sprinter's legs and pitcher's arms).[43,44]
- No change in cardiac output, blood pressure, or lactic acid accumulation during submaximal treadmill running following precompetition massage[41]
- Hinders[27] or does not remove blood lactate[25,29–31,41,42]
- Does not promote endorphin release
- No increase in arterial blood flow[25,43,44]
- No increase in muscle temperature[25]
- No better than control treatments in relieving general anxiety disorder[46]

- No better than relaxation tapes for deceasing general stress and improving sleeping following six treatment sessions[47]
- Does not cause friction between the skin and underlying fascia of the thoracic spine[48]

Indications and Contraindications

Indications for therapeutic massage include situations requiring local blood flow and increased venous return, pain relief, muscle spasm reduction, and cases in which systemic relaxation is desired.

Massage therapy appears to have few serious risks, as long as it is performed by a properly trained therapist and if appropriate cautions are followed.[4] There is little agreement, however, among professional sources (textbooks and peer-reviewed journal articles) concerning what conditions are contraindicated for massage.[49] From 3 to 86 contraindicates and precautions were identified by the 21 sources used. Such a wide range indicates the lack of scientific basis for this modality. Part of the problem is that there are a variety of massage strokes, each of which can be applied with a range of intensities. So until this is rectified by more evidence-based data, we must rely on what little data we have and common sense.

The US National Institutes of Health recommend the following[4]:

- Vigorous massage should be avoided by people with bleeding disorders or low blood platelet counts, and by people taking blood-thinning medications such as warfarin.
- Massage should not be done in any area of the body with blood clots, fractures, open or healing wounds, skin infections, or weakened bones (such as from osteoporosis or cancer), or where there has been a recent surgery.
- Although massage therapy appears to be generally safe for cancer patients, they should consult their oncologist before having a massage that involves deep or intense pressure. Any direct pressure over a tumor usually is discouraged. Cancer patients should discuss any concerns about massage therapy with their oncologist.
- Pregnant women should consult their health care provider before using massage therapy.

In addition, we suggest that massage should be performed on patients who are hypersensitive to touch, or who have arteriosclerosis, embolism, or pain of unknown origin.

Side effects of massage therapy may include temporary pain or discomfort, bruising, swelling, and a sensitivity or allergy to massage oils.[4]

Therapeutic Massage Versus a Rubdown

Therapeutic means relating to a treatment or the curing of a disease or disorder.[50] A rubdown is simply the application of friction and pressure to the body, for any purpose. So, there are two categories of massage used in sports:

1. *Therapeutic or curing*: The patient "requires" massage as part of the treatment regimen of an injury, such as chronic tendinitis or a strain.
2. *Relaxation and psychological*: The patient "desires" a rubdown because it feels good, and may help relax muscles that were overworked during activity.

Notice that in the first category, massage is required, whereas in the second category, massage is desired.

MASSAGE USE AND ABUSE

There is a fine line between what is physiologically therapeutic and what is psychologically relaxing. Therapeutic massage can be a valuable tool when it is needed. For instance, a pitcher who has thrown several fast balls in a game could benefit from an arm rubdown, followed by ice. And periodically a runner might benefit from having his or her legs rubbed down. However, some athletes abuse this tool, being too lazy to perform a proper cool-down and prefer having someone else passively move (rub out) their muscles on a regular basis. It is important that athletes perform a proper cool-down, including jogging (or easy swimming for swimmers), after each workout or competition. Clinicians must use massage when massage is indicated as part of a treatment regimen—not whenever an athlete wants a rubdown.

Massage must be considered entirely as a means to an end, the end being the restoration of function. Every movement performed during the massage should have this goal in view. Since your hands are the tools of massage, you should be able to describe and demonstrate the intended effect of each movement of the hand or finger, and what part this effect is expected to play in the restoration of function.[2]

Common Massage Strokes Used in Basic (Swedish) Massage

The primary therapeutic massage strokes are effleurage, petrissage, friction, percussion, and vibration. Massage strokes vary according to the following factors:

- Applying more or less pressure
- Using different parts of the hand

- Changing the direction of the stroke
- Changing the rhythm and speed of the application

EFFLEURAGE

Effleurage is a gliding manipulation performed with pressure (directed toward the heart) that deforms subcutaneous tissue down to the deep fascia. It is also referred to as *stroking* (Fig. 18.1).

A massage should begin and end with light effleurage. It relaxes the patient at the beginning, and at the end, it calms any nerves that were irritated during the massage.

Following are the keys for applying effleurage:

- Rhythmically stroke the skin.
- Use either light or deep pressure. Light effleurage promotes relaxation and sensory reflexes. Deep effleurage promotes mechanical effects, such as increasing superficial blood and lymphatic flow.
- When deep stroking, follow the course of veins and lymph vessels to direct fluids toward the heart.
- When superficial stroking, follow the contour of the body or the underlying tissue.
- Use the palms of both hands in a deliberate, rhythmic fashion.
- Maintain contact with the skin at all times by stroking in one direction with both hands and returning them to the beginning with light fingertip contact, in a shallow D (right hand) and reverse D (left hand)

(Fig. 18.2a). Alternatively, stagger the hands, making contact with the second before lifting the first from the body (Fig. 18.2b).

PETRISSAGE

Petrissage, from the French *petrir*, "to knead," is a group of related techniques that repetitively compress (squeeze), shear (wring), and release muscle tissue with varying amounts of drag, lift, and glide. Use petrissage when your goal is to stretch and separate muscle fiber, fascia, and scar tissue.

Following are the keys for applying petrissage:

- Lift and knead the tissues: the skin, subcutaneous tissue, and muscle.
- Lift the tissue between the thumb and fingers and palm, and then gently roll and knead the tissue in the hand (Fig. 18.3).
- Gently wring the muscle between both hands like you are wringing water out of a dishrag (Fig. 18.4).
- Petrissage can be done without lubricant or lotion.

FRICTION

Friction massage is a repetitive, specific, nongliding, shearing technique that produces movement between the fibers of dense connective tissue, increasing tissue extensibility and promoting the alignment of collagen fibers.

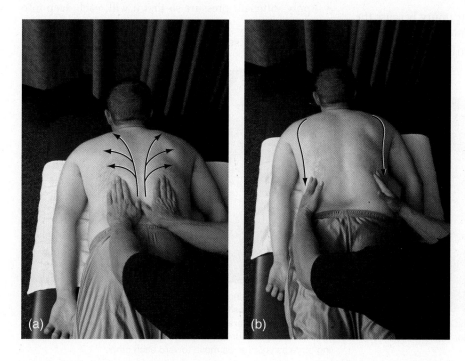

FIGURE 18.1 Effleurage uses both light and deep strokes usually beginning from the peripheral areas and moving toward the heart. **(a)** Bilateral superficial effleurage of the back, beginning at the sacrum and following different paths along the back. **(b)** The return stroke.

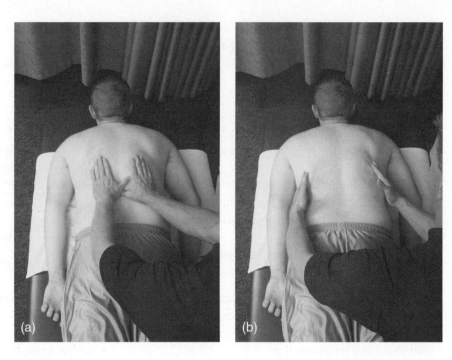

FIGURE 18.2 During effleurage, always maintain contact with the skin, by **(a)** using a D pattern with both hands, or **(b)** alternating hands.

The rationale for friction massage is to mobilize muscle and separate adhesions in muscle, tendons, or scar tissue that restrict movement and cause pain. Sometimes chronic inflammation occurs because an injury does not go through the normal stages of inflammation and healing. The purpose of friction massage is to increase inflammation ("jump start" it) to a point where the inflammatory process will run its normal course and the injury can progress to the later stages of healing. This is why cross-friction massage is often used for repetitive strain injuries such as tendinitis, where there is ongoing microtrauma, inflammation, and tissue remodeling.[2,32,51]

Do not use friction massage on acute injury, because the pressure could cause more damage. This technique is usually painful, especially when treating trigger points.

Following are the keys for applying friction massage:

- Use friction in a circular or transverse fashion. If circular, work the thumbs in a circular motion. If transverse, the thumbs stroke the tissue from opposite directions.
- Apply the strokes across fibers when treating a ligament or tendon (Fig. 18.5).
- When treating scar tissue in which the collagen has irregular organization, alternate the directions or apply the strokes in a circular motion.
- Use your elbow on large muscles.
- Place the muscle in a relaxed position.
- Apply sufficient pressure so that it will reach deep into the tissue.
- Follow it with stretching to increase ROM.

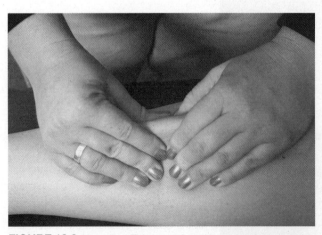

FIGURE 18.3 Kneading. This type of petrissage involves grasping the muscle between the thumb and fingers, or fingers and palm, and lifting and rolling the muscle.

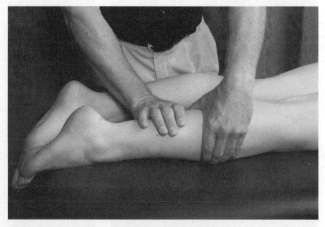

FIGURE 18.4 Wringing. This type of petrissage involves resting your hands on opposite sides of the circumference of the body segment (your hands are facing each other). You then compress the muscle between your hands and wring out the muscle with a shearing force as your hands move toward each other.

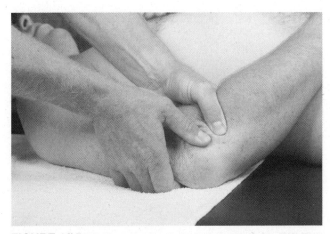

FIGURE 18.5 Friction massage being applied to the wrist extensor tendons to treat lateral epicondilitis (tennis elbow).

PERCUSSION

Percussion, also referred to as *tapotement*, is repeated, rhythmical, light striking of the skin. Techniques include gentle tapping, pounding, cupping, hacking, and slapping the skin.

The two main uses of percussion massage are for respiratory ailments to promote phlegm mobilization, and to stimulate an athlete during precompetition preparation. Following are the keys for applying percussion:

- Hack with the ulnar (pinky) side of the hand with wrist and fingers limp (karate chop) (Fig. 18.6a).

- With cupping, allow only the rim of the hand to come in contact with the body (Fig. 18.6b).
- Use raindrops, a variation to promote relaxation and desensitization of irritated nerve endings, by lightly touching the skin with the fingers in an alternating manner, like typing (Fig. 18.6c).

VIBRATION

Vibration, also referred to as *shaking*, is repetitively moving soft tissue (usually muscle) back and forth over the underlying bone with minimal joint motion (Fig. 18.7).

The main uses of vibration massage are to relax skeletal muscle and as a stimulus for precompetition and intercompetition, due to its effects of systemic arousal and enhanced awareness. Following are the keys for applying vibration:

- Apply moderate to rapid shaking strokes to the skin. Use rapid strokes for precompetition and moderate strokes after competition.
- Apply with the hands or with a machine (Fig. 18.8).

 CONCEPT CHECK 18.1. A soccer player comes into the AT clinic and tells you about a knot she has in her hamstring that won't go away. It has been bothering her for the past 2 weeks and seems to be related to an old strain. What type of massage stroke will be the most effective at relaxing the knot?

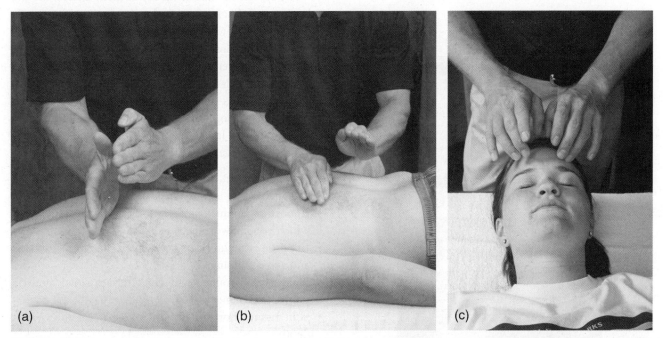

FIGURE 18.6 Percussion techniques. **(a)** Hacking is performed with the ulnar side of hand with the wrist and fingers limp (karate chop). **(b)** Cupping uses only the rim of the hand in contact with the patient's body. **(c)** Raindrops is applied by lightly touching the skin with the fingers in an alternating manner.

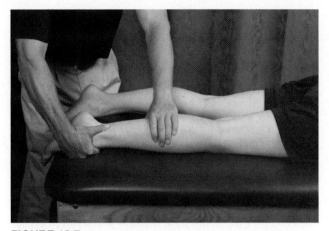

FIGURE 18.7 Vibration massage, or shaking the lower leg.

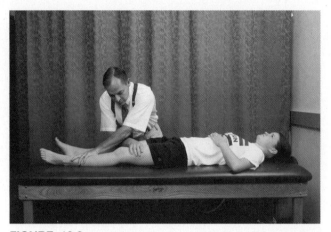

FIGURE 18.9 A myofascial release technique. This advanced method combines traction with varying amounts of stretch to produce a moderate sustained force on the muscle and associated fascia.

Myofascial Release

Myofascial release combines traction with varying amounts of stretch to produce a moderate sustained force on the muscle and its associated fascia. The goal is to produce viscoelastic lengthening and plastic deformation of the fascia[2,52] (Fig. 18.9). In other words, this technique is used to help lengthen the muscle and fascial layers and enable them to remain in the lengthened state, to restore mobility between fascial layers, and to decrease the effects of adhesions on the muscular system. This technique is indicated for a wide variety of conditions in which chronic fascial shortening results in limited joint ROM, ease of movement, and pain.[2]

Fascia is a dense connective tissue that surrounds individual muscle cells, muscle bundles, and whole muscles, and thus is inextricably linked with the muscle and is continuous with tendon.[53] Some think of it as being like the shrink wrap that surrounds meat on a styrofoam plate at the grocery store. This is simplistic, however. Fascia is not an inert substance; rather it is a dense gel (a noncellular ground substance) in which many types of cells and fibers are suspended (including fibroblasts, macrophages and mast cells, collagen and elastin). It is richly innervated with a variety of both free and encapsulated nerve endings.[54] In pathologic and post-trauma conditions, the fascia can be retracted or thickened.[55]

For athletes, the fascial tissues of main interest are the subcutaneous fascia, fascial sheaths such as retinacula at the ankle and wrist, and fascia related to the muscle. Unrestricted myofascial tissues enhance ease of movement and improve movement. The goals of MFR techniques are to make fascial tissues more pliable and to break crosslinks or adhesions. This is done by stretching tissues and applying a shearing force horizontally across the tissues that separates the fascia that has become stuck together.[56]

Tappan[57] advocated the following guidelines for MFR:

- Use observation, palpation, and knowledge of myofascial anatomy to identify areas of fascial restriction,
- Choose techniques suitable for the area and depth at which you are working.
- Use little or no lubricant so that you can feel restrictions and avoid slipping.
- Make gentle contact and enter tissues slowly until a point of resistance is felt.
- Shift tissues horizontally once you are at the correct depth.
- Hold the stretch of the tissues until they release, usually in 2–5 minutes.

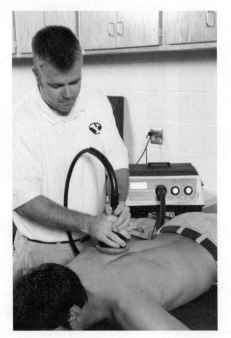

FIGURE 18.8 Vibration massage can also be performed with a machine.

- Release will feel like a melting or letting go.
- Flow with the tissues.
- Exit the tissues slowly and with awareness.
- Let fascial tissues rest and integrate change after the stretch.

Clinical training and supervised practice are critical for proper application of this technique,[2] and are beyond the scope of this book. To adequately become even a novice of myofascial massage would take too much of the semester. If you are interested in learning MFR, either enroll in a workshop or course where proper instruction and clinical skills are taught, or read texts dedicated to advanced massage techniques.[2,58–60,56,57]

Sports Massage

Sports massage is simply massage applied to athletes, and others. It uses the same strokes and techniques discussed above. Calling it a "sports massage" rather than a "massage" elevates its importance in some people's minds.

Sports massage is classified numerous ways, according to its goal or objective. All of these fit into one of two major categories; to: (a) maintain the health of the athlete or (b) enhance athletic performance.[19] Each of the major categories is divided into subgroups, again by goal.

Health maintenance sports massages include:

- Rehabilitative massage—aimed at alleviating pain due to injury and returning the body to health
- Remedial massage—to improve a debilitating condition

Performance enhancement sports massages include:

- Recovery massage—to enhance the athlete's physical and mental recovery from strenuous physical or sport activity. The hope is that this will allow the athlete to train harder and with less injury. Also known as maintenance or restorative massage.
- Pre-event massage—a short, stimulating massage 15–45 minutes before the event to help prepare the athlete physically, mentally, and emotionally for the event. It is directed toward the parts of the body that will be involved in the exertion.
- Inter-event massage—to help the athlete recover from an event while preparing for the next event, round, heat, or trial
- Postevent—given within an hour or two of the event, to help the athlete recover from an event

These techniques are questionable, however. After an extensive review in 2005, Cerapon concluded that research had not shown any clear benefit of massage on sport performance or injury prevention.[24] This does not mean they are not beneficial, only that the research to prior to 2005 had failed to demonstrate any benefit. Two studies since then indicate that massage may be helpful in reducing fatigue following short duration high intensity cycling (see Table 18.1). MFR for 40 minutes reduces HR volume and diastolic blood pressure,[11] and that 10–20 minutes of petrissage reduces fatigue.[30,31]

CASE STUDY 18.1

Erin ran three races in the high school state championship track meet—3200 m on Friday and 1600 and 800 m on Saturday. What categories of sports massage would you use on her during her 2-day ordeal?

Massage Lubricants

The purpose of a **massage lubricant** is to decrease friction and control the amount of glide and drag that occurs between the clinician's moving hands and the client's skin. Lubricants aid some techniques (e.g., where gliding is required) and are actually a hindrance for other techniques (e.g., friction massage). Lubricants should be hypoallergenic and dispensed from a squeeze bottle, pump, or shaker that prevents contamination.

There are four main types of massage lubricants: lotions, oils, creams, and powders.

LOTIONS

Massage lotions are probably the most commonly used in orthopedic injury rehabilitation. They are opaque, liquid suspensions of particles in either oil or water. They rapidly lose their ability to lubricate because they absorb into the skin quickly, and thus have to be reapplied often during a treatment. Rapid absorption, however, can be advantageous when you are preparing for more deeper or vigorous strokes when little or no lotion is desired. Lotions clean up easily with soap and water.[2]

OILS

Massage oils are not used as much in injury rehabilitation as lotions; however, they are the lubricant of choice among massage therapists.[2] Mineral oil is very popular, but any high-quality vegetable oil can be used, such as sunflower, olive, almond, safflower, coconut, or jojoba. One advantage of oil is that it does not absorb into the skin very quickly, so the clinician does not have to keep adding more. There are a few disadvantages to using oils. First, they are messy and leave a stain. It is a good idea to cover any clothing (yours or the patient's) that is in the direct vicinity of the treatment. Also, the patient will need to shower after the treatment, and the area will need to be wiped off with disposable towels, since the residue may stain the patient's clothing.[2]

CREAMS

Massage creams are thicker suspensions that fall midway between oils and lotions in their absorption rate. Some creams contain more oil to promote gliding techniques. Other creams contain sticky substances such as lanolin or beeswax to reduce glide for treating tissue release

techniques.[2] Creams often include menthol, capsaicin, or aloe vera as one of their active ingredients.

POWDERS

Powders can be used when patients prefer not to use lotions, creams, or oils. Unscented baby powder or cornstarch is commonly used. The weaknesses of using powders are that they are not very lubricating and require a lot of cleanup.[2]

 CONCEPT CHECK 18.2. What massage stroke does not require the use of a lubricant? Why?

Application of Therapeutic Massage

STEP 1: FOUNDATION

A. Definition. Therapeutic massage is a systematic manual manipulation of the body's tissues.
B. Effects
1. Depends on type, pressure, and speed of stroke. Invigorates the body prior to athletic competition, promotes relaxation, promotes blood flow in the skin, and decreases pain.
C. Advantages
1. Patients feel that you are actively involved in their healing.
2. Tactile contact by a clinician's hands can be enjoyable, relaxing, and soothing. The laying on of hands demonstrates concern, compassion, and care.
3. Requires no special equipment
4. Easily learned; extensive background is not required. The clinician can instruct individuals, family, or friends to do their own massage. However, it does require much practice to become skilled in this area.
D. Disadvantages
1. Time-consuming
2. Lotions, oils, and powders can get messy
E. Indications
1. Increase venous return
2. Break the pain-spasm-pain cycle
3. Evoke systemic relaxation
4. Improve or stimulate local blood flow

F. Contraindications
1. Acute sprains and strains. Massage can:
   a. Increase the inflammatory response
   b. Cause myositis ossificans
2. Over skin with lesions or disease conditions; may spread disease over the patient or to the clinician
3. Sites where fractures have failed to heal
4. People who are hypersensitive to touch
G. Precautions
1. Pitting edema
2. Hypertension

STEP 2: PREAPPLICATION TASKS

A. Selecting the proper modality
1. Make sure massage is the proper modality for this situation
B. Preparing the patient psychologically
1. Explain the benefits of massage. State that at no time will any private body parts be touched, or undraped.
C. Preparing the patient physically
1. Ensure a suitable environment that includes
   a. A comfortable room temperature 68–75°F (20–24°C)
   b. Upholstered table to protect pressure points and bony prominences (pelvic bones, ankles, head, etc.)
   c. A relaxed atmosphere; perhaps relaxing music
   d. Positioning the patient

i. So that both patient and clinician are comfortable

ii. With a rolled-up towel under the body parts (e.g., the ankle) to increase comfort

iii. Making sure the patient is properly draped with towels to observe modesty (if the massage involves body parts where nudity may be a concern)

D. Equipment preparation

1. Determine the type of massage you want to give, including what strokes you will use and in what order.

2. Determine whether you will use lubricants

3 STEP 3: APPLICATION PARAMETERS

A. Instead of standard procedures, a massage application is designed to meet the individual patient's needs. A "typical" sports massage application is as follows:

1. Light effleurage (superficial stroking)
2. Deep effleurage (deep stroking)
3. Petrissage (kneading, wringing, and lifting)
4. Optional friction or percussion
5. Deep petrissage (deep stroking)
6. Light effleurage (superficial stroking)

B. Dosage (varies according to patient tolerance)

1. During the treatment, seek feedback about the patient's response to your treatment by periodically asking questions such as, "How are you feeling?" "Is it tender here?" "Is this pressure OK?"

C. Length of application

1. Varies from 5 minutes for one body part to 45 minutes for the entire body

D. Frequency of application

1. Depends on the purpose of the massage. Clinicians must use massage when massage is indicated as part of a treatment regimen—not whenever an athlete wants a rubdown.

E. Duration of therapy

As long as massage continues to have a positive impact on the resolution of the injury; however, don't abuse it.

4 STEP 4: POSTAPPLICATION TASKS

A. Equipment removal

1. Remove any remaining massage lubricant.

B. Instructions to the patient

1. Schedule the next treatment.
2. Instruct the patient about the level of activity and/or self-treatment prior to the next formal treatment.

C. Record of treatment, including unique patient responses

D. Replace soiled towels and sheets with clean ones

5 STEP 5: MAINTENENCE

A. Keep your hands free of calluses.

B. Make sure massage tables are in good working order

C. Make sure you have plenty of massage lubricants on hand for future use

CLOSING SCENE

It is midway through the track and field season. Your clinical instructor over the sport approaches you and tells you she has received many compliments regarding your athletic training skills, particularly with giving massages. "I'm especially impressed," she adds, "that you don't let the athletes abuse massage as a modality. You always remind the runners to do a proper cool-down including jogging and stretching, and you limit their massages to when their muscles are tight, not just when they want a rubdown." You think to yourself, "Massage can be a great modality when it is used appropriately." You thank your supervisor for the compliment and feel good inside because you just had your ego massaged.

Chapter Reflections

1. Read and ponder each of the following points. Do you feel you have a clear understanding of each concept? If not, reread the appropriate section of the chapter.
   - Define effleurage, and explain why it is used.
   - Define petrissage, and explain why it is used.
   - Define friction massage, and explain why it is used.
   - Define MFR, and explain why it is used.
   - Define percussion, and explain why it is used.
   - Define vibration, and explain why it is used.
   - What is a typical format for a sports massage?
   - Describe the physiological effects of massage.
   - Compare and contrast the reflexive versus mechanical effects of massage.
   - List the indications for massage.
   - Name the contraindications for massage.
   - What are the advantages and disadvantages of common lubricants used during massage?
   - Explain the difference between a therapeutic massage and a rubdown.

2. Write three to five questions for discussion with your class instructor, clinical instructor, classmates, and clinical colleagues.

3. Get together with classmates and quiz each other on the concepts of this chapter. Use the points in reflection no. 1 and the questions you wrote for reflection no. 2 as a beginning. Explaining concepts out loud to others requires a deeper grasp of the material than feeling you understand it as you read.

4. Once you feel you understand the principles of application, practice applying massage, using the five-step approach, with a classmate or clinical colleague. Alternate applying each modality to each other. When it is being applied to you, listen and observe carefully to determine whether your classmate is using proper application. Consult your notes when the modality is applied to you, and during the first few times you apply the modality to another person. Continue practicing the application until you can do so without using your notes.

Concept Check Responses

CONCEPT CHECK 18.1

Petrissage, using the kneading, lifting, and wringing techniques, is the most effective stroke for relaxing the knot.

CONCEPT CHECK 18.2

Friction massage does not require a lubricant. Since the goal is to break up adhesive scar tissue, your thumbs or fingers need to remain in contact with the skin, not glide or slide over it.

REFERENCES

1. McIntyre E. Therapeutic massage: an amazing modality. *Home Health Care Mgt/Pract.* 2004;16(6):516–510.
2. Andrade C-K, Clifford P. *Outcome-Based Massage: From Evidence to Practice.* 2nd ed. Baltimore, MD: Lippincott Williams & Wilkins, 2008.
3. Massagetherapy.com. *Associated Bodywork & Massage Professionals* [web page]. Available at: http://www.massagetherapy.com/learn-more/index.php. Accessed March 2012.
4. National Center for Complementary and Alternative Medicine. *National Institutes of Health.* Available at: http://nccam.nih.gov/, March 2012.
5. Wong C. 10 Most Popular Types Of Massage Therapy. *About.com.* Available at: http://altmedicine.about.com/od/massage/a/massage_types.htm, March 2012.
6. Bond A. Top 10 Massage Techniques. *Care2 Make a Difference.* Available at: http://www.care2.com/greenliving/top-ten-massage-techniques.html. Accessed March 2012.
7. Best T, Hunter R, Wilcox A, Haq F. Effectiveness of sports massage for recovery of skeletal muscle from strenuous exercise. *Clin J Sport Med.* 2008;18(5):446–460.
8. Robb A, Sajko S. Conservative management of posterior interosseous neuropathy in an elite baseball pitcher's return to play: a case report and review of the literature. *J Can Chiroprac Assoc.* 2009;53(4):300–310.
9. Meltzer K, Cao T, Schad J, et al. In vitro modeling of repetitive motion injury and myofascial release. *J Bodyw Mov Ther.* 2010;14(2):162–171.
10. Bertolucci L. Muscle Repositioning: a new verifiable approach to neuro-myofascial release? *J Bodyw Mov Ther.* 2008;12(3):213–224.
11. Arroyo-Morales M, Olea N, Martinez M, et al. Effects of myofascial release after high-intensity exercise: a randomized clinical trial. *J Manipulative Physiol Ther.* 2008;31(3):217–223.
12. Fryer G, Morse C, Johnson J. Spinal and sacroiliac assessment and treatment techniques used by osteopathic physicians in the United States. *Osteopath Med Prim Care.* 2009;2009(3):4.
13. Black D. Treatment of knee arthrofibrosis and quadriceps insufficiency after patellar tendon repair: a case report including use of the graston technique. *Int J Ther Massage Bodywork.* 2010;3(2):14–51.
14. Hammer W. The effect of mechanical load on degenerated soft tissue. *J Bodyw Mov Ther.* 2008;12(3):246–256.

15. Rolf I. *Rolfing: Reestablishing the Natural Alignment and Structural Integration of the Human Body for Vitality and Well-Being.* Rochester, VT: Healing Arts Press, 1977.

16. Jones T. Rolfing. *Phys Med Rehabil Clin N Am.* 2004;15(4):799–509.

17. Russell J. Bodywork—the art of touch. *Nurse Pract Forum.* 1994;5(2):85–90.

18. DeLany J. Foundational platform of NMT. *International Academy of NMT.* Available at: http://www.nmtcenter.com/articles/NMT%20 Foundation%20Platform.pdf. Accessed August 2010.

19. Whedon J, Glassey D. Cerebrospinal fluid stasis and its clinical significance. *Altern Ther Health Med.* 2009;15(3):54–60.

20. Christine D. Temporal bone misalignment and motion asymmetry as a cause of vertigo: the craniosacral model. *Altern Ther Health Med.* 2009;15(6):38–42.

21. McManus V, Gliksten M. The use of craniosacral theapy in a physically impaired population in a disability service in southern Ireland. *J Altern Compelement Med.* 2007;13(9):923–930.

22. Green C, Martin C, Bassett K, Kazanjian A. A systematic review of craniosacral therapy: biological plausibility, assessment reliability and clinical effectiveness. *Complement Ther Med.* 1999;7(4): 201–207.

23. Flynn TW, Cleland JA, Schaible P. Craniosacral therapy and professional responsibility. *J Orthop Sports Phys Ther.* 2006;36(11):834–836.

24. Weerapong P, Hume P, Kolt G. The mechanisms of massage and effects on performance, muscle recovery and injury prevention. *Sports Med.* 2005;35(3):235–256.

25. Hinds T, McEwan I, Perkesm J, et al. Effects of massage on limb and skin blood flow after quadriceps exercise. *Med Sci Sport Exerc.* 2004;36(8):1308–1313.

26. Sefton J, Yarar C, Berry J, Pascoe D. Therapeutic massage of the neck and shoulders produces changes in peripheral blood flow when assessed with dynamic infrared thermography. *J Altern Complement Med.* 2010;16(7):723–732.

27. Wiltshire E, Poitras V, Pak M, et al. Massage impairs postexercise muscle blood flow and lactic acid: removal. *Med Sci Sport Exerc.* 2010;42(6):1060–1071.

28. Tiidus PM. Manual massage and recovery of muscle function following exercise: a literature review. *J Orthop Sports Phys Ther.* 1997;25(2):107–112.

29. Martin N, Zoeller R, Robertson R, Lephart S. The comparative effects of sports massage, active recovery, and rest in promoting blood lactate clearance after supramaximal leg exercise. *J Athl Train.* 1998;33(1):30–35.

30. Robertson A, Watt J, Galloway S. Effects of leg massage on recovery from high intensity cycling exercise. *Br J Sports Med.* 2002;38: 173–176.

31. Ogai R, Yamane M, Matsumoto T, Kosaka M. Effects of petrissage massage on fatigue and exercsie performance following intensive cycle pedalling. *Br J Sports Med.* 2008;42(10):834–838.

32. Sevier TL, Wilson JE. Treating lateral epicondylius. *Sports Med.* 1999;28(5):375–380.

33. Woodman R, Pare L. Evaluation and treatment of solt tissue lesions of the ankle and forefoot using the Cyraix approach. *Phys Ther.* 1982;62(8):1144–1147.

34. Cherkin D, Eisenberg D, Sherman K, et al. Randomized trial comparing traditional Chinese medical acupuncture, therapeutic massage, and self-care education for chronic low back pain. *Arch Intern Med.* 2001;161(8):1081–1088.

35. Suresh S, Wang S, Porfyris S, Kamasinski-Sol R, Steinhorn D. Massage therapy in outpatient pediatric chronic pain patients: Do they facilitate significant reductions in levels of distress, pain, tension, discomfort, and mood alterations? *Paediatr Anaesth.* 2008;18(9):884–887.

36. Sherman K, Cherkin D, Hawkes R, Miglioretti D, Deyo R. Randomized trial of therapeutic massage for chronic neck pain. *Clin J Pain.* 2009;25(3):233–238.

37. Cambron J, Dexheimer J, Coe P. Changes in blood pressure after various forms of Therapeutic massage: a preliminary study. *J Altern Complement Med.* 2006;12(1):65–70.

38. Calenda E. Massage therapy for cancer pain. *Curr Pain Headache Rep.* 2006;10(4):270–274.

39. Sagar S, Dryden T, Wong R. Massage therapy for cancer patients: a reciprocal relationship between body and mind. *Curr Oncol.* 2007;13(2):45–56.

40. Sturgeon M, Wetta-Hall R, Hart T, Good M, Dakhil S. Effects of therapeutic massage on the quality of life among patients with breast cancer during treatment. *J Altern Complement Med.* 2009;15(4): 373–380.

41. Boone T, Cooper R, Thompson WR. A physiologic evaluation of the sports massage. *Athl Train JNATA.* 1991;26(Spring):51–54.

42. Hemmings B, Smith M, Graydon J, Dyson R. Effects of massage on physiological restoration, perceived recovery, and repeated sports performance. *Br J Sports Med.* 2000;34(2):109–114; discussion 115.

43. Shoemaker JK, Tiidus PM, Mader R. Failure of manual massage to alter limb blood flow: measures by Doppler ultrasound. *Med Sci Sports Exerc.* 1997;29:610–614.

44. Tiidus PM, Shoemaker JK. Effleurage massage, blood flow flow, and long term post-exercise strength recovery. *Int J Sports Med.* 1995;1995:478–483.

45. Harmer PA. The effect of pre-performance massage on stride frequency in sprinters. *Athl Train JNATA.* 1991;26(Spring):55–59.

46. Sherman K, Ludman E, Cook A, et al. Effectiveness of therapeutic massage for generalized anxiety disorder: a randomized controlled trial. *Depress Anxiety.* 2010;27(5):441–450.

47. Hanley J, Stirling P, Brown C. Randomised controlled trial of therapeutic massage in the management of stress. *Br J Gen Pract.* 2003;53(486):20–25.

48. Bereznick D, Ross J, McGill S. The frictional properties at the thoracic skin–fascia interface: implications in spine manipulation. *Clin Biomech (Bristol, Avon).* 2002;17(4):297–303.

49. Batavia M. Contraindications for therapeutic massage: do sources agree? *J Bodyw Mov Ther.* 2004;8(1):48–57.

50. Dirckx JH. *Stedman's Medical Dictionary For The Health Professions and Nursing.* 6th ed. Baltimore, MD: Lippincott Williams & Wilkins, 2009.

51. Draper DO, Karns PB, Sokolowski MS. Chronic ankle and foot injuries in professional ice hockey players: Jumpstarting inflammation to re-direct healing. *J Athl Train.* 2001;38(2):S90.

52. Holey E, Cook E. *Evidence-Based Therapeutic Massage.* 3rd ed. London, England: Churchill Livingstone, 2011.

53. Liptan G. Fascia: A missing link in our understanding of the pathology of fibromyalgia. *J Bodyw Mov Ther.* 2010;14(1):2–12.

54. Stecco C, Porzionaato A, Macchi V, et al. Histological study of the deep fascia of the upper limb. *Ital J Anat Embryol.* 2006;111(2): 105–110.

55. Duparc F, Coquerel D, Ozeel J, et al. Anatomical basis of the suprascapular nerve entrapment, and clinical relevance of the supraspinatus fascia. *Surg Radiol Anat.* 2010;32(3):277–284.

56. Benjamin PJ, Lamp SP. *Understanding Sports Massage.* 2nd ed. Champaign, IL: Human Kinetics, 2005.

57. Benjamin P. *Tappan's Handbook of Healing Massage Techniques.* 5th ed. Upper Saddle River, NJ: Prentice, 2010.

58. Fritz S. *Fundamentals of Therapeutic Massage.* 4th ed. St. Louis, MO: Mosby-Lifeline, 1995.

59. Salvo SG. *Massage Therapy.* 3rd ed. Philadelphia, PA: WB Saunders, 2007.

60. Loving J. *Massage Therapy.* Stamford, CT: Appleton & Lange, 1999.

19

Spinal Traction

OPENING SCENE

A 47-year-old college professor has had episodes of back pain about every 6 months for the past few years. The pain would last 2 weeks and then disappear, until the last episode. After 5 weeks of pain, he had an MRI. The MRI revealed a herniated disk between vertebrae L3 and L4 and a bulging disk between L5 and S1 (Fig. 19.1). These irregularities explained the buttocks pain and radiating pain down his right leg. He was offered several solutions, including extension exercises, painkilling drugs, and traction. The medication and exercises helped, but the radiating pain still bothered him. He wondered if lumbar traction would help his situation.

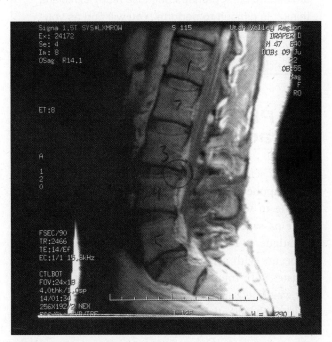

FIGURE 19.1 An MRI of the lumbar spine. Note the herniated disk between L3 and L4 and the bulging disk between L5 and S1. Manual, mechanical, and inversion traction was applied to this patient.

Cervical Pain and Lumbar Pain

The scenario in the opening scene is not uncommon; in fact, it happened to one of us (DD). As we get older, degenerative changes occur in the spine. Our intervertebral disks become thinner and lose elasticity, while calcium deposits, called **osteophytes**, form on the vertebrae. These changes often put pressure on nerve endings, resulting in neck or back pain.

Cervical pain, or neck pain and stiffness, is a common problem that affects up to 30% of people 25–29 years of age. Among working people over age 45, the percentage increases to 50%.[1] Pain that is referred to the arm may indicate irritation or entrapment of a cervical nerve root. Common causes are a bulging or herniated disk or degenerative changes,

including apophyseal joint or ligamentous hypertrophy and small bony outgrowths called osteophytes.[1]

Approximately 80% of the population will experience lumbar pain, or low-back pain, at some time in their lives; of these, 90% will resolve in 2–4 weeks, but 60–80% will recur within 1 year.[2] In the workplace, low-back pain is the leading cause of employee morbidity, disability, and lost productivity. Medical care is sought by 15–20% of those with back pain, making it the second most common reason for all physician visits.[3]

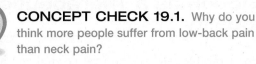

CONCEPT CHECK 19.1. Why do you think more people suffer from low-back pain than neck pain?

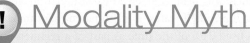

"I HAVE A SLIPPED DISK"

You may have heard someone say that she is suffering from a "slipped disk." The intervertebral disk is not one solid substance that can slip out of place like a hockey puck. Disks don't slip; they deform (bulge) or herniate (rupture or tear).

The Intervertebral Disk

Between each of our cervical, thoracic, and lumbar vertebrae is an **intervertebral disk** that functions to resist compressive forces and shock, provide flexibility, and provide adequate space between vertebrae. The outer layer of the disk is the **annulus fibrosus**, a series of interlacing cross-fibers that are attached to adjacent vertebral bodies. The inner layer is the **nucleus pulposus**, a protein gel between the cartilaginous end plates of the vertebrae and the annulus fibrosus.

The nucleus pulposus is watery, and as we age, it loses fluid (from 85 to 90% at birth to 70% by age 70) and its normal fullness. Another cause for a disk to lose its full size and normal shape is injury. The stretched or weakened annular fibers (annulus fibrosus) can protrude from the pressure of a bulging nucleus pulposus. For example, a bulging or **herniated disk** might look like what happens when you overinflate a bicycle tire inner tube that has a weak spot on it (Fig. 19.2).

If the disk is damaged and you move in a weight-bearing position, the nucleus pulposus will shift according to fluid-dynamic principles. For example, if you bend to the right side, the vertebrae squeeze the nucleus to the left. If tears develop in the annular fibers, the nucleus will tend to take the path of least resistance and move in this direction (Fig. 19.3).

Traction increases the separation of the vertebrae, decreases the central pressure in the disk space, and encourages the nucleus pulposus to return to a central position. The mechanical tension of the annulus fibrosus and ligaments surrounding the disk (especially the posterior longitudinal ligament) helps push the nucleus pulposus back into its proper place.[4]

Traction as a Therapeutic Modality

Several modalities are used to treat cervical and lumbar pain, including heat, cold, electrical stimulation, and exercise. In the United States, it is estimated that lumbar traction is used 21% of the time as part of a regimen to treat patients with low-back pain.[5]

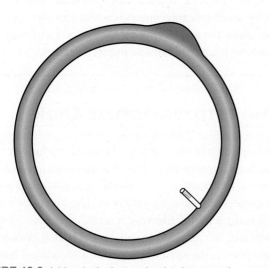

FIGURE 19.2 A bicycle tire inner tube that has a weak spot on it resembles a bulging or herniated disk.

Traction, from the Latin *tracio*, for "drawing or pulling apart,"[6] is a technique in which a pulling force is applied to body segments to stretch soft tissues and separate joint surfaces or bone fragments. Generally limited to the cervical or lumbar regions, traction has been used to treat fractures, dislocations, and spinal disorders for over 3000 years.

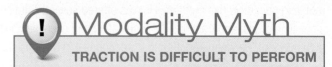

Modality Myth

TRACTION IS DIFFICULT TO PERFORM

Traction is one of the least used modalities among athletic trainers, perhaps because many clinicians think it is difficult to perform. You will find as you read this chapter that there are some methods of traction that are quite easy to perform.

The Physiological Effects of Traction

Results of scientific studies show that when 25 lb of traction are applied to the cervical spine, it elongates 2–20 mm, resulting in widening of the neural *foramen*, an opening for the passage of nerves or blood vesssels.[7] It is believed that fatigue or relaxation of the cervical paraspinal muscles occurs with cervical traction. The lumbar spine also elongates with traction when a force of about 50% of the body weight is used.[7]

Although scientists have demonstrated that traction can cause vertebral separation, it is short-lived. Once the traction force is removed and the patient sits or stands, the separation is reduced. However, traction can break the pain-spasm-pain cycle and muscle guarding and plays a valuable role in the overall treatment plan.

In one study, scientists used computed tomography to study the effects of traction on disk herniation in 30 patients.[8] The herniated nucleus pulposus material retracted during traction in 78.5% of median herniations, 66.6% of posterolateral herniations, and 57.1% of lateral herniations. Other mechanical changes were noted, including widening of disk spaces, separation of apophyseal joint facets, increase in neural foramina, and thinning of the ligamentum flavum. The authors attributed the retraction of the herniated nucleus pulposus during traction to a suction effect of negative intradiskal pressures and a pushing effect of the posterior longitudinal ligament. After 1 month of conservative treatment (heat, exercises) including traction, 28 of the 30 subjects had significant pain relief.[8]

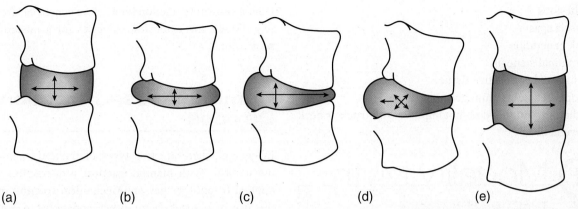

FIGURE 19.3 Intervertebral disk movement. **(a)** A disk, not bearing weight. **(b)** A normal weight-bearing disk. **(c)** A damaged disk and movement in a weight-bearing position shifts the nucleus pulposus. **(d)** Bending to the right side causes the vertebrae to squeeze the nucleus to the left. Tears in the fibers of the annulus fibrosus cause the nucleus to move in this direction. **(e)** Traction separates the vertebrae, decreases the central pressure in the disk space, and returns the nucleus pulposus to a central position. The mechanical tension of the annulus fibrosus and ligaments surrounding the disk helps push the disk back into place.

Pain relief is the main reason spinal traction is used. Traction appears to relieve pain by:[6,9–12]

- Increasing the space between vertebrae
- Separating the apophyseal joints
- Widening the intervertebral foramina
- Removing pressure or contact forces on injured tissue
- Increasing peripheral circulation
- Stretching muscles and ligaments
- Reducing muscle spasm
- Relaxing muscles
- Changing intervertebral disk pressures
- Tensing the posterior longitudinal ligament to exert force at the back of the vertebrae
- Creating suction to draw protruded disks toward their center
- Flattening of an abnormal lumbar curvature

Other than pain relief, spinal traction results in physiologic adaptations to various structures around the spine:

1. Bone. Increases spinal movement, overall and between each vertebra. Reverses immobilization-related bone weakness by increasing or maintaining bone density
2. Ligament. Creates ligament deformation, thereby increasing movement and decreasing impingement problems (long-term effects)
3. Articular facet joints. Increases the separation between joint surfaces. Decompresses articular cartilage, allowing synovial fluid exchange to nourish the cartilage. May decrease degenerative changes. May decrease pain perception
4. Muscles. Lengthens tight muscles and allows better muscular blood flow. Activates muscle *proprioceptors*, further decreasing pain
5. Nerves. Decreases compression forces on nerves

Guidelines Prior to Applying Traction

Prior to deciding on traction as a modality, a qualified clinician should study the results of the patient examination. The history, diagnostic test results, and current symptoms will determine whether or not traction is indicated or contraindicated.

It is important that you, as a student, observe several traction techniques performed by a qualified clinician before performing any techniques by yourself. You should be supervised until you become proficient at the traction techniques you employ.

Indications for Traction

Traction might be indicated for a patient when he/she presents with any or all of the following signs and symptoms: local or radiating pain, tightness, muscle spasm, weakness of limbs, or decreased deep tendon reflexes. Many of these signs and symptoms are associated with pressure on spinal nerves or connective tissue contractions. Traction is rarely used alone; it is part of a treatment regimen involving exercise, massage, electrical stimulation, and thermal modalities. The main effects of traction are mechanical. Therefore, the use of traction should be limited to conditions of the spine where the *mechanical effects* of traction would be expected to produce results. These include:

- Compression of nerve roots
- Disk protrusion
- Joint hypomobility

- Adhesions
- Muscle spasm
- Disk generation
- Foraminal stenosis
- Contracted connective tissue
- Apophyseal joint impingement
- Radiating pain that does not improve with truck or neck movement

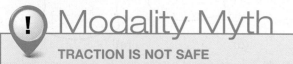

! Modality Myth

TRACTION IS NOT SAFE

Because traction involves the separation of spinal disks, many clinicians assume it is unsafe and that a patient can be easily paralyzed from traction. When used appropriately and with precaution, traction is a safe and effective modality.

Contraindications for Traction

Traction is contraindicated in some conditions. In general, traction is contraindicated following acute trauma to the neck or back. By acute, we mean that trauma caused the symptoms. Also, when traction increases **radicular pain**, or pain along the pathway of a spinal nerve, this technique should be avoided. Specific contraindications for cervical and lumbar traction include:

- Malignancy, either primary or metastatic
- Infectious diseases of the spine, such as tuberculosis

a. Uncontrolled hypertension
  - Rheumatoid arthritis
  - Spinal cord compression
  - Osteoporosis
  - Cardiovascular disease
  - Aortic aneurysm
  - Acute neck or low-back pain
  - Frail older adults
  - Severe respiratory disease
  - Hypermobile vertebrae (e.g., spondylolisthesis)
  - When traction increases radicular pain

Specific contraindications for lumbar traction include:

b. Pregnancy
  - Hiatal hernia
  - Abdominal hernia
  - Active peptic ulcers
  - Glaucoma (inversion gravity method)

Do not substitute traction for a "more beneficial" treatment (e.g., McKenzie extension exercises for a posterior disk protrusion).

Commonly Used Traction Devices

In general, there are two types of traction, manual and mechanical. With **manual traction**, a distraction force is applied by another person. **Mechanical traction** involves the use of a machine or other apparatus to apply the distractive force.

Cervical Traction

The literature shows more support for cervical traction than lumbar traction.[4,6,9,13–16] Cervical traction is generally applied with the patient in a supine or sitting position. The supine position is preferred over sitting because it eliminates the effects of gravity. This allows for increased relaxation of the patient, decreased muscle guarding, more separation between vertebral bodies, and less force having to be applied by the clinician.[13] There are three main types of cervical traction: manual cervical traction, pneumatic mechanical traction, and motorized intermittent or sustained traction.

MANUAL CERVICAL TRACTION

This technique is the one that is most readily available to the clinician because usually no equipment is needed except the hands. It enables the clinician to feel the patient's reaction to the treatment.

Manual traction should always be applied before mechanical traction when treating the neck. This approach lets you carefully control the applied force and head position to maximize the relief of symptoms. To perform this technique, have the patient lie down in a supine position on a padded treatment table. Sit or stand at the head of the table facing the patient. Cradle the head in your hands or with a towel, in a position that allows distraction of the cervical vertebrae without causing any discomfort to the patient (Fig. 19.4). Begin with gentle traction of 10–15 lb, then slowly increase the force up to 25 lb, which is necessary to overcome the resistance of the head and soft tissue structures.[7,13] As you apply traction, slowly move the head into a position of greatest relaxation and comfort as follows:

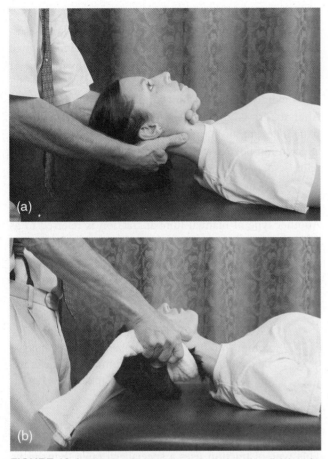

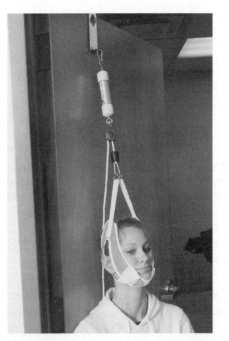

FIGURE 19.5 Mechanical traction. Note the harness, the rope, and the pulley attached to the top of the door. Pulling on the rope spreads the vertebra.

FIGURE 19.4 When performing manual traction, the clinician sits or stands at the head of the table facing the patient. The head is cradled in **(a)** the hands or **(b)** in a towel to allow distraction of the cervical vertebrae without hurting the patient. As traction is applied, the head is slowly moved to maximize relaxation and comfort.

- Neutral position for pain affecting the upper cervical vertebrae
- Flexed 30° for pain affecting the lower cervical vertebrae
- Lateral flexion for pressure on spinal nerves with radiating pain into the arms/hands

✔ APPLICATION TIP

START WITH MANUAL TRACTION

When treating the neck, always start with manual traction. If the patient tolerates it, you can then apply mechanical traction. You can stop a motion that might be troublesome to the patient more rapidly with manual traction.

MECHANICAL CERVICAL TRACTION

The simplest form of mechanical traction involves a harness, which cradles the patient's neck, a rope attached to the harness, and a pulley that is anchored to the wall or a door (Fig. 19.5) The rope runs up from the harness, through the pulley, and back down to the AT or patients hand. Pulling on the rope applies traction to the spine, separating the vertebrae. The goal is that through repeated treatments the spinal column will readjust to a normal posture, thereby reliving pain.

Pneumatic Mechanical Traction

The Posture Pump® pump is a fairly new technology that allows self-administered treatment of neck pain and postural dysfunction.[17,18] The technique, known as expanding ellipsoidal decompression (EED),[17] decompresses vertebral disks, and therefore allows them to realign.

The Cervical Posture Pump® is a pneumatic bladder device with ellipsoidal air cells that cradle the patient's head and shoulders (Fig. 19.6). The patient uses a hand pump to inflate the bladder, the force of which applies an upward pressure to the spine, gently forcing it into its natural lordotic position. In addition, the central air cell provides a milking action to the vertebra and disks.[19]

The unique action of the ellipsoidal air cells as they inflate and deflate causes joints of the cervical spine to decompress and simultaneously align the joints at the anterior and posterior aspect of the vertebral bodies and disks. In addition, the alternating action is thought to create an alternating hydration and milking of the intervertebral disks. Holding the air pressure constant over a period of 15–20 minutes has the effect of shaping or molding the spine into a curved or ellipsoidal shape. EED does not remove the normal curved

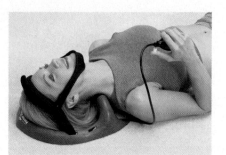

FIGURE 19.6 The Posture Pump® for the cervical region. Note the inflation pump, which is operated by repeated hand compressions. Patients should inflate the bladder to a comfortable pressure.

shape from the spine as linear traction and is therefore not harmful to the natural spinal curves.[17]

Mechanical Intermittent or Sustained Traction

This type of cervical traction uses a head harness attached to a mechanical device at the end of a table (Fig. 19.7). The device can pull sustained traction, or intermittent traction (usually 30 seconds on, 10 seconds off). Moeti and Marchetti[18] applied mechanical intermittent cervical traction to 15 patients with radiating pain from pressure on spinal nerves. Those who had been experiencing pain for 12 weeks or less demonstrated a reduction in pain and disability.[18]

 CONCEPT CHECK 19.2. A patient comes to your athletic training clinic with an MRI that shows a bulging disk at C6 and C7. She complains of radiating pain down to her thumb, index, middle finger, and the dorsal aspect of her forearm. Is this consistent with the nerve roots that are affected? What traction techniques would provide the greatest benefit to help decrease the pain and the cause? Why?

Lumbar Traction

There are more types of lumbar traction than cervical traction available to the clinician. The following are some of the most commonly used techniques.[20]

MANUAL LUMBAR TRACTION

Similar to manual cervical traction, this technique is the most readily available to the clinician, allows the clinician to feel the patient's reaction to the treatment, and can be used as an examination technique. The clinician uses his hands or a belt to pull on the patient's legs and separate the vertebrae (Fig. 19.8).

Single-Leg Traction

One type of manual traction for the lumbar area is single-leg traction (Fig. 19.9). To apply this technique, two clinicians are required. The patient can lie down prone or supine on the table. One clinician supports the patient's torso, while the other clinician pulls traction on the leg. After a series of five 30-second bouts of traction, the patient lies supine at the edge of the table and stretches the affected hip flexors which are usually tight with radicular pain.

Unilateral Leg-Pull Manual Traction

Another type of manual lumbar traction is referred to as unilateral leg-pull traction. In this technique, the patient lies supine. The clinician pulls traction on one leg with the patient's hip in 30° of flexion, 30° of abduction, and maximal outward rotation.

 CONCEPT CHECK 19.3. A patient comes into the clinic complaining of radiating pain all down her right leg from the buttocks to the foot. What type of traction might give her some immediate relief?

MECHANICAL LUMBAR TRACTION

This type of traction uses a specialized table that can be separated when adequate forces are applied. The patient's head and torso are on one half of the table, and the legs are on the other half. One end of a strap, belt, or harness is firmly attached to the patient, and the other end is attached to a mechanical device that applies a traction force that slowly elongates the lower spine (Fig. 19.10). There are two types of mechanical lumbar traction: sustained and intermittent.

Sustained Traction

Sustained traction involves a sustained force that is about 50% of the patient's body weight. The force is slightly less than intermittent traction, since there is no rest period. Treatment time is typically 10–30 minutes.

Intermittent Traction

The intensity of intermittent traction is slightly greater than sustained traction, but the treatment can last longer because there is a rest period (when the unit is off). This technique uses a mechanical device to alternately apply and release the traction force at preset intervals. The typical intervals are 30 seconds on, 30 seconds off. Longer on periods of up to 60 seconds are recommended for disk injury, whereas shorter on periods of 15 seconds are recommended for joint facet dysfunction.

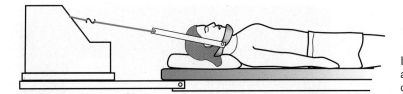

FIGURE 19.7 Cervical traction using a head harness attached to a mechanical device at the end of a table. It can provide sustained or intermittent traction.

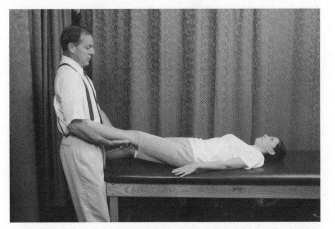

FIGURE 19.8 In manual lumbar traction, the clinician pulls, with hands or a belt, on the patient's legs to separate the vertebrae.

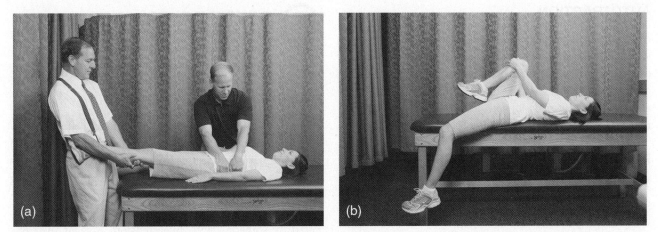

FIGURE 19.9 Manual single-leg traction. The patient lies down prone or supine on the table. **(a)** One clinician supports the patient's torso, while the other clinician pulls traction on the leg. **(b)** After the traction, the patient lies at the edge of the table and stretches the hip flexors, which are usually tight with radicular pain.

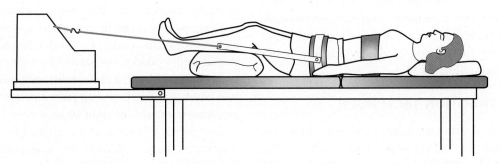

FIGURE 19.10 Mechanical lumbar traction uses a specialized table, whose top section separates, thus facilitating elongation of the lower spine when torso movement is restricted and adequate force is applied to the torso.

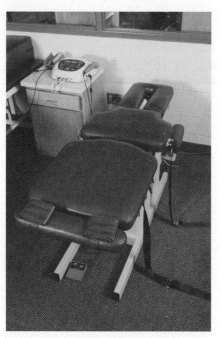

FIGURE 19.11 The two sections of an autotraction table can be individually tilted and rotated.

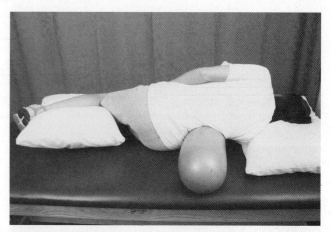

FIGURE 19.12 Positional lumbar traction. The patient is lying on the nonpainful side with a bolster under the side of the trunk, causing lateral trunk flexion. This increases the spaces between the vertebrae on the painful side, releasing pressure on the affected spinal nerve.

POOL TRACTION

Pool traction is applied in an aquatic setting and uses buoyancy of the water to reduce weight on the spine.

 CONCEPT CHECK 19.4. How could a water flotation belt or water ankle cuffs be used to assist someone who has low-back pain? Answer the question, and then look at Figure 19.13.

INVERSION TABLE TRACTION

Inversion table traction is an inexpensive, effective way to gain the benefits of traction. The patient is suspended upside down or at various angles by the ankles or thighs (Fig. 19.14). This position allows the weight of the upper body to act as a traction force. Because it causes significant increases in blood pressure, the technique is contraindicated by someone with hypertension. Also, it increases pressure to the eyes, so patients with glaucoma should not use inversion traction. Guvenol et al.[21] reported no difference between inversion traction and mechanical traction in alleviating symptoms of herniated lumbar disk patients.

One of us (DD) has used both mechanical and inversion table traction. The preference is the inversion table. It is inexpensive and can be purchased at warehouse stores for <$200, making it ideal for home use. The table is easy to use, and it works; the straps don't slip and give you a wedge like they often do on horizontal mechanical traction tables. For a step-by-step procedure on how to use an inversion traction table (Box 19.1).

Remember, when traction is applied to the low back, it increases the separation of the vertebrae and decreases the central pressure in the intervertebral disk spaces. By immediately performing prone extension following traction, the posterior longitudinal ligament helps push the

AUTOTRACTION

Autotraction uses a specially designed table divided into two sections that can be individually tilted and rotated. Patients can apply the tractive force by holding on to, or pulling on, overhead bars (Fig. 19.11). Because of the cost of the table, and the difficulty patients with low-back pain have experienced with this technique, its use has recently declined.

POSITIONAL LUMBAR TRACTION

The idea behind positional lumbar traction is to place the patient in a position where the body can pull traction on itself. This is accomplished by using bolsters or rolled-up towels to maintain flexion and rotation of the spine in order to achieve distraction of a specific vertebral segment. The goal is to alleviate pressure on an entrapped spinal nerve, thus decreasing pain and promoting muscle relaxation. The most common technique is to have the patient lie down on the non-painful side. The bolster is then placed under the side of the trunk, producing lateral trunk flexion. This should lead to increased spacing between the vertebrae on the painful side, thereby releasing pressure on the spinal nerve (Fig. 19.12).

THE 90/90 TRACTION TECHNIQUE

This technique is self-administered and convenient for home treatment. The patient is positioned with the hips and knees flexed to 90°. The patient then tilts the pelvis and flattens the lumbar lordosis by pulling on a rope that traverses the unit's frame and attaches to a pelvic harness.

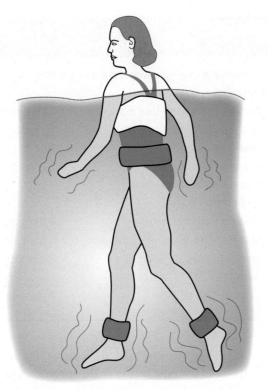

FIGURE 19.13 A flotation belt and water cuffs cause drag, resulting in traction on the lumbar vertebrae.

nuclear material of the disks back into proper position (Fig. 19.15).[4]

EXPANDING ELLIPSOIDAL DECOMPRESSION

The concept of EED with a posture pump, discussed in the cervical traction section above, can also be applied to the lumbar spine as well. The appliance used is different however (Fig. 19.16). EED does not remove the normal curved

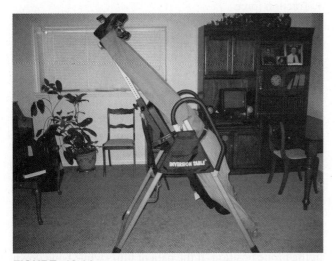

FIGURE 19.14 Inversion table traction. When the patient is suspended upside down, the weight of the upper body acts as a traction force.

BOX 19.1 USING INVERSION TABLE TRACTION

A. Set the length adjustment by pulling the spring-loaded pin at the bottom of the table and setting it at your height.

B. Adjust the strap on the bottom of the table to determine the angle at which you want to unload the spine. For example, many people find that it is difficult to start hanging directly upside down and prefer to start at a 45° or 60° angle until they get used to the table.

C. Adjust the padded leg clamps so that the ankles will slide comfortably into place.

D. Step into the padded leg clamps. Some people go barefoot; others prefer to wear shoes as extra padding.

E. Lie down supine on the table. You may place a lumbar roll into the small of your back for added support.

F. Reach both arms over your head, and the table should slowly invert. If the table inverts too quickly for your comfort, simply grasp onto the side rails and slow the table down.

G. Remember, separation of the joint surfaces is resisted by the muscles and other soft tissues surrounding the joints. While in the inverted position, try to relax your muscles and your breathing as much as possible. If you do this, you will be able to take the pressure off your nerves and intervertebral disks. At first you might be comfortable in this position for only 1–2 minutes, but eventually you can train yourself to relax and enjoy this for 10–15 minutes.

H. Slowly bring your arms back to your waist, grasp hold of the side rails, and bring the table to a horizontal position to let the blood return to your lower limbs.

I. Repeat the process. See if you can do three sets of 5 minutes each.

J. When you are finished with the last set, slowly return to the starting position. Get off the table, and lie down prone on the floor. It may help to use a 12-inch firm wedge and remain in this position for 30 minutes while reading a book.

shape from the spine as linear traction, so it not harmful to the natural spinal curves.[17]

One of us (DD) has used the posture pump on both the cervical and the lumbar regions and has found it to be one of the easiest and most effective devices for relieving the pain associated with bulging disks.

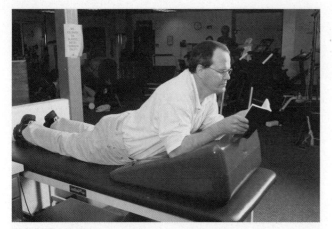

FIGURE 19.15 Lying prone and using a wedge after inversion table traction help readjust the position of the intervertebral disks.

Researchers stated that MRI changes were often dramatic—with improvement cervical and lumbar spine, widening of disk spaces, and often apparent shrinking of what appears to be disk bulges, which they thought would be physically permanent (Box 19.2). This approach appears to be the simplest, safest, and least expensive approach to date for treating chronic neck and back pain.[17]

THE EFFECTIVENESS OF LUMBAR TRACTION

Of the techniques of lumbar traction we have described, most of the research has been performed on sustained and intermittent mechanical traction. The results of the studies are mixed. For example, Beurskens[22] concluded that lumbar traction was no more effective than placebo. However, Meszaros[23] reported that when an adequate traction force was applied, lumbar traction significantly reduced pain. Harte et al.[24] performed a systematic review of randomized clinical studies on lumbar traction, concluding that the variability in the results of lumbar traction studies might be due to poorly designed studies and limited applications of traction in clinical practice.[24]

Based on the observations that many patients with intractable pain obtain rapid relief with the application of an adequate load, traction is given intermittently. In both intermittent and intermittent pulsed traction (which

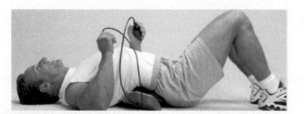

FIGURE 19.16 The Posture Pump® for the lumbar region. Note the inflation pump. When this is compressed by the hand, the bladders inflate to the desired pressure of the patient.

BOX 19.2 RESULTS AFTER ONE 20-MINUTE POSTURE PUMP® TREATMENT[17]	
The following changes were noted in the MRI's of 34 patients.	
1 or more decreased disk bulges:	20 patients
Disk lightening (increased disk hydration)	16 patients
Decreased disk bulges with decreases in spinal cord indentation	7 patients
Increased lordotic curve	6 patients
Stress vertebra alignment changes	3 patients
Changes in stair stepping of vertebra	2 patients
No visible MRI change	2 patients

allows a gradual increase and decrease of the traction force), the brief periodic nature of the application permits the use of larger loads without significant stress to the patient. No form of traction is entirely without discomfort.

 CONCEPT CHECK 19.5. A patient comes to your physical therapy clinic with weakness of hip flexion. How would you treat the most probable cause with traction techniques.

Treatment Parameters

The treatment parameters for traction are:

- Patient position
- Treatment mode
- Traction force
- Duration
- Frequency

PATIENT POSITION

For cervical traction, the patient can be sitting or supine. When lumbar traction is applied, the patient can be standing, sitting, supine, prone, and horizontal or inclined.[19] One way of determining the appropriate patient position for lumbar traction is to first find out what position decreases the pain when standing. For example, if the patient hurts while sitting but the pain goes away while he is lying or during trunk extension (such as would happen with a posterior bulging disk), he will probably respond best to traction in the prone position. If the patient hurts while lying down or in trunk flexion but the pain decreases while sitting, he will probably respond best to traction in the supine position. The most important thing to remember is that muscle relaxation is considered essential to achieving the optimal effects of traction.[18] Therefore, the patient should be positioned so that muscle relaxation is maximized.

TREATMENT MODE

Treatment mode refers to applying traction in either the sustained or the intermittent mode. There are varied opinions regarding which mode is better to use. Some believe that sustained traction is essential to fatiguing the muscles and allowing the traction force to act on the joints, whereas intermittent traction creates a stretch reflex and is ineffective in reducing disk problems.[9]

Others are of the opinion that the same result can occur with both modes of traction, although patients are more able to tolerate higher forces when traction is intermittent. Still others state that the diagnosis should determine which mode to follow.[6] For example, if the diagnosis is a disk protrusion, the sustained method (or longer hold-rest periods) should be employed. If the diagnosis is degenerative disk disease or joint hypomobility, the intermittent mode (with shorter hold-rest periods) should be used.[6]

TRACTION FORCE

A force of sufficient magnitude and duration must be exerted to separate the vertebrae. This can be done by weights and pulleys, mechanical devices, or manually. The direction of the traction force may be either vertical, horizontal, or at an angle.

The magnitude of the needed force depends on the frictional resistance to traction and the resistance to stretch by the muscles and soft tissues. A small additional force will bring about separation of the vertebrae. During traction, movement of the body by the external force must be resisted by an equal and opposite force—either body weight or friction with the surface that is in contact with the body. The friction force is approximately equal to one half the body weight. Gravity may either assist or resist traction.[25] When frictional resistance is not sufficient to prevent movement, an additional counterforce must be added. This force also dissipates some of the desired traction force and hence some of the effectiveness. The part of the force that is lost as a stretch force must be reclaimed by applying a heavier traction force unless the frictional resistance can be overcome or eliminated. This can be done with a split traction table or by applying the force in a vertical position.

Separation of the joint surfaces is also resisted by the muscles and other soft tissues surrounding the joints. The traction force must then be increased by a force sufficient to overcome this additional resistance to stretch before distraction of the joint surfaces can take place. In clinical practice, the patient's tolerance and response to stretch must be the ultimate guide in the therapeutic use of traction.

The minimum traction force to get separation in the cervical spine is about 25 lb, although there is general disagreement about the minimum force needed for effective treatment. The angle of pull also plays a significant role in the cervical spine. For example, when the neck is flexed to 20–30°, the anterior curve of the cervical spine is decreased. Traction force applied at between 20° and 30° of flexion has been shown to give moderate to complete pain relief.

For lumbar traction, there are similar disagreements about the necessary and sufficient force to obtain clinical relief. Meszaros[23] studied patients with low-back pain and found significant decreases in pain when 30% and 50% of the patient's body weight was used as the traction force. When only 10% of the patient's body weight was used as a traction force, there was no reduction in pain.[23]

The lumbar muscles resistance to stretch is considerable. We recommend starting with 25% of the body weight, and if this is easily tolerated, increase the force to 50% of the patient's weight. Elimination of the lumbar lordosis has been suggested as a method of reducing the traction force needed to obtain separation of the vertebrae. It is apparent, then, that the proper angle of pull is just as important in lumbar traction as it is in cervical traction.

✔ APPLICATION TIP

USE THE ONE-THIRD GUIDELINE WHEN SETTING UP INTERMITTENT TRACTION FORCE CYCLES

With intermittent traction, the force applied at rest is typically one third of the force applied during the on setting. For example, if the force during the on cycle is set at 90 lb, the force during the off cycle should be set at 30 lb.

DURATION

Recommended treatment times for sustained or intermittent traction range from a few minutes to 40 min. The important thing to remember is during the first session, apply traction for just a short time, and then assess the patient's response to the treatment.[25]

FREQUENCY

Although some scientists advocate daily treatment sessions, there have been no scientific studies to suggest that traction performed daily is any better than traction performed every other day. Because many health insurance companies limit the number of reimbursable visits, many clinicians schedule their patients to be treated every other day.

Application of Spinal Traction

As previously stated, traction should not be administered until a full evaluation has been completed, a definitive diagnosis has been made, and specific indications for traction have been established.[25] Careful history taking, a physical examination, and diagnostic x-rays of the spine are all necessary. Traction is usually administered in conjunction with heat, massage, and immobilization. Exercises may also be used if indicated.[25]

Space will not allow us to describe how to apply all of the several types of traction. Thus, we have limited our scope to one manual and one mechanical traction technique of the cervical and lumbar spine:

- Manual cervical traction
- Mechanical cervical traction (intermittent or sustained)
- Manual lumbar traction (unilateral leg pull)
- Mechanical lumbar traction (intermittent or sustained)

STEP 1: FOUNDATION

A. Definition. Traction is a technique in which a pulling force is applied to body segments to stretch soft tissues and separate joint surfaces or bone fragments.
B. Effects
   1. Spinal movement
      a. Increases spinal movement, overall and between each vertebra
   2. Bone
      a. Reverses immobilization-related bone weakness by increasing or maintaining bone density
   3. Ligament
      a. Creates ligament deformation, thereby increasing movement and decreasing impingement problems (long-term effects)
   4. Articular facet joints
      a. Increases separation of joint surfaces
      b. Decompresses articular cartilage, allowing synovial fluid exchange to nourish the cartilage
      c. May decrease degenerative changes
      d. May decrease pain perception
   5. Muscular system
      a. Lengthens tight muscles
      b. Allows better muscular blood flow
      c. Activates muscle proprioceptors, further decreasing pain
   6. Nerves
      a. Decreases compression forces on nerves
C. Advantages
   1. See Effects, above

D. Disadvantages
   1. Manual traction can become physically tiring for the clinician to perform.
   2. For some techniques, special equipment is required.
   3. Once the traction force is removed and the patient sits or stands, the vertebral separation is reduced.
E. Indications
   1. Compression of nerve roots
   2. Disk protrusion
   3. Joint hypomobility
   4. Adhesions
   5. Muscle spasm
   6. Disk generation
   7. Foraminal stenosis
   8. Contracted connective tissue
   9. Apophyseal joint impingement
   10. Radiating pain that does not improve with truck or neck movement
F. Contraindications
   1. Cervical and lumbar traction
      a. Malignancy, either primary or metastatic
      b. Infectious diseases of the spine, such as tuberculosis
      c. Uncontrolled hypertension
      d. Rheumatoid arthritis
      e. Spinal cord compression
      f. Osteoporosis
      g. Cardiovascular disease
      h. Aortic aneurysm
      i. Acute neck or low-back pain
      j. Frail older adults
      k. Severe respiratory disease
      l. Hypermobile vertebrae (e.g., spondylolisthesis)
      m. When traction increases radicular pain
   2. Lumbar traction
   3. Pregnancy
   4. Hiatal hernia
   5. Abdominal hernia
   6. Active peptic ulcers
   7. Glaucoma (inversion gravity method)
G. Precautions
   1. Do not substitute traction for a "more beneficial" treatment (e.g., extension exercises for a posterior disk protrusion).

STEP 2: PREAPPLICATION TASKS

A. Make sure traction is the proper modality for this situation.

1. Reevaluate the injury/problem. Make sure you understand the patient's condition.
2. Check for contraindications.
3. Confirm that the objectives of therapy are compatible with the use of traction.

B. Preparing the patient psychologically
   1. Explain that a "pulling" sensation should be felt, but it should not cause discomfort.
   2. The force should relieve pressure and decrease any radiating pain due to pressure on nerves.

C. Preparing the patient physically
   1. Remove clothing, earrings, bandages, tape, braces, etc., as necessary.
   2. Secure the head harness (cervical traction) or chest and pelvic harness (lumbar traction) to the patient.
   3. Position the patient.
      a. Manual cervical traction
         i. Supine on padded treatment table
         ii. Head is cradled in the clinician's hands by placing one hand under the patient's chin and the other hand supporting the back of the head starting at the occiput.
         iii. Head is flexed 20–30°.
      b. Mechanical cervical traction
         i. Supine on padded treatment table
         ii. Attach the harness to the mechanical unit so the maximum pull is placed on the occiput, not the chin.
         iii. Neck is flexed 20–30°.
      c. Unilateral leg-pull manual traction (lumbar)
         i. Supine
         ii. 30° hip flexion
         iii. 30° hip abduction
         iv. Maximal outward rotation
      d. Mechanical lumbar traction
         i. Depends on technique used

D. Equipment preparation
   1. For mechanical traction, see the user manual for specific setups.
   2. Make sure the machine is operating properly.
   3. Make sure the displayed traction is correct.
   4. Make sure the duty cycle is operating properly, if using intermittent traction.

3 STEP 3: APPLICATION PARAMETERS

A. Procedures
   1. Manual cervical traction
      a. With the head supported, the clinician gently applies a force (20–25 lb) toward her.
      b. An intermittent force is applied lasting 5–10 seconds on with a very short rest period.
      c. Total treatment time is 3–10 minutes.

   2. Mechanical cervical traction
      a. With the head supported in the harness, the machine gently applies a force (20–25 lb).
      b. An intermittent force is applied with an on-off ratio of 3:1 or 4:1. For example, if the on time was 12 seconds, the off time would be 3 or 4 seconds.
      c. Total treatment time is 20–25 minutes.
   3. Manual lumbar traction (unilateral leg pull)
      a. A steady pull is applied until a noticeable distraction is felt.
   4. Mechanical lumbar traction
      a. Intermittent or sustained
      b. Select force of traction.
      c. Select duty cycle (if intermittent).
      d. Select number of progressive steps (if intermittent).
      e. Select treatment time.

B. Dosage
   1. Cervical
      a. Sustained: up to 25 lb
      b. Intermittent: up to 25 lb
   2. Lumbar
      a. Sustained: Start with 25% of body weight, then work up to 50% of body weight
      b. Intermittent: Start with 25% of body weight, then work up to 50% of body weight

C. Length of application
   1. Cervical
      a. Sustained: 10 minutes
      b. Intermittent: 20 seconds on, 5 seconds off for 20–25 minutes
   2. Lumbar
      a. Sustained: 4 minutes or more
      b. Intermittent: 15 seconds on, 10 seconds off for 20–25 minutes

D. Frequency of application
   1. Every day, if possible

E. Duration of therapy
   1. Traction can be used daily, as long as it helps to decrease pain.

4 STEP 4: POSTAPPLICATION TASKS

A. Equipment removal
   1. Remove harness or belts from the patient.
   2. Make sure the machine is turned off.

B. Instructions to the patient
   1. Schedule the next treatment.
   2. Instruct the patient about the level of activity and/or self-treatment prior to the next formal treatment.
   3. Instruct the patient about what he/she should feel following treatment.

C. Record of treatment, including unique patient responses
D. Clean up
   1. Clean off the table (if used).

5 **STEP 5: MAINTENANCE**

A. Periodic check of belts, harnesses (etc.) to ensure they are in good working order.

CLOSING SCENE

The professor in the chapter opening scene had a herniated disk and a bulging lumbar disk that were causing pain. He tried extension exercises, walking, cardio-glide at the gym, intermittent traction tables, and massage. Each of these provided only temporary relief from the radiating pain. After 3 months, he purchased an inversion table traction unit for his home. He used this two or three times a day for 5–10 minutes each time, and ended each session with extension exercises. This routine provided him the most relief, and slowly (over 4 weeks) the radiating pain began to centralize (returned to the origin) and diminish.[26,27] He did end up having a partial surgical removal of the disk between L3 and L4. However, the disk between L5 and S1 was saved, probably due to traction, extension, exercise, and luck.

Chapter Reflections

1. Read and ponder each of the following points. Do you feel you have a clear understanding of each concept? If not, reread the appropriate section of the chapter.
   • Define traction.
   • List the physiological effects of traction.
   • Describe the difference between manual and mechanical traction.
   • Identify the parameters for delivering cervical traction.
   • Name the parameters for delivering lumbar traction.
   • List the indications for traction.
   • List the contraindications for traction.
2. Write three to five questions for discussion with your class instructor, clinical instructor, classmates, and clinical colleagues.
3. Get together with classmates and quiz each other on the concepts of this chapter. Use the points in #1 and the questions you wrote for #2 as a beginning. Explaining concepts out loud to others requires a deeper grasp of the material than feeling you understand it as you read.

4. Once you feel you understand the principles of application, practice applying massage, using the five-step approach, with a classmate or clinical colleague. Alternate applying each modality to each other. When it is being applied to you, listen and observe carefully to determine whether your classmate is using proper application. Consult your notes when the modality is applied to you, and during the first few times you apply the modality to another person. Continue practicing the application until you can do so without using your notes.

Concept Check Responses

CONCEPT CHECK 19.1

People have low-back and neck pain for a couple of reasons. One reason is poor mechanics from lifting; we should bend more at the knees and use our legs, not our back. A simple reason is that our lumbar region supports much more weight than the cervical spine.

CONCEPT CHECK 19.2

Yes this is consistent with the dermatomes of C6 and C7. Possible traction techniques that would provide her the greatest benefit to help decrease the pain and the cause are using the Posture Pump® and manual traction.

The Posture Pump® would provide for separation of the joints at the anterior and posterior aspect of the vertebral bodies and disks in a ratio coinciding with their natural wedged spacing. Continuous expansion and contraction of the air cells to create alternating hydration and milking of the intervertebral disks. Holding the air pressure constant over a period of 15–20 minutes has the effect of shaping or molding the spine into a curved or ellipsoidal shape.

CONCEPT CHECK 19.3

An irritation of the sciatic nerve is probably causing the pain to radiate from the buttocks down the patient's entire right leg. Manual single-leg traction applied to the right leg can increase intervertebral disk space of the lumbar vertebrae and decrease pressure on this nerve.

CONCEPT CHECK 19.4

A flotation belt or ankle cuffs could be worn as the patient swims in a horizontal position, causing drag and thereby creating traction on the vertebrae.

CONCEPT CHECK 19.5

- Strain of the hip flexor muscles (rectus femoris, iliopsoas, and sartorius)
- Contusion of the origin of the hip flexor muscles
- Bulging disks at L1, L2, L3, and L4

The two most probable traction techniques are inversion table traction and EED (Posture Pump®). The reason for inversion table traction is it provides very good continuous separation of the vertebrae that put pressure on the disks. After a 5- to 10-minute treatment, the patient could lie in a prone position with the back extended, which will help the posterior longitudinal ligament to push the bulging disk back into the central part of the disk.

The reason for using EED via the (Posture Pump®) is for separation in which joints of the lordotic spinal region are decompressed and simultaneously aligned in a curved or lordotic configuration. Using a handheld pump, ellipsoidal air cells expand and contract from within the lordotic spinal concavity separating the joints at the anterior and posterior aspect of the vertebral bodies and disks in a ratio coinciding with their natural wedged spacing. Continuous expansion and contraction of the air cells can be employed to create alternating hydration and milking of the intervertebral disks. Holding the air pressure constant over a period of 15–20 minutes has the effect of shaping or molding the spine into a curved or ellipsoidal shape.

REFERENCES

1. Shakoor MA, Ahmed MS, Kibria G, et al. Effects of cervical traction and exercise therapy in cervical spondylosis. *Bangladesh Med Res Counc Bull.* 2002;28(2):61–69.
2. Hides JA, Richardson CA, Jull GA. Multifidus muscle recovery is not automatic after resolution of acute, first-episode low back pain. *Spine.* 1996;21(23):2763–2769.
3. Cypress BK. Characteristics of physician visits for back symptoms: a national perspective. *Am J Public Health.* 1983;73(4):389–395.
4. Ellenberg MR, Honet JC, Treanor WJ. Cervical radiculopathy. *Arch Phys Med Rehabil.* 1994;75(3):342–352.
5. Jette AM, Delitto A. Physical therapy treatment choices for musculoskeletal impairments. *Phys Ther.* 1997;77(2):145–154.
6. Saunders H, Saunders R. *Evaluation, Treatment and Prevention of Musculoskeletal Disorders: Spine.* Vol 1. 3rd ed. Bloomington: Educational Opportunities, 1995.
7. Geiringer SR, deLateur BJ. Physiatric therapeutics. 3. Traction, manipulation, and massage. *Arch Phys Med Rehabil.* 1990;71 (4-S):S264–266.
8. Onel D, Tuzlaci M, Sari H, Demir K. Computed tomographic investigation of the effect of traction on lumbar disc herniations. *Spine.* 1989;14(1):82–90.
9. Cyriax J, Russell G. *Textbook of Orthopaedic Medicine, vol. 2: Treatment by Manipulation, Massage and Injection.* 10th ed. London: Bailliere Tindall, 1980.
10. Cailliet R. *Low Back Pain Syndrome.* Philadelphia, PA: F.A. Davis Co., 1988.
11. Goldish G. Lumbar Traction. *Interdisciplinary Rehabilitation of Low Back Pain.* Baltimore, MD: Williams and Wilkins, 1989:305–321.
12. Krause M, Refshauge KM, Dessen M, Boland R. Lumbar spine traction: evaluation of effects and recommended application for treatment. *Man Ther.* 2000;5(2):72–81.
13. Cameron M. *Physical Agents in Rehabilitation: From Research to Practice.* St. Louis, MO: Saunders, 2003.
14. Swezey RL, Swezey AM, Warner K. Efficacy of home cervical traction therapy. *Am J Phys Med Rehabil.* 1999;78(1):30–32.
15. Tekeoglu I, Adak B, Bozkurt M, Gurbuzoglu N. Distraction of lumbar vertebrae in gravitational traction. *Spine.* 1998;23(9):1061–1063; discussion 1064.
16. Lee MY, Wong MK, Tang FT, Chang WH, Chiou WK. Design and assessment of an adaptive intermittent cervical traction modality with EMG biofeedback. *J Biomech Eng.* 1996;118(4):597–600.
17. Shealy NC. Expanding ellipsoidal decompression (EED™) for cervical pain. 2006 IRB approved study. http://www.chiropractic-biophysics.com/clinical_chiropractic/2010/1/14/cervical-decompression-treatment.html
18. Moeti P, Marchetti G. Clinical outcome from mechanical intermittent cervical traction for the treatment of cervical radiculopathy: a case series. *J Orthop Sports Phys Ther.* 2001;31(4):207–213.
19. Marovino T. Expanding ellipsoidal decompression (EED) of the spine. *Pract Pain Manage.* 2010;10(2):75–77.

20. Pellecchia GL. Lumbar traction: a review of the literature. *J Orthop Sports Phys Ther.* 1994;20(5):262–267.

21. Guvenol K, Tuzun C, Peker O, Goktay Y. A comparison of inverted spinal traction and conventional traction in the treatment of lumbar disc herniations. *Physiother Theory Pract.* 2000;16:151–160.

22. Beurskens AJ, de Vet HC, Koke AJ, et al. Efficacy of traction for nonspecific low back pain. 12-week and 6-month results of a randomized clinical trial. *Spine.* 1997;22(23):2756–2762.

23. Meszaros TF, Olson R, Kulig K, Creighton D, Czarnecki E. Effect of 10%, 30%, and 60% body weight traction on the straight leg raise test of symptomatic patients with low back pain. *J Orthop Sports Phys Ther.* 2000;30(10):595–601.

24. Harte AA, Baxter GD, Gracey JH. The efficacy of traction for back pain: a systematic review of randomized controlled trials. *Arch Phys Med Rehabil.* 2003;84(10):1542–1553.

25. Hinterbuchner C. Traction. In: Basmajian J, ed. *Manipulation, Traction and Massage.* Baltimore, MD: Williams and Wilkins, 1985.

26. Draper D. Inversion table traction as a therapeutic modality, part 1. *Athl Ther Today.* 2005;10(3):42–43.

27. Draper D. Inversion table traction as a therapeutic modality, part 2. *Athl Ther Today.* 2005;10(4):40–42.

20

Laser and Light Therapy

BY KENNETH L. KNIGHT AND TY HOPKINS

Chapter Outline

OPENING SCENE

Alex was stumped when his professor asked, "What do an athletic trainer, a cancer surgeon, a plastic surgeon, an Air Force general, a computer printer, a robot in a Detroit auto factory, a college professor, a telephone, and a TV have in common?" He was more stumped by the answer: "Each uses lasers to do its job." Surely, he thought, the simple-looking device he saw in the athletic training clinic was not the same as the devices that are used to shoot down missiles in outer space, point to important (and sometimes dull) elements on a lecture room screen, print computer-generated text and pictures, carry telephone and television signals in an optic fiber, weld car parts, and so on. And how could the same device be used in medicine to perform microsurgery, cauterize ruptured blood vessels, assist in a variety of diagnostic tasks, and reduce pain and stimulate healing?

Light Therapy

Light therapy, also known *as photopherapy*, is a broad term that refers to the application of light for a variety of devices for a variety of therapeutic purposes. Devices include lasers, light-emitting diodes (LEDs), super-luminous diodes (SLDs), fluorescent lamps, infrared lamps, ultraviolet (UV) lamps, diachronic lamps, and very bright incandescent light bulbs. They are used to treat orthopedic injuries, skin conditions, and psychological problems such as depression and seasonal affective disorder and to tan the skin. In this chapter we are concerned only with the therapeutic use of lasers and LEDs but will briefly mention UV radiation.

Light therapy began with lasers in the 1970s. **Laser**, an acronym for light amplification by stimulated emission of radiation, is a device that transforms electromagnetic energy of various frequencies, in or near the range of visible light, into an extremely intense, small, and nearly nondivergent beam of monochromatic radiation with all its waves in phase. The therapeutic theory is that specific wavelengths of laser light, when absorbed, cause specific physiological responses in the body. Although the therapeutic value of these responses has been debated, the industry continues to grow. Numerous factors, including technological advances, have led to the use of nonlaser devices, such as LEDs, SLDs, and polarized polychromic light, to deliver light of specific wavelengths to the body.[1]

As with any emerging technology, there is much confusion in terminology.[1,2] Light therapy is today where electrotherapy was in the early 1980s (see Chapter 18). Terms and acronyms used to describe light therapy include phototherapy, cold laser, soft laser, low-energy laser, low-level laser therapy (LLLT), low-energy laser therapy (LELT), low-intensity laser activated biostimulation (LILAB), low-power laser irradiation (LPLI), low-power laser therapy (LPLT), low-intensity lasers (LIL), and monochromic infrared energy. It is easy for clinicians to become confused when reading the professional literature. Leaders in the field are now calling for clinicians, scientists, and corporate professionals to begin using the terms *light therapy* or *phototherapy*.[1,2]

LASERS AND NONLASER DEVICES

Both lasers and nonlaser devices (LEDs/SLDs) deliver light of specific wavelengths, although the way the light is generated, and some of its characteristics, are different. There is no consensus about the relative merits of these two technologies, and it is difficult to discuss their therapeutic value. The major problem is with terminology. Some lasers use LEDs, so the discussion cannot be lasers versus LEDs. Some scientists use the terms *laser* and *nonlaser light*,[1] whereas others use *coherent* and *noncoherent light*[3] to distinguish the two technologies. To understand the difference, you must understand how each is produced.

Characteristics of Lasers

To produce laser radiation, a laser device must have an energy source, a mechanical structure, and a **lasing medium**, which can be gas, liquid, crystal, chemical, or semiconductors (such as LEDs). The difference in lasing medium will result in differing wavelengths, levels of light coherence, and levels of light divergence.

Laser light is very different from normal light. Laser light is monophasic, monochromatic, coherent, and nondivergent (directional)—meaning it is composed of particles of light with equal energy and of a single phase and color that move in step with each other (Fig. 20.1). The following list of terms and definitions further describes the characteristics of lasers.

- **Light**: Electromagnetic radiation that can produce a visual sensation
- **Amplify**: To increase in size, volume, or significance
- **Stimulate**: To excite or invigorate; to encourage or provoke something to grow, develop, or become more active
- **Emission**: A flowing forth, such as the release of electrons from parent atoms
- **Radiation**: The transfer of energy in the form of rays, waves, or particles, often from a central source; also called radiant energy

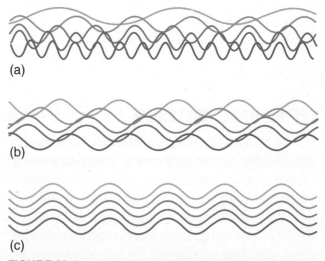

FIGURE 20.1 Wave patterns of three types of light. (**a**) Light from a common light bulb is composed of waves with different frequencies and phases. (**b**) An LED emits light with waves of the same frequency (monochromatic) but out of phase (incoherent). (**c**) A laser emits light with waves of the same frequency (monochromatic) and in phase (coherent).

- **Electromagnetic energy**: One of the fundamental forms of energy in the universe. Its characteristics change radically depending on frequency and wavelength, which tend to correlate closely with each other (see Chapter 10).
- **Frequency**: The rate of vibration of a force or wave, usually measured relative to local time
- **Visible light**: An electromagnetic wave that is divergent, multichromatic, incoherent, and multiphasic
- **Nondivergent**: Incapable of separating or widening. Contrast the light from a laser pointer (nondivergent) with that coming from a flashlight (divergent). Nondivergent light is also known as directional light (Fig. 20.2).
- **Monochromatic**: Having a single frequency and a single color (if it is in the light spectrum (see Fig. 20.1)
- **Coherent**: Logically ordered or integrated; a quality of electromagnetic waves that have the same wavelength and a fixed phase relationship (see Fig. 20.1)
- **Fixed phase**: The unified launching of the wave fronts of all light particles of a laser beam

A laser is not a single device, but rather a variety of devices, each with a specific frequency, amplification, and focus of its emitted beam. The therapeutic modality used to treat wounds cannot be used to control your TV or weld car parts, and vice versa. Some therapeutic lasers have applicator heads with a variety of diodes (laser-emitting devices) so they can deliver a variety of frequencies or laser beams simultaneously.

The word laser is used as part of several related concepts:

- **Laser device**: A machine or device that produces, or generates, and emits a laser beam. This is generally what is meant when *laser* is used by itself.
- **Laser beam**: The output of a laser device; highly amplified, single-frequency, single-colored, nondivergent, coherent light
- **Laser light**: The light of a laser beam
- **Laser energy**: The energy of a laser beam

THE NATURE OF LIGHT

Lasers are possible because of the dual nature of light; it is both a wave and a particle.[4] In most situations, including when it travels from one point to another, light acts as a wave of oscillating electrical and magnetic fields (see Fig. 10.3). When it is absorbed or emitted by atoms, however, it acts as a particle. The particles, or packets of energy, are called **photons**. The amount of energy of a given photon is a function of its wavelength, or frequency, since each photon has a unique wavelength and a unique frequency (see Chapter 10).

LASER ENERGY PRODUCTION

Laser energy production requires four components (Fig. 20.3):

- An amplifying chamber or resonating cavity in which the stimulation and amplification take place
- A lasing medium (gas, liquid, crystal, chemical, or semiconductor) placed in the amplifying chamber
- An external source of energy (electrical, chemical, or optical)
- A pair of mirrors at either end of the amplifying chamber, one of which is **half-silvered**, meaning it reflects only half the light and allows the other half to pass through.

When external energy is applied to a lasing medium, some of the lasing medium atoms absorb the energy. The absorbed energy excites the atoms, causing them to move to higher-energy orbits. This is an abnormal or unstable state, however, so the electrons return to their normal state. As they do, the absorbed energy is released as a photon, a particle of light.

Photons are part of our daily life. Atoms release energy as photons of light all the time. The light from light bulbs, TV picture tubes, fire, and the heating coils on electric

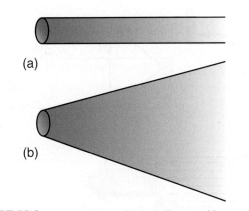

FIGURE 20.2 The divergence of light is illustrated by contrasting (**a**) a nondivergent beam with (**b**) a divergent beam.

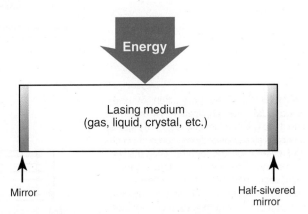

FIGURE 20.3 The basic components of a laser.

stoves, ovens, and toasters are all caused by the release of photons as atoms change orbits. Unlike laser energy, however, these photons are released at a variety of wavelengths and therefore appear and behave very differently than laser energy.

Lasers are designed to control the excitation (stimulation) of atoms, and the subsequent release (emission) of this stimulated energy. Identical atoms with identical states of excitation will emit photons of identical wavelengths. Thus, by using a specific lasing medium and controlling the process, the released photons are monochromatic and coherent.

The majority of photons in the lasing medium are lost. As shown in Figure 20.4, photons P1, P2, and P3 exit the amplifying chamber without striking either of the mirrors on the right and left ends of the amplifying chamber. Photons P4 and P5 strike a mirror and are reflected out of the chamber. Photon P6, however, strikes the right mirror at a right angle and is reflected back toward the second mirror, where it will strike and bounce back toward the first mirror.

As photons bounce back and forth between the two mirrors, through the lasing medium, they stimulate electrons of excited atoms to return to their normal state, giving up energy in the form of additional photons. Some are lost, but others bounce back and forth. Half of the bouncing photons pass through the half-silvered mirror and become the laser beam (light). Thus, a cascade effect occurs in which more and more photons are emitted.

This process may be affected by the type of lasing medium. For example, lasers with a semiconductor medium do not emit purely monochromatic light and the coherence length is shorter than lasers with a chemical medium. So although LED-based lasers produce light at a wavelength in a therapeutic range, the differences in the energy and other light characteristics (i.e.,

coherence) cause some to question the effectiveness of semiconductor-based lasers.

ENERGY LEVEL DETERMINES EFFECTS

The effects of a laser are largely determined by the amount of energy it emits. High-energy lasers produce great amounts of heat, which is useful in welding and shooting down satellites. In the human body, tissue is destroyed if high levels of energy are applied. While this may be desirable to a surgeon, it is not the goal of ATs or other rehabilitation specialists.

Therapeutic modality lasers emit low levels of energy (<500 mW) that do not heat body tissue. These are called **low-level lasers**, also referred to as *cold lasers* or *soft lasers* (Fig. 20.5).

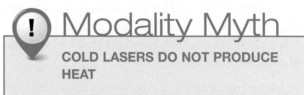

Modality Myth

COLD LASERS DO NOT PRODUCE HEAT

It is only partially true that cold lasers do not produce heat. They are said to be athermic, meaning they do not directly heat tissues. However, because low-level lasers increase blood flow to the treated area, there is a slight measurable increase in tissue temperature as a result of their use.

LASER CLASSIFICATION

The wide variety of lasers are commonly classified in two ways: according to the type of lasing medium they employ (Table 20.1) and according to their safety (Table 20.2).

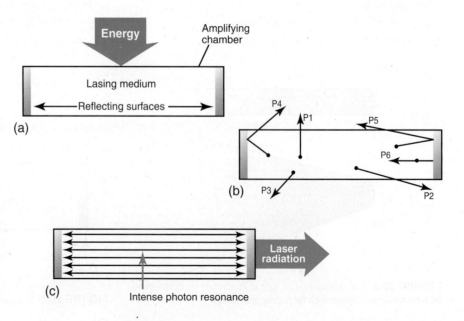

FIGURE 20.4 The production of laser energy. (**a**) The application of external energy to the medium causes (**b**) the spontaneous release of photons, some of which (P6) reflect back and forth between the two mirrors. (**c**) This leads to intense photon resonance, part of which is released as laser light through the half-silvered mirror at one end of the chamber. (Source: Adapted from Baxter.[10])

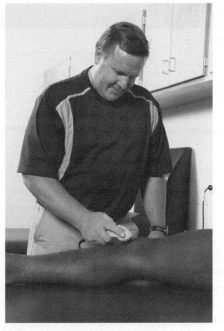

FIGURE 20.5 A low-level laser, or cold laser.

The following list summarizes the five types of lasers and their lasing medium:

- *Gas lasers*: Use gas as a lasing medium. Helium and helium-neon (HeNe) are the most common gas lasers.
- *Diode or semiconductor lasers:* Use semiconductors as the lasing medium. They can be either small and low-powered or large and high-powered. Low-powered semiconductor lasers are those used in laser pointers, laser printers, and compact disc players. In fact, the 780-nm aluminum gallium arsenide (AlGaAs) laser diode, used in CD players, is the most common type of laser in the world. Large industrial diode lasers are capable of generating great amounts of heat and are used for cutting and welding.

- *Dye lasers*: Use large-molecule organic dyes in a liquid solution as the lasing medium. They can be "tuned" to produce laser beams over a broad range of wavelengths.
- *Solid-state lasers*: Use various minerals as their lasing medium. Examples are the ruby and neodymium:yttrium-aluminum garnet (Yag) lasers.
- *Excimer lasers*: Use a dimer as the lasing medium. (A dimer is a pseudo-molecule created by electrically stimulating a mixture of reactive gases, such as chlorine and fluorine, with inert gases, such as argon, krypton, or xenon.)

Safety is determined by the amount of energy applied to the lasing medium and the subsequent amount of energy released in the form of light—in other words, the power of the laser. The greater the power of the laser, the greater the potential danger (see Table 20.2).

Two other factors to consider when discussing types of lasers are wavelength and color. Although neither wavelength nor color is used to classify lasers, these terms are important when discussing and applying lasers. The body's response to laser application is specific to the laser's wavelength. A laser of one specific wavelength will cause a certain tissue reaction, whereas a laser of another wavelength will cause a different reaction or no reaction at all. This specificity of response makes understanding and using lasers complex and at times confusing. Clinicians must always identify the specific wavelength of a laser when discussing its effects.

Lasers are often referred to by their color, such as a red laser or a violet laser. This practice is imprecise, though, and we recommend against it. For example, all lasers with wavelengths of 150–380 nm are ultraviolet (Table 20.3). But the tissue response to a 150-nm laser is different than to a 380-nm laser, so each laser should be referred to by its specific wavelength rather than calling them both ultraviolet lasers.

TABLE 20.1 TYPES OF LASERS CLASSIFIED BY LASING MEDIUM			
LASER TYPE	**LASING MEDIUM**	**WAVELENGTH (NM)**	**SAFETY CLASSIFICATION**
Gas	HeNe	633	I–IV
Gas	CO_2	10,600	IIIb–IV
Gas	Argon	488–514	IV
Diode or Semiconductor	AlGaAs	600–1000	IIIb
Dye	Tunable dye	577	IV
Solid state	Ruby	694	IV
Solid state	HdYag	1060	IV
Excimer	Dimer	351	IV

TABLE 20.2	SAFETY CLASSIFICATIONS OF LASERS		
CLASS	**POWER (MW)**	**VISIBILITY***	**SAFETY CONCERNS**
I	<0.5	Either	None
II	<1	Visible	Safe for momentary viewing
IIIa	<5	Either	Photochemical effect
IIIb	<500	Either	Photobiomodulation, no photothermal effect, no harm to skin or clothing, potential damage to eye
IV	>500	Either	Photothermal effect; harmful to skin, eyes, and clothing; use with extreme caution

Either means there are both visible and nonvisible laser beams in this class.

Characteristics of LEDs and SLDs

A **light-emitting diode (LED)** is a special type of semiconductor diode that emits visible light when an electric current passes through it.[4,5] As its name implies, a **superluminous diode (SLD)** is a brighter LED. Like normal diodes, it consists of a semiconducting material such as silicone or germanium that is impregnated, or *doped*, with impurities to create a structure called a p-n junction. In crystalline form, silicone and germanium are electrical insulators, but the impurities turn them into electrical conductors. Although they are not strong conductors like metal, they will conduct electricity adequately.

The p-n junction of the diode consists of two pieces of a semiconductor material, each doped with a different substance (Fig. 20.6). After the doping material on the n-side of the junction chemically bonds with the semiconductor material, there are extra free electrons. This results in the semiconductor being negatively charged, hence the *n*.

The doping material on the p-side does not have enough electrons to fully bond with the semiconductor material, so the result is a positively charged material, hence the p. The interaction of the two sides of the p-n junction gives the diode some unique characteristics, such as allowing electrical current to flow in one direction but blocking it in the opposite direction, and generating light.

As electricity passes through it, the diode gives off energy in the form of photons. The wavelength of the energy given off, and thus the color of the emitted light, is determined by the chemical composition of the doping materials. LEDs and SLDs typically are covered by plastic cases of varying colors. The plastic case has no bearing on the color of the light; it simply is used to indicate the specific wavelength of energy emitted by the diode, and therefore the color of the light.

Light emitted from an LED or SLD is monochromatic but not coherent. This means their light will be more scattered than that of a laser, and therefore less of the light will strike the target. Thus, less energy is imparted to the tissue.

DIFFERENCES BETWEEN LIGHT THERAPY LASERS AND LEDs

Since both semiconductor-based lasers and diode devices use LEDs and SLDs, one might think that the light delivered from the two devices is the same. Not true. The p-n junction of the diode device emits energy directly to the

TABLE 20.3	TISSUE PENETRATION OF VARIOUS WAVELENGTHS	
WAVELENGTH (NM)	**COLOR RANGE**	**DEPTH OF PENETRATION (MM)**
150–380	Ultraviolet	<0.1
390–470	Violet to deep blue	~0.3
475–545	Blue to green	~0.3–0.5
545–600	Yellow to orange	~0.5–1.0
600–650	Red	~1.0–2.0
650–1000	Deep red to infrared	2.0–3.0
1000–1350	Near to mid-infrared	3.0–5.0
1350–12,000	Infrared	<0.1

Adapted with permission from Baxter.[10]

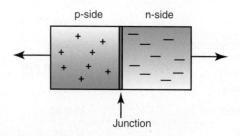

FIGURE 20.6 The p-n junction of a diode.

patient.[4] With a semiconductor laser, however, the emission from the diode is further processed by the laser to stimulate additional photons. When the photons escape via the laser's half-silvered mirror they are coherent but also have a greater photon density—that is, more photons per area. The clinical implications are that diode devices will take much longer to deliver the same amount of energy to the target tissue, and the energy they deliver probably will not penetrate the tissue as effectively as laser light.

Although many insist that coherence is essential for clinical effectiveness, others argue that light is light, and it is the wavelength and the dose that matter.[6] It also should be noted that SLDs and/or clusters of SLDs have been effective in the treatment of some cells and tissues.[1]

Lasers in Medicine

Various forms of lasers are used in medicine.[7,8] Applications include surgery (cutting tissue or cauterizing bleeding vessels), diagnosis, imaging, and physical medicine and rehabilitation. The lasers, LEDs, and SLDs used in rehabilitation are very different from the laser therapies used in other areas of medicine—primarily, the power is much lower. The maximal output of these devices is <500 mW.

The relatively low power output of light therapy makes it athermic (lacking heat). This does not mean that no thermal reactions take place in treated tissues, but rather that the temperature rise is so small that it is virtually undetectable.

The U.S. Food and Drug Administration (FDA) has not approved light therapy for rehabilitation, but it has cleared specific machines for specific therapeutic uses. The FDA believes that more evidence (from controlled clinical trials) is necessary for approving light therapy. To date, light therapy has been cleared for use in the temporary relief of neck and shoulder pain of musculoskeletal origin, wrist and hand pain associated with carpal tunnel syndrome, and iliotibial band syndrome pain.[9] Light therapy devices may also be used in controlled clinical trials with approval from the Institutional Review Board, a committee at universities and research institutions that reviews research proposals involving human subjects to ensure that the research does not expose research subjects to undue risk or harm and that their rights are protected.

Many clinicians feel that once a low-level laser has been purchased it can be used to treat about any medical condition.[9] There are no "laser police" to prevent such actions, but this does not relieve the clinician of liability for any damages that might result from the improper use of the device.[9] Use lasers with caution.

When used properly, light therapy is relatively safe. While many electrical modalities have extended lists of contraindications and precautions, light therapy appears to be safe for patients who have pins, metal plates, plastic implants, growth plates, and pacemakers, and for treating the gonads.[10]

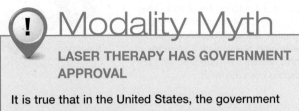

Modality Myth

LASER THERAPY HAS GOVERNMENT APPROVAL

It is true that in the United States, the government has given limited approval for laser therapy. The FDA has cleared specific models of low-level lasers from certain manufactures for treating particular musculoskeletal conditions. Thus, the use of lasers other than the specifically approved models is illegal. In addition, the use of an approved model for treating of any condition other than the approved condition is illegal.

THE EFFECTS OF LIGHT THERAPY ON TISSUE

Laser and nonlaser devices vary in the depth of penetration, the type of tissue that is affected, and the types of molecules within the tissue that are affected. Water and organic molecules, such as amino acids, nucleic acid bases, hemoglobin, and melanin, account for absorption rates of radiation in body tissues. Skin color may, therefore, play a role in how much light is absorbed by the tissue and to what depth it penetrates during treatment.

Photobiomodulation
Photobiomodulation is the act of modifying biological processes with light. That's exactly what laser therapy does—it stimulates tissue in a way that modifies pain and/or the healing processes. Some clinicians continue to use an older term, *biostimulation*, but this term is only half right.[9] Lasers sometimes inhibit biological processes, as in reducing pain.

Mechanisms of Action
When light is absorbed by tissues, it acts at the molecular level by one or a combination of the following three mechanisms (Fig. 20.7):

1. Excitation of electron bonds within molecules, which can result in molecules breaking or undergoing structural changes
2. Excitation of atoms to higher levels of oscillation (movement) in relation to each other within the molecule, which could lead to low levels of heat production
3. Rotational changes of atoms within the molecule, which could also lead to changes in temperature

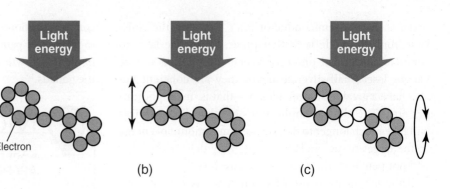

FIGURE 20.7 Three possible mechanisms by which molecules absorb light. (**a**) Excitation of molecular electron bonds, (**b**) excitation of atoms to higher levels of oscillation (movement), and (**c**) rotational changes of atoms within the molecule. (Source: Adapted from Baxter.[10])

The exact mechanisms by which laser light affects tissues have not been decisively determined. The energy of any electromagnetic wave is a photon. The accepted theory is that photons are absorbed by photoreceptors in tissue cells,[11] causing a change in the photoreceptors' molecular configuration (called the primary reaction). This change in configuration alters the cells' molecular processes (called secondary reactions).

In vitro studies, in which cellular or tissue cultures in laboratory vessels are used to model living human tissue, support this theory, including these secondary reactions:

• Photobiomodulation of cellular events
• Stimulated/optimized tissue repair
• Pain relief

More research is needed to confirm that these effects occur **in vivo**—within actual patients when lasers are applied to the body directly.

Many components of the body's metabolic pathway may be primary photoreceptors, absorbing laser light and inducing changes in cellular homeostasis, ultimately enhancing healing by promoting the synthesis of ATP molecules for energy and numerous cellular activities related to the proliferation (spread or increase) of new cells.[11,12] Fibroblasts do increase following He-Ne irradiation of tissue cultures.[13–16] Furthermore, light therapy seems to increase collagen production by fibroblasts.[17] The conversion of fibroblasts to myofibroblasts also appears to be a positive effect of light therapy.[18] (Myofibroblasts are modified fibroblasts that help contract or pull the margins of wounds closer together during wound healing.) While these findings support the use of light therapy, the results have not always been duplicated due to variations in treatment parameters and tissue culture types.[19,20] Therefore, more research is needed to support these positive effects of light therapy and identify the specific mechanisms that mediate these effects.

Light therapy may be effective in increasing lymphocyte proliferation[21] and their ability to bind pathogens.[22,23] However, results of other studies suggest that light therapy has the opposite effect, a decrease or inhibition of lymphocyte proliferation.[24,25] It appears that these effects may depend on the wavelength and power output used in treatment. The data may help support the idea that lasers assist in healing chronic wounds by suppressing the immune system. Again, more research is needed to support these potential effects of light therapy on the immune system.

Tissue Healing

The cellular and molecular effects just described help explain why light therapy may strengthen tissue healing. Enhanced ATP synthesis would lead to increased fibroblast proliferation; so fibroblasts would produce increased levels of collagen, and as a result, fibroplasia (production of fibrous tissue) would theoretically be facilitated and wounds would contract more quickly.

This idea is supported in the research. Light therapy enhances wound contraction of experimental wounds on human skin,[26] the healing of skin ulcerations in humans,[27–29] peripheral nerve regeneration,[30] and various skin injuries in animals.[22,31] It should also be noted again that other studies using animal and human wounds have shown light therapy to have no effect on healing.[32–34] In fact, there is a much greater discrepancy in these studies than in the previously reported *in vitro* studies.

It is possible that light therapy enhances tissue healing during three phases of tissue healing as follows:[10]

1. Cellular phase: increased mast cell release, interleukin-6 (an inflammatory regulatory substance) formation, and decreased dermal necrosis
2. Collegenization phase: enhanced collagen formation, degranulation, myofibroblast conversion
3. Remodeling phase: wound contraction, tensile strength/stress

With an increase in fibroblast proliferation and collagen activity during the repair phase of healing, some clinicians suggest that light therapy may result in oversized scarring. While this is certainly something the clinician should pay attention to, there is currently no evidence to suggest that light therapy results in hypertrophic scars or keloids. In fact, light therapy has been shown to flatten and soften existing keloids.[13]

Pain Relief

- Opinions are varied concerning the effect of light therapy on acute and chronic pain. Much of the support for reducing pain with light therapy is from anecdotal claims rather than from controlled, blinded investigations or randomized clinical trials, although there have been at least five randomized clinical trials of neck pain.[35] Controlled research has been split, some indicating light therapy is effective in reducing pain[1,35] and others indicating it is not.[36–38] Much of the debate centers on the optimal parameters for the application of light therapy to reduce pain and the elusive mechanism by which light therapy occurs.

  Several well-conducted studies have supported the use of light therapy in treating the following painful conditions:

- Acute musculoskeletal trauma[39]
- Myofascial pain[40,41]
- Rheumatoid arthritis[42]
- Carpal tunnel syndrome[43]
- Low-back pain[44]
- Trigger points[40,41]
- Neck pain[35]

Conversely, other controlled studies indicated that light therapy had no effect on the following conditions:

- Musculoskeletal pain[38]
- Lateral ankle sprains[37]
- Plantar fasciitis[45]
- Delayed-onset muscle soreness[46]

Several theories have been suggested to explain how light therapy works to relieve pain. While there is no concrete evidence supporting one specific mechanism of action, these theories collectively point to some possibilities:

- Increased serotonin[37] that, if released in the central nervous system (CNS), may inhibit pain transmission
- Decreased cholinergic release,[10] and therefore reduced pain transmission in the CNS
- Inhibition of prostacyclin,[47] a key player in pain during the inflammatory process of healing
- Increased sensory nerve transmission time of superficial nerves,[48,49] potentially decreasing overall pain transmission over time; however, other studies have failed to replicate these findings[50]
- Increased CNS pain perception threshold[51]
- Placebo effect

Treatment Parameters

The treatment parameters for light therapy are:

- Delivery technique
- Dosage and duration
- Tissue penetration

DELIVERY TECHNIQUE

Light therapy can treat a variety of different sites, including a lesion, wound, or area of pain; nerve roots and trunks; trigger points or acupressure points; and lymphatic and blood vessels.

Most lasers use a **single laser probe** to deliver light of a specific wavelength to tissues.

However, in recent years **cluster probes** have been used to apply multiple wavelengths to a larger area during treatment (Fig. 20.8).

For optimum delivery of laser light, the laser probe should be in contact with the skin, to minimize divergence and reflection. In the case of open wounds, the probe may be held close (<1 cm) to the wound without touching it. Some clinicians place a sterile transparent film over the open wound so that the probe can be placed in contact with the damaged tissue.

Obviously the cluster head is the best option for treating a large area. When a cluster head is not available, however, a single probe can be used in one of two ways: sequential application to multiple areas of tissue, called **grid application**, or moving the head across the area like an ultrasound head, a technique called **scanning**.

To use the grid application, imagine the treatment area as a series of 1-cm² segments. Systematically treat each segment with the appropriate dosage for the condition. Scanning consists of moving the laser probe back and forth over the treatment area at a slow and steady rate. Each pass progresses across the wound until the treatment area has been covered. Then treat the entire area a second time, at 90° to the first pass. The entire treatment area and the machine's output should be considered to formulate the duration of treatment. Dosage is much less accurate using the scanning method.

For treatment over trigger points or acupressure points, slowly move the laser probe and apply more pressure for a massage effect. Ask the patient to tell you if the pressure is too great.

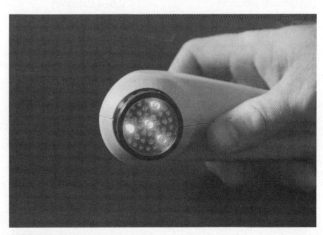

FIGURE 20.8 A cluster probe.

DOSAGE AND DURATION

The dosage depends on three factors: average output power, time of light exposure, and treatment area. These factors are represented in the following formula (Tx stands for treatment):

$$\text{Dosage} = (\text{average power} \times \text{Tx time}) / \text{Tx area}$$

where dosage is given in joules per centimeter squared (J/cm^2); average power is the average output power of the machine (in mW); Tx time is the length of treatment (in min); and Tx area is the area of the laser beam or area to be treated (in cm^2).

The power output of a laser is fixed, and the only way to alter the dosage is to alter the time of application. Treatment time must be computed for each specific device, because the output differs among devices. Treatment time is computed from the total output of the specific device.

Manufacturers report the total output power of their individual devices, and many of those who offer multiple pulse rates report the average power for each of their pulse rates. If, however, average power is not given, you must compute it using the following formula:

$$\text{Average power} = \text{pulse rate (Hz)} \times \\ \text{peak power (mW)} \times \text{pulse width (sec)}$$

Dosage ranges for specific conditions have been derived from available research and mathematical theory. Some of these are presented in Tables 20.4 and 20.5. The differences in these two tables reflect the lack of precise knowledge about this modality. Consult your laser application manual for additional dosages.

Compute treatment time using the following formula:

$$\text{Tx time} = (\text{Dosage} \times \text{Tx area}) / \text{Power}$$

where dosage is the value (in J/cm^2) obtained from a table; Tx area is the area (in cm^2) you want to treat; and power is peak power (if you are treating with a continuous wave) or average power (if you are treating with a pulsed wave), per the manufacturer's data, or your computed average power using the formula above.

For example, if the desired dosage for a specific condition is 1.5 J/cm^2, the average power of the laser is 0.5 mW, and the surface area of the laser beam is 0.1 cm^2, then:

$$\text{Tx time} = (1.5 \, J/cm^2 \times 0.5 \, cm^2) / 0.5 \, mW$$

Because 1 J = 1 W*sec and 0.5 mW = 0.0005 W, the formula can be rewritten as:

$$\text{Tx time} = (1.5 \, W^* \sec / cm^2 \times 0.5 \, cm^2) / 0.0005 \, W$$
$$\text{Tx time} = 300 \text{ seconds or 5 minutes}$$

To deliver 1.5 J/cm^2 it would take 5 minutes. However, if the treatment area were larger than the laser probe, then the time to treat the entire area could be computed using a scanning method. If the grid application were to be used, then treatment would be delivered using the treatment time calculated for the laser probe, and each grid would be treated for that time period.

TISSUE PENETRATION

Depth of penetration is a major issue with light therapy. No matter how effective the light is on specific tissue, its effect is of no value if it does not reach the target tissue

TABLE 20.4	MUSCULOSKELETAL CONDITIONS AND THEIR APPROXIMATE LASER DOSAGES	
CONDITION	**DOSAGE***	**NOTES***
Superficial wounds	0.5–4.0 J/cm^2	Increase dosage as the wound bed develops over time
Trigger points	8 J/cm^2	Use a laser probe; treat each trigger point with 1 J
Nerve root application	8–24 J/cm^2	Use a laser probe (1–3 J/point)
Tendinitis	1–3 J/point	
Capsulitis	1 J/point	
Epicondylitis	2–3 J/point	
Muscle strain	1–2 J/point	
Patellofemoral problems	1–2 J/point	
Ligament strain	2–4 J/point	
Plantar fasciitis	1–3 J/point	

Point denotes an area the size of the laser probe.

Adapted with permission from Baxter.[10]

TABLE 20.5   BASIC RECOMMENDATIONS FOR LASER TREATMENT DOSAGES

CONDITION	ACUTE (J)		CHRONIC (J)	
	Per Point	Dosage Total	Per Point	Dosage Total
Muscle strain	3–4	25–35	5–6	35–45
Tendinitis	3–6	24–30	5–8	35–45
Ligament sprain	3–4	25–30	5–6	35–45
Stress fracture	7–8	25–30	8–10	35–40
Open wounds	0.5–1.5	*	1.0–4.0	*
Myofascial trigger point	1.0	†	1.0	†

*Depends on the size of the wound.

†Because of their focalized nature, myofascial trigger points are treated once at the most tender location.

Reproduced with permission from McLeod.[9]

with appropriate dosage. As light is absorbed by various tissue cells, the depth of penetration is reduced.

Laser penetration is a function of its wavelength and power. Although wavelength is probably the most important factor in determining depth of penetration, there must also be a driving force. The driving force is the power or amount of energy that is being applied. A good analogy is that of a short nail and a long nail. The shorter nail represents a shorter wavelength and hence a lower depth of penetration; the longer nail represents a longer wavelength. If we were to drive the shorter nail into a piece of wood with a heavy blow and were to gently tap the longer nail, common sense dictates that the shorter nail would be driven deeper into the piece of wood. Despite the fact that the longer nail is capable of penetrating more deeply, the lack of force results in a shallower depth of penetration. Keep in mind that no matter how hard either nail is hit, the total depth of penetration is limited. The same is true for lasers—for any given wavelength, there is a maximum depth of penetration, and in order to elicit responses up to and including the maximum depth of penetration, an appropriate amount of energy must be used.

Tissue penetration of lasers is only superficial, at best 5 mm (see Table 20.3). It is even less with LED and SLD devices. Most wavelengths penetrate <1 mm, however. This partly accounts for the difference between results of *in vitro* studies (outside the body) and *in vivo* studies of tissues in the body; cells in a culture dish are irradiated directly, while those in tissue are irradiated only after the beam is partially absorbed in skin and other tissues.

Depth of penetration is wavelength-dependent. The near- to mid-infrared spectrum (1000–1350 nm) appears to penetrate deepest, 3–5 mm.[10] These depths may be affected by the power or intensity of the incident light, however, so it is debatable whether light therapy has enough dosage to treat deeper tissues.

It appears from the literature that light therapy may be beneficial to superficial wounds and pain originating from superficial tissues. Since light energy is absorbed by only superficial tissues, its use is limited.

 CONCEPT CHECK 20.1 Compare and contrast diathermy and laser therapy. In what ways are they alike? In what ways are they different?

Skin Color

Melanin, a pigment that contributes to skin color, absorbs light in the visible spectrum very well.[10] Therefore, patients with darker skin may absorb more light in the cutaneous layers, preventing light from penetrating to deeper tissues. In addition, the production of melanin is triggered by light in the near-ultraviolet range. This could result in darkening of skin or scar tissue as more melanocytes are produced.

Obesity

Considering the issues related to depth of penetration of therapeutic light, the thickness of subcutaneous fat should be considered when treating conditions that exist deep to the subcutaneous layers. It seems debatable whether light therapy can reach deeper tissues at a dosage appropriate for treatment. When the subcutaneous fat layer is excessively thick, the likelihood of therapeutic dosages reaching deeper tissues is even more questionable.

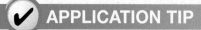 **APPLICATION TIP**

WEAR SAFETY GOGGLES

Even with the low power output of therapeutic lasers, the light is sufficient to cause damage to the eyes. You and your patients must wear protective goggles during laser applications to prevent accidental exposure of the eyes to the light. Goggles are equipped with light filters aimed at reducing the incident light.

Application of Light Therapy

 ### STEP 1: FOUNDATION

A. Definition. Light therapy is the application of light for therapeutic purposes.
B. Effects
   1. Photobiomodulation of tissue healing
   2. Pain relief
C. Advantages
   1. Relatively safe
      a. No side effects
      b. Athermic
   2. Easy to use
   3. Cost-effective
      a. Therapist time
      b. Patient recovery
D. Disadvantages
   1. Limited depth of penetration
   2. Light density can damage eyesight
E. Indications
   The indications for light therapy are numerous. Although conclusive data do not exist to support all reported indications for light therapy, the following are supported:
   1. Activating cells into a healing mode
   2. Wound healing
   3. Pain relief
   4. Increasing tensile strength of scar tissue
F. Contraindications
   1. Irradiation directly into the eye
   2. Irradiation of the uterus during pregnancy
   3. Cancer
   4. Organ transplant patients
G. Precautions
   1. Be cautious when applying light therapy to a patient who:
      a. Is photosensitive
      b. Suffers from epilepsy
   2. Has had a recent steroid injection
   3. Is taking anti-inflammatory medication
   4. Has an acute infection
   5. Suffers from a thyroid condition

STEP 2: PREAPPLICATION TASKS

A. Make sure light therapy is the proper modality for this situation
   1. Reevaluate the injury/problem. Make sure you understand the patient's condition.
      a. Question the patient about any abnormalities following the previous treatment.
   2. Check for contraindications.

   3. Confirm that the objectives of therapy are compatible with the use of light therapy.
B. Preparing the patient psychologically
   1. Explain that no sensation should be felt.
   2. Describe expected outcomes.
C. Preparing the patient physically
   1. Remove clothing, earrings, bandages, tape, braces, etc. as necessary.
   2. Clean and dry the skin of the treatment area.
D. Equipment preparation
   1. Check the manual for the average power output of the unit.
   2. Calculate the treatment time based on desired dosage, average power output, and the area to be treated.
   3. Make sure the machine is operating properly.
   4. Make sure the displayed time is correct.
   5. If applicable, make sure the pulse rate is set appropriately for the treatment.

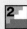 ### STEP 3: APPLICATION PARAMETERS

A. Procedures
   1. Turn on the machine (if necessary).
   2. Adjust the output parameters as needed (pulse rate and treatment time).
   3. Wear safety goggles.
   4. Application technique.
      a. Direct contact with the skin, with the exception of an open wound.
      b. Treat large areas with one of the following:
         i. Cluster probe.
         ii. Grid application, treating 1-cm^2 areas consecutively.
         iii. Scanning technique, crisscrossing the wound area.
B. Dosage
   1. Tables 20.4 and 20.5 provide approximate dosages for various musculoskeletal conditions.
   2. Consult owners' manual for more recommendations on dosages.
C. Length of application
   1. Treatment time is calculated from:
      a. Desired dosage
      b. Average power output
      c. Area to be treated
D. Frequency of application: Daily
E. Duration of therapy: As long as discernable progress is being made.

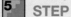 STEP 4: **POSTAPPLICATION TASKS**

A. Equipment removal; patient cleanup
B. Instructions to the patient. These should be written if they are extensive or complicated.
   1. Schedule the next treatment.
   2. Instruct the patient about the level of activity and/or self-treatment prior to the next formal treatment.
   3. Instruct the patient about what she should feel following treatment.

C. Record of treatment, including unique patient responses
D. Equipment replacement; area cleanup

STEP 5: **MAINTENANCE**

A. Regular equipment cleaning
   1. Clean the laser head with a disinfectant if it was applied directly to the skin.
B. Routine maintenance
C. Simple repairs

Ultraviolet Radiation

Ultraviolet modalities were once part of athletic training clinics, but this is no longer the case. It now is generally applied by dermatologists. This brief section is intended to inform you of the effects so you understand the treatment given when one of your patients sees a dermatologist.

Ultraviolet (UV) radiation is a portion of the electromagnetic spectrum that produces chemical reactions in microorganisms, epidermis, and dermis. Its effects are superficial and mainly chemical, and it is used therapeutically to destroy superficial infectious organisms and other microorganisms.

UV radiation is easy to misuse. Incorrect application can lead to numerous dermatitis conditions, such as local ulceration, impetigo, folliculitis, and herpes simplex. Overexposure can lead to increased sensitivity to ordinary sunlight. It can also lead to cancer.

Caution must be exercised when treating patients with a generalized dermatitis (eczema, psoriasis, herpes simplex, etc.), freckles atrophy, keratoses, or prematurely senile skin; diabetes or hyperthyroidism; and those who are highly nervous.

CLOSING SCENE

Alex now understands how lasers are used by a variety of people for a variety of reasons, and that although they are similar in principle, they differ in the type of lasing medium they use to produce their beam, and in the wavelength and power of their output. He understands that the laser a surgeon uses to burn tissue generates more power than the one an AT uses to stimulate tissue healing. Alex also knows that although light therapy appears to be powerful therapy for some conditions, it is no more than a placebo for others. He is eager to follow the future writings of scientists and master clinicians as they more fully determine when it is most appropriate to use lasers.

Chapter Reflections

1. Read and ponder each of the following points. Do you feel you have a clear understanding of each concept? If not, reread the appropriate section of the chapter.
   • Describe what laser means.
   • Describe how a laser beam is generated.
   • Define each of the following terms as they relate to lasers: light, amplify, stimulate, emission, radiation, electromagnetic energy, frequency, visible light, nondivergent, monochromatic, coherent, fixed phase, lasing medium, half-silvered mirror, photon.
   • Explain what is meant by this statement: Lasers are not a single device, but rather a variety of devices.
   • Describe how lasers are classified, and name some of the levels within the classification.

- Explain how laser safety is determined.
- Explain the roles of wavelength, color, and energy level in the body's response to laser therapy.
- Explain the difference between laser therapy and light therapy using an LED or SLD. What are the implications of this difference?
- Explain the differences between the lasers used by surgeons and athletic trainers.
- Describe what happens at the molecular level when lasers are applied to the tissue.
- What is photobiomodulation, and what role does it play in laser therapy?
- Differentiate between in vitro and in vivo research, and relate these concepts to laser therapy.
- What does light therapy mean; and how is it related to laser therapy?
- What are the primary indications for laser therapy?
- Define the three primary delivery techniques used to apply laser therapy.
- Explain how dosage is determined for treating orthopedic injuries with laser therapy.

- Discuss the depth of penetration of lasers in human tissue, and explain the implications this has on laser therapy.

2. Write three to five questions for discussion with your class instructor, clinical instructor, classmates, and clinical colleagues.

3. Get together with classmates and quiz each other on the concepts of this chapter. Use the points in #1 and the questions you wrote for #2 as a beginning. Explaining concepts out loud to others requires a deeper grasp of the material than feeling you understand it as you read.

4. Once you feel you understand the principles of application, practice applying light therapy using the five-step approach, to a classmate or a clinical colleague. Once you have applied it, allow the classmate to apply the modality to you, listening and observing carefully to determine if your classmate is applying it properly. You should use your notes when the modality is applied to you, and during the first few times you apply the modality. Continue practicing the application until you can do so without your notes.

Concept Check Response

CONCEPT CHECK 20.1

Diathermy and laser therapy are alike because both are electromagnetic and the photon is the basic unit of both modalities. Differences include diathermy generates heat, laser does not; diathermy penetrates deep, laser is only superficial; laser waves are visual, diathermy waves are not.

REFERENCES

1. Enwemeka CS. Low level laser therapy is not low. *Photomed Laser Surg.* 2005;23:529–530.
2. Smith KC. Laser (and LED) therapy is phototherapy. *Photomed Laser Surg.* 2005;23:78–80.
3. Vladimirov YA, Osipov AN, Klebanov GI. Photobiological principles of therapeutic application of laser radiation. *Biochemistry (Moscow).* 2004;69:81–90.
4. Quimby RS. *Photonics and Lasers.* Hoboken, NJ: John Wiley and Sons, 2006.
5. Harris T, Fenton W. How Light Emitting Diodes Work. *How Stuff Works.* Available at: http://www.howstuffworks.com/led.htm. Accessed July 2012.
6. Enwemeka CS. Light is light. *Photomed Laser Surg.* 2005;23:159–160.
7. Müller GJ. Laser Applications in Medicine, Biology, and Environmental Science. Paper presented at: International Conference on Lasers, Applications, and Technologies, 2002; Moscow, Russia.
8. Berlien H-P, Müller G, eds. *Applied Laser Medicine.* New York: Springer-Verlag, 2005.
9. McLeod IA. Low-level laser therapy in athletic training. *Athl Ther Today.* 2004;9(5):17–21.
10. Baxter GD. *Therapeutic Lasers: Theory and Practice.* Edinburgh: Churchill Livingstone, 1994.
11. Karu TI. Molecular mechanism of the therapeutic effect of low intensity laser irradiation. *Lasers Life Sci.* 1988;2:53–74.
12. Karu T, Pyatibrat L, Kalendo G. Irradiation with He-Ne laser increases ATP level in cells cultivated in vitro. *J Photochem Photobiol B.* 1995;27(3):219–223.
13. Abergel RP, Meeker CA, Lam TS, et al. Control of connective tissue metabolism by lasers: recent developments and future prospects. *J Am Acad Dermatol.* 1984;11:1142–1150.
14. Boulton M, Marshall J. He-Ne laser stimulation of human fibroblast proliferation and attachment in vitro. *Lasers in Life Sci.* 1986;1:125–134.
15. Poon VK, Huang L, Burd A. Biostimulation of dermal fibroblast by sublethal Q-switched Nd:YAG 532 nm laser: Collagen remodeling and pigmentation. *J Photochem Photobiol B.* 2005;81(1):1–8.
16. Pourzarandian A, Watanabe H, Ruwanpura SM, Aoki A, Ishikawa I. Effect of low level Er:YAG laser irradiation on cultured human gingival fibroblasts. *J Periodontol.* 2005;76(2):187–193.
17. Lyons RF, Abergel RP, White RA. Biostimulation of wound healing in vivo by helium neon laser. *Ann Plast Surg.* 1987;18:47–50.
18. Pourreau-Schneider N, Ahmed A, Soudry M, et al. Helium-neon laser treatment transforms fibroblasts into myofibroblasts. *Am J Pathol.* 1990;137:171–178.

19. Colver GB, Priestly GC. Failure of HeNe to affect components of wound healing in vitro. *Br J Dermatol.* 1989;121:179–186.

20. Hallman HO, Basford JR, O'Brien JF. Does low energy HeNe laser irradiation alter in vitro replication of human fibroblasts? *Lasers Surg Med.* 1988;8:125–129.

21. Stadler I, Evans R, Kolb B, et al. In vitro effects of low-level laser irradiation at 660 nm on peripheral blood lymphocytes. *Laser Surg Med.* 2000;27:255–261.

22. Mester E, Mester A, Mester A. The biomedical effects of laser application. *Lasers Surg Med.* 1985;5(1):31–39.

23. Young S, Bolton P, Dyson M, Harvey W, Diamantopoulos C. Macrophage responsiveness to light therapy. *Lasers Surg Med.* 1989;9:497–505.

24. Inoue K, Nishioka J, Hukuda S. Altered lymphocyte proliferation by low dosage laser irradiation. *Clin Exp Rheumatol.* 1989;7:521–523.

25. Oath A, Abergel RP, Vitto J. Laser modulation of human immune system: inhibition of lymphocyte proliferation by Gallium-Arsenide laser at low energy. *Laser Surg Med.* 1987;7:199–201.

26. Hopkins JT, McLoda TA, Seegmiller. Low-level laser therapy facilitates superficial wound healing. *J Athl Train.* 2004;39(3):223–229.

27. Chromey PA. The efficacy of carbon dioxide laser surgery for adjunct ulcer therapy. *Clin Podiat Med Surg.* 1992;9:709–719.

28. Gogia PP, Hurt BS, Zirn TT. Wound management with whirlpool and infrared cold laser treatment. A clinical report. *Phys Ther.* 1988;68:1239–1242.

29. Schindl A, Schindl M, Schindl L. Successful treatment of a persistent radiation ulcer by low power laser therapy. *J Am Acad Dermatol.* 1997;37(4):646–648.

30. Gigo-Benato D, Geuna S, Rochkind S. Phototherapy for enhancing peripheral nerve repair: a review of the literature. *Muscle Nerve.* 2005;31(6):694–701.

31. Dyson M, Young S. Effect of laser therapy on wound contraction and cellularity in mice. *Lasers Med Sci.* 1986;1:126–130.

32. Allendorf JD, Bessler M, Huang J, et al. Helium-neon laser irradiation at fluences of 1, 2, and 4 J/cm2 failed to accelerate wound healing as assessed by wound contracture rate and tensile strength. *Lasers Surg Med.* 1997;20:340–345.

33. Hunter J, Leonard L, Wilson R, Snider G, Dixon J. Effects of low energy laser on wound healing in a porcine model. *Lasers Surg Med.* 1984;3:285–290.

34. Lundberg T, Malm M. Low-power HeNe laser treatment of venous leg ulcers. *Ann Plast Surg.* 1991;27:537–539.

35. Chow R, Barnsley L. Systematic review of the literature of low-level laser therapy (LLLT) in the management of neck pain. *Lasers Surg Med.* 2005;37(1):46–52.

36. Beckerman H, de Bie R, Bouter L, De Cuyper H, Oostendorp R. The efficacy of laser therapy for musculoskeletal and skin disorders: a criteria-based meta-analysis of randomized clinical trials. *Phys Ther.* 1992;72:483–491.

37. de Bie RA, de Vet HCW, Lenssen TF, van den Wildenberg FAJM, Koostra G, Knipschild PG. Low-level laser therapy in ankle sprains: a randomized clinical trial. *Arch Phys Med Rehabil.* 1998;79:1415–1420.

38. Gam AN, Thorson H, Lonnberg F. The effect of low-level laser therapy on musculoskeletal pain: a meta analysis. *Pain.* 1993;52:63–66.

39. Enwemeka CS, Parker JC, Dowdy DS, Harkness EE, Sanford LE, Woodruff LD. The efficacy of low-power lasers in tissue repair and pain control: a metanalysis. *Photomed Laser Surg.* 2004;22(4):323–329.

40. Simunovic Z. Low level laser therapy with trigger points technique: a clinical study on 243 patients. *J Clin Laser Med Surg.* 1996;14(4):163–167.

41. Simunovic Z, Trobonjaca T, Trobonjaca Z. Treatment of medial and lateral epicondylitis-tennis and golfer's elbow-with low level laser therapy: a multicenter double blind, placebo-controlled clinical study on 324 patients. *J Clin Laser Med Surg.* 1998;16(3):145–151.

42. Brosseau L, Welch V, Wells G, et al. Low level laser therapy for osteoarthritis and rheumatoid arthritis: a metaanalysis. *J Rheumatol.* 2000;27:1961–1969.

43. Naeser MA, Hahn KK, Lieberman BE, Branco KF. Carpal tunnel syndrome pain treated with low-level laser and microamperes trancutaneous electric nerve stimulation: a controlled study. *Arch Phys Med Rehabil.* 2002;83:978–988.

44. Basford JR, Sheffield CG, Harmsen WS. Laser therapy: a randomized, controlled trial of the effects of low-intensity Nd:YAG laser irradiation on musculoskeletal back pain. *Arch Phys Med Rehabil.* 1999;80(6):647–652.

45. Basford JR, Malanga GA, Krause DA, Harmsen WS. A randomized controlled evaluation of low intensity laser therapy: plantar fascitis. *Arch Phys Med Rehabil.* 1998;79(3):249–254.

46. Craig JA, Barlas P, Baxter GD, Walsh DM, Allen JM. Delayed-onset muscle soreness: lack of effect of combined phototherapy/low-intensity laser therapy at low pulse repetition rates. *J Clin Laser Med Surg.* 1996;14(6):375–380.

47. Gür A, Karakoc M, Nas K, et al. Efficacy of low power laser therapy in fibromyalgia: a single-blind, placebo-controlled trial. *Lasers Med Sci.* 2002;17:57–61.

48. Snyder-Mackler L, Bork CE. Effect of Helium-Neon laser irradiation on peripheral sensory nerve latency. *Phys Ther.* 1988;68:223–225.

49. Vinck E, Coorevits P, Cagnie B, et al. Evidence of changes in sural nerve conduction mediated by light emitting diode irradiation. *Lasers Med Sci.* 2005;20(1):35–40.

50. Basford JR, Daude JR, Hallman HO. Does low intensity Helium-Neon laser irradiation alter sensory nerve action potentials or distal latencies? *Laser in Surg Med.* 1990;10:35–39.

51. Ferreira DM, Zangaro RA, Villaverde AB, et al. Analgesic effect of He-Ne (632.8 nm) low-level laser therapy on acute inflammatory pain. *Photomed Laser Surg.* 2005;23(2):177–181.

Review Questions

Part VI

Chapter 18

1. Which massage technique is also known as kneading?
   a. tapotement
   b. vibration
   c. pétrissage
   d. Rolfing
   e. effleurage

2. Which of the following is *not* a physiological effect of massage?
   a. wringing out lactic acid
   b. decreasing pain
   c. increasing flexibility
   d. stimulating circulation
   e. facilitating healing

3. Which of the following is a contraindication for massage?
   a. postacute edema
   b. pain
   c. muscle spasm
   d. embolism
   e. sore muscles

4. Which of the following is *not* a reflexive effect of massage?
   a. decreased pain
   b. elongated fascia
   c. increased circulation
   d. increased metabolism
   e. relaxation

5. Which massage stroke is used to stimulate the muscles for competition?
   a. pétrissage
   b. friction
   c. effleurage
   d. percussion
   e. tapotement

6. Which type of massage technique is used to break up adhesions?
   a. pétrissage
   b. friction
   c. effleurage
   d. tapotement
   e. raindrops

7. Which of the following is *not* a contraindication for massage?
   a. fractures
   b. arteriosclerosis
   c. pain of no known origin
   d. acute edema
   e. none of the above

8. Which massage technique is used to relieve soft tissue from the abnormal grip of surrounding tissue?
   a. pétrissage
   b. friction massage
   c. Hoffa technique
   d. myofascial release
   e. deep effleurage

Chapter 19

1. Which of the following is *not* a treatment parameter for traction?
   a. patient position
   b. treatment mode
   c. traction force
   d. device needed
   e. frequency

2. Which of the following refers to whether or not the traction is sustained or intermittent?
   a. patient position
   b. treatment mode
   c. traction force
   d. device needed
   e. frequency

3. In general, what percentage of the patient's weight should be applied when performing lumbar traction?
   a. 30
   b. 40
   c. 50
   d. 60
   e. 70

4. In general, no more than how many pounds of force should be applied when performing cervical traction?
   a. 25
   b. 35
   c. 45
   d. 55
   e. one quarter of the body weight

5. Which of the following requires a special split table to apply traction?
   a. manual traction
   b. autotraction
   c. single-leg manual traction
   d. pneumatic mechanical traction
   e. inversion-table traction

6. Which of the following is contraindicated by someone with glaucoma?
   a. manual traction
   b. autotraction
   c. single-leg manual traction
   d. pneumatic mechanical traction
   e. inversion-table traction

7. Which of the following is a contraindication for traction?
   a. adhesions
   b. apophyseal joint impingement
   c. muscle spasm
   d. radiating pain that does not improve with trunk movement
   e. acute neck pain

8. Which of the following is not a way in which traction appears to relieve pain?
   a. widening the intervertebral foramen
   b. creating suction to draw protruded disks toward their center
   c. relaxing muscles
   d. decreasing space between vertebrae
   e. two of the above

9. Benefits of the inversion-table traction device include which of the following?
   a. It can be purchased at a wholesale outlet store for about $200.00.
   b. It is easy to use.
   c. There are no belts to slip; thus constant traction is applied the whole time.
   d. The patient can control the level (in degrees) of traction desired.
   e. all of the above

Chapter 20

1. Light therapy is a form of _____.
   a. electromagnetic energy
   b. mechanical energy
   c. superficial heat
   d. deep heat
   e. none of the above

2. Which of the following is not a characteristic of laser?
   a. monophasic
   b. monochromatic
   c. radiant
   d. coherent
   e. divergent

3. Lasers are commonly classified according to _____.
   a. the type of lasing medium they use
   b. their safety
   c. the intensity of their color
   d. both a and b
   e. both b and c

4. The safety of a laser is primarily a function of its _____.
   a. color
   b. divergence
   c. energy
   d. lasing medium
   e. coherence

5. The difference between a surgical laser and a therapeutic laser is primarily owing to its _____.
   a. color
   b. divergence
   c. energy
   d. lasing medium
   e. coherence

6. Therapeutic lasers are also known as low-level lasers. What does *low level* refer to?
   a. frequency
   b. wavelength
   c. divergence
   d. energy
   e. coherence

7. All of the following are techniques of applying light therapy *except* _____.
   a. single-probe application
   b. tricorder-probe application
   c. cluster-probe application
   d. grid application
   e. scanning

8. Altering the dosage of a laser is done by altering the _____.
   a. total power
   b. average power
   c. divergence
   d. coherence
   e. treatment time

9. Which of the following would be most likely to benefit from light therapy?
   a. deep muscle strain
   b. subscapular bursitis
   c. forearm abrasion
   d. blurred vision
   e. nosebleed

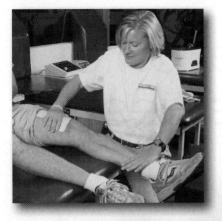

Putting It All Together

The two brief chapters of Part VII set the stage for a successful and productive career providing health care to people with musculoskeletal injuries. We will help you pull everything together so you can make proper decisions about what modality is best for specific situations.

The philosophy in Chapter 21 is totally different than the philosophy of the majority of this book. The perspective of the individual modality chapters has been to present a specific modality, including its scientific and theoretical base, how the body reacts to it, the types of injuries you can treat with it, and expected outcomes from using it. Although this is the standard, and probably the best, way to teach each of the modalities, it is not the perspective of a clinician using the modalities.

In Chapter 21, we turn your thinking around a bit—try to get you thinking from the perspective of a clinician who sees a patient with pain and loss of function, often specific, but sometimes general and indistinct. Thinking about individual modalities is the farthest from her mind at this point. She must evaluate the patient, determine the patient's specific needs, develop a treatment plan with performance goals, and then select the modality that is best suited for achieving the most immediate short-term goals. The emphasis is on what the patient needs, not what a specific modality can do.

Chapter 22 is a series of case studies, presented as referral sheets from a physician. Working through the case studies will help you make the transition we introduce in Chapter 21.

Differential Application of Therapeutic Modalities

OPENING SCENE

During Thanksgiving break, Andrew sprained his ankle during a pickup game of basketball with friends. He thought the injury was minor and did nothing to care for it. A week later, it is now swollen and painful when he walks. Knowing you have almost completed a therapeutic modalities course, your clinical instructor asks your advice about a treatment plan. He agrees with you that your first goals are to reduce swelling and restore pain-free range of motion. Then he asks you how you plan to accomplish these goals, what therapeutic modality you should use. Many modalities are indicated for treating ankle sprains—is one better than another? How do you decide which to use?

Differential Application of Modalities

Differential application of modalities refers to the process of determining the optimal modality to use under specific circumstances. Knowing when to use a particular modality, or knowing what modality is best under certain circumstances, is one of the most important concepts you need to grasp. If you introduce the wrong modality at the wrong time, your patients will fail to respond to the treatment, or their injuries might become worse (e.g., using heat as a modality too early after an acute injury). As a result, recovery will be compromised.

LEARNING ABOUT VERSUS USING THERAPEUTIC MODALITIES

In writing this book, we have followed the standard approach to teaching therapeutic modalities—presenting a specific single modality at a time. For each modality we discussed what it was, what it does, and indications (conditions) for using the modality (Table 21.1). The approach is correct for teaching but the exact opposite of how therapeutic modalities are used in real life. Patients generally do not approach you saying, "I have a strained flexor carpi ulnaris and need an ultrasound treatment." Rather, they say, "My elbow hurts." You must diagnose the specific problem, establish treatment goals, and then select the most effective modality for reaching those goals (Table 21.2).

In Chapter 1, we presented criteria for selecting a therapeutic modality, which are to:

1. Have a correct diagnosis.
2. Have a definite concept of the pathological and physiological changes associated with the injury.
3. Know what you want to accomplish with the modality; in other words, have a therapeutic goal.
4. Understand the modality's effects, indications, and contraindications.
5. Match your therapeutic goal with a modality that will help you achieve that goal.

You start with the patient and injury, select a goal, and then select the appropriate modality.

 CONCEPT CHECK 21.1. What do you think will be the biggest stumbling block to your full use of the differential application process in choosing therapeutic modalities?

TABLE 21.1 SPECIFIC INDICATIONS FOR SELECTED THERAPEUTIC MODALITIES

MODALITY	CONDITION
Connective tissue stretch	Connective tissue contractures
	Stretching collagen-rich tissues
	Ankle sprains
	Edema
	Sprains
	Swelling
Contrast baths	(do not use)
Cryokinetics	Ankle and other joint sprains
	Edema and swelling reduction
	Blood flow stimulation
Cryostretch	Contusions
	Muscle spasm
	Muscle stiffness
	Muscle strain
Diathermy	Bursitis
	Joint contractures
	Muscle strain
	Myofascial trigger points
	Pain
	Subacute inflammation
	Tendinitis
	Tenosynovitis
High-volt pulsed current (HPVC) stimulation	Chronic muscle spasm
	Edema (control and reduction)
	Muscle spasm
	Pain
	Wound healing (pressure sores, incisions)
Hot packs	Local heat
	Blood flow stimulation
	Supplement to other treatment.
Interferential current (IFC)	Pain; acute and chronic
	Muscle spasm
Iontophoresis	Anesthesia
	Inflammation
	Injection alternative
	Pain

(Continued)

TABLE 21.1 SPECIFIC INDICATIONS FOR SELECTED THERAPEUTIC MODALITIES (Continued)

MODALITY	CONDITION
Laser	Pain
	Superficial wounds
Lymphedema pump	Post-traumatic edema
	Swelling
	Venous stasis ulcers
	Relaxation, systemic
	Swelling
Neuromuscular electrical stimulation (NMES)	Chronic muscle spasm
	Disuse atrophy
	Immobilization
	Muscle strain
	Neuromuscular function impaired
	Pain
Paraffin	Local heat, feet and hands Supplement to other treatment
Phonophoresis	Tendinitis, bursitis Myofascial trigger points
RICES	Acute injury
Spinal traction	Adhesions
	Apophyseal joint impingement
	Connective tissue contractures
	Disk degeneration
	Disk protrusion
	Foraminal stenosis
	Joint hypomobility
	Muscle spasm
	Nerve root compression
	Radiating pain unresponsive to movement
Transcutaneous electrical nerve stimulation (TENS)	Pain, acute; pain, chronic
Ultrasound	Bone spurs
	Bursitis
	Plantar warts
	Sprains, strains, and contusions
	Tendinitis
Ultraviolet radiation	Skin conditions involving microorganisms
Whirlpool	Stiffness, general
	Supplement to other treatment

TABLE 21.2 SELECTED CONDITIONS AND THERAPEUTIC MODALITIES FOR TREATMENT

CONDITION	MODALITY
Adhesions	Spinal traction
Anesthesia	Iontophoresis
Ankle sprains	Cryokinetics
Apophyseal joint impingement	Spinal traction
Blood flow stimulation	Cryokinetics
	Diathermy
	Hot packs
	Massage
Bone spurs	Ultrasound
Bursitis	Diathermy
	Phonophoresis
	Ultrasound
Chronic muscle spasm	HVPC stimulation
	NMES
Chronic pain	IFC
	TENS
Connective tissue contractures	Connective tissue stretch
	Spinal traction
Contusions	Cryostretch
Disk degeneration	Spinal traction
Disk protrusion	Spinal traction
Disuse atrophy	NMES
Edema control	HVPC stimulation
	RICES
Edema reduction	Cryokinetics
	HVPC stimulation
	Lymphedema pump
Foraminal stenosis	Spinal traction
Immobilization	NMES
Inflammation	Iontophoresis
Injection alternative	Iontophoresis
Joint contractures	Diathermy
Joint hypomobility	Spinal traction
Local heat	Hot packs
Local heat, feet and hands	Paraffin

(Continued)

TABLE 21.2 SELECTED CONDITIONS AND THERAPEUTIC MODALITIES FOR TREATMENT (*Continued*)

CONDITION	MODALITY
Muscle spasm	Cryostretch
	HVPC stimulation
	IFC
	Massage
	NMES
	Spinal traction
Muscle stiffness	Cryostretch
Muscle strain	Cryostretch
	Diathermy
	NMES
Myofascial trigger points	Diathermy
	Phonophoresis
Nerve root compression	Spinal traction
Neuromuscular function impaired	NMES
Pain	Diathermy
	HVPC stimulation
	IFC
	Iontophoresis
	Laser
Pain, acute	IFC
	TENS
Pain, chronic	TENS
Pain, muscle spasm	Massage
	NMES
Plantar warts	Ultrasound
Post-traumatic edema	cryokinetics
	Lymphedema pump
	Massage
Radiating pain unresponsive to movement	Spinal traction
Relaxation, systemic	Massage
Skin conditions involving microorganisms	Ultraviolet radiation
Sprains	Cryokinetics
Sprains, strains, and contusions	Ultrasound
Stiffness, general	Whirlpool

TABLE 21.2 SELECTED CONDITIONS AND THERAPEUTIC MODALITIES FOR TREATMENT (*Continued*)

CONDITION	MODALITY
Stretching collagen-rich tissues	Connective tissue stretch
Subacute inflammation	Diathermy
Swelling	Cryokinetics
	Lymphedema pump
	Massage
Tendinitis	Diathermy
	Phonophoresis
	Ultrasound
Tenosynovitis	Diathermy
Venus stasis ulcers	Lymphedema pump
Wound healing (pressure sores, incisions)	HVPC stimulation
Wound healing, surface	Laser

TREATMENT GOALS

Treatment goals are the guiding light to all therapeutic modality use. Long-term, midrange, and daily short-term goals should be articulated, and treatment protocols, including the judicious use of therapeutic modalities, should be selected to achieve those goals. Review the section on treatment goals in Chapter 1, and refer to Table 21.3. Remember that therapeutic modalities are just one part of a comprehensive therapy plan to rehabilitate the patient to full, pain-free activity.

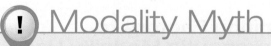

! Modality Myth

SHORT-TERM GOALS FOCUS ON REDUCING SYMPTOMS RATHER THAN TREATING THE INJURY

Some clinicians have claimed that long-term treatment goals should focus on treating the cause of the injury, whereas short-term treatment goals often include modality use to reduce the symptoms.[1] This is short-sighted. Although modality use can reduce symptoms, which is beneficial, they should be used primarily to promote healing and resolution of the injury. Rarely, if ever, should your goal be merely to reduce symptoms.

TABLE 21.3	MODALITY APPLICATION BASED ON PHASE OF INJURY AND HEALING		
PHASE	**SYMPTOMS**	**MODALITY**	**RATIONALE**
Immediate care	Swelling, pain to touch and motion	RICES	↓metabolism and pain
Transition care	As above; discoloration	RICES	↓pain
		Cryokinetics	↓pain; restore function
		Cryostretch	↓pain; restore function
		NMES	↓pain and spasm
		Ultrasound, nonthermal	↑healing
		Lymphedema pump	↓swelling
		Laser	↓pain
		Iontophoresis	↓pain
Subacute care	Swelling subsides; pain to touch and motion decreases then disappears	Cryokinetics	↓pain; restore function
		Cryostretch	↓pain; restore function
		Thermal modalities	↑heat; ↑circulation
		NMES	↓pain; muscle pumping
		Ultrasound, continuous	↑heat; ↑circulation
		Laser	↓pain
		PSWD	↑heat; ↑circulation
Post-acute and chronic	Stiffness, pain	NMES	ROM and strength
		Ultrasound, continuous	↑heat; ↑circulation; ↑tissue extensibility*
		Laser	↓pain; ↓adhesions
		PSWD	↑heat; ↑circulation; ↑tissue extensibility*
		Iontophoresis	↓pain; ↓adhesions
		Thermal modalities	↑heat; ↑circulation

*When combined with stretching or joint mobilization.

Limiting Factors to Therapeutic Modality Use

Following are five factors that could prevent you from using a specific modality, even if it is the most appropriate:

- Availability of the modality
- Time available for treatment
- Evidence supporting the modality
- Patient compliance
- Clinician compliance

AVAILABILITY OF THE MODALITY

The ideal setting for the treatment and rehabilitation of orthopedic injuries would include several possible modalities at your disposal. This, however, is more often the exception than the rule. Thus, many clinicians have to make do with the modalities that are available to them.

Suppose a patient is lacking full range of motion in the shoulder and you want to apply deep heat to the area prior to stretching. In this situation, the ideal modality would be pulsed shortwave diathermy (PSWD; it heats deeply and covers a large area). Unfortunately, not many athletic training or physical therapy clinics house a PSWD unit. If this is your situation, you will need to use what is available. You could try ultrasound because it heats deeply into the tissue. However, this solution is not ideal, as ultrasound will heat only small areas and therefore is not appropriate for heating the entire glenohumeral joint. You could use a hot pack because it will heat a large area such as the shoulder. Unfortunately, hot pack application will result in only minimal heating (1.8°F, or 1°C, at 3 cm deep).[2] You will have to make do with what is available, and if hot packs are your only source of heat that will cover a large area, that's the modality you will need to use.

Some clinic directors lease equipment that they otherwise wouldn't be able to afford. Shortwave diathermy has been used on a "cost-by-use" basis. The machine is equipped with a timer that bills the clinic a predetermined amount for each hour the unit is used. You might want to consider the lease option if the budget in your facility is not high enough to purchase an expensive piece of equipment.

Another consideration is the number of duplicate modalities available. For example, if your facility has only one ultrasound machine and that unit is traveling with another sports team, a different modality will have to be substituted for ultrasound. Or if another clinician is using the ultrasound machine when you need it, you might have to substitute another modality. Regardless of the reason, availability plays a big role in determining when to use certain modalities.

TIME AVAILABLE FOR TREATMENT

A key consideration when determining what modality to use is the optimal treatment times for each modality. Remember, one of the purposes for using modalities is to prepare the tissues to perform a specific function. If the goal is increased range of motion, a 10-minute hot pack application prior to exercise or stretching is not sufficient to relax tissues or promote tissue extensibility. A modality must be applied long enough to deliver the benefits.

For example, during rehabilitation after back surgery, one of us (DD) had ice packs applied for only 10 minutes after exercise. If the goal was to reduce postexercise pain, it worked. However, a 20–30 minute-ice pack application is more appropriate to curb the effects of microtrauma that might have occurred during exercise. Table 21.4 lists the approximate treatment times for several therapeutic modalities.

Another key consideration when determining what modality to use is how much time the patient has for each individual treatment. Treatment sessions using therapeutic modalities typically take an hour (20–30 minutes of application and an additional 20–30 minutes of teaching, therapeutic exercise, and assessment).[3] Therefore, it might be important to schedule patients when you know that a particular modality is available. Giving a shorter treatment time than is optimal borders on being unethical. For example, it is unethical to bill an insurance company for an ultrasound treatment that only lasted 5 minutes, when a 12-minute treatment would have been optimal for the condition.

By contrast, treatments that last too long may actually add to the muscle guarding secondary to tension, with

TABLE 21.4 APPROXIMATE TREATMENT TIMES FOR THERAPEUTIC MODALITIES	
MODALITY	**TREATMENT TIMES (MIN)**
Ice pack (RICES)	30–45
Ice massage	10–15 (until numb)
Ice immersion	10–15 (until numb)
Lymphedema pump	15–30
Whirlpool (cold)	10–15 (until numb)
Whirlpool (hot)	15–20
Hot packs	15–20
Paraffin bath	10–15
Ultrasound (pulsed)	5–10
Ultrasound (3 MHz)	5–8
Ultrasound (1 MHz)	10–15
PSWD	15–30
TENS	15–30
HVPC stimulation	15–30
IFC	15–30
NMES	20–30
Iontophoresis	8–12
Microcurrent	10–15
LASER	2–6

an increased pain perception.[3] Long treatments can also add to a patient's boredom, or the idea that she is being cheated. The patient might feel that she should be paying to be worked on by a clinician, not a machine.

It is not necessary to use every modality that could possibly be employed to treat a patient. Because of overlapping responses, using a variety of modalities is redundant. Also, few ATs have spare time to apply redundant treatments. Assess the situation, establish therapeutic goals that you think will alleviate the problem, and limit the choices of modalities to those that will accomplish the goal(s). Assess the outcome of a modality, and then, if necessary, add an additional modality to address any symptoms the modality did not relieve.

The approach taken may be more effective if the patient is involved in the process. For example, if a patient recently read an article in a magazine about the benefits of icing for pain reduction, he might respond better to ice treatments than electrical stimulation. Or if a patient saw an advertisement on television about the benefits of portable, long-lasting heat, she might use the product at home as an adjunct to heat used in the clinic.

EVIDENCE SUPPORTING THE MODALITY

Before you employ any modality, ask yourself: Is there evidence to support the use of this modality in this situation? Perhaps the most important consideration is whether or not a modality actually does what the product brochure claims it does. Search the evidence-based databases (see Table 2.2). If there is little or no evidence to support the use of the modality, don't waste your time and the patient's money in a purely placebo treatment. Familiarize yourself with the research regarding those modalities you use the most. Also, if there is ample support for the use of a particular modality, consider sharing these positive research results with the patient. This may lead to not only improved treatment outcomes but also better patient compliance.

COMPLIANCE

Compliance is a manifestation of the old adage that *you can lead a horse to water, but you can't make him drink*. No matter how effective a given intervention is for a specific injury or illness, unless it prescribed and then administered properly, it is of limited value. Noncompliance can result from either failure of the clinician to initiate proper interventions or failure of the patient to follow the recommended intervention.[4] Noncompliance is a major medical issue.[5,6]

Patient Compliance

Patient compliance (also known as patient adherence[7,8]) means consistently and accurately following the treatment orders or instructions given by the clinician. **Patient noncompliance** is the failure to fully follow the treatment orders or instructions given by the clinician, including home treatment and returning for clinic treatments. Many factors are involved in whether or not a patient will comply with your treatment orders. Compliance by the patient's family or spouse is also important.

Research in a variety of health professions clearly indicates a direct relationship between patient compliance and rate of or degree of recovery.[6,9] In some situations, noncompliance can be devastating. Consider the mallet finger; no matter how careful you are in protecting it with special splints and taping during and after practices for weeks after the injury, a single episode of flexing the finger will negate everything you have done.[10]

Despite its importance, however, compliance remains a major problem in medicine. As one author questioned: "Why, after 40 years of intensive research, is adherence to treatment still an issue?"[5]

An example of noncompliance to a home treatment is a junior high school basketball player who suffered an acute ankle sprain in Friday's game. The athletic trainer prescribed RICES over the weekend. Unfortunately, the athlete found the cold treatment to be uncomfortable. His parents give in to his complaints and allow him to omit the ice treatments. In this way, noncompliant parents support a noncompliant patient. The result is that the athlete returns to school on Monday with an ankle that is more swollen and painful than it should have been.

Poor treatment in the clinic often results in noncompliance—the patient fails to return for follow-up treatments. If the clinician doesn't seem to take much of an interest in the patient,[4] or if the treatments are painful, the patient might not return as often as necessary to obtain optimal results. For example, when one of us (DD) was running cross-country at a junior college, I had knee surgery that required my left leg to be in a straight-leg cast for 4 weeks. The week the cast was removed, I reported to physical therapy. The therapist noted very little ROM in knee flexion, and attempted to restore it in one treatment. The therapist had me lie down on the table and said, "Now this is going to hurt." She then grabbed the leg and tried to flex it as far as possible in one quick motion. I cried out in pain as I slid forward on the table. I never returned to that physical therapist or clinic. Patient compliance could have been achieved if the therapist provided some form of heat therapy to my knee and then performed graded joint mobilizations.

Following are suggestions for improving patient compliance:

- Communication.[6,11,12] Develop the following four habits when communicating with patients[6]: (1) Invest in the beginning–engage the patient, develop a rapport. (2) Elicit the patients perspective; invite the patient to become a partner in resolving the injury/illness. (3) Demonstrate empathy; encourage the patients to share feelings and emotions, and respond in a way that validates their emotions. (4) Invest in the end; focus on sharing information, establishing goals, inviting questions. (See Table 21.5 and Abgood[6,12] for further explanation and examples of these habits.)
- Educating patients about their disorder and about healthy lifestyle behaviors helps increase their compliance.[4,6–8] Make sure they understand how to perform assigned self-care activities. Education is not enough; however, a large proportion of patients remain noncompliant despite awareness of risk.[13]

TABLE 21.5 EFFECTIVE COMMUNICATION SKILLS FOR HEALTH CARE PROVIDERS

- Ability to assess the emotional state of the patient
- Ability to evaluate the patient's knowledge and understanding of the situation
- Ability to ask open-ended questions (responses are not simply "yes" or "no")
- Active listening to patient responses (rather than rushing to ask another question)
- Ability to accurately interpret verbal cues, such as silence
- Recognize nonverbal cues from patient's body language
- Provide clear, unambiguous instructions

Source: Adapted from Abood[12]

- Give written instructions for self-care activities and behaviors (Table 21.6). The more complex instructions are, the less likely they will be performed properly. Think of how compliant you would be if your professor gave you three ranges of pages to read for the next class, and you were unable to write them. You might have a specific sheet of instructions for the most common conditions that can be copied and given to patients.
- Prepare a DVD of specific interventions, such as common exercise programs that you can give to patients, or upload to their iphone.[14]

TABLE 21.6 SELF-CARE ACTIVITIES AND BEHAVIORS INSTRUCTIONS

Injury _____

GOAL:

_____ Promote Healing	_____ Inc M Speed
_____ Reduce Pain	_____ Inc skill
_____ Inc ROM	_____ Inc Power
_____ Inc Strength	_____ Inc Agility
_____ Inc M. Endurance	_____ Inc CR Endurance

SPECIFIC INTERVENTION:

Frequency: Days _____, Times/day _____

Protocol (how to) & Specific Instructions:

ACTIVITIES TO AVOID:

NEXT FORMAL TREATMENT:

Clinician _____ ph # _____

- In-depth follow-up of behaviors since last formal treatment. Patients usually are assigned specific behaviors to follow between formal treatments, such as taking medication at specific times, refraining from certain activities, performing *x* repetitions of other activities. Carefully follow up by asking specific questions about each assigned behavior. Simply asking a patient if they did what they were supposed to is not enough, they often overstate their compliance. For example, in one study, only 34% of patients who perceived themselves as compliant exhibited a good level of compliance when specific behaviors were investigated.[13]

CLINICIAN COMPLIANCE

Another component of therapeutic intervention leading to patient compliance or noncompliance is **clinician compliance**–the reliability, knowledge, confidence, and professionalism of the clinician. If the clinician approaches the patient with an unsure attitude such as, "Well, I'm not sure if this piece of equipment will help, but let's give it a try," the patient loses faith in the clinician. Also, if several modalities are used in a shotgun manner, the patient might question whether the clinician knows what he or she is doing. A patient who is made to feel a like guinea pig will often refuse to return for follow-up treatment.

Another reason for noncompliance in returning for treatment is improper use of modalities. If the treatment protocol doesn't make sense to the patient (and isn't helping the condition improve), the patient may not return for follow-up treatments. For example, a 14-year-old girl was diagnosed with temporomandibular joint (TMJ) syndrome. The physician prescribed a heat-and-stretch routine for the jaw, and referred her to a nearby clinic. Ultrasound was correctly applied with the proper protocol to heat the tissues (3 MHz; continuous; 1 W/cm^2; 5–6 minute). Unfortunately, the therapist did not begin to stretch the mandible until 30 minutes after the ultrasound treatment. By that time, the tissue was cooled, and the modality had little effect on the stretching. After two additional similar sessions, the parents took the girl out of therapy. The therapist either did not understand the role of the ultrasound treatment in preparing the tissues for the stretching or was too complacent to care.

It is imperative that clinicians have a firm knowledge of therapeutic modalities. Those who understand the modalities tend to use them to the patient's benefit. On the other hand, clinicians whose only modality is their hands probably do not understand how these valuable tools can prepare tissues for the therapist's hands.

CLOSING SCENE

Recall from the chapter opening scene that you were seeing Andrew, who sprained his ankle; because he thought it was a minor injury, he did nothing to care for it. A week later, it is swollen and painful when he walks. Your clinical instructor asks you what your first goals are. Then she asks you how you plan to accomplish these goals and what therapeutic modality should you use. Differential application of modalities refers to the process of determining the optimal modality to use under specific circumstances. You decide that your first goal should be to remove swelling and restore pain-free range of motion. You employ a lymphedema pump and elevation twice a day to help remove the edema. When the athlete is not in the pump, he wears a compression sock on the ankle.

Chapter Reflections

1. Read and ponder each of the following points. Do you feel you have a clear understanding of each concept? If not, reread the appropriate section of the chapter.
   - What is meant by differential application of therapeutic modalities? How does this concept differ from the way modalities have been taught in this book? How is it more like real life than the approach taken in the previous chapters of this book?
   - Describe several situations where you would use certain modalities in different phases of injury.
   - List several treatment goals, and what modalities would be appropriate to use to reach those goals.
   - Provide several examples of patient compliance.
   - Provide several examples of patient noncompliance.
   - Provide several examples of clinician compliance.
   - Provide several examples of clinician noncompliance.
   - Describe keys to good clinician-patient communication.
2. Write three to five questions for discussion with your class instructor, clinical instructor, classmates, and clinical colleagues.
3. Get together with classmates and quiz each other on the concepts of this chapter. Use the points in no. 1 and the questions you wrote for no.2 as a beginning. Explaining concepts out loud to others requires a deeper grasp of the material than feeling you understand it as you read.

Concept Check Response

CONCEPT CHECK 21.1

The following are factors that could hinder you from properly using the differential application process in choosing therapeutic modalities:
- Inadequate understanding of the anatomy, pathophysiology, and mechanism of specific injuries. Each of these elements is necessary to make a correct diagnosis. And without a correct diagnosis, you cannot develop a proper treatment plan.
- Inadequate understanding of the indications, contraindications, and limitations of each modality. Constant reading of the latest research, including randomized clinical trials, is a prerequisite to properly selecting and using therapeutic modalities.
- Limited availability of a specific therapeutic modality. Knowing that a specific modality is the best modality for the job is of no value if you don't have access to the modality.

REFERENCES

1. Behrens BJ, Michlovitz SL. *Physical Agents: Theory and Practice for the Physical Therapist Assistant*. 2nd ed. Philadelphia, PA: FA Davis, 2008.
2. Draper DO, Harris ST, Schulthies SS, et al. Hotpack and 1 mhz ultrasound treatments have an additive effect on muscle temperature increase. *J Athl Train*. 1998;33:1–2.
3. Behrens BJ, Michlovitz SL. *Physical Agents: Theory and Practice for the Physical Therapist Assistant*. Philadelphia, PA: FA Davis, 1996.
4. Suzuki T, Saito I, Adachi M, Shimbo T, Sato H. Influence of patients' adherence to medication, patient background and physicians' compliance to the guidelines on asthma control. *Yakugaku Zasshi*. 2011;131(1):129–138.
5. Leibing A. Inverting compliance, increasing concerns: aging, mental health, and caring for a trustful patient. *Anthropol Med*. 2010;17(2):145–158.
6. Abood S. Increasing adherence in practice: making your clients partners in care. *Vet Clin North Am Small Anim Pract*. 2007;37(1):151–164.
7. Hacihasanoglu R, Gözüm S. The effect of patient education and home monitoring on medication compliance, hypertension management, healthy lifestyle behaviours and BMI in a primary health care setting. *J Clin Nurs*. 2011;20(5-6):692–705.
8. Deccache A, van Ballekom K. From patient compliance to empowerment and consumer's choice: evolution or regression? An overview of patient education in French speaking European countries. *Patient Educ Couns*. 2010;78(3):282–287.
9. Miyamoto T, Kumagai T, Lang M, Nunn M. Compliance as a prognostic indicator. II. Impact of patient's compliance to the individual tooth survival. *J Periodontol*. 2010;81(9):1280–1288.
10. Anderson D. Mallet finger–management and patient compliance. *Aust Fam Phys*. 2011;40(1/2):47–48.
11. Hahn M. Patient compliance; wherefore art thou? *Am J Bioeth*. 2010;10(11):13–14.
12. Abood S. Effectively communicating with your clients. *Top Companion Anim Med*. 2008;23(3):143–147.
13. Bui T, Cavanagh H, Robertson D. Patient compliance during contact lens wear: perceptions, awareness, and behavior. *Eye Contact Lens*. 2010;36(6):334–339.
14. Kingston G, Gray M, Williams G. A critical review of the evidence on the use of videotapes or DVD to promote patient compliance with home programmes. *Disabil Rehabil Assist Technol*. 2010;5(3):153–163.

Case Studies Using Therapeutic Modalities

Chapter Outline

Clinical Case Studies

The case studies in this chapter will help you apply the differential application principles introduced in Chapter 20. In these case studies, we present a brief history (Hx) and diagnosis (Dx) as they would come to you on a referral slip. (See Table 22.1 for common abbreviations physicians use on therapy referral slips.) Based on this information, decide what therapeutic modality would be best suited in each situation, and why you feel it is best. As you read each case, keep in mind the pathology, the effects of each physical agent, and the precautions that must be addressed. Our opinions about the preferred modality are presented later in the chapter.

If there are differences between your opinions and ours, try to determine why by doing the following:

- Refer to the chapter(s) in which the modalities are presented.
- Discuss the differences with fellow students, your professor, and a clinical instructor.

CASE STUDY 1: LUMBOSACRAL PAIN

REFERRAL	
Hx:	22 y/o overweight offensive lineman, c/o diffuse LBP × 2 wk. Pain is nonradiating and increases c̄ strenuous lifting.
Dx:	Lumbosacral muscle spasm c̄ 1° strain of quadratus lumborum.

Rx: What modalities would be best suited in this situation? Why?

CASE STUDY 2: PIRIFORMIS SYNDROME

REFERRAL	
Hx:	20 y/o ♀ volleyball player c/o (L) buttocks and LBP, × 6 wk.
Dx:	Piriformis syndrome c̄ sciatica.

Rx: What modalities would be best suited in this situation? Why?

CASE STUDY 3: CHRONIC SUPRASPINATIS TENDINITIS

REFERRAL	
Hx:	44 y/o ♂ painter, c/o pain in R shoulder, and limited shoulder ROM due to pain.
Dx:	Chronic supraspinatis tendinitis.

Rx: What modalities would be best suited in this situation? Why?

CASE STUDY 4: HYPOMOBILE RADIAL CARPAL JOINT

REFERRAL	
Hx:	22 y/o ♂ soccer goalie, × 3 mo p/o bone graft for avascular necrosis of the (L) scaphoid.
Dx:	Hypomobile radial carpal joint in all motions due to prolonged cast immobilization.

Rx: What modalities would be best suited in this situation? Why?

TABLE 22.1 ABBREVIATIONS COMMONLY USED ON REFERRALS

ABBREVIATION	DEFINITION	ABBREVIATION	DEFINITION
AA	active assistive	MMT	manual muscle test
Bil	bilateral	NN	nerve
c̄	with	OA	osteoarthritis
c̄/o	complains of	p	post
Dx	diagnosis	p/o	post-operation
ER	emergency room	pt	patient
EXER	exercise	RA	rheumatoid arthritis
♀ or F	female	ROM	range of motion
fx	fracture	RUE	right upper extremity
Hx	history	Rx	prescription
LBP	low-back pain	s	without
LLE	left lower extremity	s/p fx	status post-fracture
L-S	lumbosacral	Tx	treatment
♂ or M	male	×6 mo	for 6 months (or 6 months' duration)
MM	muscle	y/o	year-old

CASE STUDY 5: FIRST-DEGREE INVERSION ANKLE SPRAIN

REFERRAL	
Hx:	16 y/o ♀ basketball player c/o pain on R lateral ankle, c̄ swelling 24 hours post-injury.
Dx:	1° inversion sprain of R ankle.

Rx: What modalities would be best suited in this situation? Why?

CASE STUDY 6: CARPAL TUNNEL SYNDROME

REFERRAL	
Hx:	37 y/o R-handed ♀ employed as a computer operator, c/o tingling and numbness in R hand c̄ loss of ROM and grip strength.
Dx:	Early stages of carpal tunnel syndrome in R hand.

Rx: What modalities would be best suited in this situation? Why?

CASE STUDY 7: ACHILLES TENDINITIS

REFERRAL	
Hx:	30 y/o ♂ marathon runner, c/o chronic pain in area of (L) Achilles tendon.
Dx:	Achilles tendinitis.

Rx: What modalities would be best suited in this situation? Why?

CASE STUDY 8: MILD SPASM OF R/L UPPER TRAPEZIUS

REFERRAL	
Hx:	40 y/o ♂ c/o pain in the cervical region, c̄ muscle spasms. X-rays ruled out fx.
Dx:	1° spasm of R/L upper trapezius.

Rx: What modalities would be best suited in this situation? Why?

CASE STUDY 9: SECOND-DEGREE QUADRICEPS STRAIN

REFERRAL	
Hx:	20 y/o ♂ soccer player c/o pain on L midportion of quadriceps, c̄ swelling 30 min post-injury.
Dx:	2° strain to the L quadriceps.

Rx: What modalities would be best suited in this situation? Why?

CASE STUDY 10: PATELLAR TENDINITIS

REFERRAL	
Hx:	20 y/o ♂ collegiate miler, c/o chronic pain in area of (R) patellar tendon.
Dx:	Patellar tendinitis.

Rx: What modalities would be best suited in this situation? Why?

CASE STUDY 11: LATERAL EPICONDYLITIS

REFERRAL	
Hx:	18 y/o ♀ tennis player, c/o chronic pain in area of (R) elbow.
Dx:	Lateral epicondylitis.

Rx: What modalities would be best suited in this situation? Why?

CASE STUDY 12: ACROMOCLAVICULAR (AC) SEPARATION

REFERRAL	
Hx:	21 y/o ♀ rugby player c/o pain on R AC joint, c̄ swelling 2 hours post-injury. No visible or palpable step-off deformity.
Dx:	1° AC sprain of R shoulder.

Rx: What modalities would be best suited in this situation? Why?

CASE STUDY 13: HAMSTRING CONTUSION

REFERRAL	
Hx:	20 y/o ♂ soccer player c/o pain on L midportion of hamstring, c̄ swelling 30 min post-injury.
Dx:	Moderation contusion to the L hamstring.

Rx: What modalities would be best suited in this situation? Why?

Possible Treatment Regimens

Following are possible treatment regimens for the case studies outlined above. Compare your suggestions with the ones below. Are there differences? If so, does that mean that you (or we) are wrong? Not necessarily. Discuss these cases with classmates, clinical instructors, or your professor. If differences exist, try to determine why.

CASE STUDY 1: LUMBOSACRAL PAIN

REFERRAL	
Hx:	22 y/o overweight offensive lineman, c/o diffuse LBP × 2 wk. Pain is nonradiating and increases c̄ strenuous lifting.
Dx:	Lumbosacral muscle spasm c̄ 1° strain of quadratus lumborum.

Rx: This injury is chronic. Goal: Decrease muscle spasm and increase circulation to assist healing. Possible modalities to decrease muscle spasm:

- Interferential current. (Setting of 5–10 seconds on, 5–10 seconds off, intensity adjusted to contraction level to fatigue the muscle spasm. This large treatment area can easily be bracketed with four electrodes.)
- Pulsed shortwave diathermy. (Deep heat may help relax the muscle spasm, plus this modality will cover a large area.)
- Massage. (Especially petrissage; the kneading will help reduce the spasm.)
- Traction. (Lumbar traction may help decrease the spasm.)

Possible modalities to increase temperature and blood flow and assist with healing:

- Pulsed shortwave diathermy (provides deep heat to a large area). If you don't have access to PSWD:
- Warm whirlpool (superficial heat, yet the warm water will surround the entire area).
- Hot packs (superficial heat, yet a large pack will cover the entire area).

CASE STUDY 2: PIRIFORMIS SYNDROME

REFERRAL	
Hx:	20 y/o ♀ volleyball player c/o (L) buttocks and LBP, × 6 wk.
Dx:	Piriformis syndrome c̄ sciatica.

Rx: This injury is chronic. Goal: Decrease muscle spasm and pain, and increase hip internal rotation by stretching the piriformis. Possible modalities to decrease muscle spasm and pain are:

- Interferential current. (Setting of 5–10 seconds on, 5–10 seconds off, intensity adjusted to contraction level to fatigue the muscle spasm. This large treatment area can easily be bracketed with four electrodes.)
- TENS. (Setting of 5–10 seconds on, 5–10 seconds off, intensity adjusted to contraction level to fatigue the muscle spasm.)
- Massage. (Especially petrissage; the kneading will help reduce the spasm.)

Possible modalities to heat the area prior to stretch:

- Pulsed shortwave diathermy (provides deep heat to a large area). If you don't have access to PSWD:
- Warm whirlpool (superficial heat, yet the warm water will surround the entire area).
- Hot packs (superficial heat, yet a large pack will cover the entire area).

CASE STUDY 3: CHRONIC SUPRASPINATIS TENDINITIS

REFERRAL	
Hx:	44 y/o ♂ painter, c/o pain in R shoulder, and limited shoulder ROM due to pain.
Dx:	Chronic supraspinatis tendinitis.

Rx: This injury is chronic. Goal: Decrease muscle spasm and pain. Possible modalities to decrease muscle spasm and pain are:

- Interferential current. (For muscle spasm: setting of 5–10 seconds on, 5–10 seconds off, intensity adjusted to contraction level to fatigue the muscle spasm. For pain: Continuous setting with intensity adjusted to sensory level for stimulation of large myelinated nerve fibers. This large treatment area can easily be bracketed with four electrodes.)
- TENS. (For muscle spasm: setting of 5–10 seconds on, 5–10 seconds off, intensity adjusted to contraction level to fatigue the muscle spasm. For pain: Continuous setting with intensity adjusted to sensory level for stimulation of large myelinated nerve fibers.)
- Pulsed shortwave diathermy. (Provides deep heat to a large area which may help relax the muscle and reduce the spasm.)
- Massage. (Especially petrissage; the kneading will help reduce the spasm.)
- Hot packs. (Superficial heat, yet a large pack will cover the entire area.)

CASE STUDY 4: HYPOMOBILE RADIAL CARPAL JOINT

REFERRAL	
Hx:	22 y/o ♂ soccer goalie, × 3 mo p/o bone graft for avascular necrosis of the (L) scaphoid.
Dx:	Hypomobile radial carpal joint in all motions due to prolonged cast immobilization.

Rx: Goal: Increase ROM of radial carpal joint. A heat and stretching regimen or heating the area prior to joint mobilizations are the best options. To heat the tissues prior to stretching or joint mobilization:

• 3 MHz ultrasound (Continuous setting to patient tolerance; the wrist structures are superficial, which is in the heating range for 3 MHz ultrasound.)
• Paraffin. (Superficial heat that will form a glove surrounding the treatment area.)
• Hot pack. (Superficial heat, applied to the dorsal aspect of the hand to focus on schapoid.)
• Whirlpool. (Superficial heat, yet the warm water will surround the entire area.)

CASE STUDY 5: FIRST-DEGREE INVERSION ANKLE SPRAIN

REFERRAL	
Hx:	16 y/o ♀ basketball player c/o pain on R lateral ankle, c̄ swelling 24 h post-injury.
Dx:	1° inversion sprain of R ankle.

Rx: Goal: Immediate care, reduce pain, and prevent secondary metabolic injury. Decrease swelling and increase function during transition care. To prevent secondary metabolic injury and reduce pain:

• RICES. (30 minutes). Reevaluate the injury. If the diagnosis is still a first-degree sprain, begin transition care. If the injury seems more severe, continue RICES until the next day.

To decrease swelling and increase function:

• Cryokinetics (increase in function as per patient progress).

To decrease swelling during transition care:

• Interferential current. (This small treatment area can easily be bracketed with four electrodes. For muscle pumping to get rid of edema: setting of 5–10 seconds on, 5–10 seconds off, intensity adjusted to contraction level.)
• Sequential lymphedema pump (will assist with lymphatic drainage).

CASE STUDY 6: CARPAL TUNNEL SYNDROME

REFERRAL	
Hx:	37 y/o R-handed ♀, employed as a computer operator, c/o tingling and numbness in R hand c̄ loss of ROM and grip strength.
Dx:	Early stages of carpal tunnel syndrome in R hand.

Rx: Goal: Reduce pain and inflammation on median nerve. Possible modalities:

• Ice pack (when applied to the ventral and dorsal aspects of the wrist, it will cover the entire treatment target).
• Ice water immersion (will cover the entire treatment target, and allow for active ROM exercises).
• Cold whirlpool (will cover the entire treatment target, and allow for active ROM exercises).

CASE STUDY 7: ACHILLES TENDINITIS

REFERRAL	
Hx:	30 y/o ♂ marathon runner, c/o chronic pain in area of (L) Achilles tendon.
Dx:	Achilles tendinitis.

Rx: Goal: Break up scar tissue and stretch triceps surae. A heat-and-stretch regimen, to breaking up adhesions, is best here. To heat the tissues prior to joint movement:

• 3 MHz ultrasound. (Continuous setting to patient tolerance. The Achilles tendon is superficial, which is in the heating range for 3 MHz ultrasound.)
• Paraffin (superficial heat that will form a glove surrounding the treatment area).
• Warm whirlpool (superficial heat, yet the warm water will surround the entire area).
• Hot packs (superficial heat, yet a large pack will cover the entire area).

To break up adhesions:

• Cross-friction massage (going perpendicular to the fibers will aid in breaking up scar tissue).

CASE STUDY 8: MILD SPASM OF R/L UPPER TRAPEZIUS

REFERRAL	
Hx:	40 y/o ♀ c/o pain in the cervical region, c̄ muscle spasms. X-rays ruled out fx.
Dx:	Mild spasm of R/L upper trapezius.

Rx: Goal is to reduce muscle spasm. Appropriate modalities:

- Cryostretch. (After several minutes of cold application the area will become numb, thus reducing the pain and muscle spasm.)
- Cervical traction. (Gentle distraction will take pressure off of nerves and help reduce muscle spasm.)
- TENS. (This small treatment area is easily targeted with TENS. For muscle spasm: setting of 5–10 seconds on, 5–10 seconds off, intensity adjusted to contraction level to fatigue the muscle spasm. For pain: Continuous setting with intensity adjusted to sensory level for stimulation of large myelinated nerve fibers.)
- Interferential current. (This small treatment area can easily be bracketed with four electrodes. For muscle spasm: setting of 5–10 seconds on, 5–10 seconds off, intensity adjusted to contraction level to fatigue the muscle spasm. For pain: Continuous setting with intensity adjusted to sensory level for stimulation of large myelinated nerve fibers.)

CASE STUDY 9: SECOND-DEGREE QUADRICEPS STRAIN

REFERRAL	
Hx:	20 y/o ♀ soccer player c/o pain on L mid-portion of quadriceps, c̄ swelling 30 min post-injury.
Dx:	2° strain to the L quadriceps.

Rx: Goal: Reduce pain and swelling and prevent further secondary metabolic injury, then transition into functional activity.

- RICES (30 minutes) Treatment repeated every 2 hours. Keep compression wrap on and limb elevated during and between ice pack applications.

To increase function during transition care:

- Cryostretch (cold applications and stretching will break the muscle spasm).
- Cryokinetics (transition into after muscle spasm is reduced).

In addition:

- Intereferential current. (This small treatment area can easily be bracketed with four electrodes. For muscle pumping to get rid of edema: setting of 5–10 seconds on, 5–10 seconds off, intensity adjusted to contraction level.)
- Sequential lymphedema pump (will assist with lymphatic drainage).

CASE STUDY 10: PATELLAR TENDINITIS

REFERRAL	
Hx:	20 y/o ♂ collegiate miler, c/o chronic pain in area of (R) patellar tendon.
Dx:	Patellar tendinitis.

Rx: Goal: Break up adhesions associated with condition. Increase pain-free ROM. A heat-and-stretch regimen, or heating the tissues prior to breaking up adhesions are good options. To heat the tissues prior to joint movement:

- 3 MHz ultrasound. (Continuous setting to patient tolerance. The patellar tendon is superficial, which is in the heating range for 3 MHz ultrasound.)
- Warm whirlpool (superficial heat, yet the warm water will surround the entire area).
- Hot pack (superficial heat, and a small pack will cover the entire area).

To break up adhesions:

- Cross-friction massage (going perpendicular to the fibers will aid in breaking up scar tissue).

CASE STUDY 11: LATERAL EPICONDYLITIS

REFERRAL	
Hx:	18 y/o ♂ tennis player, c/o chronic pain in area of (R) elbow.
Dx:	Lateral epicondylitis.

Rx: Goal: Break up adhesions associated with condition. Increase pain-free ROM. A heat-and-stretching regimen, and heating the area prior to breaking up adhesions, are good options. To heat the tissues prior to joint movement:

- 3 MHz ultrasound. (Continuous setting to patient tolerance. The attachment of the wrist extensors on the lateral epicondyle are superficial, which is in the heating range for 3 MHz ultrasound.)
- Warm whirlpool (superficial heat, yet the warm water will surround the entire area).
- Hot pack (superficial heat, and a small pack will cover the entire area).

To break up adhesions:

- Cross-friction massage (going perpendicular to the fibers will aid in breaking up scar tissue).

CASE STUDY 12: ACROMOCLAVICULAR (AC) SEPARATION

REFERRAL
Hx: 21 y/o ♀ rugby player c/o pain on R AC joint, c̄ swelling 2 hours post-injury. No visible or palpable step-off deformity.
Dx: 1° AC sprain of R shoulder.

Rx: Goal: Immediate care, reduce pain, and prevent secondary hypoxic injury. Decrease swelling in the area during transition care. To prevent secondary hypoxic injury and reduce pain:

- RICES (30 minutes). Treatment repeated every 2 hours. Keep compression wrap on and limb elevated during and between ice pack applications.
- TENS. (This small treatment area is easily targeted with TENS. Continuous setting with intensity adjusted to sensory level for stimulation of large myelinated nerve fibers.)

To decrease swelling in the area during transition care:

- Intereferential current. (This small treatment area can easily be bracketed with four electrodes. For muscle pumping to get rid of edema: setting of 5–10 seconds on, 5–10 seconds off, intensity adjusted to contraction level.)

CASE STUDY 13: HAMSTRING CONTUSION

REFERRAL
Hx: 20 y/o ♂ soccer player c/o pain on L mid-portion of hamstring, c̄ swelling 30 min post-injury.
Dx: Moderation contusion to the L hamstring.

Rx: Goal: Immediate care, reduce pain, and minimize secondary metabolic injury. Decrease swelling in the area during transition care. To minimize secondary hypoxic injury and reduce pain:

- RICES (30 minutes). Treatment repeated every 2 hours. Keep compression wrap on and limb elevated during and between ice pack applications.

To decrease swelling in the area during transition care:

- Intereferential current. (This treatment area can easily be bracketed with four electrodes. For muscle pumping to get rid of edema: setting of 5–10 seconds on, 5–10 seconds off, intensity adjusted to contraction level.)
- Sequential lymphedema (will assist with lymphatic drainage).

Review Questions

Chapter 21

1. The process of determining the optimal modality to use under certain circumstances is referred to as _____.
   a. indication
   b. contraindication
   c. differential application
   d. compliance
   e. noncompliance

2. A patient following the treatment orders given by the therapist is an example of _____.
   a. indication
   b. contraindication
   c. noncompliance
   d. compliance
   e. differential application

3. Which of the following would be the *best* modality to use to heat a large joint (such as the knee) before stretching?
   a. shortwave diathermy
   b. ultrasound
   c. whirlpool
   d. hot packs
   e. cryokinetics

4. Which of the following is *not* a limiting factor to modality use?
   a. availability of the modality
   b. time available for treatment
   c. evidence supporting the modality
   d. patient compliance
   e. none of the above; all are limiting factors

5. *Clinician compliance* refers to the _____.
   a. reputation of the clinician
   b. clinician reporting to work on time
   c. reliability and professionalism of the clinician
   d. clinician using the same modality day after day
   e. applying as many modalities as possible so as to give the greatest chance of resolving the problem

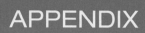

Answers to Review Questions

PART I

Chapter 1
1. d
2. b
3. b
4. a
5. c

Chapter 2
1. e
2. e
3. a
4. e
5. d
6. b
7. e
8. d
9. c

Chapter 3
1. b
2. d
3. e
4. b

Chapter 4
1. e
2. e
3. b
4. d
5. d
6. b

PART II

Chapter 5
1. a
2. b
3. e

4. e
5. d
6. e
7. a

Chapter 6
1. c
2. c
3. c
4. d
5. a
6. e

Chapter 7
1. c
2. e
3. e
4. b
5. e
6. e

PART III

Chapter 8
1. b
2. b
3. a
4. d
5. a
6. d
7. a
8. a
9. d

Chapter 9
1. c
2. e
3. b
4. e

5. a
6. c
7. c

PART IV

Chapter 10
1. a
2. c
3. b
4. a
5. a
6. e
7. c
8. d
9. a
10. d

Chapter 11
1. b
2. e
3. e
4. b
5. b
6. e
7. b
8. a

Chapter 12
1. b
2. e
3. b
4. a
5. c
6. a
7. b
8. a

Chapter 13
1. a
2. d
3. d
4. d
5. c
6. b

Chapter 14
1. b
2. a
3. c
4. b
5. e
6. e
7. a
8. e
9. a
10. c
11. d
12. b

Chapter 15
1. b
2. c
3. e
4. e
5. b
6. e
7. c
8. e
9. a
10. b

PART V

Chapter 16
1. a
2. d

3. b
4. c
5. d
6. c
7. a
8. c
9. a
10. d
11. b
12. b

Chapter 17
1. d
2. e
3. a
4. e
5. a
6. a
7. b
8. e
9. e
10. b

PART VI

Chapter 18
1. c
2. a
3. d
4. a
5. d
6. b
7. e
8. d

Chapter 19
1. d
2. b
3. c

4. a
5. b
6. e
7. e
8. d
9. e

Chapter 20
1. a
2. e
3. a
4. c
5. d
6. d
7. b
8. e
9. c

PART VII

Chapter 21
1. c
2. d
3. a
4. e
5. c

Glossary

absorption The action of electromagnetic waves being immersed or taken in by a substance.

AC train A continuous repetitive series of pulses at a fixed frequency (or a segment of AC).

acoustic microstreaming The unidirectional movement of fluids along the boundaries of cell membranes resulting from ultrasonically induced pressure waves.

acoustic waves Waves produced by sound and ultrasound. Also known as sound waves.

action potential A change in electrical potential between the inside and outside of a nerve cell membrane.

active electrode The electrode under which the current density is great enough to elicit the desired response. See also DISPERSIVE ELECTRODE.

acute care Treatment of an acute injury during the first 4 days after the injury.

acute injury An injury of sudden onset, caused by high-intensity, short-duration forces; examples are sprains, strains, and contusions.

acute pain Rapid-onset pain of brief duration, caused by the activation of nociceptors from external sources, such as a contusion, or internal sources, such as a muscle strain.

A-delta fiber A peripheral nerve that carries sensations, including nociceptive stimuli that result in acute pain; larger and faster-acting than C fibers.

adenosine triphosphate (ATP) The major source of energy in muscles.

advantages In the context of the five-step application procedure, the benefits of a specific modality that make it more effective in treating a specific injury than other modalities.

affective dimension of pain The emotional or autonomic response to the pain stimulus, such as crying or being very anxious or depressed due to painful experiences. It makes you determined to do something. Also known as *affective/motivational*.

afferent nerve A sensory nerve; it enters the spinal cord via the dorsal horn.

A fiber The largest (1–22 μm in diameter) nerve fiber; conducts action potentials the most rapidly (5–120 m/sec). Some A fibers are sensory; others have a motor function.

agility A combination of speed of movement and coordination; developed as skill patterns are performed quickly, usually with sport-specific team drills.

alternating current (AC) A continuous flow of electrons that rhythmically changes direction because the two generator terminals alternatively change from positive to negative.

ampere (amp) A unit of current flow, equal to the passage of 1 coulomb (i.e., 6.28×10^{18} electrons) per second.

amplify To increase in size, volume, or significance.

amplitude The amount of current flowing through the circuit; also known as intensity.

ammeter A device to measure the rate of current flow in amperes.

analgesic balm An externally applied drug that has a topical analgesic, anesthetic, or anti-itching effect by depressing cutaneous sensory receptors or a topical counterirritant effect by stimulating cutaneous sensory receptors.

angiogenesis Growth of new blood vessels.

annulus fibrosus The outer layer of an intervertebral disk, consisting of a series of interlacing cross-fibers attached to adjacent vertebral bodies.

Arndt-Schultz principle There is an optimal amount of energy absorption per unit of time that is beneficial. Less than this amount will not cause a reaction, and more than this amount will be detrimental.

arthrogenic muscle inhibition (AMI) An ongoing reflex inhibition of muscles surrounding a joint, caused by distension or damage to that joint.

artificial ice pack A vinyl pouch filled with water and enclosed in a nylon covering, frozen in a freezer at 1°F (~17°C).

asymmetrical pulse A pulse with differing phases.

atom A single unit of an element; composed of protons, electrons, neutrons, and other smaller substances.

attenuation A decrease in energy as an ultrasound wave is transmitted through various tissues owing to scattering and dispersion.

autonomic motor nerve A nerve that transmits impulses from the CNS to the periphery of the body and terminates in smooth muscle, cardiac muscle, glands, and organs; controlled involuntarily.

autonomic nervous system (ANS) The part of the peripheral nervous system that regulates smooth muscle, cardiac muscle, organs, and glands; consists of sympathetic and parasympathetic branches.

average current The average magnitude of a pulse.

average patient One who exists only in a research study, as the composite of all the research subjects in the study. Although research is indispensable in directing clinical practice, never assume that any specific patient will respond exactly as the average of research subjects.

balanced pulse A pulse containing equal phase charges.

beam nonuniformity ratio (BNR) An indicator of the amount of intensity variability within an ultrasound beam: the ratio between the average intensity of the ultrasound beam across the soundhead divided by the highest intensity of the ultrasound beam.

beat frequency An adjustable frequency; the difference between two intersecting currents of different frequencies.

Bedside Sports Rehabilitation Laboratory Sports competition is calendared and generally immovable. Therefore, time is crucial to sports injury rehabilitation, and the patients are more highly motivated to return to participation. Consequently, new therapies often stem from innovative clinicians. See KNOWLEDGE TRANSLATION.

best practice (*standard of care, standard therapy*) Treating a specific patient's specific condition in the way that will lead to resolution of the condition in the most complete and expedient manner possible; treatment that experts agree is appropriate, accepted, widely used, and reproducible.

best practice statements See CLINICAL PRACTICE GUIDELINES.

B fiber Between A and C fibers in size (1–3 μm) and in rate of conduction (3–14 m/sec); autonomic motor nerve.

bidirectional knowledge translation The concept that clinicians are responsible to share new or unique clinical discoveries with scientists so the clinical knowledge can be refined through formal scientific investigation. See KNOWLEDGE TRANSLATION.

biofeedback A process of measuring a biological mechanism using an objective means and then telling the patient his scores. The feedback helps the patient progress more quickly.

biphasic A pulse with two phases; current flows in both directions.

bipolar technique The application of electrodes of equal size, resulting in essentially equal current density under them; both electrodes are, therefore, active.

BNR See BEAM NONUNIFORMITY RATIO (BNR).

bodywork Various forms of touch therapies that may use manipulation, movement, and/or repatterning to affect structural changes to the body. Related to therapeutic massage.

brief-intense TENS A modality used to treat chronic pain before rehabilitation by stimulating C fibers; beat frequency varies between low and high and changes periodically; intensity higher than sensory mode TENS (to the patient's tolerance). The patient reports a burning, needling sensation and twitch and tetanic muscle contractions. Also known as noxious TENS.

burst A finite series of pulses (or a finite interval of AC at a specific frequency) flowing for a limited time period, followed by no current flow (e.g., turning a pulse train or AC on and off).

burst interval The time during which a burst occurs, usually measured in milliseconds.

CAP See CRITICALLY APPRAISED PAPER.

capillary arcade A series of capillary arches that eventually develop throughout the entire wound area, providing abundant circulation, which is necessary to support collagenization.

capillary arch The process in which adjacent capillary bud sprouts migrate toward one another, meet, and form together creating an arch.

capillary budding A process where endothelial cells of existing vessels at the edge of the wound begin to divide.

The new cells crawl away from, but keep contact with, the existing vessel. New cells force themselves between existing cells, thus forcing the end cells to advance into the wound area.

capillary filtration pressure   The mathematical sum of a number of forces, known as Starling forces.

capillary hydrostatic pressure (CHP)   Pressure that forces fluid out of the capillary.

capillary oncotic pressure (COP)   Pressure that pulls fluid into the capillary.

capsaicin   A derivative of the hot pepper plant; an irritant included in analgesic balms to provide a sensation of heat.

cardiorespiratory endurance   The ability of the heart and lungs to supply exercising muscles with adequate oxygen to produce the energy needed to maintain the activity.

carrier frequency   The preset frequency built into a machine.

case series   Observational research. A case study involving multiple patients with the same injury or illness. It may be prospective or retrospective. Also known as a cohort study.

case studies   Observational research involving carefully recorded details of specific interventions in a single patient, or preferably, in multiple patients with the same injury/illness. They identify patient responses to a specific intervention for a specific injury/illness.

case-control study   Observational research. Two groups of patients are selected based on the presence or absence of an outcome, and examined concerning their involvement with the intervention of interest.

CATS   See CRITICALLY APPRAISED TOPICS.

cavitation   The formation of gas-filled bubbles that expand and contract owing to ultrasonically induced pressure changes in tissue fluids.

cellular phase   In the repair process, the same as leukocyte migration and phagocytosis in the inflammatory response. Macrophages scavenge the cellular debris. The circulatory and lymphatic systems (mostly lymphatic) drain away the liquefied cellular remains, which are mostly small particles of free protein.

central control   A theory that previous experiences, emotional influences, sensory perception, and other factors influence the response of the brain to nociceptors and thus the perception of pain. Central control collects and stores information related to pain and mediates the body's response to noxious stimuli. Previous experiences and other sensory input influence pain via central control.

central control   A theory that previous experiences, emotional influences, sensory perception, and other factors could influence the transmission of pain signals and thus the perception of pain.

central control trigger theory   A modification of the gate control theory of pain.

central nervous system (CNS)   The brain and spinal cord.

cerebral cortex   The outer part of the brain; coordinates pain signals and determines pain location and intensity. The cerebral cortex initiates descending pain control mechanisms.

C fiber   A peripheral nerve that carries sensations, including nociceptive stimuli that result in chronic pain; smaller and slower-acting than A fibers. The smallest (<1 μm) and slowest (<2 m/sec) nerve fiber; sensory nerves.

chemical mediators   Chemicals, such as histamine, bradykinin, and cytokines, that mobilize the body's resources after injury to neutralize the cause of the injury and to begin removing the cellular debris so that repair can take place. Chemical mediation is one of eight events in the inflammatory response.

chronic inflammation   A cellular response to long-term, low-intensity forces; not to be confused with recurring acute inflammation.

chronic injury   *(1)* An injury caused by low-intensity, long-duration forces, in tendinitis or bursitis. *(2)* A recurring acute injury, such as a chronic sprained ankle.

chronic pain   Pain that lasts a month beyond the usual course of an acute disease or a reasonable time for an injury to heal; also associated with a chronic pathological process that causes continuous pain or in which the pain recurs at intervals for months to years.

CINAHL   The Cumulative Index to Nursing and Allied Health Literature database indexes articles from 1981 and from more than 3000 nursing and allied health journals.

circuit breaker   A safety device that protects equipment and body structures against excess current by opening the circuit when too much current is flowing.

clinical and translational science   A medical discipline of getting evidence into the hands of medical practitioners, by translating knowledge from the scientist to the practitioner, commonly referred to as "from the laboratory to the bedside." See also KNOWLEDGE TRANSLATION, KNOWLEDGE BROKER, BIDIRECTIONAL KNOWLEDGE TRANSLATION, BEDSIDE SPORTS REHABILITATION LABORATORY.

clinical decision making The process of making a diagnosis and developing a specific plan for treating the patient.

clinical guidelines See CLINICAL PRACTICE GUIDELINES.

clinical outcomes The end result (pathophysiological, social, or psychological) of specific health care practices and interventions.

clinical practice guidelines Systematically developed statements that describe best and achievable practice in specific areas of care; they reflect current scientific knowledge of practices and expert clinical judgment on the best ways to prevent, diagnose, treat, or manage injury or diseases. They are written in a clinician-friendly format, ready to be integrated into health care decisions; also known as *clinical guidelines, best practice statements, recommendation statements, CMSG (Cochrane Musculoskeletal Group) Guidelines,* or *health care guidelines.*

clinical practice statements Summaries, reviews, and critique of available clinical practice guidelines, usually written by professional groups, such as the American College of Physicians.

clinical trials research A cross between observational and laboratory research. They are controlled research of a specific medical intervention on patients with a specific injury or disease. They are called *clinical or controlled trials (CTs)* if patients are not randomly assigned to treatment groups or *randomized clinical trials (RCTs)* when they are randomly assigned to treatment groups. The RCT is considered the gold standard of *evidence-based medicine* because they are likely to provide much more reliable information than other sources of evidence.

clinician compliance The reliability, knowledge, confidence, and professionalism of a clinician.

closed circuit A complete circuit, allowing flow; there are no breaks in the circuit.

clotting A multistage process that results in fibrin and platelets closing a damaged blood vessel.

cluster probe A laser applicator with multiple probes that can apply multiple wavelengths to a larger area during treatment.

CMSG (Cochrane Musculoskeletal Group) guidelines See CLINICAL PRACTICE GUIDELINES.

COCH See COCHRANE DATABASE OF SYSTEMATIC REVIEWS.

cochrane See COCHRANE DATABASE OF SYSTEMATIC REVIEWS.

cochrane database of systematic reviews (COCH) A worldwide endeavor to collect, evaluate, synthesize, and maintain a database of Randomized Clinical Trials in all areas of medicine. Also known as the Cochrane Collaboration.

Cochrane Musculoskeletal Group (CMSG) guidelines See CLINICAL PRACTICE GUIDELINES.

cognitive behavioral strategies A set of psychologic behaviors used to modulate a patients perception or interpretation of a pain sensation or situation. These strategies include meditation, distraction, relaxation, fear, depression, former pain experiences, and family and cultural influences.

coherent Logically ordered or integrated; a quality of electromagnetic waves that have the same wavelength and a fixed phase relationship.

cohort study Observational research. A case study involving multiple patients with the same injury or illness. It may be prospective or retrospective. Also known as a case series.

cold The absence of heat or something that has less heat than one would desire; the sensation produced by low temperatures.

cold hypersensitivity Intense pain during ice or cold pack application.

cold pack A generic term that refers to crushed ice packs, gel packs, artificial ice packs, and crushable chemical packs.

cold water immersion (CWI) Immersion of arms or legs in a crushed ice and water bath.

cold-induced vasodilation (CIVD) An increase in the circumference of blood vessels as a result of cold applications.

collagen A fibrous protein found in all types of connective tissue; the primary solid substance of ligaments, tendons, and scar tissue.

collagen synthesis See COLLAGENIZATION.

collagenization The process of manufacturing and laying down collagen in the wound space.

collimated beam A focused, less-divergent beam of energy. Both ultrasound and laser energy are transmitted as collimated beams.

compliance The extent to which a patient follows a prescribed treatment regimen. Also called adherence or maintenance.

comprehensive literature search A literature search that involves searches of a multitude of databases, including *PubMed, Cochrane, National Clearing House, PEDro, CINAHL*. It is of utmost importance to a *meta-analysis*.

compression A region of high molecular density and high pressure as the molecules in a longitudinal wave are squeezed together. See also RAREFACTION.

conduction A process of heat transfer that occurs when two objects of uneven temperatures come into contact with each other. Heat is transferred from the object with the higher temperature to the object with the lower temperature, causing the warmer object to cool and the cooler object to warm.

conductor A substance that can transport electrical charge (or current) from one point to another; it must have free electrons that can be pushed along (e.g., metal, water).

connective tissue stretch A combination of heat application, long-term passive stretch, and cold applications, used to increase joint flexibility after prolonged immobilization during which connective tissue contractures have developed.

Consolidated Standards of Reporting Trials (CONSORT) Standards developed by a group of scientists and editors to facilitate critical appraisal and interpretation of RCTs.

CONSORT See CONSOLIDATED STANDARDS OF REPORTING TRIALS.

constant stimulation pattern Stimulation in which amplitude of successive pulses (or cycles) is the same.

continuous ultrasound An ultrasound mode in which the sound intensity remains constant throughout the treatment and the ultrasound energy is being produced 100% of the time.

contraction Collapsing of the capillary arcade toward the end of repair. Makes the scar smaller and paler.

contraction and restructuring phase In the repair process, two processes that cause scar tissue to become smaller and paler (in light-skinned people); a new scar will appear red (in a light-skinned person) and mounded or raised above the surrounding tissue.

contraindications Situations in which a specific modality should not be used—that is, situations in which it may do more harm than good.

contrast bath therapy The alternating immersion of an injured body part in hot and cold water baths.

control group One of two or more groups of subjects in a research study. Its purpose is to minimize the effects of variables other than the treatment variable(s), and this increase the reliability of the results.

controlled trials (CT) See CLINICAL TRIALS RESEARCH.

convection The transfer of heat to or from an object by the passage of a fluid or air past its surface.

conversion A process that occurs when a form of energy other than heat (electricity, chemical, mechanical, etc.) is converted to heat within the body.

cookbook approach to rehabilitation A treatment approach in which the clinician follows a specific "recipe" or protocol for each injury, consisting of phases with specific time periods and therapeutic interventions. All patients with the same or similar injury are treated the same, without regard for individual patient differences.

cosine or right-angle law The optimum radiation occurs when the source of the radiation is perpendicular to the center of the surface of the area to be radiated.

coulomb The basic unit of charge, produced by 6.28×10^{18} displaced electrons (6280 quadrillion).

counterirritant A substance that irritates the skin, causing mild skin inflammation, which causes a gating effect and thereby relieves mild pain in muscles, joints, and internal organs.

coupling medium In ultrasound, a substance that facilitates the transmission of ultrasound energy by decreasing impedance at the air–skin interface. In electrotherapy, a substance that facilitates the transmission of electrical current from the electrodes to the skin; also called couplant.

craniosacral therapy (CST) A gentle, hands-on method of enhancing the craniosacral system—the spine and the membranes and cerebrospinal fluid that surround and protect the brain and spinal cord. Also known as cranial sacral therapy.

critical thinker approach to rehabilitation An organized procedural outline that includes fairly broad guidelines to help the clinician choose the most appropriate modality and mode of applying that modality.

critical thinking A process that requires explanation rather than a definition. See Chapter 2 for its characteristics and components.

critically appraised paper (CAP) Summary of a single research study providing evidence regarding a clinical question. It's similar to a CAT, differing only in that it summarizes a single study, as opposed to multiple studies.

critically appraised topics (CATs) Short summaries of evidence on a topic of interest, usually focused around a clinical question. It's a shorter and less rigorous version of a systematic review, summarizing the best available research evidence on a topic. Usually more than one study is referenced in a CAT.

cross-sectional study Observational research. A group of patients is examined at a single time during, or following, an intervention concerning their current and past history regarding the effects of an intervention on the outcomes of interest.

crushable chemical pack A thin-walled vinyl pouch of a liquid packaged within a stronger, larger vinyl pouch of dry crystals. Squeezing breaks the smaller pouch, and fluid leaks into the larger, outer pouch. Fluid and crystals combine in a chemical reaction that cools the fluid.

crushed ice pack Crushed ice, typically from an ice machine, in a plastic or cloth bag.

crutch palsy A temporary or permanent loss of either sensation or the ability to move or control movement.

cryokinetics Alternating cold application and active graded exercise for rehabilitating acute joint sprains.

cryostretch Alternating cold application, passive stretch, and resistive muscle contraction for rehabilitating acute muscle strains.

cryosurgery A surgical technique that uses ultralow-temperature probes (–4 to –94°F [–20 to –70°C]) to freeze tissue and thereby destroy it.

cryotherapy The therapeutic use of cold; the application of a device or substance with a temperature less than body temperature, thus causing heat to pass from the body to the cryotherapy device.

crystal An ultrasound transducer.

cultural stagnation Resistance to new ideas that require changing behavior. One of the major impediments to evidence-based practice is that people need to change their professional behavior.

cumulative index to nursing and allied health See CINAHL.

current density A measure of the quantity of charged ions moving through a particular cross-sectional area of an electrode.

current electricity A stream of loose electrons passing along a conductor.

current flow The flow of electrical charge from one point to another, from an area of higher electron concentration (the negative pole or cathode) to an area lacking electrons (the positive pole or anode).

current modulation Manipulating, regulating, and adjusting of the input current to create a variety of specific output wave forms.

cycle In an alternating current, two impulses: current flowing from the baseline to the maximum in one direction and back to the baseline.

daily adjustable progressive resistive exercise (DAPRE) technique An aggressive, four-set system of isotonic weight lifting that takes advantage of the fact that strength can be redeveloped more quickly than it was developed initially. Patients perform maximal repetitions during their third and fourth sets, and the number of repetitions performed is used as a basis for adjusting the resistance during the fourth set and on the next day, respectively.

data synthesis The process of combining and summarizing results and opinions from many related individual studies and commentary. The multiple forms of data synthesis of medical literature include *narrative reviews, meta-analysis, systematic reviews, clinical practice guidelines, clinical practice statements, critically appraised topics (CATS)*.

decay time The time from maximal amplitude to the end of a phase.

deep thermotherapy The application of modalities that cause a tissue temperature rise (TTR) in deeper tissues.

dermatome The area of skin innervated by a particular spinal nerve.

descending endogenous opiate system (DEOS) A system operating at supraspinal levels that contains opiate secreting neurons to assist in pain control.

diathermy The therapeutic use of high-frequency electromagnetic waves to heat deep tissues.

differential application of modalities The process of determining the optimal modality to use under specific circumstances.

direct (galvanic) wave form Pure DC, used for iontophoresis.

direct current (DC) A steady or continuous, unidirectional flow of electrons between the anode and the cathode of a battery; also known as galvanic current.

direct pain relief Focuses on the pain itself.

direction of current flow The flow of current from the positive pole to the negative pole.

disability A poorly defined, misunderstood, and difficult-to-measure concept. It is an umbrella term covering impairments, activity limitations, and participation restrictions. It can be physical, cognitive, mental, sensory, emotional, developmental, or a combination of these. It is also a legal or social judgment, based in part on medical judgments.

disadvantages In the context of the five-step application procedure, the possible negative effects a specific modality might cause or the benefits that might be lost by not using another modality.

discharge note A type of SOAP note written when treatment is discontinued.

dispersive electrode The electrode under which the current density is not great enough to elicit the desired response. See also ACTIVE ELECTRODE.

dopamine A neurotransmitter in the brain used by the body to synthesize norepinephrine and epinephrine; affects brain processes that control movement, emotional response, and the ability to experience pleasure and pain.

dorsal horn The posterior portion of the gray matter of the spinal cord; also called posterior horn.

dry cell A battery that uses electrolyte paste rather than a solution. One example is a zinc-carbon battery in which a zinc tube is filled with electrolyte paste and a carbon rod is inserted into the middle.

duty cycle The percentage of time that ultrasound is being generated (pulse duration) over one pulse period.

dynamic vector In IFC therapy, two intersecting, moving currents used to treat large areas.

edema An accumulation of the fluid portion of blood in the tissues.

effective radiating area (ERA) The part of the surface area of a soundhead in an ultrasound device that transmits a sound wave from the crystal to the tissues.

effects In the context of the five-step application procedure, the physiological and/or pathological changes the modality evokes, both locally and systemically (throughout the body).

efferent nerve A motor nerve; it exits the spinal cord via the ventral horn.

effleurage A gliding manipulation performed with light or heavy pressure (directed toward the heart) that deforms subcutaneous tissue down to the deep fascial layers; also called stroking.

electrical charge The net sum of the charges of electrons and protons in an atom or molecule; the difference between the number of protons and electrons.

electrical circuit A system of conductors that allows electrons to move between the two poles of a battery or generator.

electrolyte A substance that contains ions and can, therefore, conduct electricity.

electromagnetic energy One of the fundamental forms of energy in the universe; consists of electrical and magnetic waves.

electromagnetic induction The process of converting mechanical power into electrical power (electrical generator) and for converting electrical power into mechanical power (electrical motor).

electromagnetic wave A combination of oscillating electric and magnetic fields at right angles to one another that travel in wave-like fashion through space at a speed of about 186,000 mi./sec (300,000 km/sec); also known as radiation. Forms include heat, light, electricity, x-rays, and cosmic rays.

electron A subunit of an atom, orbiting the nucleus, with a negligible mass and an electrical charge of −1.

element The primary substance of matter (e.g., oxygen, copper, carbon).

emergency care Care given after a serious or life-threatening injury, such as CPR or transportation to a hospital.

emission A flowing forth, such as the release of electrons from parent atoms.

endogenous Developed or produced within the body.

endorphin A drug that inhibits pain signal transmission and decreases the amount of chemical irritants present in the CNS.

endothelium The wall of a blood vessel.

enkephalin A drug that blocks pain by interfering with A-delta and C fiber signal transmission to T cells.

epinephrine A hormone secreted by the adrenal glands in response to stress; a neurotransmitter that stimulates the fight-or-flight response. Also known as adrenaline.

epithelialization The process of developing a membranous tissue covering (epithelium) over exposed tissue or organs.

evaluative dimension of pain The conscious thought processes concerning the pain stimulus. It causes you to think carefully about the pain before making a judgement about its importance or quality A patient compares noxious stimulus with past experiences and assigns a meaning to the experience. Also known as *cognitive/evaluative*.

evidence Anything used to establish a fact, or give a reason to believe something. It may be tradition, experience, research, or theory.

evidence repositories Web-based searchable sites of scientific literature in biomedical and life sciences. It grew from the online Entrez PubMed biomedical literature search system. PubMed Central was developed by the U.S. National Library of Medicine (NLM) as an online archive of biomedical journal articles and data bases.

evidence-based medicine Medicine based on the latest and most rigorous scientific evidence, integrated with clinical experience and patient preferences and circumstances. It approaches patient care from a biomedical perspective, based solely on scientific facts; a cognitive-rational enterprise. It is a doctor-oriented, disease-centered model that focuses on gathering, synthesizing, and providing clinicians with the best available scientific evidence for how to treat specific diseases.

evidence-based practice Health care that is based on scientific evidence rather than tradition and experience alone. Its goal is to improve the quality and effectiveness of health care.

evidence-based practice The application of the principles of evidence-based medicine to patient care; health care that is based on scientific evidence and patient preferences. Its goal is to improve the quality and effectiveness of health care.

experience The result of successes and failures in treating similar patients and similar conditions in the past. It ranges from solid factual reality to unfounded opinion, rumor, and fiction.

extracellular space The space between cells.

extrapyramidal system A neural network in the brain that controls and coordinates movement.

facilitation Enabling a neural response.

faradic wave form Induced asymmetrical AC.

five-step application procedure A standardized framework for applying any therapeutic modality. It is rigid enough for quality control, yet flexible enough to allow the clinician to use modalities in the context of a critical thinking approach to rehabilitation.

fixed phase The unified launching of the wave fronts of all photons of a laser beam.

fluid dynamics The movement of fluid between capillaries and tissue.

fluidotherapy A convection-type heating modality that uses circulating ground-up corn cobs (or an artificial substitute)—a dry whirlpool of sorts—that is used to treat the extremities.

frequency *(1)* The rate of passage of crests on a wave form, expressed in cycles per second or hertz (Hz). *(2)* The rate of vibration of a force or wave, usually measured relative to local time.

friction massage A repetitive, specific, nongliding, shearing technique that produces movement between the fibers of dense connective tissue, increasing tissue extensibility and promoting the alignment of collagen fibers.

functional progression The performance of functional activities in an ordered sequence, beginning with unloaded, single-plane, slow-speed, slow-transition activity and progressing to overloaded, multiple-plane, high-speed, quick-transition activities. Accomplished by graded exercise, it facilitates the acquisition or reacquisition of skills needed for the safe, effective performance of complex skills. Also known as progressive reorientation.

fused response A sustained sensory response that feels like pins and needles, in response to moderate-amplitude, high-frequency pulsed or AC stimulation.

galvanometer A device that measures the electromagnetic effects of currents.

gate control theory of pain A theory that proposes a gating mechanism in the dorsal horn of the spinal cord that allows only one sensation at a time to pass through to the brain.

gel pack A reusable type of cold pack, made with water, antifreeze, and a gel in a vinyl pouch. Cooled in a freezer at 1°F (~17°C), but does not freeze.

generator A device that converts an input electrical current (AC or DC) into various output currents (AC, DC, or pulsed).

glycolysis The conversion of glucose to lactic acid when sufficient oxygen is not available. The primary mechanism of anaerobic metabolism.

GRADE See GRADING QUALITY OF EVIDENCE AND STRENGTH OF RECOMMENDATIONS.

graded exercise A series of exercises of increasing complexity and difficulty used to progressively reorient a patient to full functional activity following injury. See also FUNCTIONAL PROGRESSION.

grading quality of evidence and strength of recommendations (GRADE) A system of classification types of evidence, based on the integration of quality of evidence and strength of recommendations.

graphic rating scale A pain-rating scale that uses a horizontal line with anchor points at each end and descriptors spread along the line, administered and scored the same as the VAS.

graston An instrument-assisted soft tissue mobilization method that requires specific training and certification.

grid application A technique of applying a single laser probe to a large area by dividing the treatment area into a grid and treating each area separately.

ground-fault interrupter (GFI) A device that senses very small ground-fault currents, such as current flowing through the body of a person standing on damp ground while touching a hot AC line wire. The GFI quickly trips the circuit breaker, thereby limiting the total energy flow through the body to a safe value.

half-slivered mirror A mirror that reflects only half the light and allows the other half to pass through.

health care guidelines See CLINICAL PRACTICE GUIDELINES.

health-related quality of life (HRQoL) research Measurement of patients feelings of the quality of their life. It is an emerging field of rehabilitation evidence generation. See QUALITY OF LIFE.

heat The kinetic energy of atoms and molecules; a form of energy that is transferred by a difference in temperature. All substances with a temperature above absolute zero (–273°C) possess heat.

heat sink An area of the body that can accept and dissipate great amounts of heat.

hemarthrosis The presence of blood in a joint.

hematoma An accumulation of hemorrhaged blood and cellular debris.

hemodynamic changes Vascular changes that mobilize and transport defense components of the blood to the injury site and secure their passage through the vessel wall into the tissue.

hemorrhaging Bleeding.

hemostasis The arrest or stoppage of bleeding; the opposite of *hemorrhaging*.

herniated disk Disruption of the annulus fibrosus of an intervertebral disk.

high-volt pulsed current (HVPC) A twin-peak, monophasic, pulsed current driven by a high electromotive force or voltage for the purpose of pain modulation, edema reduction, muscle reeducation, spasm reduction, and wound healing.

hot pack A form of moist superficial heat that can be heated and reused.

hot spot An area at tissue interfaces that is overheated from too much energy being concentrated in one area.

HRQoL See HEALTH-RELATED QUALITY OF LIFE RESEARCH.

hunting response An oscillation in surface temperature during prolonged (>15 min) ice water immersion. It is caused by the buildup and interruption of a thermal gradient—not to cold-induced vasodilation.

hydrocollator pack A canvas pack that encases silica gel and that can be heated and reused.

hydrostatic pressure Pressure exerted by a column of water.

hyposkilliac A medical practitioner with deficient skills, caused by overdependence on science without critical thinking.

hypothalamus The brain's central monitoring and control station; regulates autonomic nervous system functions, and plays a role in mood and motivational states.

hypoxia Inadequate oxygen in body tissue, often resulting from prolonged ischemia. Not as severe as anoxia, a total lack of oxygen.

ice massage Stroking a body part (usually a muscle) with a large ice cube or ice cup (ice pop).

ice water immersion The use of a container filled with cold water and ice 32–34°F (0–1°C) for numbing extremities before exercise; also called ice bath immersion and sometimes inappropriately called ice water submersion.

idiopathic pain Pain of unknown origin, meaning there is no identifiable pathology associated with it.

immediate care Treatments within the first 12 hours after an orthopedic injury; a subset of acute care.

impedance Resistance or opposition to the flow of AC.

implementation science See KNOWLEDGE TRANSLATION.

impulse AC current flow in a single direction.

in vitro In cellular or tissue cultures.

in vivo Within the tissues.

indications In the context of the five-step application procedure, situations in which a specific modality should be used; conditions that would benefit from application of a certain modality.

indirect pain relief Focuses on removing the cause of pain.

inflammation The local, or tissue, response of the body to an injury or irritant. Also known as the inflammatory response.

infrared (IR) lamp A form of superficial heat that radiates from a heat lamp.

inhibition Restraining or repressing a neural response.

initial note A type of SOAP note written after the initial assessment.

insulator A nonconductor; something that resists the flow of electrons because they have no free electrons to move (e.g., rubber, glass, wood).

intensity A measure of the rate at which energy is being delivered per unit area.

interburst interval The time between bursts, usually measured in milliseconds.

interferential current (IFC) therapy The interference or superimposition of at least two separate medium-frequency sinusoidal currents on one another, mainly used to relieve pain.

interferential wave form Symmetrical, sinusoidal, high-frequency (2000–5000 Hz) AC. Two channels, with different frequencies, used simultaneously, causes a current amplitude modulation in the tissue.

interim note A type of SOAP note that includes periodic documentation of the results of the treatment plan. Also known as progress note.

interpulse interval The time between successive pulses.

interrupted DC wave form Unidirectional current flow caused by rapid and repeated turning of the current on and off.

intervention A medical treatment; an action taken to improve a medical disorder.

intervertebral disk A structure between two vertebrae that functions to resist compressive forces and shock, provide flexibility, and provide adequate space between vertebrae.

inverse square law ($I - 1/d^2$) The intensity (I) of radiation is inversely proportional to the distance squared (d^2).

ion An atom or molecule that has lost or gained one or more electrons and is, therefore, positively or negatively charged.

ion migration Ions move through the tissue in response to continuous DC stimulation.

iontophoresis The application of a mild direct electrical current (DC) to transport negatively or positively charged ions from a drug solution into a patient's skin and underlying tissues.

ischemia A deficit in blood supply to an organ or body part, usually owing to functional constriction or actual obstruction of a blood vessel. If prolonged, ischemia leads to tissue hypoxia.

joint flexibility The ability of a joint to move through its full range of motion.

keloid A larger-than-normal scar, caused by excessive protein in the wound.

knobology A tongue-in-cheek term referring to the study of application without theory. Knobologists are students and clinicians who want to know only which knobs on a therapeutic modality to turn but are uninterested in why they are doing so.

knowledge broker Those who facilitate *knowledge translation*, the transfer of research and other evidence between researchers and practitioners.

knowledge brokering See KNOWLEDGE TRANSLATION.

knowledge diffusion See KNOWLEDGE TRANSLATION.

knowledge exchange See KNOWLEDGE TRANSLATION.

knowledge mobilization See KNOWLEDGE TRANSLATION.

knowledge transfer See KNOWLEDGE TRANSLATION.

knowledge translation The process of translating clinically relevant science from the research lab to the clinician; of putting knowledge into action. It is the link between knowledge developers and knowledge users, also known as *knowledge exchange, knowledge transfer, knowledge mobilization, knowledge brokering, knowledge diffusion, research utilization, knowledge utilization, implementation science,* and over 85 other terms.

knowledge utilization See KNOWLEDGE TRANSLATION.

laboratory research Conducted in a laboratory. It is the least expensive and easiest to do, and allows the greatest control over interventions.

laboratory research Typically assesses the effects of specific treatment interventions on the physiological response of healthy, uninjured humans or pathophysiological response of injured animals.

laser Acronym for light amplification by stimulated emission of radiation, a device that produces and emits a highly amplified single-frequency and single-colored beam of nondivergent coherent light.

lasing medium A substance (gas, liquid, crystal, chemical, or semiconductor) that is activated and subsequently gives off photons during laser light production.

latent heat of fusion The amount of heat energy needed to convert a substance from a solid state to a liquid state without changing its temperature.

law of Grotthus-Draper Electromagnetic waves must be absorbed to be beneficial.

learned pain A conditioned response that develops from a patient's "pain memories" of physiological and emotional elements of pain experiences. Pain stimuli from events such as injury, organic disease, or surgery is indirectly paired with any of an infinite number of environmental or sociological stimuli, even inactivity. Eventually these secondary stimuli elicit a pain experience although there is no traditional pain stimuli.

leukocyte A white blood cell; contains and kills foreign substances and cellular debris.

leukocyte migration The movement of leukocytes from blood vessels to the injury site.

level of evidence A function of the type of research design used to generate the evidence; the degree to which it maximizes the validity of the results by minimizing opportunities for the results to be influenced by bias and other confounding factors.

light Electromagnetic radiation that produces a visual sensation.

light therapy The application of light by a variety of devices for a variety of therapeutic purposes; also known as phototherapy.

light-emitting diode (LED) A special type of semiconductor diode that emits visible light when an electric current passes through it; used in both laser and nonlaser devices.

lock and key A metaphor for the way neurotransmitter shapes fit specific receptors on dendrites.

longitudinal wave The primary wave form in which ultrasound energy travels in soft tissue, with molecular displacement along the direction in which the wave travels. See also TRANSVERSE WAVE.

low-level laser A low-power laser, also referred to as a cold laser or soft laser.

lymphedema pump A device consisting of a pump attached to a boot or sleeve that intermittently forces air or chilled water into the sleeve for the purpose of decreasing lymphedema; formerly known as intermittent compression device, cold compression device, and pneumatic compression pump.

lysosome A cellular organelle containing enzymes that digest foreign matter.

macrophage A long-lived leukocyte that is the primary scavenger after tissue damage occurs.

macrotrauma An injury that results in immediate tissue disruption. Also called impact injury or contact injury. Injuries that result from macrotrauma are classified as acute injuries.

magnetic field The force field that develops between the two poles.

manual traction A distraction force applied by another person.

massage lubricant A lotion, oil, cream, or powder used to decrease friction and control the amount of glide and drag that occurs between the clinician's moving hands and the client's skin.

massage The application of soft-tissue manipulation techniques to the body, generally intended to reduce stress and fatigue while improving circulation. Also called **therapeutic massage**.

matter Anything that has weight and occupies space.

McGill Pain Questionnaire A pain-rating scale that uses pictures, scales, and words to help patients describe the sensory and affective aspects, as well as magnitude and changes, in their pain.

mechanical nociceptor A lightly myelinated A-delta fiber, activated primarily by strong mechanical displacement of the skin; also called high-threshold mechanoreceptor.

mechanical traction A distraction force applied by a machine or other apparatus.

medline A database of journal citations and abstracts for biomedical literature from around the world. It is accessed via PubMed®, which provides free access to MEDLINE and links to full text articles when possible. It is maintained by the US National Library of Medicine, National Institutes of Health.

menthol An alcohol obtained from oil of peppermint and derived from mint plants; an irritant included in analgesic balms to provide a sensation of cold, or cool burning.

meta-analysis The use of statistical tools to systematically combine and summarize the results of several individual/independent primary studies on a specific topic (such as *RTC's*). They attempt to identify consistent patterns and sources of disagreements among the results of individual studies, and therefore provide a stronger conclusion than provided by individual studies. They are the primary tool of systematic reviews. They are also known as *data synthesis* or *quantitative overview*.

methyl salicylate Wintergreen oil, produced synthetically or from distilled sweet birch leaves; an irritant that causes redness on the skin, included in analgesic balms to provide a sensation of heat.

microcurrent electrical nerve stimulation (MENS) The therapeutic use of constant (direct) and pulsed (interrupted) currents by which the stimulus amplitude is in the microamperage (millionth of an ampere) range.

microtrauma An injury caused by overuse, cyclic loading, or friction. Injuries that result from microtrauma are classified as chronic injuries.

microwave diathermy (MWD) The therapeutic use of high-frequency (usually 2450 MHz) electromagnetic waves, similar to radar, to heat tissues.

mirror therapy An exercise to reset a distorted mental body image, and thus reduce chronic pain. A mirror hides the patients injured or amputated limb and projects the image of their uninjured limb to appear as the injured limb. Thus exercising the uninjured limb appears as exercising both limbs. Watching what appears as normal exercise of the injured limb removes the distorted mental image. Also known as motor imagery.

modified square wave form Monophasic, rectangular, pulsed current.

molecule Two or more atoms held together in a chemical bond.

monochromatic Having a single frequency and a single color (if it is in the light spectrum).

monophasic A pulse with one phase; current flows in one direction only.

morphine A drug that blocks pain by filling receptors so that neurotransmitters cannot occupy them.

motor imagery See MIRROR THERAPY.

motor point The point at which a motor nerve enters a muscle, usually located at the beginning of the muscle belly; the place where a given amount of current will elicit the greatest muscular contraction.

motor skill The integration and coordination of many muscles acting in concert to produce a desired movement; developed only by practicing sport-specific skill patterns.

motor TENS A TENS application used to treat chronic pain by stimulating small-diameter afferent nerves; beat frequency is low (1–5 pps) and intensity higher than sensory TENS (to the patient's tolerance). The patient reports some burning, needling sensation, and a slight muscle twitch.

motor unit A motor nerve and all the muscle fibers with which it synapses.

muscle cramp A sudden, intense, painful, tetanic muscle contraction that is short lived, usually lasting <20 sec; commonly called charley horse.

muscle guarding An involuntary process of splinting an injured limb by inducing a low-grade (mild) muscle spasm of antagonistic muscle groups.

muscle spasm *(1)* A muscle tightness of gradual onset, usually not very painful. *(2)* A sudden, involuntary contraction of one or more muscles. A low-grade spasm manifests as tightness, as opposed to a muscle cramp or charley horse.

muscular endurance The ability of a muscle to contract repeatedly without becoming fatigued.

muscular power The combination of strength and speed of movement; must be developed after those performance attributes.

muscular speed The speed at which a muscle contracts. Explosive-type activities (short duration, maximal power) develop muscular speed.

muscular strength A measure of the ability of a muscle to exert force. Regularly performed progressive resistive exercises will increase muscular strength.

myofascial release (MFR) Light sustained pressure applied in opposite directions to gently stretch and release myofascia restrictions that inhibit movement or cause pain.

myofascial release A technique that combines traction with varying amounts of stretch to produce a moderate sustained force on the muscle and its associated fascia.

myoglobin An oxygen-transporting and storage protein in muscle cells. Similar in function to hemoglobin in the blood.

naloxone A drug that reverses the effect of morphine.

narrative reviews A standard literature review that typically is nonsystematic and therefore subject to bias. See DATA SYNTHESIS.

national guideline clearinghouse A public resource for evidence-based clinical practice guidelines and related documents. It is maintained by the Agency for Healthcare Research and Quality of the US Department of Health and Human Services.

negative feedback Activity on a nerve fiber that eventually is returned through a neural network, thereby inhibiting further activity on that neuron.

negative terminal The terminal into which the current enters the battery or generator from the body.

nerve A bundle of nerve fibers that transmits information via electrical signals among the brain, spinal cord, and other parts of the body.

nerve excitability The amount of electrical current applied to the surface necessary to elicit an action potential in a specific nerve.

nerve fiber An axon of a single neuron, or nerve cell, and its multiple dendrites.

nerve palsy The partial loss of motor function in a local area; may be permanent or temporary.

neural inhibition The decreasing or stopping of neural activity, thus retarding or preventing normal musculoskeletal functioning. (Derived from the Latin *hibitus*, "to keep back.")

neuromatrix theory of pain A theory of pain that involves a gating mechanism in the spinal cord, as in the gate control theory, but that emphasizes a much larger role of the brain in interpreting and responding to painful stimuli. It is regarded as the most complete explanation of pain and pain management.

neuromuscular electrical stimulator (NMES) A therapeutic device that delivers current to the body to cause sensory and motor nerve depolarization. Its purpose is to cause muscle contraction.

neuromuscular therapy (NMT) A variety of techniques, claimed to improve functioning of the immune system, glands, joints, muscles, and related soft tissues.

neuron The basic functional unit of the nervous system; main components are the cell body, dendrites, the axon, and branches that end in axon terminals. Also called nerve cell.

neuropathic pain A complex, chronic pain state that often shows up in illogical ways. It usually is accompanied by tissue damage to the nerve fibers themselves, which become dysfunctional and send incorrect signals to the brain and other pain centers.

neurotransmitter A chemical released by axon terminals that transmits an impulse across a synapse. Neurotransmitters fit into receptors on the cell body or dendrites of the postsynaptic neuron, where they either stimulate or inhibit a response.

neutron A subunit of an atom, located in the nucleus, with a mass of 1 and an electrical charge of 0.

neutrophil A short-lived leukocyte that forms the first line of defense against pathogens. Also called a polymorph.

nociception The ability to feel pain; also known as pain sense, algesia, algesthesia, and nociperception.

nociceptor A peripheral nerve that receives and transmits painful or other noxious stimuli.

nociceptive pain Pain that occurs in response to injury or illness to bodily structures.

nondivergent Incapable of separating or widening. Contrast the light from a laser pointer (nondivergent) with that coming from a flashlight (divergent). Nondivergent light is also known as directional light.

non-weight-bearing gait A crutch walking gait used when the objective is to completely remove weight from one leg or foot. The injured limb is lifted and the patient walks alternatively on the good leg and the two crutches. Also known as the swing-through gait.

norepinephrine A hormone secreted by the adrenal glands; the principal neurotransmitter of sympathetic nerves supplying the major organs and skin. It increases heart rate, blood pressure, the rate and depth of breathing, and blood sugar level, and decreases digestive functions. Also known as noradrenaline.

noxious stimulus A harmful, unhealthy stimulation. Pain is caused by noxious stimuli.

noxious TENS TENS applied with a high enough intensity to be painful.

nucleus pulposus The inner layer of an intervertebral disk, composed of a protein gel between the cartilaginous end plates of the vertebrae and the annulus fibrosus.

number scale A tool for measuring pain intensity that consists of a range of numbers and descriptors. Patients select the number that best describes their pain.

observational research In context observations of people as they go about routine activities in their natural environment. It may be prospective (designed before data are collected) or retrospective (designed to study existing data). The dependent (or measurement) variable of these is determined by clinical practice rather than a scientific protocol.

ohm A unit of resistance or opposition to the flow of DC: 1 ohm (Ω) is equal to the resistance caused by a column of mercury 1 mm^2 in cross-section, 106 cm high at a temperature of 0°C. It is equal to 1 V/amp.

Ohm's law The relationship between current, force, and resistance (current = force/resistance; amp = volt/ohm).

ohmmeter A device that measures resistance to current flow.

oncotic pressure Pressure resulting from the attraction of fluid by free protein. Also called colloid osmotic pressure.

onion skin model of pain Describes the pain experience as being comprised of four elements (nociception, pain perception, suffering, and pain behavior), depicted as nested concentric circles, like the layers of an onion, arranged from the inside outward. Together, the neuromatrix theory and onion skin model are regarded as the most complete explanation of pain and pain management.

open circuit An interrupted or broken circuit; flow ceases.

opiate A substance that numbs or decreases pain; its synthetic form is known as an opioid.

organelle A specialized structure within tissue cells.

orthopedic injury A sprain, strain, fracture, or contusion caused by excessive stress.

osteophyte A small, bony calcium deposit that forms on the vertebrae.

overload The concept of challenging the body to greater function by pushing it beyond its comfort zone to near its limits. The body adapts by increasing its capacity.

pain An unpleasant sensory and emotional experience associated with actual or potential tissue damage or described in terms of such damage.

pain perception The attributes or characteristics of the pain experience as interpreted by the brain.

paraffin bath A form of moist superficial heat applied by forming a wax glove around the affected body part.

parasympathetic nervous system The branch of the ANS that regulates the "rest and digest" responses, such as decreased heart rate and secretion of digestive enzymes.

partial conductor A substance that allows some flow of electricity under certain conditions (e.g., dry wood, paper, tap water, moist air, kerosene).

partial-weight-bearing gait A crutch walking gait in which the patient walks as with a normal gait, except for using the crutches to remove just enough weight from the injured limb to eliminate pain and limping. Also called the three-point gait.

patient compliance The act of following the treatment orders or instructions given by a clinician.

patient noncompliance The failure to fully follow the treatment orders or instructions given by a clinician.

patient-centered medicine A humanistic, biopsychosocial approach. Its focus is on patient participation in clinical decision making, using in-depth patient communication to understand patients' complaints, unique needs in the context of their lives, preferences, culture, beliefs, backgrounds, behaviors, and emotional status; in essence, who the patient is. It moves care from clinician control to patient empowerment.

peak area of the maximum BNR (PAMBNR) An ultrasound beam profile.

peak current The highest magnitude of a pulse.

PEDro The *Physiotherapy Evidence Database* of randomized trials, systematic reviews, and clinical practice guidelines in physiotherapy. It is sponsored by the Australian Physiotherapy Association.

percussion Repeated, rhythmical, light striking of the skin. Techniques include gentle tapping, pounding, cupping, hacking, and slapping the skin; also called tapotement.

performance attributes Specific neuromuscular functions necessary for sport or work performance, such as pain-free movement, muscular strength, and motor control. Injury disrupts one or more of the performance attributes, and rehabilitation should systematically reestablish them.

periaqueductal gray (PAG) matter Gray matter in the brain whose neurons are excited by endorphins and opiate analgesics. It plays a role in the descending modulation of pain and in defensive behavior.

peripheral nervous system (PNS) The cranial nerves and spinal nerves.

pétrissage A group of related techniques that repetitively compress (squeeze), shear (wring), and release muscle tissue with varying amounts of drag, lift, and glide.

phagocytosis The process of digesting cellular debris and other foreign material into pieces small enough to be removed from the injury site via lymph vessels.

phagolysosome A sac in a leukocyte, formed by lysosomes spilling their digestive enzymes into a phagosome; digests pathogens and debris from an injury site.

phagosome A sac within a leukocyte, formed as the leukocyte engulfs pathogens or debris from an injury site.

phantom limb pain Pain that a person interprets as coming from an amputated limb.

phase A period of unidirectional charged particle movement (current flow).

phase change A change from one state (solid or liquid or gas) to another without a change in chemical composition.

phase charge The total electrical charge of a single phase, expressed as coulombs (microcoulombs for MNES). It is the time interval (area under the curve); the result of both amplitude and width (duration).

phase duration The time during which current flows in a single direction.

phase shape The shape of an output current after being modulated (e.g., rectangular, spike, triangular, sawtooth).

phonophoresis A technique in which ultrasound is used to help move a topical medication into the tissues. See also SONOPORATION.

photobiomodulation The act of modifying biological processes with light.

photon A particle of light; the basic unit of radiant energy. The amount of its energy is a function of the frequency of the electromagnetic wave.

physiatrist A physician who specializes in physical medicine, the medical subspecialty relating to the treatment of injury and disease by physical agents, such as heat, cold, light, electricity, and exercise.

physical agent An external form of energy, such as heat, cold, light, electricity, or exercise.

physical medicine and rehabilitation The medical subspeciality relating to the treatment and rehabilitation of physical conditions.

physical medicine Treating injury or disease by physical agents, such as heat, cold, light, sound, electricity, and exercise.

Physiotherapy Evidence Database See PEDro.

piezoelectric effect The contracting and expanding of a crystal, when an alternating electrical current is passed through it.

placebo A medicinally inactive substance or mock intervention administered to bring about a desired response and satisfy the patient's demand for medicine.

placebo effect The measurable, observable, or felt improvement in health not attributable to treatment; occurs in response to many types of interventions.

plateau The time during which electrical pulses remain at maximum preset intensity.

polarity The positive or negative voltage on an active electrode compared to the voltage on a dispersive electrode. Polarity applies only when a unipolar placement technique is used.

polymodal nociceptor An unmyelinated C fiber, activated by several different types of stimuli, such as heat, mechanical pressure, or inflammatory chemical mediators produced by tissue injury.

polyphasic A pulse with many phases. Current flow with many phases.

positive feedback Activity on a neuron that eventually is returned through a neural network, thereby facilitating further activity on that neuron.

positive terminal The terminal from which the current leaves the battery or generator to enter the body.

postacute care Treatment of an acute injury after 14 days after the injury.

power A function of both pulse width and pulse frequency, measured in watts. Also called intensity.

precautions Situations that could cause harm if the clinician is not careful. For example, failure to move the soundhead during ultrasound treatment could damage tissue or cause extreme pain.

primary injury Cellular damage caused by an acute traumatic force.

progress note A type of SOAP note that includes periodic documentation of the results of the treatment plan. Also known as interim note.

progression The practice of inducing incremental increases in a performance attribute by sequentially overloading the body as it adapts to a training load.

progressive reorientation See FUNCTIONAL PROGRESSION.

proliferation phase of healing Three major events: *angiogenesis* (growth of new blood vessels), *collagen synthesis*, and *wound contraction* (the drawing together of the wound edges).

proprioceptive neuromuscular facilitation (PNF) Techniques that help maintain joint flexibility, such as hold-relax (static stretch interspersed with isometric contraction of the involved muscle) and contract-relax (static stretch interspersed with isometric contraction of the antagonistic muscle).

prospective research Designed before data are collected.

prospectus A research plan written prior to data collection. Also known as a research design.

protocol A plan or a set of specific steps to be followed in an investigation or intervention that provides a strict

process for monitoring and taking care of a patient. They provide a practical, step-by-step framework for implementing guidelines.

proton A subunit of an atom, located in the nucleus, with a mass of 1 and an electrical charge of +1.

pseudounipolar neuron A sensory neuron in the PNS; similar to a neuron, but without dendrites. They are sometimes called a **specialized neuron**, or simply a neuron.

PubMed See MEDLINE.

pulse A finite period of charged particle movement separated from other pulses by a limited time during which no current flows. Consists of one or more phases.

pulse charge balance The relationship between the charges of two phases of a biphasic pulse, independent of whether or not the phases are symmetrical.

pulse charge The amount of electrical charge of a single pulse; the sum of phase charges.

pulse period The beginning of a pulse to the beginning of the subsequent pulse; pulse duration plus interpulse interval.

pulse rate The number of pulses per second (pps).

pulse symmetry The relationship between the shapes of the two phases of a biphasic pulse.

pulse width The time required for each pulse to complete its cycle; also known as pulse duration.

pulsed current Interrupted or noncontinuous electron flow.

pulsed shortwave diathermy (PSWD) The therapeutic use of high-frequency (10–100 MHz) electromagnetic waves, in pulsed form, to produce nonthermal and thermal effects in deep tissues.

pulsed ultrasound An ultrasound mode in which the intensity is periodically interrupted, with no ultrasound energy being produced during the off period. With pulsed ultrasound, the average intensity of the output over time is reduced.

quadripolar technique The application of four electrodes of equal size; generally they crisscross the target tissue.

quality of evidence The quality of care depends on the quality of evidence used to direct the care. It is the core of evidence-based medicine.

quality of life A broad, multidimensional, patient-centered concept that measures a person's general feeling of personal well-being or satisfaction with life. It helps identify the effects of individual experiences, beliefs, values, expectations, and perceptions on physical and psychosocial dimensions of life.

quantitative overview See META-ANALYSIS.

radiating pain Pain that originates from an irritated nerve root and travels along that particular nerve's dermatome.

radiation Energy that is transmitted in the form of rays, waves, or particles, often from a central source; also called radiant energy. See also ELECTROMAGNETIC WAVE.

radicular pain Pain along the pathway of a spinal nerve.

ramp down The time during which the intensity of an electrical surge decreases.

ramp up The time during which the intensity of an electrical surge increases.

randomized clinical trial (RCT) A controlled research study of a specific medical intervention on patients with a specific disease or injury. Also called Randomized Controlled Trials. See CLINICAL TRIALS RESEARCH.

randomized controlled trial (RCT) Also called Randomized Clinical Trials. See CLINICAL TRIALS RESEARCH.

raphe nucleus A group of neurons in the center of the brainstem that release serotonin, making them part of brain's pain relief system.

rarefaction A region of lower molecular density in a longitudinal wave, as the molecules are pulled apart. See also COMPRESSION.

Raynaud disease A circulatory disorder caused by cold or emotion, in which the hands, and less commonly the feet, become discolored and painful.

recommendation statements See CLINICAL PRACTICE GUIDELINES.

reconditioning Conditioning again. Often improperly used as a synonym for *injury rehabilitation*. Although rehabilitation and conditioning share many principles, there are fundamental differences. Rehabilitation is much more than conditioning again, and the terms should not be used synonymously.

reconstitution The process of replacing damaged cells with healthy cells of the same type as those that were injured.

record keeping The process of writing and storing accurate and detailed information about individual injuries, treatments given, and how the patient responded to the treatments.

recovery cryotherapy The use of extremely cold whole-body cryotherapy (WBC) or cold water immersion (CWI) of arms or legs to help athletes recover from the rigors of their workout or competition more quickly.

recurring inflammation Acute inflammation that is reinitiated before the previous episode of acute inflammation has finished.

referred pain Pain at a site other than the location of a trauma; usually projects outward from the torso and distally along the extremities.

reflection The bending back of electromagnetic waves when they hit a substance. The angle of reflection is determined by the angle of the strike.

reflexology The application of finger and thumb pressure to specific reflex areas of patients' hands and feet that are thought to correspond to all of the glands, organs, and parts of the body.

refraction The bending of electromagnetic waves when they pass through a substance. The amount of bending depends on the frequency of the waves.

refractory period The time during which the nerve membrane repolarizes; divided into relative and absolute refractory periods.

rehabilitation The process of restoring an individual to a normal or optimal state of health. (Derived from the Latin *rehabilitare*, "to make fit again.")

repair The process of replacing dead or damaged cells with healthy ones.

replacement The process of replacing damaged cells with simpler cells, as in connective tissue, muscle tissue, and CNS tissue and in any area where the damage is extensive enough to disrupt the basic cellular framework. Replacement results in scar tissue formation. Also called repair by connective tissue.

research The result of scientific investigation.

research design A research plan written prior to data collection. Also known as a prospectus.

research evidence See LABORATORY, OBSERVATIONAL, AND CLINICAL TRIALS.

research utilization See KNOWLEDGE TRANSLATION.

residual pain Pain that develops after an unaccustomed activity, generally occurring the next day. It indicates that the previous day's activity was too rigorous.

resistance Opposition to the flow of electricity, caused by a conductor.

response A reaction, such as contraction of a muscle or secretion of a gland, that results from stimulation.

restructuring Collagen fibers are reorganized from the haphazard way they were laid down to a parallel arrangement, causing the scar to become more compact. Occurs near the end of repair.

retrospective research Designed to study existing data.

RICES Acronym for rest, elevation, ice, compression, elevation, and stabilization: the prescription for immediate care.

rifle approach Treating a patient with one or two specific modalities, targeted to achieve a particular goal. It is more focused than the shotgun approach.

rise time The time from the beginning of a phase until it reaches maximal amplitude.

rolfing Vigorous deep tissue massage with the fingers, thumb, fist, and/or elbow, combined with myofascial release to restore normal body alignment, structure, and function. Also known as Structural Integration.

RCT An abbreviation for both *Randomized Clinical Trials* and *Randomized Control Trials*.

Russian wave form A medium-frequency polyphasic, symmetrical, sinusoidal, burst wave form generated in 50 bursts/sec envelopes.

SAID principle Acronym for specific adaptation to imposed demands. The body responds to a given demand with a specific and predictable adaptation. Specific adaptation *requires* that *specific* demands be imposed.

scanning A technique of applying a single laser probe to a large area by moving the head across the area like an ultrasound head.

secondary enzymatic injury Tissue damage resulting from enzymes, such as those in lysosomes, released from damaged cells.

secondary injury Cellular injury caused by enzymatic action and metabolic deficiency.

secondary metabolic injury Tissue damage resulting from a metabolic imbalance secondary to an acute traumatic orthopedic injury.

semiconductor A substance with poor conductivity at low temperatures; conductivity increases when other substances are added, or by the application of heat, light, or voltage. Used to regulate the flow of electricity (e.g., carbon, silicone, germanium).

sensory dimension of pain What you feel–the source of the pain. It involves distinguishing it from other sensations and locations. Also known as *sensory/ discriminative*.

sensory nerve A nerve that transmits impulses from the periphery of the body to the CNS.

sensory TENS A TENS application with a high beat frequency (80–200 pps) and intensity adjusted to the point at which the patient reports a buzzing or tingling sensation; used to treat acute pain by stimulating large-diameter sensory nerves.

sensory twitch Repetitions of brief isolated sensory ticks in response to moderate-amplitude, low-frequency pulsed stimulation. This response is not used therapeutically.

sequela An effect that follows, or results from, an injury, disease, or treatment.

serotonin A biochemical messenger and regulator, found primarily in the CNS, GI tract, and blood platelets; mediates several physiological functions, including neurotransmission.

shiatsu A form of Japanese pressure point therapy, similar to *trigger point therapy* but concentrating on application of pressure to acupuncture points.

shortwave diathermy (SWD) The therapeutic use of high-frequency (10–100 MHz) electromagnetic waves, similar to radio waves, to heat deep tissues.

shotgun approach Treating a patient with every possible modality, with the hope that one will be effective. It gives the impression that the clinician's only goal is to reduce the patient's symptoms. See also RIFLE APPROACH.

single laser probe An applicator of laser light.

sinusoidal wave form Pure AC. A biphasic, symmetrical, balanced wave form with a gradual rise in the amplitude followed by a gradual decline in the amplitude.

SOAP note A type of problem-oriented medical record. S = subjective, information gathered primarily from questioning the patient on his present condition; O = objective, reproducible information from tests or evaluative measures; A = assessment, the clinician's professional judgment or impression of the injury; P = plan, the course of action to rehabilitate the patient.

somatic A term used to denote a body/mind or whole-body approach therapy. Related to therapeutic massage.

somatic motor nerve A nerve that transmits impulses from the CNS to the periphery of the body and terminates in skeletal muscle; controlled voluntarily.

somatic nervous system (SNS) The somatic motor nerves and sensory nerves.

sonoporation A process in which ultrasound increases cell membrane permeability, thereby facilitating the delivery of molecules of a medication to precise locations in the body. See also PHONOPHORESIS.

SORT See STRENGTH OF RECOMMENDATION TAXONOMY.

soundhead A ceramic, aluminum, or stainless-steel plate attached to the crystal that transfers the acoustic energy (sound waves) from the crystal to the tissues.

spatial average intensity (SAI) The intensity of an ultrasound beam averaged over the area of the soundhead.

spatial peak intensity The highest intensity in an ultrasound beam across the soundhead's surface.

spatial summation Summed over space; occurs when a number of subthreshold stimuli from different axons converge on one cell body simultaneously.

specific heat The amount of heat energy required to raise 1 kg of a substance 1°C.

spinal adaptation syndrome A theory that nociceptive impulses from traumatized tissue inhibit motor functions and tissue repair but that voluntary activity can reestablish central control and prevent this inhibition. Prolonged inactivity after an injury will lead to neural inhibition that could become permanent.

sports massage Application of swedish massage techniques to athletes, and others involved in physical activity.

stabilization The act of supporting or holding steady, with or as if with a brace. After injury, it allows surrounding muscles to relax.

standard of care See BEST PRACTICE.

standard operating procedures (SOPs) Specific guidelines and protocols for performing a specific task. Having SOPs is a form of quality control because they promote consistency. They help you remember the

specific steps and ensure that all essential elements are performed.

standard therapy See BEST PRACTICE.

Starling forces Forces that cause capillary filtration: capillary oncotic, capillary hydrostatic, tissue oncotic, and tissue hydrostatic.

static electricity Frictional electricity created by rubbing two objects together; one object gains electrons and the other one loses electrons.

static vector A vector that stays centered where two interferential currents cross.

stimulate To excite or invigorate; to encourage or provoke something to grow, develop, or become more active.

stimulation pattern The structure of the pulses used in the current.

stimulus The action of one agent on another (e.g., nerve, muscle) that evokes activity in the receiving structure or agent.

strength of evidence The credibility, clinical significance, and applicability of evidence. The confidence you have that it represents the "truth." It is a combination of quality and level of evidence.

strength of recommendation taxonomy (SORT) A rating of the strength of the clinical recommendations made in review and clinical technique articles by the editors of the journals in which the articles are published.

stretching window The time period of vigorous heating when tissues will undergo their greatest extensibility and elongation.

structural integrity The health of a patient's anatomical structures, such as bones, muscles, ligaments, and tendons.

subacute care Treatment of an acute injury during days 4–14 after the injury. An injury in this stage is moving beyond acute but is still somewhat or bordering on acute.

subacute pain Pain that lasts for 1 to 3–6 months. It usually starts as acute pain.

substantia gelatinosa (SG) The location of the pain gate in the dorsal horn of the spinal cord, according to the gate control theory of pain.

subthreshold stimulus Stimulation below the threshold level; does not evoke a response but causes a change in the electrical activity of the tissue.

suffering A state of severe distress, associated with events that threaten to harm the person; a cognitive-social behavior that the brain assigns to the pain signal.

summation A process by which subthreshold stimuli add together to evoke a response.

superficial thermotherapy The application of modalities that heat primarily the surface tissues.

super-luminous diode (SLD) A very bright LED.

surged stimulation pattern Stimulation in which amplitude of successive pulses (or cycles) gradually increase from zero to a maximum preset intensity.

swedish massage Classic, traditional, or basic massage for both relaxation and injury rehabilitation. It uses a variety of strokes, including effleurage, petrissage, friction, tapotement, and vibration.

swelling An increase in tissue volume owing to extra fluid and cellular material in the tissue.

symmetrical pulse A pulse with identical phases.

sympathetic nervous system The branch of the ANS that regulates the body's fight-or-flight responses, such as increased heart rate.

synapse The junction between two neurons; the space between the axon terminal of a presynaptic neuron and the cell body or dendrite of a postsynaptic neuron.

systematic reviews A type of literature review that aims to circumvent bias by using a predefined, rigorous, and explicit methodology See DATA SYNTHESIS.

systems approach to rehabilitation An approach to rehabilitation based on the philosophy that each patient and each injury is unique, so treatment must be individualized, dynamic, and interactive. Intervention is based on the patient's initial signs and symptoms and is altered according to patient progress. The systems approach is based on 11 principles of rehabilitation and consists of 10 core goals related to performance attributes.

T cell Transmission cell; a group of cells in the dorsal horn of the spinal cord that determines which impulse will continue up or down the spinal cord and to other parts of the body.

temperature The measure of an object's ability to spontaneously give up energy; indicates the level of molecular motion associated with heat.

temporal average intensity (TAI) The power of ultrasonic energy over a given period of time.

temporal summation Summed over time; occurs when a number of subthreshold stimuli from the same axon are repeated one after another before the effect of the previous stimulus has dissipated.

TENS See TRANSCUTANEOUS ELECTRICAL NERVE SIMULATOR (TENS).

tensile strength The amount of longitudinal stress a wound can withstand before tearing apart.

terminal (pole) The output device of a battery or generator.

tetanic contraction A sustained muscular contraction in response to repetitive high-frequency, high-amplitude pulsed or AC stimulation of at least 20–30 pulses per second; occurs in individual muscle fibers or in entire muscle groups.

tetany The point at which muscle fibers, as a result of increased frequency of stimulation, do not have time to relax between stimuli so that the contraction becomes steady, as opposed to a series of individual twitches; occurs when stimulation exceeds 20–30 pps, depending on the type of muscle fiber.

thalamus The brain's relay center. Signals from the sense organs (except the nose) are sent to the thalamus, which relays the information to the cerebral cortex.

theory The best guess of what is going on based on a logical evaluation of evidence.

therapeutic goal An aim or desired result of a therapeutic regimen.

therapeutic massage The systematic manual manipulation of the body's tissues to restore normal function.

therapeutic modality A device or application that delivers a physical agent (heat, cold, light, electricity, exercise) to the body for therapeutic purposes.

therapeutic purpose A goal of using physical agents in treating orthopedic injuries; examples are promoting wound healing, relieving pain, and increasing flexibility or range of motion.

thermal gradient A gradual change in temperature from the interior of one object to the interior of the other object as heat is exchanged by conduction; also known as temperature gradient.

thermoreceptor A sensory receptor that responds to heat and cold.

thermotherapy The therapeutic use of heat; the application of a device or substance with a temperature greater than body temperature, thus causing heat to pass from the thermotherapy device to the body.

threshold The minimal point at which a stimulus begins to produce a gross response (psychological or physiological).

time off The time during which the current does not flow; the time between surges.

time on The time during which the current flows from the beginning to the end of a surge.

tissue hydrostatic pressure (THP) Pressure that forces fluid into the capillary.

tissue oncotic pressure (TOP) Pressure that pulls fluid out of the capillary.

tract A bundle of nerve fibers with a common origin, termination, and function; also called pathway.

traction A technique in which a pulling force is applied to body segments to stretch soft tissues and separate joint surfaces or bone fragments.

tradition Theories, techniques, and procedures that have been handed down from one clinician to the next. It ranges from solid factual reality to unfounded opinion, rumor, and fiction.

transcutaneous electrical nerve stimulator (TENS) A therapeutic device that delivers current to the body to cause sensory nerve depolarization. Its purpose is to stimulate sensory nerves to modulate pain.

transducer A device that converts variations in a physical quantity (such as pressure or brightness) into an electrical signal, or vice versa.

transition care Treatment of an acute injury between 12 hour and 4 days after the injury; a subset of acute care.

transmission The action of an electromagnetic wave passing through a substance.

transverse wave A wave form occurring only in bone, in which the molecules are displaced in a direction perpendicular to the direction in which the ultrasound wave is moving. See also LONGITUDINAL WAVE.

trauma A physical injury caused by physical force.

trigger point pain A hypersensitive area or site in muscle or connective tissue; usually associated with myofascial pain syndromes.

trigger point The site of referred pain.

trigger point therapy. Repetitive cycles of isolated pressure and release over a trigger point, a painfully tight area in a muscle caused by muscle overuse or injury.

triphasic A pulse with three phases of current flow.

twin pulse wave form Monophasic, pulsed, twin spiked form; common wave form of high-volt muscle simulators.

twitch contraction Repetitions of isolated brief muscular contraction followed by relaxation in response to low-frequency, high-amplitude pulsed stimulation; occurs in individual muscle fibers or in entire muscle groups.

ultrasound applicator The housing for the crystal and soundhead plus a handle that facilitates application of the ultrasound to patients.

ultrasound Inaudible, acoustic vibrations of high frequency that produce thermal and/or nonthermal physiologic effects.

ultrastructural changes The breakdown and disruption of cell membranes and cellular organelles.

ultraviolet (UV) radiation A portion of the electromagnetic spectrum that produces chemical reactions in microorganisms, epidermis, and dermis; usually used therapeutically to kill microorganisms.

unbalanced pulse A pulse containing unequal phase charges.

unipolar technique The application of electrodes of unequal size, thus creating active and dispersive electrodes; the active electrode(s) is (are) applied to the treatment area and the dispersive electrode is applied to a remote location.

urticaria A noncontagious, short-lived allergic reaction characterized by wheals on the skin. It is caused by cold or exercise or from eating certain foods or taking certain medicines. Also known as hives.

vascular phase In the repair process, a transient phase of 4–6 days during which new blood vessels are formed to deliver oxygen and nutrients to the wound area.

ventral horn The anterior portion of the gray matter of the spinal cord; also called anterior horn.

verbal rating scale A pain-rating scale that consists of a group of descriptors but no numbers. Patients rate their pain as absent, mild, moderate, or severe, and their pain relief as none, slight, moderate, or good.

vibration Repetitively moving soft tissue (usually muscle) back and forth over the underlying bone with minimal joint motion; also called shaking.

visible light An electromagnetic wave that is divergent, multichromatic, incoherent, and multiphasic.

visual analog scale (VAS) A pain-rating scale that consists of a line of specific length, usually 100 mm (4 in.), with contrasting descriptors ("no pain" and "severe pain") on the two ends. Patients make a vertical slash on the line indicating pain level. The clinician measures from the left side of the scale to the slash to assess pain level.

volt A unit of force required to push a current of 1 amp through a resistance of 1 ohm.

voltage The force created by an accumulation of, or an absence of, electrons on an atom or body.

voltmeter A device that measures voltage.

wave form The shape of an electrical current, created when the current is graphed with amplitude on the vertical axis and time on the horizontal axis.

wavelength The distance of one repetition of a sinusoidal wave, expressed in meters or centimeters; often defined as the distance from the crest of one repetition to the crest of the next repetition of the wave.

wet cell A battery that consists of two metals and an electrolyte solution; also called a galvanic cell.

wheal A smooth, slightly raised, rounded, or flat-topped area of skin, usually accompanied by burning or intense itching. Also known as a welt or a hive.

whirlpool A large body of either hot or cold water that is forcibly circulated or "whirled" about in its container.

whole-body cryotherapy (WBC) Used for recovery cryotherapy. It consists of a brief exposure (2–3 minutes) to very cold air (–110° to –140°C; –166° to –220°F) in a temperature-controlled chamber.

wound contraction The drawing together of the wound edges.

Index

(Note: Page numbers in italics denote figures; those followed by t denote tables; those followed by b denote boxes.)

460